THE NEUROLOGY
OF VISION

CONTEMPORARY NEUROLOGY SERIES

SID GILMAN, M.D., SERIES EDITOR

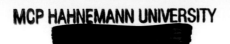
THE NEUROLOGY
OF VISION

JONATHAN D. TROBE, M.D.

Professor of Neurology and Ophthalmology
University of Michigan Medical Center
Ann Arbor, Michigan

Illustrations by Tanya K. Leonello, M.F.A.

OXFORD
UNIVERSITY PRESS
2001

OXFORD
UNIVERSITY PRESS

Oxford   New York
Athens   Auckland   Bangkok   Bogotá   Buenos Aires   Calcutta
Cape Town   Chennai   Dar es Salaam   Delhi   Florence   Hong Kong   Istanbul
Karachi   Kuala Lumpur   Madrid   Melbourne   Mexico City   Mumbai
Nairobir   Paris   São Paulo   Shanghai   Singapore   Taipei   Tokyo   Toronto   Warsaw

and associated companies in
Berlin   Ibadan

Color plates reproduced courtesy of the
Kellogg Eye Center, Ann Arbor, Michigan.

Published by Oxford University Press, Inc.
198 Madison Avenue, New York, New York 10016

Oxford is a registered trademark of Oxford University Press

Library of Congress Cataloging-in-Publication Data
Trobe, Jonathan D., 1943–
The neurology of vision / Jonathan D. Trobe ; illustrations by Tanya K. Leonello.
p. ; cm. — (Contemporary neurology series ; 60)
Includes bibliographical references and index.
ISBN 0-19-512978-4 (cloth)
1. Neuroophthalmology. I. Title. II. Series.
[DNLM: 1. Vision Disorders. 2. Eye—innervation. 3. Eye—physiopathology. 4. Ocular
Physiology. WW 140 T843n 2001]
RE725.T76 2001
617.7—dc21   00-055052

The science of medicine is a rapidly changing field. As new research and clinical experience broaden our knowledge, changes in treatment and drug therapy do occur. The author and the publisher of this work have checked with sources believed to be reliable in their efforts to provide information that is accurate and complete, and in accordance with the standards accepted at the time of publication. However, in light of the possibility of human error or changes in the practice of medicine, neither the author, nor the publisher, nor any other party who has been involved in the preparation or publication of this work warrants that the information contained herein is in every respect accurate or complete. Readers are encouraged to confirm the information contained herein with other reliable sources, and are strongly advised to check the product information sheet provided by the pharmaceutical company for each drug they plan to administer.

1 2 3 4 5 6 7 8 9

Printed in Hong Kong
on acid-free paper

To Joan Holly, Rebecca, Dana, Julian, Noah, Krish, Susie, Ruth and Hilly, Bronia and Ralph

ACKNOWLEDGMENTS

I am deeply grateful to Dan Jacobson and David Kaufman for critical review of the manuscript; Roy Beck, Ron Burde, Charles Butter, Jim Corbett, Wayne Cornblath, Joel Glaser, Jonathan Horton, Jeff Odel, Valerie Purvin, Peter Savino, Norman Schatz, Jim Sharpe, Mike Wall, Helmut Wilhelm, and Jackie Winterkorn for shaping my views; and Lauren Enck and Sid Gilman for editorial assistance.

CONTENTS

Part V   Nonorganic Visual Disturbances

Part VI   Problem Cases

THE NEUROLOGY
OF VISION

INTRODUCTION

The function of the visual system (Fig. I-1) is to locate objects in space, decide if they are moving, and determine if they are familiar. Light is focused onto an array of retinal receptors and converted to neural signals that are sent to primary visual cortex, where elementary features such as color, form, depth, and motion are separately encoded. Motion and depth information is conveyed to the occipitoparietal cortex, where spatial percepts are derived. Color and form information is conveyed to the occipitotemporal cortex, where it is interpreted as familiar or unfamiliar. Many other neocortical regions contribute attentional and motivational inputs that help to select and bind relevant features into meaningful visual symbols.

THE THREE COMPONENTS OF THE VISUAL SYSTEM

When vision fails, the best way to approach problem-solving is to divide the system into three components:

- **Optical:** the eye's focusing elements. They must present a clear and faithful image to the retina (Fig. I-2).
- **Retinocortical:** the segment extending from the retina to the primary visual cortex. Neural signals must travel from one end to the other without interruption and only in response to external visual stimuli. The primary visual cortex must perform correct elementary encoding (Fig. I-3).
- **Integrative:** the segment extending from the primary visual cortex to the parietal and temporal vision-related cortex. Encoded elementary features must reach these association cortex regions and be converted into meaningful percepts (Fig. I-4).

This segmentation of the visual pathway is clinically useful because it lends itself to a proper divison of labor among the specialists involved in vision care. If a problem is optical in nature, an optometrist or ophthalmologist will take charge. If a problem is retinocortical, a neurologist, ophthalmologist, and neurosurgeon may have to collaborate in localizing and managing the pathologic process. If the problem lies at the integrative level, detailed cognitive evaluation by a neurologist or neuropsychologist may be necessary.

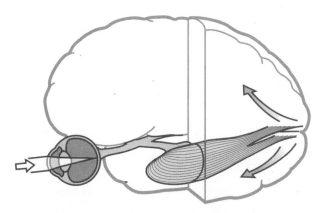

Figure I–1. The Visual Pathway. There are three functional components: optical (cornea to retina), retinocortical (retina to primary visual cortex), and integrative (primary visual cortex to vision-related parietal and temporal cortex).

HOW THIS BOOK IS ORGANIZED

The Neurology of Vision is organized according to the three components of the visual system described above.

Part I, "How the Human Visual System Works," is an overview of how each component works, linking current scientific and clinical concepts.

Part II, "Symptoms of a Failing Visual System," differentiates the symptoms of optical, retinocortical, and integrative disorders.

Part III, "Measures of a Failing Visual System," reviews the tests used to assess visual function, with an emphasis on rationale, technique, and interpretation, especially in terms of localization to the three components.

Part IV, "Topographic Disorders," provides information about vision-impairing conditions according to anatomic site, from the retina to the primary visual cortex.

Part V, "Nonorganic Visual Disturbances," deals with visual signs and symptoms generated by behavioral and psychiatric disorders.

Part VI presents real cases that can be solved only by incorporating the principles and facts presented in the text.

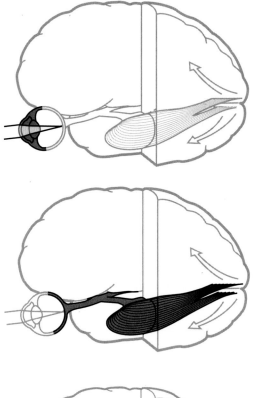

Figure I–2. The Optical Component. The cornea and lens refract light in order to bring it to a point focus on the retina.

Figure I–3. The Retinocortical Component. Retinal photoreceptors convert light into neural signals that are sent to primary visual cortex for elementary encoding.

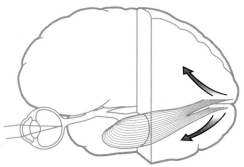

Figure I–4. The Integrative Component. The occipitoparietal pathway integrates motion and depth information into spatial percepts ("where" pathway). The occipitotemporal branch integrates form and color information into recognizable symbols ("what" pathway).

Part I

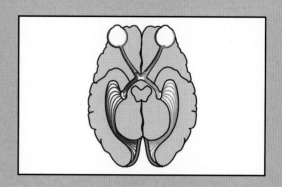

How the Human Visual System Works

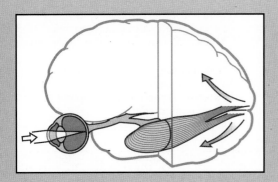

Chapter 1

THE OPTICAL, RETINOCORTICAL, AND INTEGRATIVE COMPONENTS

The visual pathway consists of an optical, a retinocortical, and an integrative component.

THE OPTICAL COMPONENT

The purpose of the optical component of the visual pathway is to present a clear, undistorted image to the retina. For this to take place, three conditions should be met: (*1*) *emmetropia,* where the refracting (focusing) power of the cornea and crystalline lens must match the anteroposterior (axial) length of the eye, so that parallel light rays emanating from a distant target come to a point focus on the retina; (*2*) *accommodation,* where the eye must be able to increase its refractive power enough to bring diverging light rays emanating from a near target (situated at reading distance) into focus on the retina; and (*3*) *ocular media transparency,* where the eye's transparent tissues, located between the cornea and the retina, must be free of imperfections or opacities (Table 1-1).

5

Table 1–1. **How the Optical Component Works and Fails**

	Normal Function	**Abnormal Function**
Refraction	Converges parallel light rays from distant objects to a point focus on the retina	Deficient refractive power: hyperopia Excessive refractive power: myopia Abnormal corneal curvature: astigmatism
Accommodation	Converges diverging light rays from near objects to a point focus on the retina	Deficient accommodation: presbyopia, accommodation paresis Excessive accommodation: spasm of accommodation
Ocular media	Provide smooth surfaces and transparent tissues	Surface irregularities and tissue opacities

Emmetropia

When the eye's optical system is able to bring light rays from distant objects to a point focus on the retina without the need for an refractive aid, the eye is said to be in a state of "emmetropia" (Fig. 1-1). Emmetropia is present in about 30% of the adult population;[1] the remaining 70% have a refractive error, or *ametropia,* in which light rays come to a point focus either behind the retina (hyperopia) (Fig. 1-2*a*) or in front of it (myopia) (Fig. 1-3*a*). In hyperopia, the eye's deficient refractive power must be enhanced with a convex spherical lens, which converges light rays, in order to bring parallel light rays from an object viewed at far distance onto a retinal focus (Fig. 1-2*b*). In myopia, the eye's excess refractive power must be reduced with a concave spherical lens, which diverges light rays, in order for parallel light rays to focus on the retina (Fig. 1-3*b*).[2]

At birth, the eyeball is relatively short (18 mm), so that light rays are focused behind the retina, creating hyperopia. The eye

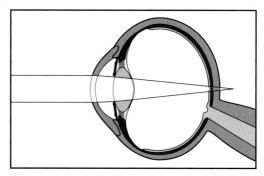

a

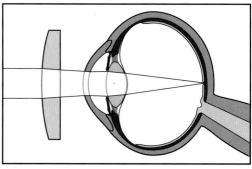

b

Figure 1–2. Hyperopia. (*a*) Uncorrected hyperopia. The hyperopic eye has deficient refractive power for its relatively short axial length, so light rays from distant objects come to a focus behind the retina. (*b*) Corrected hyperopia. A convex lens placed before the eye increases refractive power and allows light rays from a distant target to come to a focus on the retina.

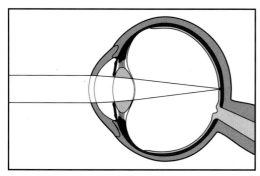

Figure 1–1. Emmetropia. The eye's focusing elements and its axial length are perfectly balanced. Parallel light rays emanating from objects viewed at a distance of 20 feet or more are focused on the retina.

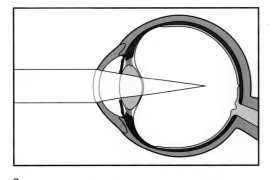 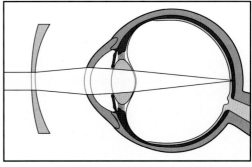

a   b

Figure 1–3. Myopia. (*a*) Uncorrected myopia. The eye's refractive power is too great for its long axial length, so that light rays from distant objects come to a focus in front of the retina. (*b*) Corrected myopia. A concave lens is placed before the eye to reduce its refractive power and allow light rays from a distant target to come to a focus on the retina.

grows 5 mm in the first 3 years of life, and then about 1.5 mm up to age 14, when adult size (24–25 mm) is reached.[3] Were there no change in the eye's refractive power during this growth period, the increase in its axial length would result in a relatively long eyeball, and light rays would be focused in front of the retina, creating myopia. But a compensatory reduction in crystalline lens power occurs concurrently as part of an active process called "emmetropization," in which deviations from emmetropia alter the release of retinal neurotransmitters and growth factors, which, in turn, mediate changes in growth of the lens, sclera, and choroid.[4–7]

The failure of emmetropization, which creates a mismatch between refractive power and axial length, is genetically determined and arises within the first two decades of life. Refractive errors may also occur later in life as the result of a an aging change in lens protein, displacement of the lens, swelling of the retina, or deformation of the globe (Chapter 2).

Patients who have myopia or hyperopia often have an accompanying refractive aberration called *astigmatism,* in which the corneal curvature is warped. Without optical correction, the astigmatic eye cannot focus light rays to a single point (Fig. 1-4*a*). Unlike myopia and hyperopia, which are corrected with a spherical lens, astigmatism is corrected with a cylinder, which adds focusing power only in the optical plane where refraction is deficient (Fig. 1-4*b*).

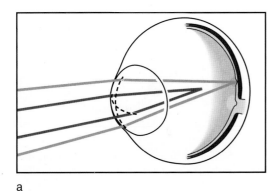 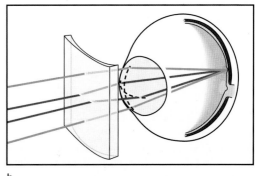

a   b

Figure 1–4. Astigmatism. (*a*) Uncorrected astigmatism. The corneal curvature is warped, so that light rays in two different planes do not come to a point focus on the retina. (*b*) Corrected astigmatism. A cylindrical lens placed before the eye refracts light in only one plane (here the horizontal plane) and thereby brings light rays to a point focus on the retina.

Accommodation

Emmetropia and the correction of hyperopia, myopia, and astigmatism apply to the task of focusing objects viewed at a distance of 20 feet or greater from the eye. Light rays reaching the eye from such remote distances are parallel. By contrast, light rays emanating from objects located within 20 feet of the eye are diverging. To focus diverging light rays on the retina, the eye must be able to "crank up" additional convergence power. This is accomplished by means of accommodation, an increase in the refractive power of the crystalline lens triggered by an attempt to view an object placed within reading distance (Fig. 1-5a). Parasympathetic innervation originating in parietooccipital regions bihemispherically produces concentric contraction of the ciliary muscle, which loosens the muscle's filamentous attachments to the lens. Freed of this restraint, the lens assumes its natural convex shape, which allows greater convergence of light rays (Fig. 1-5b).

Physiologic decline in the accommodative power of the lens with increasing age is called presbyopia (Fig. 1-5c). It usually becomes noticeable in the fifth decade, when one's arms seem to be too short to hold the telephone directory at a clear reading distance. Degeneration of crystalline lens protein during aging stiffens the lens, so that it cannot assume its natural convexity as the ciliary muscle contracts during accommodation. Poor lens responsiveness only intensifies accommodative effort, which gives rise to ciliary muscle spasm and a deep eye and brow ache. A properly

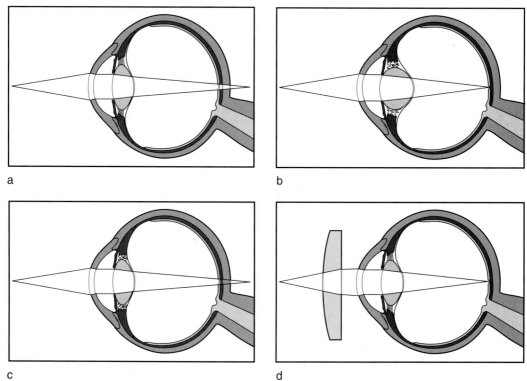

a   b

c   d

Figure 1–5. Accommodation. (*a*) Unaccommodated state. Light rays emanate from a target viewed at reading distance, so that they are diverging when they reach the eye. Unless the eye's ciliary muscle contracts, the image will come to a focus behind the retina (and appear blurred). (*b*) Normal accommodation. The eye's ciliary muscle undergoes concentric contraction, which loosens the zonular connections to the lens. Freed of zonular restraints, the lens assumes its natural convex shape, increases its refractive power, and focuses the target on the retina. (*c*) Uncorrected presbyopia. With advancing age, lens protein stiffens so that the lens cannot assume its convex shape, despite loosening of the zonules by ciliary muscle contraction. Targets viewed at reading distance cannot be focused on the retina. (*d*) Corrected presbyopia. A convex lens placed before the eye replaces its lost accommodative power and allows light rays from near targets to be focused on the retina.

fitted reading spectacle (or bifocal) corrects the problem (Fig. 1-5d).

Apart from presbyopia, other causes of accommodation failure are systemically administered anticholinergic agents, ciliary nerve or muscle damage due to trauma or inflammation, and surgical removal of a cataractous lens (Chapter 2).

Accommodation may also occur inappropriately (or excessively) when distant objects are being viewed (Chapter 2). Such "accommodative spasm" causes the image to come to a focus in front of the retina, creating an artificial myopia. Inappropriate accommodation is usually a manifestation of anxiety, depression, or malingering, but it may also occur with topically administered cholinergic agents or after severe brainstem trauma (Chapter 2).

Ocular Media Transparency

In reaching the retina, refracted light rays must pass through the refracting elements—the cornea and lens—and the nonrefracting space occupied by the aqueous and vitreous. Together, these refracting and the nonrefracting elements make up the *ocular media.* Even if refractive errors have been corrected, viewed objects will not come to a clear focus on the retina if there are ocular media imperfections, such as surface irregularities or opacities. These imperfections do not generally block light; they redirect it in a disorderly fashion, preventing a coherent focus on the retina (Fig. 1-6a,b). The only media abnormality that blocks light is a dense vitreous opacity. If it lies immediately in front of the retina, it will cast a discrete shadow on the retina and cause the patient to report a gray or black speck "in front of my vision" (positive scotoma) (Fig. 1-6c). Glasses cannot eliminate the blurred vision created by media imperfections. However, if the defect lies in the superficial cornea, a contact lens often dramatically corrects the problem by providing a smooth optical surface.

The Pinhole Effect

Even if there are ocular media imperfections, light rays passing through a narrow

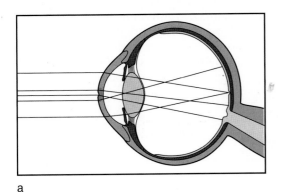

a

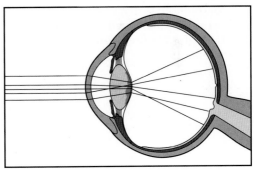

b

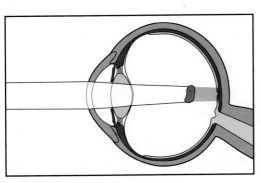

c

Figure 1–6. Media imperfections. (*a*) A corneal scar scatters light so that no coherent image forms on the retina. (*b*) A lens opacity (cataract) scatters light and precludes a clear retinal image. (*c*) A posterior vitreous opacity casts a shadow on the retina that is perceived as a speck or blob that blocks vision (positive scotoma).

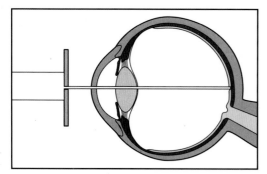

Figure 1–7. The pinhole effect. By narrowing the aperture to light rays, the pinhole bypasses the refractive aberrations in eyes with refractive errors or media imperfections. Vision becomes astoundingly clear. This principle is the basis of the pinhole test used in differentiating optical from neural causes of vision loss (Chapter 6).

channel may "get through" coherently if the channel is located in a portion of the ocular media where there are no optical imperfections.[2] Called the "pinhole effect," this phenomenon is the basis for a useful clinical maneuver called the pinhole test (Fig. 1-7 and Chapter 6). After visual acuity has been tested, an occluder perforated with multiple 2.5 mm diameter holes is placed before the eye. Marked improvement in visual acuity with the pinhole is diagnostic of an optical cause of subnormal visual acuity—either an uncorrected refractive error or a media imperfection.

THE RETINOCORTICAL COMPONENT

The retinocortical component of the visual pathway extends from the retina to the primary visual cortex (Fig. 1-8). The retina converts focused light rays into neural signals and enhances the contrast between viewed objects and their surroundings. These enhanced signals are then transmitted via the lateral geniculate body to the primary visual cortex, where luminance, color, and position features are separately processed.

Retina

The retina is a mosaic of photoreceptors connected by interneurons to long-range message transmitters, the retinal ganglion cells (Fig. 1-9).[8] This "vertical transmission" is modified by a network of horizontal cells and amacrine cells that enhance contrast between signals derived from adjacent retinal segments. Glial (Mueller) cells protect signal transmission by buffering extracellular ions and neurotransmitters.

In primates, the retina has two functions: to mediate form and color vision at the point of fixation (the foveal region) and to mediate motion vision away from the fovea (Box 1-1; Fig. 1-10).[9] These functions are actuated

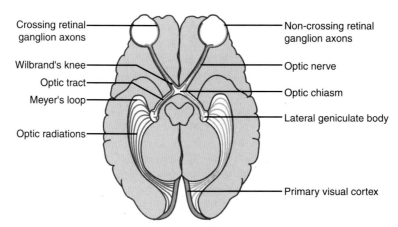

Crossing retinal ganglion axons · Non-crossing retinal ganglion axons · Wilbrand's knee · Optic nerve · Optic tract · Optic chiasm · Meyer's loop · Lateral geniculate body · Optic radiations · Primary visual cortex

Figure 1–8. The retinocortical component. Focused light rays undergo transduction to neural signals in the retinal photoreceptors. Signals transmitted via retinal ganglion cell axons synapse in the lateral geniculate body and are then conveyed to primary visual cortex. The brain's view of visual space changes from an ocular to a hemifield representation at the optic chiasm.

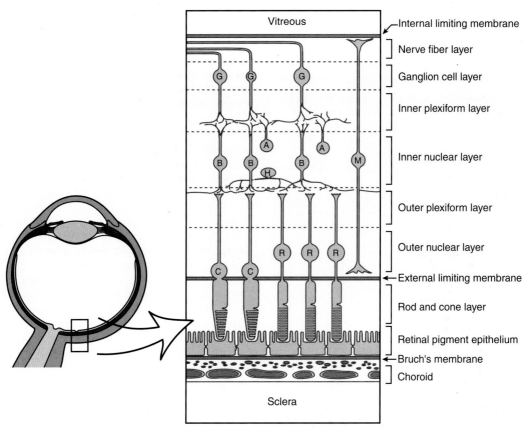

Figure 1–9. The retina. This cross-sectional view emphasizes synaptic connections. Light is absorbed by photopigments in the rods (R) and cones (C). Light causes a graded decrease in glutamate release from photoreceptors, which results in a graded change in signal transmission from bipolar cells (B). Bipolar cells connect to ganglion cells (G), which, when depolarized, fire long-range action potentials to the lateral geniculate body, midbrain, and hypothalamus. Small (parvocellular) ganglion cells subserve visual acuity and color vision, and large (magnocellular) ganglion cells subserve motion detection. Horizontal cells (H) and amacrine cells (A) modify transmission of surrounding impulse traffic in order to enhance visual contrast. Muller cells (M) are glial cells that protect signal transmission by buffering extracellular ions and neurotransmitters.

by two types of photoreceptors, the rods and the cones.

PHOTORECEPTORS

The photoreceptors are suspended on a monolayer of retinal pigment epithelium (RPE), which provides critical metabolic support. Rods outnumber cones by 20 to 1 and are designed for low light, low resolution, and slow motion detection. Absent from the fovea, they are present throughout the peripheral retina, with heaviest concentration in the parafoveal region. Rods lack sensitivity to color, but their vast stores of photopigment amplify achromatic light signals by absorbing photons over long reaction times. Their light detection capability is further enhanced by the fact that they converge on retinal ganglion cells in a ratio that varies from 1 to 50 parafoveally to 1 to 1500 in the peripheral retina.

Cones are designed to detect color and fine detail in high light levels. Heavily concentrated in the fovea, they react quickly and converge on retinal ganglion cells with a ratio that is as low as 2 to 1 in the fovea but increases with greater distance from the fovea. The most peripheral 10% of the retina contains no cones—it is completely color blind. There are three kinds of cones, which are distinguished by photopigments that have unique spectral sensitivities. The inter-

Box 1-1

THE CENTRAL RETINA

In describing the central retina, the terms "fovea" and "macula" are often used interchangeably. Moving outward, the correct anatomic designations are:

- **Foveola:** 0.35 mm diameter concavity in the center of the fovea that contains only cone photoreceptors.
- **Fovea:** 1.5 mm diameter area in the center of the macula. It has denser pigment than surrounding retina
- **Macula:** round area of retina 6 mm in diameter centered 4 mm temporal and 0.8 mm inferior to the optic disk. It contains two or more layers of ganglion cells.

play between these three kinds of cone is responsible for conveying color vision.

Photon capture and conversion into neural signals (transduction) takes place in the retinal photoreceptors.[10] Both types of photoceptors use an identical transduction mechanism (Fig. 1-11). In darkness (Fig. 1-11 left), photoreceptors prepare themselves to absorb light. All-trans retinaldehyde is converted to all-trans retinol (vitamin A), which is shunted from the outer segment to the RPE. There it is replenished with additional vitamin A from the choroidal arterioles, transformed into 11-*cis*-retinaldehyde, and conveyed to the photoreceptor outer segment. It links with opsins to form photopigment (rhodopsin in rods, iodopsins in cones). A deficiency of vitamin A or dysfunction of either photoreceptors or RPE interrupts this process. The patient experiences delayed recovery of vision following exposure to bright light, a prolonged afterimage, and an impaired ability to detect low light in darkness (nyctalopia).

When the retina is exposed to light (Fig. 1-11 right), the opsin's 11-*cis*-retinaldehyde is converted to its all-trans isomer, or "bleached." This transformation decreases intracellular cyclic guanosine monophosphate (cGMP), closes cGMP-gated membrane sodium channels, and hyperpolarizes the photoreceptors from a standing potential of −40 mV toward −70 mV. The increase in resting potential leads to a decrease in glu-

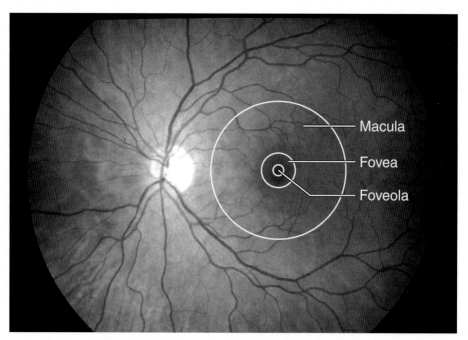

Figure 1-10. The central retina (ophthalmoscopic view).

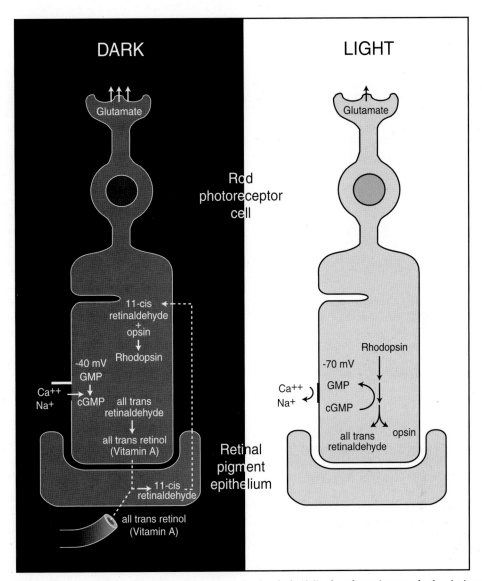

Figure 1–11. Phototransduction in rod photoreceptors. In the dark (*left*), the photopigment rhodopsin is generated in the retinal pigment epithelium (RPE). The photoreceptor calcium–sodium cell membrane channel is open, generating cyclic GMP and setting the intracellular potential at −40 mV, which causes large glutamate release. In the light (*right*), rhodopsin is converted to all-trans retinaldehyde and opsin. This bleaching process converts cyclical GMP to GMP, closes the calcium–sodium channel, raises intracellular potential to −70 mV, and reduces glutamate release. The reduced glutamate release stimulates bipolar cells and eventually influences the firing rate of retinal ganglion cells.

tamate release, which stimulates bipolar cells and eventually ganglion cells. The decline in glutamate release is graded. That is, it is proportional to the intensity of light, the amount of available 11-*cis*-retinaldehyde, and calcium currents. Under constant high illumination, healthy cones slowly extrude

calcium, thereby raising the level of cGMP, reopening some sodium channels, and allowing the cones to react to additional light stimuli. This "light adaptation" process fails in cone dysfunction syndromes and the patient experiences a persistent dazzling blindness in bright light called *hemeralopia*.

GANGLION CELLS

Rods and cones communicate with ganglion cells through horizontal and amacrine cells. These interneurons enhance contrast within the ganglion cell's receptive field—the region of visual space from which a light stimulus will alter the cell's firing rate. All retinal ganglion cells have concentric receptive fields with disk-shaped centers and doughnut-shaped surrounding areas. The inputs to these two portions of the receptive field have antagonistic effects, one excitatory, the other inhibitory. The effect of this arrangement is to permit the visual system, in its earliest neural portion, to detect local differences in light intensity, which later become the basis for perceiving form, color, position, and movement.

Unlike retinal receptors, which have graded potentials, retinal ganglion cells have all-or-nothing signal properties. Once threshold is reached, ganglion cells fire action potentials with a frequency that depends on the degree of excitation. There are at least two types of ganglion cell, a small-cell (parvocellular), small–receptive field class designed for color and form vision perception, and a large-cell (magnocellular), large–receptive field class designed for motion and depth perception. The small ganglion cells receive primarily cone transmission. A subset of small cones designed for color vision subtract the transmissions from three types of cones to derive spectral information. The subset of cones designed for form vision summate the cone inputs and signal high-contrast achromatic information.

Small ganglion cells react slowly and specialize in transmitting information related to identifying static objects, whereas large ganglion cells are capable of rapid firing in order to detect the rate of change in local light intensities, which will later be interpreted as motion. The large ganglion cells receive both cone and rod inputs and carry low-contrast visual information.

Form and color vision are mediated by a tiny 1.5 mm diameter retinal region called the *fovea*, (Box 1-1), which contains only cone photoreceptors. Away from the fovea, the rods and cones primarily serve the large ganglion cells for motion and position de-

tection, with the cones working in high- and the rods in low-light environments.

RETINAL NERVE FIBER BUNDLES

Between the photoreceptors and their ganglion cells, the retinal architecture is vertical (Fig. 1-9). That is, the receptive fields of ganglion cells correspond to patches of receptors lying immediately underneath them. A lesion deep within the retina causes a visual field defect whose shape corresponds exactly to the shape of the lesion. In the superficial retina, between the ganglion cells and the optic nerve, the topography turns horizontal, according to the geography of the axons of the retinal ganglion cells (Fig. 1-12). A lesion in this region causes a visual field defect whose configuration is based on the configuration of the axon (nerve fiber) bundles as they sweep across the retinal surface to converge on the optic disk. Three compartments of nerve fiber bundles are distinguished by their shape and differential vulnerability to disease:[11]

- **Papillomacular.** Axons of ganglion cells located in the macula and the area be-

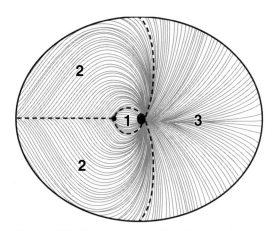

Figure 1–12. The retinal nerve fiber layer (right eye). The inner retinal surface consists of the retinal nerve fiber layer, made up of axons of retinal ganglion cells. The large oval is the optic disk; the small dot is the fovea. There are three functional compartments: papillomacular bundle (1), carrying macular axons; superior and inferior arcuate bundles (2), carrying extramacular axons in the temporal retina; nasal radial bundle (3), carrying axons emanating from the retina nasal to the optic disk. Lesions of the optic nerve, nerve fiber layer, and retinal ganglion cells give rise to visual field defects that have a shape corresponding to the compartment that has been damaged.

tween the macula and the optic disk project directly toward the optic nerve head (papilla = optic nerve head). Damage to them produces *central scotomas*, round defects centered at fixation (Fig. 1-13*a*), and *cecocentral scotomas*, oval or cigar-shaped defects that span the area between fixation and the physiologic blind spot (Fig. 1-13*b*). Injury to this bundle is caused most commonly by optic nerve compression, inflammation, nutritional deprivation, mitochondrial DNA mutations, and toxins (Chapters 12, 13).

- **Arcuate.** Axons that loop above and below the papillomacular bundle make up the ar-

cuate bundles. They originate either above or below a border that extends horizontally from the fovea to the temporal periphery of the retina. Lesions limited to the more peripheral arcuate axons cause podlike defects in the nasal field that are aligned to the horizontal meridian (Fig. 1-14*a*). Lesions affecting both the peripheral and central axons within the arcuate region produce scimitar-shaped arcuate visual field defects (Fig. 1-14*b*). Destruction of the entire arcuate compartment above or below this horizontal line produces an altitudinal visual field defect (Fig. 1-14*c*). Common causes are glaucoma and isch-

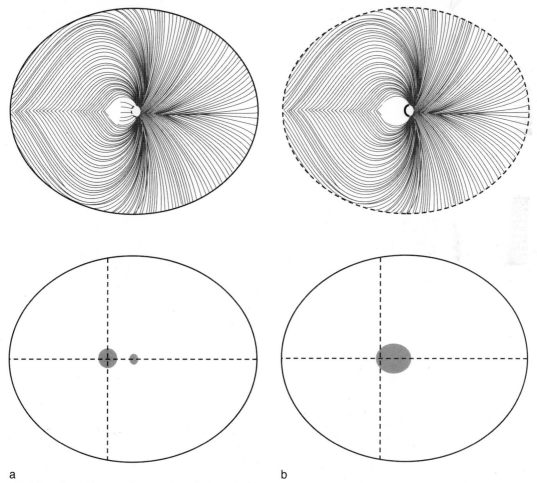

a   b

Figure 1–13. Papillomacular nerve fiber lesions and their visual field defects. (*a*) Central scotoma. A lesion destroying macular axons—either on the retina or in the optic nerve—(*top*) causes a central scotoma, pictured as the large gray circle at the intersection of the horizontal and vertical fixational meridians (*bottom*). (*b*) Cecocentral scotoma. A lesion destroying the axons emanating from the macula and the region between the macula and the optic disk (*top*) causes a centrocecal scotoma (*bottom*).

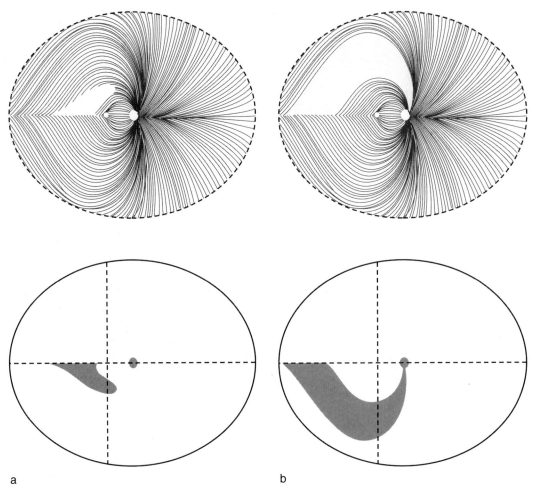

a   b

Figure 1–14. Arcuate nerve fiber bundle lesions and their visual field defects. (*a*) Nasal step. A lesion destroying the terminal axons in some upper arcuate bundles (*top*) causes a podlike visual field defect (*bottom*) with its foot attached to the horizontal meridian. (*b*) Arcuate scotoma. A lesion destroying all axons in some upper arcuate bundles (*top*) causes an inferior scimitar-shaped visual field defect (*bottom*). (*continued*)

emic, inflammatory, dyplastic, and drusen optic neuropathies (Chapters 12, 13).

- **Nasal radial.** Unlike the axons in temporal retina, those in nasal retina take a converging linear and radial course toward the optic disk. In the visual field, damage to these fibers appears as a temporal wedge scotoma that usually emerges from the physiologic blind spot (Fig. 1-15). This relatively uncommon scotoma occurs in dysplastic and inflammatory optic neuropathies (Chapters 12, 13).

BLOOD SUPPLY

The blood supply of the RPE and photoreceptors comes from the choroidal arteries, which form one branch of the ophthalmic artery (Fig. 1-16). The retinal ganglion cells and their axons, as well as the bipolar cells, are nourished by the other branch of the ophthalmic artery, the central retinal artery.

Optic Nerve

The optic nerve is a cylindrical diencephalic white matter tract. Retinal ganglion cell axons, unmyelinated on the retinal surface, take on oligodendroglial myelin within the optic nerve. As the nerve approaches the chiasm, axons coming from the nasal and temporal retina begin to segregate (Fig. 1-8). Posterior optic nerve lesions therefore cause

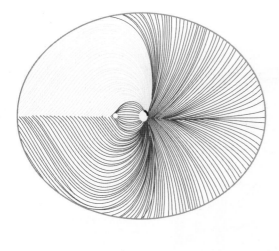

ized and very tiny, the twigs that nourish this part of the optic nerve branch off a ring around the optic nerve called the circle of Zinn-Haller. These branches are particularly vulnerable to occlusion in hypoperfusion states, arteriosclerosis, and increased intracranial pressure.

The intraorbital optic nerve segment is supplied by pial branches of the ophthalmic artery. These pial penetrators supply mainly the rim of the nerve; small collaterals of the central retinal artery contribute marginally to the core of the distal 1–1.5 cm of the intraorbital segment. Thus the core of the intraorbital optic nerve segment is another region vulnerable to infarction, particularly in patients with acute hypotension and anemia.

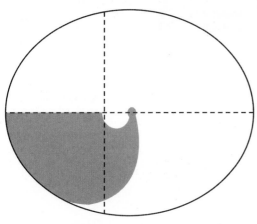

c

Figure 1–14. (*continued*) (*c*) Altitudinal scotoma. A lesion destroying all of the upper arcuate bundles (*top*) causes an inferior visual field defect with an extensive border at the horizontal meridian (*bottom*).

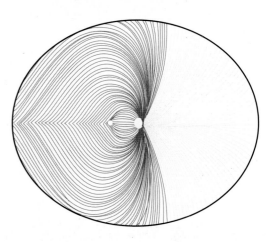

visual field defects that have hemianopic features suggestive of chiasmal lesions.

Familiarity with the blood supply of the optic nerve (Figs. 1-16, 1-17) is critical to understanding its pathophysiology.[12–14] The main points follow.

The surface of the optic nerve (prelaminar segment) is supplied jointly by choroidal arterioles and branches of the central retinal and short posterior ciliary arteries. This rich vascular system protects against infarction.

The optic nerve segment that lies within the scleral lamina cribrosa (laminar segment) and behind the scleral lamina (postlaminar segment) is supplied by the short posterior ciliary arteries. Poorly collateral-

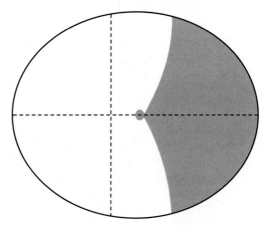

Figure 1–15. Nasal radial nerve fiber bundle lesion and its visual field defect. A lesion destroying some of the nasal radial axons (*top*) causes a temporal wedge visual field defect with its apex at the physiologic blind spot (*bottom*).

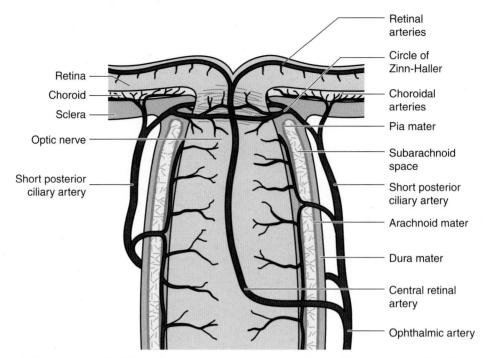

Figure 1–16. Arterial supply of the retina and optic nerve. The retinal nerve fiber, ganglion cell, and bipolar layers are supplied by the central retinal artery; the pigment epithelium and photoreceptor layers are supplied by the ciliary circulation via the choroidal arteries. The distal optic nerve is supplied mainly by the ciliary circulation. The intraocular portion of the optic nerve is supplied by the circle of Zinn-Haller. This poorly collateralized circle competes with the choroid for ciliary blood and is particularly vulnerable to occlusion. The orbital portion of the optic nerve is supplied by pial penetrators from the ciliary circulation. The intracanalicular and intracranial portions are supplied jointly by ophthalmic and internal carotid arteries.

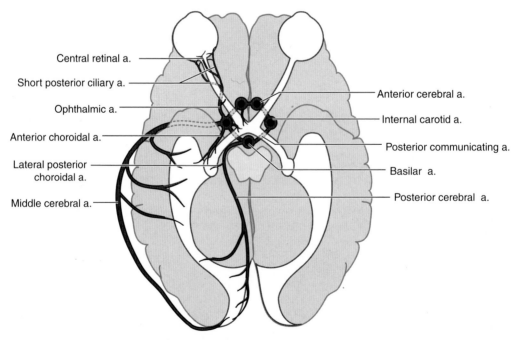

Figure 1–17. Arterial supply of the retinocortical component.

The intracanalicular and intracranial optic nerve segments are supplied jointly and richly by ophthalmic and internal carotid arteries. These segments are rarely infarcted, except in compressive or traumatic lesions.

Optic Chiasm

At the optic chiasm, the brain's view of visual space changes from an ocular to a hemifield representation. This change is accomplished by routing axons according to whether they come from nasal or temporal retina. About 55% of axons emanate from nasal retina; they cross within the chiasm to the opposite optic tract.[15] The 45% of axons that come from temporal retina join the ipsilateral optic tract. The slight excess of crossing fibers accounts for the low-intensity afferent pupil defect found contralateral to an optic tract lesion (Chapter 8).

Chiasmal crossing fibers are especially vulnerable to damage, perhaps because their blood supply is relatively tenuous.[16] Although ample supply from many branches of the internal carotid and anterior cerebral arteries (Fig. 1-17) protects against infarction, the median bar of the chiasm, where the crossing fibers lie, is particularly vulnerable to compression. As a result, mass lesions typically cause loss of temporal fields (bitemporal hemianopia; Fig. 1-18*a*), *no matter what their anatomic relationship to the chiasm may be.*

Lesions at the junction between the optic chiasm and optic nerve produce visual field defects that are hybrids of nerve fiber bundle defects and hemianopic defects. There are two "junctional" patterns.

Type 1 consists of a combination of a nerve fiber bundle defect and an incomplete temporal hemianopic defect in the ipsilateral eye[15a] (Fig. 1-18*b*). The field of the contralateral eye is normal. This pattern results from optic nerve lesions located 2 to 4 millimeters anterior to the chiasm. The partial temporal hemianopia reflects the segregation of nasal and temporal optic nerve axons at this point and the relative vulnerability of nasal fibers.

Type 2 consists of a nerve fiber bundle de-

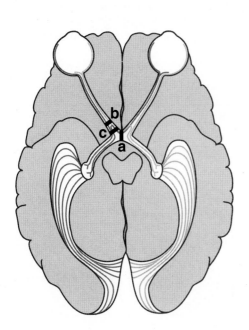

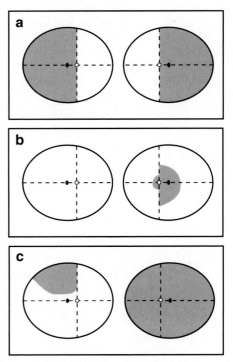

Figure 1–18. Lesions of the optic chiasm and their visual field defects. (*a*) Lesion of the optic chiasm: bitemporal hemianopia. (*b*) Anterior lesion of the optic nerve-chiasm junction: ipsilateral nerve fiber bundle defect and incomplete temporal hemianopia. (*c*) Posterior lesion of the optic nerve-chiasm junction: ipsilateral nerve fiber bundle defect and contralateral superior temporal hemianopia.

fect in the visual field of the ipsilateral eye and a superior temporal hemianopic defect in the field of the contralateral eye (Fig. 1-18*c*). This pattern results from optic nerve lesions situated within 1.5 millimeters of the chiasm. The contralateral hemianopic defect is attributed to damage to crossing fibers emanating from the contralateral inferior retina that loop anteriorly 1 to 1.5 millimeters into the ipsilateral optic nerve (Wilbrand's knee).[17,18] Histologic studies in monkeys and humans have challenged the existence of Wilbrand's knee, so perhaps the correct anatomic explanation for the Type 2 junctional defect is still to be found.

Some retinal axons bifurcate at the optic chiasm and send collaterals to the preoptic nucleus of the hypothalamus.[20] This pathway probably mediates certain vegetative functions that depend on light and dark (circadian) cycles.

Optic Tract

The optic tract is the segment of the visual pathway that connects the optic chiasm to the lateral geniculate body.[21] Within the optic tract, the retinal axons from the corresponding retinal regions of the two eyes are not adjacent to one another. As a result, in-

complete lesions give rise to incongruous homonymous hemianopias, or defects that are not identical in size, shape, or depth in the two eyes (Fig. 1-19*a*).

The optic tract sends the bulk of its fibers to the lateral geniculate body (LGB), the remainder going to the mesencephalon via the brachium of the superior colliculus. The mesencephalic branch leaves the tract immediately rostral to the LGB, providing light input to the pupillary reflex pathway and visual spatial input to the superior colliculus. Input to the superior colliculus mediates rudimentary detection vision and reflex visually guided eye movements. The two anatomic offshoots of the optic tract account for three clinical phenomena:

1. Pupillary reactions to light are preserved in patients with visual pathway lesions situated posterior to the optic tract.
2. Reflex eye movements to the sudden appearance of a light in the peripheral field are preserved when cerebral lesions destroy pathways for generating eye movements.
3. Subconscious ability to detect light may be preserved in a field rendered blind by a visual cortex lesion ("blindsight").[22–25]

The optic tract is supplied by the anterior choroidal artery (Fig. 1-17).[26] Spontaneous

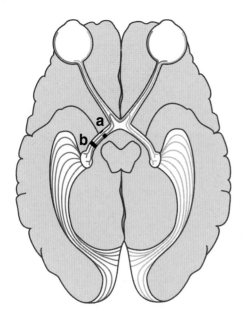

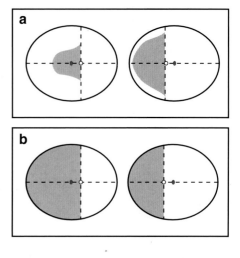

Figure 1–19. Lesions of the optic tract and their visual field defects. (*a*) Incomplete lesion. The field loss is an incongruous homonymous hemianopia. (*b*) Complete lesion. The field loss is a complete homonymous hemianopia.

strokes are uncommon, but surgical trauma or compressive lesions may infarct the tract by injuring its blood supply. Contralateral hemiparesis and hemisensory loss are accompanying manifestations of anterior choroidal artery stroke.

Lateral Geniculate Body

The lateral geniculate body, a posterolateral division of the thalamus, contains synaptic connections with retinal axons (Fig. 1-20), as well as inputs from many other cerebral sources (see below).[21] Axons from ipsilateral and contralateral eyes are segregated in layers. Numbered from ventral to dorsal, layers 1, 4, and 6 are the terminus of axons from the contralateral eye, whereas layers 2, 3, and 5 contain the axons coming from the ipsilateral eye. Layers 1 and 2 contain large (magnocellular) cells and receive inputs from large retinal ganglion cells. The other four layers contain small (parvocellular) cells and receive inputs from small ganglion cells.

The receptive fields of LGB neurons resemble those of the retinal ganglion cells in being bull's-eye, center-surround antagonistic. Exactly how the visual message is modified at the LGB is not known. However, the fact that 80% of inputs to LGB come from nonretinal sources, including the mesencephalic reticular formation, other thalamic nuclei, posterior parietal cortex, and occipital cortex, suggests that the *LGB may screen relevant from irrelevant visual information before it is sent on to visual cortex.*[21]

Although each layer of the LGB contains a retinotopic map of the contralateral hemifield, retinal space is not represented isometrically. The foveal region, which occupies less than 10% of the retinal surface, projects to 50% of the surface area in the LGB. This "magnification factor" reflects both the volume and importance of foveal projections. It has no clinical relevance in the LGB, where subtotal lesions are exquisitely rare. But this magnification of the foveal region is perpetuated in the visual cortex, which occupies a much larger brain volume and where subtotal lesions are common (see "Primary Visual Cortex," below).

The LGB is supplied peripherally by the anterior choroidal artery and centrally by the lateral posterior choroidal artery (Fig. 1-21a).[26,27] Occlusive disease of either vessel, which is rare, produces distinctive visual field defects (Fig. 1-21b,c, and Chapters 7, 14).[28] Because the LGB is such a small structure and the two vascular supplies are contiguous, large lesions often interrupt both circulations (Fig. 1-21d).

Optic Radiations

The optic radiations are cerebral hemispheric white matter tracts that course from the LGB to the primary visual cortex (Figs. 1-8, 1-22a).[29] After they leave the LGB, the radiations occupy the hind end of the posterior limb of internal capsule. The root of the radiations is fed by the anterior choroidal artery (Fig. 1-22b) and is vulnerable to occlusion, often causing the "capsular triad"—contralateral hemianopia (Fig. 1-23), hemiplegia, and hemianesthesia.

The fibers carrying inferior visual field information sweep directly backward toward the occipital lobe, but those carrying superior visual field information arch anteroinferiorly around the temporal horn of the lateral ventricle before turning backwards. This forward loop, named after the anatomist

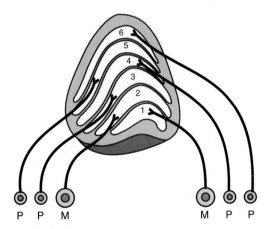

Figure 1–20. Retinal inputs to the (right) lateral geniculate body. Inputs from ipsilateral and contralateral eyes are segregated. Layers 1, 4, and 6 are the terminus of axons from the contralateral (left) eye, whereas layers 2, 3, and 5 are the terminus of axons from the ipsilateral (right) eye. Layers 1 and 2 receive input only from large (magnocellular) retinal ganglion cells (M), carrying contrast and motion information; layers 4–6 receive input only from small (parvocellular) ganglion cells (P), carrying acuity and color information.

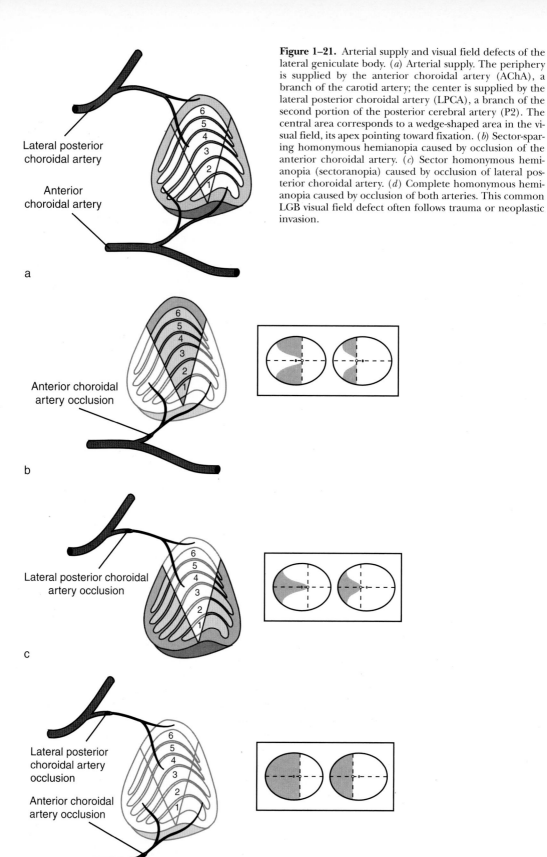

Figure 1–21. Arterial supply and visual field defects of the lateral geniculate body. (*a*) Arterial supply. The periphery is supplied by the anterior choroidal artery (AChA), a branch of the carotid artery; the center is supplied by the lateral posterior choroidal artery (LPCA), a branch of the second portion of the posterior cerebral artery (P2). The central area corresponds to a wedge-shaped area in the visual field, its apex pointing toward fixation. (*b*) Sector-sparing homonymous hemianopia caused by occlusion of the anterior choroidal artery. (*c*) Sector homonymous hemianopia (sectoranopia) caused by occlusion of lateral posterior choroidal artery. (*d*) Complete homonymous hemianopia caused by occlusion of both arteries. This common LGB visual field defect often follows trauma or neoplastic invasion.

Lateral posterior
choroidal artery

Anterior
choroidal artery

a

Anterior choroidal
artery occlusion

b

Lateral posterior choroidal
artery occlusion

c

Lateral posterior
choroidal artery
occlusion

Anterior choroidal
artery occlusion

d

Meyer ("Meyer's loop"),[30] reaches within 1 mm of the anterior tip of the ventricle, approximately 4–5 cm behind the anterior temporal pole. Lesions that extend more than 5 cm posteriorly into temporal lobe typically interrupt Meyer's loop to cause a wedge-shaped "pie-in-the-sky" visual field defect (Fig. 1-23).[31,32] Perfused by middle cerebral branches, this segment is rarely infarcted except in complete proximal stem occlusions. Meyer's loop defects are, however, particularly common after anterior temporal lobectomy for intractable partial seizures.

As the optic radiations sweep around the lateral ventricle, they are pancaked along its lateral surface, medial to the corona radiata and far from the cortical mantle. Fibers from the inferior retina remain inferior and those from the superior retina remain superior. Once the optic radiations reach the ventricular trigone, the fibers are so compact that lesions often produce complete homonymous hemianopias (Fig. 1-23). Because retinal axons from the corresponding retinal regions of the two eyes lie adjacent to one another, incomplete lesions cause congruous homonymous hemianopias, in which the defects in the two hemifields are identical in size, shape, and depth (Fig. 1-24a).

As the radiations pass beyond the trigone, they bifurcate to enter the upper and lower banks of the calcarine fissure. These branches are anatomically separate and are served by different calcarine artery branches. Accordingly, lesions here often cause lower (Fig. 1-24b) or upper homonymous quadrantanopias (Fig. 1-24c).

The majority of fibers in the optic radiations do not actually come from the LGB but from other thalamic nuclei and the visual cortex. They may play a role in visually guided eye movements and in visual attention.

Primary Visual Cortex

The optic radiations reach a destination in the primary visual cortex (striate cortex, V1; Fig. 1-25). The term "striate" derives from the prominent white line visible on gross anatomic sections that is caused by a dense myelinated fiber plexus.[33] In humans, 85% of primary visual cortex (V1) is buried within the interhemispheric fissure, its anterior border reaching the parietooccipital fissure.[34,35] With its posterior border extending out onto the occipital convexity 1 to 1.5 cm, V1 occupies between 25 and 40 cm² of cortex. The visual field is mapped onto V1 with a magnification factor for the fixational region similar to that found in LGB. Based on correlation of visual fields with MRI lesions[36,37] and functional MRI,[38] there are three clinically relevant divisions to the topography of the primary visual cortex (Fig. 1-26):

1. The caudal 50% of primary visual cortex encodes transmissions from the central 10 degrees of the visual field (fixational area).
2. The middle 40% of primary visual cortex encodes transmissions from 10 to 60 degrees eccentric to fixation (nonfixational binocular field).
3. The rostral 10% of primary visual cortex encodes transmissions from 60 to 90 degrees in the monocular field (temporal crescent).

Based on this mapping pattern, large lesions of the posterior visual cortex cause small, elusive, but visually troublesome defects restricted to the fixational area of the visual field (hemianopic paracentral scotomas). Lesions confined to the anterior and middle portions of visual cortex cause defects in the nonfixational binocular field and spare the fixational area (macular sparing; Fig. 1-27b). Rare lesions confined to the anterior 10% of visual cortex cause a defect in the monocular temporal crescent (Fig. 1-27a).

The primary visual cortex is supplied predominantly by the posterior cerebral artery—its occipitotemporal, parieto-occipital, and calcarine branches (Figs. 1-17, 1-22b). In some individuals, the portion of visual cortex that lies on the exposed brain surface receives collateral supply from posterior branches of the middle cerebral artery. This dual supply may account for preservation of posterior visual cortex (and macular sparing in the visual field) following posterior cerebral artery occlusions.[39]

Primary visual cortex, or V1, is organized into vertical columns that extend through the full thickness of cortex, from the pial surface to the underlying white matter (Fig. 1-28). Neurons in each column are tuned (fire most rapidly) to edges of a particular

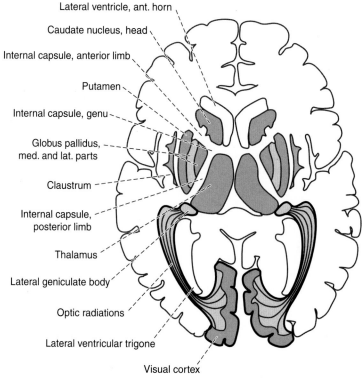

- Lateral ventricle, ant. horn
- Caudate nucleus, head
- Internal capsule, anterior limb
- Putamen
- Internal capsule, genu
- Globus pallidus, med. and lat. parts
- Claustrum
- Internal capsule, posterior limb
- Thalamus
- Lateral geniculate body
- Optic radiations
- Lateral ventricular trigone
- Visual cortex

a

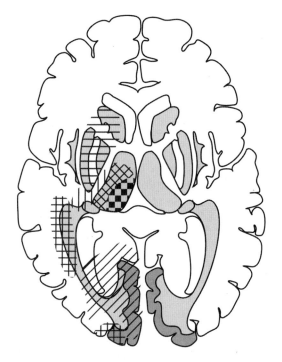

≡	Lenticulostriate arteries (middle cerebral artery)
⧆	Thalamogeniculate and lateral posterior choroidal arteries (posterior cerebral artery)
‖	Anterior choroidal artery (carotid artery)
▦	Middle cerebral artery–convexity branches
▨	Calcarine, parieto-occipital, occipito-temporal arteries (posterior cerebral artery)
▩	Thalamoperforating arteries (posterior cerebral artery)

b

Figure 1–22. Optic radiations and visual cortex. (*a*) Anatomic relationships. (*b*) Arterial supply.

24

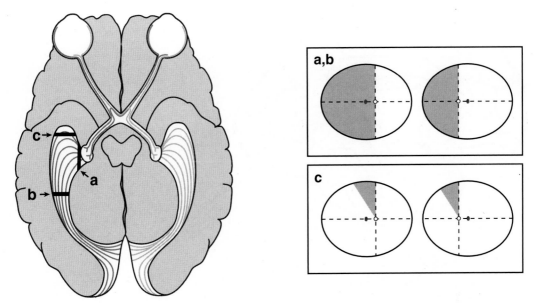

Figure 1–23. Lesions and visual field defects of the anterior and midoptic radiations. (*a*) Root lesion causing a complete homonymous hemianopia. (*b*) Anterior trigone lesion also causing a complete homonymous hemianopia. (*c*) Meyer's loop lesion cauing a wedge-shaped homonymous hemianopia with one border aligned to the vertical meridian ("pie-in-the-sky" defect).

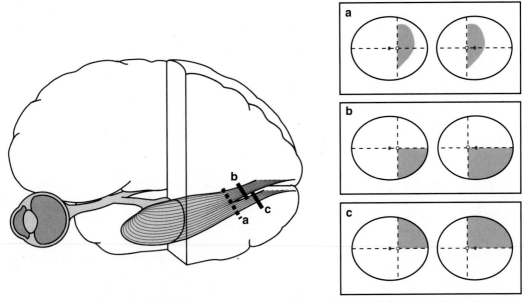

Figure 1–24. Lesions and visual field defects associated with the posterior optic radiations. (*a*) Incomplete posterior trigone lesion causing a congruous homonymous hemianopia. (*b*) Lesion of the superior bifurcation of posterior optic radiations causing an inferior homonymous quadrantanopia. (*c*) Lesion of the inferior bifurcation causing a superior homonymous quadrantanopia.

25

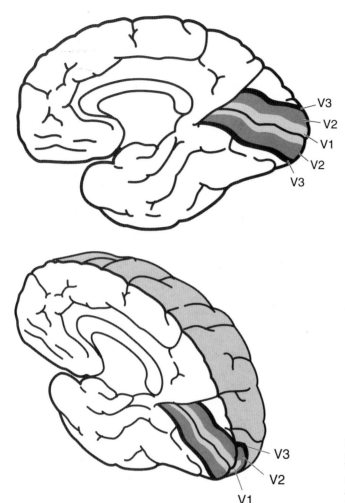

Figure 1–25. Primary visual cortex (striate cortex, V1). Surrounded by V2 and V3, two association visual cortices, V1 receives most of the input from the LGB. All but one-sixth lies buried within the interhemispheric fissure.

orientation.[29,35] There is a separate column for every 10 degree difference in orientation. Hypercolumns are aggregates of columns sensitive to all possible orientations of a stimulus located in a particular region of visual space.

Inputs from the right and left eye terminate in alternating hypercolumns, creating a checkerboard of "ocular dominance columns."[40] The synaptic input to the hypercolumns is not hard-wired at birth, in that axons coming from the right and left eye compete for cortical hookups. Thus if one eye of neonatal cats or monkeys is occluded, its ocular dominance and inputting LGB neurons shrink.[41] Cortical cells are then driven entirely by light signals from the non-occluded eye. In macaque, visual deprivation does not cause column shrinkage if it commences after age 12 weeks.[42] In humans, if one eye does not receive a clearly focused image on its fovea within the first weeks of life—owing to ocular misalignment, uncorrected refractive error, or media opacity—the deprived eye develops a loss of visual acuity called *amblyopia*.[43] If amblyopia develops later, these anatomic changes may not occur. For example, a postmortem study demonstrated that uniocular amblyopia resulting from accommodative esotropia with onset after age 2 years did not cause column shrinkage.[44] An intriguing fact is that amblyopia is the only *retrochiasmal* cause of monocular visual acuity loss (Chapter 15).

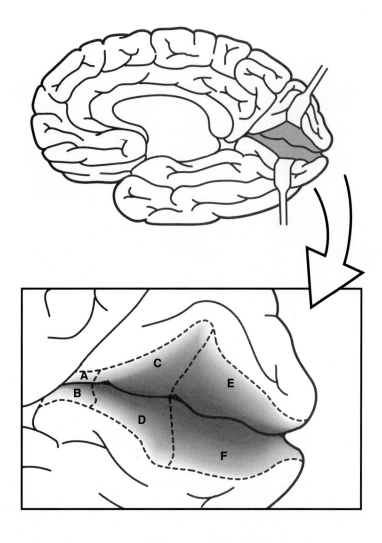

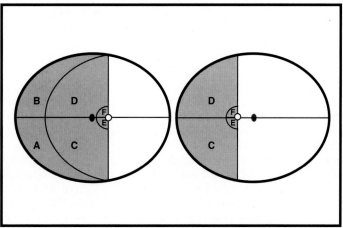

Figure 1–26. Mapping the visual field onto primary visual cortex. The posterior 50% of primary cortex (E, F) encodes the central 10% of the visual field. The middle 40% (C, D) encodes the peripheral field except the unpaired temporal crescent of the visual field, which is encoded by the anterior 10% of visual cortex (A, B).

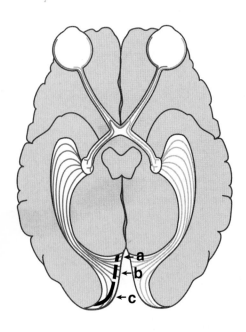

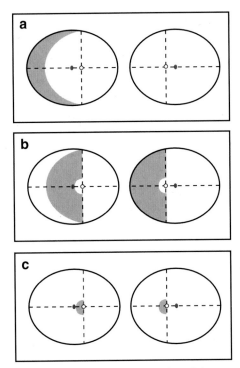

Figure 1–27. Incomplete lesions of the primary visual cortex and their visual field defects. (*a*) Lesion of the anterior 10% of visual cortex causes monocular crescent defect. (*b*) Lesion of the middle 40% of visual cortex causes macular-sparing homonymous hemianopia (and spares the monocular temporal crescent). (*c*) Lesion of the posterior 50% of visual cortex causes homonymous paracentral scotomas.

In the macaque, visual impulse traffic flows from V1 to V2 and then to V3, visual areas that closely resemble V1 but process slightly more complex information. The human pathway is uncertain, but for purposes of clinical correlation, V1, V2, and V3 are combined because their small receptive fields are similar and because lesions produce identical visual field defects.[36] In Brodmann's nomenclature, V1 corresponds to area 17; V2 and V3 to area 18. Four visual features are processed in V1 (Fig. 1-28):

- **Form.** Spots are converted to line segments. Output is primarily to pale stripes in V2 and from there to V3 or V4.
- **Color.** Encoded by wavelength within "blobs," regions suspended within hypercolumns that stain intensively with cytochrome oxidase. Output is primarily to cytochrome oxidase–staining thin dark stripes in V2 and from there to V4.
- **Motion.** Encoded by luminance changes of line segments in particular orientations. Output is primarily to cytochrome oxidase–staining dark thick stripes in V2 and from there to the middle temporal (MT) area (V5).
- **Depth.** Encoded by merging the slightly disparate images from the two eyes in "binocular disparity–sensitive" neurons on column borders that receive inputs from adjacent ocular dominance columns.[40] Because the eyes are separated, objects that are situated away from points of fixation are focused on noncorresponding regions of the two retinas. If these noncorresponding retinal points are within a certain proximity range, the visual system is able to fuse their information in the disparity-sensitive neurons in V1 and at higher integrative levels. This process subserves binocular depth perception, or stereopsis. The early childhood conditions associated with unclear retinal focus that cause amblyopia also

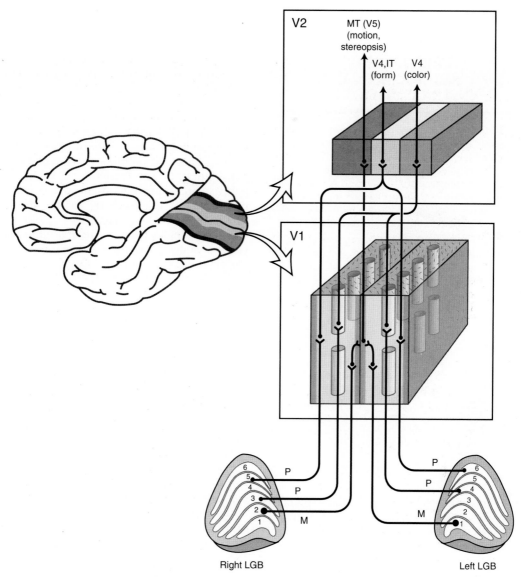

Figure 1–28. Feature processing in visual cortex. Form, color, motion detection, and depth perception (stereopsis) are encoded in separate channels. For form, input to V1 is parvocellular, and output is to pale stripes in V2 and from there to V3 or V4. For color, input is parvocellular to cylindrical "blobs," regions suspended within hypercolumns that stain intensively with cytochrome oxidase. Output is to cytochrome oxidase–staining thin dark stripes in V2 and from there to V4. For motion, input is magnocellular and output is mainly to cytochrome oxidase–staining dark thick stripes in V2 and from there to MT (V5). For stereopsis, input is mainly magnocellular to "binocularity disparity-sensitive" neurons located on the border zones of the ocular dominance columns. Output is mainly to cytochrome oxidase–staining dark thick stripes in V2, which is later conveyed to MT (V5).

cause a loss of stereopsis and a disappearance of V1 cells sensitive to visual stimuli from both eyes.[45] Output is mainly to cytochrome oxidase–staining dark thick stripes in V2 and from there to MT (V5).

In reviewing retinocortical transmission, one discerns three guiding principles: retinotopic mapping, parallel processing, and hierarchical processing (Box 1-2). *Retinotopic mapping* is the transmission of vi-

Box 1–2

PRINCIPLES OF RETINOCORTICAL TRANSMISSION

- **Retinotopic mapping.** Each point in visual space is neurologically represented on a specific geographic region of the retina, a specific bundle of retinocortical axons, and a specific portion of V1, V2, and V3. Therefore, lesions produce discrete topographic (retinotopic) sensory deficits called *scotomas*—depressions in luminance and crude form detection.

- **Parallel processing.** Separate processing of form and/or color and spatial information begins at the retina and is carried out in distinct channels.[105] Spatial channels may be selectively damaged in glaucoma,[106] amblyopia,[107] dyslexia,[108] and Alzheimer's disease.[109]

- **Hierarchical processing.** Uncoding of visual information proceeds from a primitive to a more complex level. Retinal receptors encode an array of spots of different light intensities; retinal ganglion cells enhance edge contrasts and encode spectral information; the primary visual cortex encodes orientation of line segments.

sual information to brain regions spatially corresponding to each point in visual space. *Parallel processing* indicates that visual features (form, color, motion, depth) are processed in separate neural channels beginning at the retinal ganglion cell level. *Hierarchical processing* is the extraction of progressively more complex and global features at higher levels of the visual pathway. Parallel and hierarchical processing persist within the integrative component of the visual pathway, but retinotopic mapping is sacrificed to allow for global feature processing.

THE INTEGRATIVE COMPONENT

After reaching V3, visual information is carried along two functionally separate pathways, as seen in Table 1-2:

1. The occipitoparietal ("where") pathway, which signals where an object is in space, how fast it is moving, and where it is going (Table 1-3). It also mediates how attention is to be distributed across items in visual space.
2. The occipitotemporal ("what") pathway, which identifies objects, symbols, and colors (Table 1-4). Largely dependent on foveal parvocellular inputs, it is phylogenetically newer than the occipitoparietal pathway.

Evidence for the existence of these two pathways in humans comes, in part, from extrapolation of single-cell recordings and lesional studies in the macaque.[46–50] But the close homologies between the macaque and human brain,[51] together with human psychophysical,[52,53] lesional,[54] functional magnetic resonance imaging (MRI),[55–57] magnetoencephalographic,[58] and positron emission tomographic (PET) studies[59–61] support the inference that humans have similar physiology. Although two parallel integrative visual pathways clearly exist in humans, there is equally firm evidence that the two pathways converge and interact in the perceptual process.[62–64] Indeed, some investigators interpret the experimental data as showing relatively little specificity of neural channels within the visual system.[65,66]

Hierarchical processing that begins in the retinocortical component reaches greater intricacy in the integrative component. As visual signals travel farther from the primary visual cortex, receptive fields become larger, and more complex features are processed. In the occipitotemporal pathway, for example, the orientation of an object in space becomes secondary to its shape. In the occipitoparietal pathway, more complicated motion is processed, and retinotopic spatial coordinates are converted to craniotopic coordinates. At higher levels of both pathways, processing is strongly influenced by attentional and motivational factors.[67,68]

Occipitoparietal Pathway

The occipitoparietal pathway extends dorsolaterally from the occipital pole, passing through superolateral temporal structures along the way (Fig. 1-29). The standard nomenclature for anatomic stations is de-

Table 1–2. **Integrative Visual Processing**

Anatomic Region*	Form	Color	Motion	Depth
V4 (Anterior lingual gyrus; Brodmann 19, 37)	Length, width, and orientation in patterns	Relative color ("Color constancy")		Binocular disparity
MT (V5)/MST complex (Occipito-parieto-temporal junction; Brodmann 39, 19, 37)			Fast motion of objects in all planes Relative motion Rotational motion	Binocular disparity
Inferior parietal area 7a/LIP (Posterior inferior parietal lobule; Brodmann 39)			Motion in relation to head position Motion toward or away from fixation Visual attention	Binocular disparity
Lateral intraparietal area (LIP) (Intraparietal sulcus; junction of Brodmann 39 and 7)			Uncertain	Binocular disparity
Posterior inferior temporal cortex (Fusiform gyrus; Brodmann 37)	Large patterns			
Anterior inferior temporal cortex (Fusiform gyrus; Brodmann 20)	Complex patterns			

*Macaque areas. Human homologues listed in parentheses.

Table 1–3. **How the Occipitoparietal Integrative Segment Works and Fails**

Anatomic Region*	Working	Failing
MT (V5)–MST complex (Occipito–parieto–temporal junction, Brodmann 39, 19, 37)	Appreciates motion	Cannot appreciate motion[†] Cannot pursue visual target[†] Makes inaccurate saccades to moving targets[†]
	Appreciates depth	Lacks stereopsis
Inferior parietal area 7A (Angular gyrus; Brodmann 39)	Converts retinotopic to craniotopic coordinates	Misreaches to visual targets
	Explores visual space	Visually inattentive
Lateral intraparietal area (LIP) (Intraparietal sulcus, junction of inferior and superior parietal lobules)	Delivers to superior colliculus the error signal between position of currently fixated target and that of eccentric stationary target to be viewed	Has no visually guided saccades

*Macaque areas. Human homologues listed in parentheses.
[†]In hemifield contralateral to lesion.

rived from the macaque brain, with putative homologies to the human brain.

THE MIDDLE TEMPORAL AREA

The magnocellular neurons in V1, V2, and V3 send most of their output to MT, or V5. The term MT, "middle temporal," derives from the region in owl monkey where it was first described.[48] In the macaque, MT is located within the superior temporal sulcus at the occipitotemporoparietal junction. The homologous area in humans lies at the junction of Brodmann's areas 19, 37, and 39, im- mediately ventral to the angular gyrus in the inferior parietal lobule.[69] The MT differs from V1 and V2 in being more sensitive to higher speeds, directional movement of large patterns rather than small components, motion toward or away from the viewer rather than just in the orthogonal plane, and relative rather than absolute motion.

Damage to MT impairs the monkey's ability to detect motion within the contralateral hemifield ("no notion for motion").[70] The animal cannot pursue or make accurate fast eye movements (saccades) to targets moving in any direction within that field.[71] Similar

Table 1–4. **How the Occipitotemporal Integrative Segment Works and Fails**

Anatomic Region*	Working	Failing
V4 (Posterior fusiform gyrus; Brodmann area 37)	Appreciates color constancy	Loses binocular color vision without losing visual acuity (cerebral achromatopsia)
	Recognizes patterns	Cannot recognize or copy drawings of objects (apperceptive visual object agnosia)
Inferior temporal area (IT) (Anterior fusiform gyrus; Brodmann area 20)	Recognizes complex patterns (including faces)	Cannot recognize familiar or famous faces (prosopagnosia)
		Cannot recognize but can copy drawings of objects (associative visual object agnosia)

*Macaque areas. Human homologues listed in parentheses.

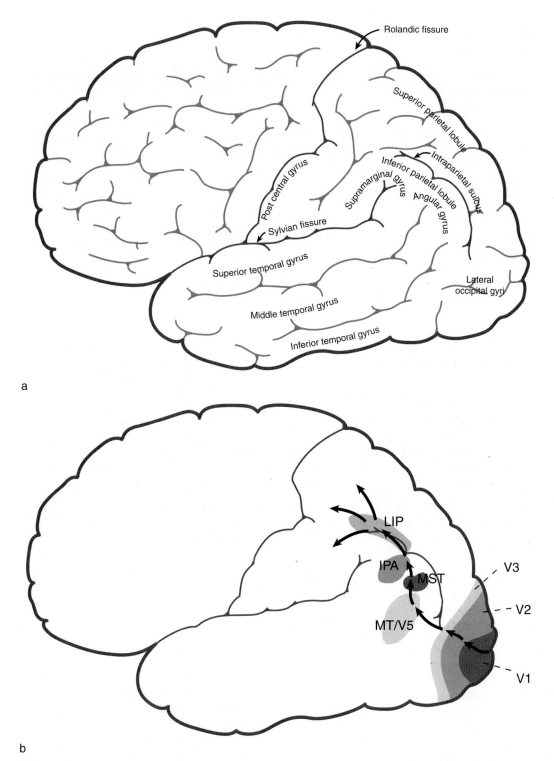

Figure 1–29. The occipitoparietal ("where") pathway. (*a*) The important cortical landmarks. (*b*) The occipitoparietal pathway. V1 = primary visual cortex; V2, V3 = association visual cortex; MT = middle temporal area (in macaque); MST = medial superior temporal area (in macaque); IPA = inferior parietal area, also known as area 7a (in macaque); LIP = lateral intraparietal area (in macaque).

deficits have been reported from bilateral lesions in the equivalent region in humans.[46,72–74] Damage to this region is also associated with loss of stereopsis.[75]

MEDIAL SUPERIOR TEMPORAL AREA

The middle temporal area projects to the medial superior temporal (MST) area, a part of the monkey's inferior parietal lobule that lies dorsally adjacent to MT. Unlike MT, MST appears to code for rotational movement. This area represents a transition between sensory and motor processing, in that MST neurons increase their firing rate during eye movements without a stimulus present. Lesions in this region cause two pursuit defects: (1) an omnidirectional defect within the contralateral hemifield; and (2) a unidirectional defect when a stimulus is moved toward the side of the lesion within the ipsilateral hemifield.[76,77]

INFERIOR PARIETAL AREA 7a

The medial superior temporal area projects dorsally to macaque 7a, a posterior inferior parietal region equivalent to human angular gyrus, or Brodmann area 39. Populations of neurons in 7a are differentially sensitive to motion toward and away from fixation. Others are tuned to eye position in space, converting retinotopic to craniotopic spatial coordinates.[78] In other words, these neurons compute the position of an image in space by adding a correction factor based on the degree to which the eyes are shifted away from straight-ahead gaze. This correction allows subjects to properly gauge movement in space. When it fails, they will misreach for objects (optic ataxia; Chapters 3, 16).[79,80]

Area 7a also contains neurons that show enhanced responses when rewarding stimuli appear in their receptive fields, regardless of whether the monkey makes an eye movement in that direction.[81] This enhanced firing is the neurophysiologic correlate of selective attention. Damage to area 7a could explain inattention or neglect (Chapter 16).

LATERAL INTRAPARIETAL AREA

Apart from 7a, the other major target of MST output is the lateral intraparietal area (LIP), situated slightly dorsal to 7a within the intraparietal sulcus that separates the inferior and superior parietal lobules. This area is associated with saccadic eye movements to visual and remembered targets.[82] It delivers to the superior colliculus an error signal between the position of the fixated target and that of an eccentrically placed stationary target that the individual intends to fixate with a saccade. Patients with lesions in the homologous region (intraparietal sulcus) cannot make visually guided saccades.[83]

The parietal vision–related cortex distributes signals for coordination of eye and body movements not only to the superior colliculus, but also to the frontal eye fields, primary motor cortex, and supplementary motor cortex. Projection to the prefrontal cortex may play a critical role in the retrieval of visual spatial memories.

Occipitotemporal Pathway

Unlike the occipitoparietal pathway, the occipitotemporal pathway (Fig. 1-30) extends inferomedially along the undersurface of the occipital and temporal lobes, probably as far forward as the amygdala.

AREA V4

The visual form and color signals that emerge from V1–V3 are sent to V4, located in the ventral occipitotemporal region. The human homologue is uncertain, although the posterior fusiform gyrus—Brodmann area 37—is proposed on the basis of physiologic and pathologic studies.[84,85]

Originally V4 was believed to specialize entirely in color processing, but it has since been shown to have two populations of neurons, one wavelength-sensitive, the other shape-, size-, and texture-sensitive. The receptive fields of V4 range from 20-fold to 100-fold larger than those of V1 and V2, and they predominantly represent the fixational area of the visual field. The larger receptive fields allow coding of much larger features. Achromatic neurons are tuned for length and width but not position of stimuli. This position-independence means that objects can be recognized on the basis of their inherent features even if they are shifted about

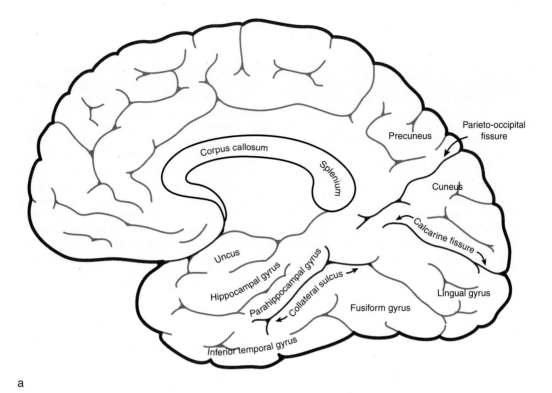

a

b

Figure 1–30. The occipitotemporal ("what") pathway. (*a*) The important cortical landmarks. (*b*) The occipitotemporal pathway. IT = inferior temporal area.

in space. Another characteristic of V4 neurons is that their firing rate is reduced if an identically shaped or textured stimulus falls within surrounding receptive fields. Shape and texture enhancement allows the visual system to differentiate figure from ground.[86] Failure of this process could explain loss of pattern recognition found in patients with apperceptive visual object agnosia (Chapter 17).[87]

The chief contribution of V4 to color processing is the ability to perceive color as invariant even if the ambient illumination changes (color constancy). Color constancy is achieved in the same way as figure/ground enhancement, by altering the neuron's firing rate to a fixated stimulus according to the wavelength signals arriving in the surrounding receptive fields.[49] Damage to V4 has been invoked in cases of acquired binocular color vision loss with sparing of visual acuity (cerebral achromatopsia; Chapter 17).[53,84]

INFERIOR TEMPORAL AREA

Area V4 is the highest integrative center for color-sensitive neurons, but the achromatic V4 neurons send signals anteriorly to the inferior temporal (IT) cortex. The human homologue could be the anterior fusiform gyrus—Brodmann area 20. Receptive fields in IT are much larger than in V4 and are not restricted to hemifield boundaries, implying strong intercallosal connections. Activation studies in humans have shown that matching tasks become more specific in the anterior direction along inferior temporal lobe. For example, separating faces by gender activates the posterior temporal lobe region; identifying a face as unique activates the anterior region.[59]

The IT has extensive interconnections with the hippocampus/amygdala and prefrontal cortex, and there is increasing evidence that these regions participate in various components of visual memory. The ability to recall the names and uses of visual objects is stored near the highest order IT neurons associated with perception of those objects, according to PET and MRI activation studies in humans.[59] The hippocampus and amygdala may mediate the consolidation of new memories, but their safekeeping is in IT. The prefrontal cortex has been implicated in retrieval of visual memories.[88] Intriguingly, a dorsal prefrontal region appears to be active during tasks requiring visual spatial discriminations, while a ventral prefrontal region is active during tasks that require differentiating objects by their features rather than their location.[59,88,89] A current hypothesis is that long-term visual memory may consist of IT neural networks that have been constructed by perception, primed by hippocampus and amygdala, and placed in widespread storage in IT. When an object is newly presented, the stored representation is retrieved from IT by prefrontal cortex and compared with the challenge sensation.[90] A match results in a synchronous discharge that is interpreted as familiarity.[91,92]

These findings begin to explain the genesis of human recognition deficits, called *agnosias*. Lesions producing visual object and face agnosias are located in the inferior occipitotemporal white matter and cortex (Chapter 16). In some patients, a failure to copy or match (apperceptive agnosia) suggests that the recognition process is disturbed at a relatively primitive stage of visual processing, perhaps at V4 or earlier. In others, where copying and matching are closer to normal (associative agnosia), subtle perceptual deficits might impair activation of the primed areas located throughout IT. Face agnosia may result from direct damage to anterior IT, or from a disconnection between primary visual cortex and the anterior IT areas where distinctions are based on subtle feature differences and where, in monkeys, a small proportion of IT neurons fire intensely when the animal is exposed either to side views or profiles of whole faces, parts of faces, or faces with certain expressions.[93,94] Perhaps this phenomenon reflects the adaptive value of face recognition for monkeys. Whether a limited face-selective region also exists in humans is uncertain.[95] Surface[96] and depth electrode[97] studies and PET scanning[98] have shown participation of wide areas in both hemispheres, suggesting that the human cortex analyzes by grouping shared features rather than by recognizing predetermined entities.

Attention and Object Recognition

The interdependence of occipitoparietal and occipitotemporal pathways is evident when one examines the way that attention mediates object recognition.[99,100]

PREATTENTION

Recognizing objects requires the selection of relevant (or salient) signals from irrelevant background noise. Elements that differ from distractors in simple properties like color or line orientation are instantaneously extracted from an array with a single glance, a phenomenon called "preattention." Preattention is an example of perceptual parallel processing—simultaneous awareness of elements scattered across an array.

SELECTIVE ATTENTION

By contrast, picking out more complicated elements from distractors requires serial processing—shifting attention from one element to another, or "selective attention".[101] The roving spotlight of selective attention settles on behaviorally relevant targets and filters out unimportant ones. For example, if behaviorally effective and ineffective stimuli are placed in the receptive field of a V4 or IT neuron and a monkey is instructed to fixate the effective stimulus, the neuron fires rapidly. But if the monkey is then trained to look at the ineffective stimulus still displayed within the receptive field, the neuron's firing rate sharply declines, as if the receptive field had shrunk so that the effective stimulus were no longer inside it.[86]

DISENGAGEMENT OF ATTENTION

Other experiments illustrate the importance of task-related factors on attention.[86] Inferior temporal neurons fire more rapidly when a monkey performs a matching task to a familiar than unfamiliar stimulus,[102] and when the task is one of discrimination rather than detection.[103] The fact that neurons from V1 to IT along the occipitotemporal pathway fire faster to an eccentric target if the fixational target is removed first ("gap task") demonstrates that attention cannot be engaged without first being *disengaged*.[103] Among patients with parietal lesions, removal of a fixation target may miraculously "open up" their peripheral field to visual targets.

ENGAGEMENT OF ATTENTION

If the critical center for disengagement of attention is posterior parietal lobe, it is the pulvinar, in the posterior thalamus, that is responsible for mediating *engagement* of attention, or orienting toward meaningful stimuli and screening out irrelevant noise.[104] Thus damage to thalamic and paralimbic inputs, as well as to posterior parietal cortex, can be responsible for disturbances to various components of selective attention.

SUMMARY

The purpose of the optical component of the visual system is to present a clear, undistorted image to the retina. The eye does this by using two refracting elements—the cornea and lens—to focus light rays through transparent media.

In one-third of the population, refractive power and axial length are perfectly matched, and the eye is able to bring light from distant objects to a point focus on the retina (emmetropia). In the remainder, there is a power–length mismatch, and a refractive error is created. Refractive errors include myopia, hyperopia, and astigmatism. In patients with myopia, the eye's refractive power is excessive; in those with hyperopia, it is deficient. Astigmatism (warpage of the cornea) precludes a point focus. Refractive errors may be corrected by placing appropriate glasses or contact lenses in front of the eye.

Objects viewed at a close distance may be unclear if the eye's accommodative apparatus fails. The most common cause is presbyopia, an age-related degeneration in lens protein which impairs lens reactivity to ciliary muscle contraction. Accommodation may also be recruited inappropriately in viewing distant objects, creating an artificial myopia. Such inappropriate accommodation is usually a psychogenic manifestation (anxiety, malingering), but it may also occur after topical cholinergic medication or severe brainstem trauma.

Even if the eye has no refractive error, a clear image will not form on the retina if the ocular media contain imperfections such as surface irregularities or opacities. Glasses cannot overcome these aberrations, but contact lenses often improve vision in patients with corneal imperfections.

By limiting the entry of light to a narrow beam, the pinhole occluder bypasses the eye's refractive apparatus. Marked improvement in visual acuity when the pinhole device is placed before the eye is diagnostic of an optical abnormality—either an uncorrected refractive error or a media imperfection.

The retinocortical segment, extending from the retina to the primary visual cortex, transduces light into neural signals and extracts local features related to form, color, motion, and depth.

The retina has two functions: mediating color and form vision largely in the foveal region and mediating motion vision in the extrafoveal region. Form and color vision is initially processed by cones, motion vision by both rods and cones.

Although rods and cones share the same transduction mechanism, they have fundamentally different properties. Rods function in low light conditions and are insensitive to color, form details, or rapid changes in luminance. Cones function in high light conditions and are fast-reacting and sensitive to color and fine discrimination.

Form and color signals are transmitted by small (parvocellular) retinal ganglion cells, whereas motion signals are transmitted by large (magnocellular) retinal ganglion cells.

The organization of the nerve fiber layer of the retina (the axons of retinal ganglion cells) accounts for the shape of visual field defects produced by optic nerve and superficial retinal lesions.

The optic chiasm converts the representation of visual space from a monocular to a hemifield pattern. This tranformation is accomplished in humans by having axons emanating from nasal retina cross to the opposite side and having axons emanating from temporal retina remain on the same side. Lesions of the optic chiasm typically damage the crossing fibers to produce bitemporal hemianopia.

Each optic tract contains retinal axons from one hemifield, but the fibers from the two eyes are not adjacent. This explains why optic tract lesions give rise to homonymous hemianopias that are incongruous, or nonidentical in size, shape, and depth. The retinocortical and retinomesencephalic visual systems bifurcate in the posterior optic tract. Thus lesions caudal to this point spare the pupillary reflex pathways and may allow unconscious detection vision (blindsight).

The lateral geniculate body (LGB) is divided into six stacked layers, three for the inputs of each eye. The signals do not appear to be altered at this level, except that their transmission to visual cortex may be gated by incoming inhibitory pathways. Lesions limited to the LGB are rare.

The optic radiations pass through the posterior internal capsule where they are vulnerable to infarction producing contralateral hemianesthesia, hemiplegia, and hemianopia—the capsular triad. Inferior fibers swing anteriorly into the temporal lobe as Meyer's loop, where they may be extirpated in epilepsy surgery. Midportions of the optic radiations are apposed to the lateral ventricle and are vulnerable to deep temporoparietal lesions. The posterior optic radiations are often infarcted together with primary visual cortex in posterior cerebral artery occlusions.

The primary visual cortex (striate cortex, V1, Brodmann area 17) converts spots into bars of light in vertical columns that are alternately arranged to receive inputs from each eye (ocular dominance columns). The columns are ordered with each sensitive to a slightly different bar orientation. On the borders of the ocular dominance columns lie binocular disparity–sensitive neurons that are sensitive to the differences between signals coming from noncorresponding points in the two retinas. Output of these disparity-sensitive neurons eventually allows the sensation of stereopsis. Color information is processed separately in "blobs" suspended within the columns.

The output of V1 is largely to V2 and V3, regions that surround V1 and correspond to Brodmann area 18. Receptive fields here are larger than in V1, but otherwise visual processing is only minimally altered.

The clinical deficits associated with V1 lesions are visual field (luminance and crude form) defects and unformed hallucinations. The location of the visual field defects is explained by the retinotopic mapping onto V1, which can be divided into three portions: (*1*) the caudal 50%, which encodes the central 10 degrees of field; (*2*) the middle 40%, which encodes the rest of the binocular field; and (*3*) the rostral 10%, which encodes the 30 degree monocular temporal crescent.

The guiding principles of retinocortical transmission are retinotopic mapping, parallel processing, and hierarchical processing. Retinotopic mapping refers to the fact that features pertaining to each point in visual space are processed in brain regions spatially corresponding to them. Parallel processing indicates that these features are processed in separate neural channels beginning at the retinal ganglion cell level. Hierarchical processing indicates that progressively more complex and global features are extracted at higher levels of the visual pathway. To allow for global feature processing, retinotopic mapping is lost in the integrative component of the visual pathway.

Two interdependent visual integrative pathways extract the complex features of viewed objects. The occipitoparietal ("where") pathway analyzes motion and depth; the occipitotemporal ("what") pathway analyzes form and color.

In the occipitoparietal pathway, signals proceed from V3 to MT (or V5), which lies at the temporo–parieto–occipital junction, the interface of Brodmann's areas 19, 37, and 39. The MT (V5) processes fast and relative motion and depth; it projects to MST, an adjacent region located in the posterior angular gyrus, which analyzes rotational motion. Lesions in the MT or MST cause an inability to recognize motion, a failure of ocular pursuit, inaccurate saccades to moving targets, and astereopsis.

The MST projects to monkey inferior parietal area 7a, corresponding to human angular gyrus, where retinotopic coordinates are converted to craniotopic spatial coordinates. If this system fails, visually guided misreaching (optic ataxia) occurs. Area 7a probably mediates attentional mechanisms in general; breakdown could account for inattention (neglect).

In the occipitotemporal pathway, signals proceed from V1–V3 to V4, whose human homologue is anterior lingual gyrus. Here colors are recognized by comparing wavelengths in and around receptive fields (color constancy). Damage could explain acute, binocular loss of color vision in the presence of normal visual acuity (cerebral achromatopsia). Area V4 also analyzes achromatic forms as large patterns rather than small fragments. Damage could lead to the impaired pattern recognition found in patients with apperceptive visual object agnosia.

The output of V4 is directed anteriorly to monkey inferior temporal (IT) area, equivalent to human fusiform gyrus. Here, complex patterns—including faces—are analyzed. Direct damage or impaired transmission to this region could explain face agnosia (prosopagnosia) and associative visual object agnosia.

Attentional mechanisms originating in posterior inferior parietal lobe and its limbic connections refine and enhance object recognition. This phenomenon is an example of the interdependency of the two branches of the integrative component of vision.

Visual memory for object features is probably stored in IT regions responsible for complex pattern perception. Memories are laid down with the cooperation of hippocampus/amygdala and called up with the help of prefrontal cortex.

REFERENCES

1. Duke-Elder S, Abrams D. *System of Ophthalmology.* Vol 5 . St. Louis: Mosby; 1970:227–250.
2. Michaels DD. *Visual Optics and Refraction: A Clinical Approach.* St. Louis: Mosby; 1985.
3. Sorsby A. Biology of the eye as an optical system. In: Tasman W, Jaeger EA, eds. *Duane's Clinical Ophthalmology.* Vol 1. Philadelphia: Lippincott; 1998: pp. 1–15.
4. Troilo D. Neonatal eye growth and emmetropisation—a literature review. *Eye.* 1992;5:154–160.
5. Van Alphen GW. Emmetropization in the primate eye. *Ciba Found Symp* 1990;155:115–120.
6. Daw NW. *Visual Development.* New York: Plenum Press; 1995:193–201.
7. Phelps N, Koretz JF, Bron AJ. The development and maintenance of emmetropia. *Eye.* 1999;13: 83–92.

8. Rodieck RW. *The First Steps in Seeing*. Sunderland, Mass: Sinauer Associates; 1998.

9. Ogden TE. Topography of the retina. In: Ryan SJ, ed. *Retina*. Vol 1. St. Louis: Mosby; 1989:32–36.

10. Rando RR. Molecular mechanisms of visual pigment regeneration. *Photochem Photobiol*. 1992;56:1145–1156.

11. Trobe JD, Glaser JS. *The Visual Fields Manual. A Practical Guide to Testing and Interpretation*. Gainesville, Fla: Triad; 1983.

12. Johnson MW, Kincaid MC, Trobe JD. Bilateral retrobulbar optic nerve infarction after blood loss and hypotension: a clinicopathologic case study. *Ophthalmology*. 1987;94:1577–1584.

13. Hayreh SS, Zimmerman MB, Podhajsky P, Alward WLM. Nocturnal arterial hypotension and its role in optic nerve head and ocular ischemic disorders. *Am J Ophthalmol*. 1994;117:603–624.

14. Hayreh SS. The blood supply of the optic nerve. *Ophthalmologica*. 1996;210:285–295.

15. Kupfer C, Chumbley L, Downer J. Quantitative histology of optic nerve, optic tract and lateral geniculate nucleus of man. *J Anat*. 1967;101:393–401.

15a. Traquair HM. An Introduction to Clinical Perimetry. 6th Edition. London, Kimpton, 1949.

16. Bergland RM, Ray BS. The arterial blood supply of the human optic chiasm. *J Neurosurg*. 1969;31:327–334.

17. Hoyt WF, Luis O. The primate chiasm: details of visual fiber organization studied by silver impregnation techniques. *Arch Ophthalmol*. 1963;70:69–85.

18. Breen LA, Quaglieri FC, Schochet SS. Neuroanatomical feature photo. *J Clin Neuroophthalmol*. 1993;3:283–284.

19. Horton JC. Wilbrand's knee of the primate optic chiasm is an artifact of monocular enucleation. *Trans Am Ophthalmol Soc*. 1997;95:579–609.

20. Sadun AA, Schaechter J, Smith LE. A retinohypothalamic pathway in man: light mediation of circadian rhythms. *Brain Res*. 1984;302:371–377.

21. Kline LB. Anatomy and physiology of the optic tracts and lateral geniculate nucleus. In: Miller NR, Newman NJ, eds. *Walsh & Hoyt's Clinical Neuro-ophthalmology*. 5th ed. Vol 1. Baltimore: Williams & Wilkins; 1998:101–120.

22. Weiskrantz L. *Blindsight: A Case Study and Implications*. Oxford: Oxford University Press; 1986.

23. Sahraie A, Weiskrantz L, Barbur JL, Simmons A, Williams SCR, Brammer MJ. Pattern of neuronal activity associated with conscious and unconscious processing of visual signals. *Proc Natl Acad Sci USA*. 1997;94:9406–9411.

24. Danziger S, Fendrich R, Rafal RD. Inhibitory tagging of locations in the blind field of hemianopic patients. *Conscious Cogn*. 1997;6:291–307.

25. Stoerig P, Cowey A. Blindsight in man and monkey. *Brain*. 1997;120:535–559.

26. Lindenberg R, Walsh FB, Sacks JG. *Neuropathology of Vision: An Atlas*. Philadelphia: Lea & Febiger; 1973:315–334.

27. Frisen L, Holmegaard L, Rosencrantz M. Sectorial optic atrophy and homonymous horizontal sectoranopia: a lateral choroidal artery syndrome? *J Neurol Neurosurg Psychiatry*. 1978;4:374–380.

28. Frisen L. Quadruple sectoranopia and sectorial optic atrophy—a syndrome of the distal anterior choroidal artery. *J Neurol Neurosurg Psychiatry*. 1979;42:590–594.

29. Wall M. Optic radiations and occipital cortex. Miller NR, Newman NJ, eds. *Walsh & Hoyt's Clinical Neuro-ophthalmology*. 5th ed. Vol 1. Baltimore: Williams & Wilkins; 1998:121–151.

30. Meyer A. The connections of the occipital lobes and the present status of the cerebral visual affections. *Trans Assoc Am Physicians*. 1907;22:7–15.

31. Tecoma ES, Laxer KD, Barbaro NM. Frequency and characteristics of visual field deficits after surgery for mesial temporal sclerosis. *Neurology*. 1993;43:1235–1238.

32. Hughes TS, Abou-Khalil B, Lavin PJM, Fakhoury T, Blumenkopf B, Donahue SP. Visual field defects after temporal lobe resection: a prospective quantitative analysis. *Neurology*. 1999;53:167–172.

33. Lund JS. Organization of neurons in the visual cortex, area 17, of the monkey (Macaca mulatta). *J Comp Neurol*. 1973;147:455–463.

34. Van Essen DC, Drury HA, Joshi S, Miller MI. Functional astructural mapping of human cerebral cortex: solutions are in the surfaces. *Proc Natl Acad Sci USA*. 1998;95:788–795.

35. Tootell RBH, Hadjikhani NK, Vanduffel W, et al. Functional analysis of primary visual cortex (V1) in humans. *Proc Natl Acad Sci USA*. 1998;95:811–817.

36. Horton JC, Hoyt WF. The representation of the visual field in human striate cortex: a revision of the classic Holmes map. *Arch Ophthalmol*. 1991;109:816–824.

37. Wong AM, Sharpe JA. Representation of the visual field in the human occipital cortex: a magnetic resonance imaging and perimetric correlation. *Arch Ophthalmol*. 1999;117:208–217.

38. Kollias SS, Landau K, Khan N, et al. Functional evaluation using magnetic resonance imaging of the visual cortex in patients with retrochiasmal lesions. *J Neurosurg*. 1998;89:780–790.

39. Gray LG, Galetta SL, Siegal T, Schatz NJ. The central visual field in homonymous hemianopia: evidence for unilateral foveal representation. *Arch Neurol*. 1997;54:312–317.

40. Horton JC, Hocking DR. Monocular core zones and binocular border strips in primate striate cortex revealed by the contrasting effects of enucleation, eyelid suture, and retinal laser lesions on cytochrome oxidase activity. *J Neurosci*. 1998;18:5433–5455.

41. Hubel DH, Wiesel TN, LeVay S. Functional architecture of area 17 in normal and monocularly deprived macaque monkeys. *Cold Spring Harb Symp Quant Biol*. 1975;40:581–589.

42. Horton JC, Hocking DR. Timing of the critical period for plasticity of ocular dominance columns in macaque striate cortex. *J Neurosci*. 1997;17:3684–3709.

43. Daw NW. *Visual Development*. New York: Plenum Press; 1995:123–138.

44. Horton JC, Hocking DR. Pattern of ocular dominance columns in human striate cortex in strabismic amblyopia. *Vis Neurosci*. 1996;13:787–795.

45. Rizzo M. Astereopsis. In: Boller F, Grafman J, eds. *Handbook of Neuropsychology*. Vol 2. Amsterdam: Elsevier; 1989:415–427.

46. Marcar VL, Zihl J, Cowey A. Comparing the visual deficits of a motion blind patient with the visual deficits of monkeys with area MT removed. *Neuropsychologia*. 1997;35:1459–1465.

47. Ungerleider LG, Mishkin M. Two cortical visual systems. In: Ingle DJ, Goodale MA, Mansfield RJW, eds. *Analysis of Visual Behavior*. Cambridge, Mass: MIT Press; 1982:549–586.

48. Felleman DJ, Van Essen DC. Distributed hierarchical processing in the primate cerebral cortex. *Cereb Cortex*. 1991;1:1–47.

49. Maunsell JHR, Newsome WT. Visual processing in monkey extrastriate cortex. *Ann Rev Neurosci*. 1987;10:363–401.

50. Andersen RA. Visual and eye movement functions of the posterior parietal cortex. *Ann Rev Neurosci*. 1989;12:377–403.

51. Kaas JH. Theories of visual cortex organization in primates. *Cereb Cortex*. 1997;12:91–125.

52. Livingstone MS, Hubel DH. Psychophysical evidence for separate channels for the perception of form, color, movement, and depth. *J Neurosci*. 1987;7:3416–3468.

53. Merigan W, Freeman A, Meyers SP. Parallel processing streams in human visual cortex. *Neuroreport*. 1997;8:3985–3991.

54. Damasio H, Damasio A. *Lesion Analysis in Neuropsychology*. New York: Oxford University Press; 1989.

55. Van Essen DC, Drury HA. Structural and functional analyses of human cerebral cortex using a surface-based atlas. *J Neurosci*. 1997;17:7079–7102.

56. Courtney SM, Ungerleider LG. What fMRI has taught us about human vision. *Curr Opin Neurobiol*. 1997;7:554–561.

57. Tootell RBH, Mendola JD, Hadjikhani NK, Liu AK, Dale AM. The representation of the ipsilateral visual field in human cerebral cortex. *Proc Natl Acad Sci USA*. 1998;95:818–824.

58. Holliday IE, Anderson SJ, Harding GF. Magnetoencephalographic evidence for non-geniculostriate visual input to human cortical area V5. *Neuropsychologia*. 1997;35:1139–1146.

59. Ungerleider L. Functional brain imaging studies of cortical mechanisms for memory. *Science*. 1995; 270:769–775.

60. Haxby JV, Grady CL, Horwitz B, et al. Dissociation of object and spatial visual processing pathways in human extrastriate cortex. *Proc Natl Acad Sci USA*. 1991;88:1621–1625.

61. Watson JDG, Myers R, Frackowiak RSJ, et al. Area V5 of the human brain: evidence from a combined study using positron emission tomography and magnetic resonance imaging. *Cereb Cortex*. 1993;3: 79–94.

62. Shipp S. Visual processing: the odd couple. *Curr Biol*. 1995;5:116–119.

63. Bullier J, Nowak LG. Parallel versus serial processing: new vistas on the distributed organization of the visual system. *Curr Opin Neurobiol*. 1995;5: 497–503.

64. Kraut M, Hart J Jr, Soher BJ, Gordon B. Object shape processing in the visual system evaluated using functional MRI. *Neurology*. 1997;48:1416–1420.

65. Lamme VA, Super H, Spekreijse H. Feed forward, horizontal, and feedback processing in the visual cortex. *Curr Opin Neurobiol*. 1998;8:529–535.

66. Schiller PH. Past and present ideas about how the visual scene is analyzed by the brain. *Cereb Cortex*. 1997;12:59–90.

67. Maunsell JHR. The brain's visual world: representation of visual targets in cerebral cortex. *Science*. 1995;270:764–768.

68. Luck SJ, Ford MA. On the role of selective attention in visual perception. *Proc Natl Acad Sci USA*. 1998;95:825–830.

69. Zeki S, Watson JDG, Lueck CJ, Friston KJ, Kennard C, Frackowiak RSJ. A direct demonstration of functional specialization in human visual cortex. *J Neurosci*. 1991;11:641–649.

70. Newsome WT, Paré EB. A selective impairment of motion perception following lesions of the middle temporal visual area (MT). *J Neurosci*. 1988;8: 2201–2211.

71. Newsome WT, Wurtz RH, Dursteler MR, Mikami A. Deficits in visual motion perception following ibotenic acid lesions of the middle temporal visual area of the macaque monkey. *J Neurosci*. 1985;5: 825–840.

72. Zihl J, Von Cramon D, Mai N. Selective disturbance of movement vision after bilateral brain damage. *Brain*. 1983;106:313–340.

73. Pierrot-Deseilligny C, Gray F, Brunet P. Infarcts of both inferior parietal lobules with impairment of visually guided eye movements, peripheral visual inattention and optic ataxia. *Brain*. 1986;109:81–97.

74. Thurston SE, Leigh RJ, Crawford T, Thompson A, Kennard C. Two distinct deficits of visual tracking caused by unilateral lesions of cerebral cortex in humans. *Ann Neurol*. 1988;23:266–273.

75. Rizzo M, Damasio H. Impairment of stereopsis with focal brain lesions. *Ann Neurol*. 1985;18:147–.

76. Morrow MJ, Sharpe JA. Cerebral hemispheric localization of smooth pursuit asymmetry. *Neurology*. 1990;40:284–292.

77. Lekwuwa GU, Barnes GR. Cerebral control of eye movements: I. The relationship between cerebral lesion sites and smooth pursuit deficits. *Brain*. 1996;119:473–480.

78. Andersen RA, Essick GK, Siegel RM. Encoding of spatial location by posterior parietal neurons. *Science*. 1985;230:456–458.

79. Perenin MT, Vighetto A. Optic ataxia: a specific disruption in visuomotor mechanisms: I. Different aspects of the deficit in reaching for objects. *Brain*. 1988;111:643–674.

80. Graff-Radford NR, Bolling JP, Earnest F, Shuster EA, Caselli RJ, Brazis PW. Simultanagnosia as the initial sign of degenerative dementia. *Mayo Clin Proc*. 1993;68:955–964.

81. Bushnell MC, Goldberg ME, Robinson DL. Behavioral enhancement of visual responses in monkey cerebral cortex: I. Modulation in posterior parietal cortex related to selective visual attention. *J Neurophysiol*. 1981;46:755–772.

82. Barash S, Bracewell RM, Fogassi L, Gnadt JW, Andersen RA. Saccade-related activity in the lateral intraparietal area. *J Neurophysiol*. 1991;66:1095–1108.

83. Pierrot-Deseilligny C, Gautier JC, Loron P. Acquired ocular motor apraxia due to bilateral frontoparietal infarcts. *Ann Neurol*. 1988;23:199–202.

84. Zeki S. A century of cerebral achromatopsia. *Brain*. 1990;113:1721–1777.

85. McKeefry DJ, Zeki S. The position and topography of the human colour centre as revealed by functional magnetic resonance imaging. *Brain*. 1997;120:2229–2242.

86. Desimone R, Ungerleider LG. Neural mechanisms of visual processing in monkeys. In: Boller F, Grafman J, eds. *Handbook of Neuropsychology*. Vol 2. Amsterdam: Elsevier; 1989:pp 267–300.

87. Rizzo M, Nawrot M, Blake R, Damasio A. A human visual disorder resembling area V4 dysfunction in the monkey. *Neurology*. 1992;42:1175–1180.

88. Wilson FAW, Scalaidhe SP, Goldman PS. Dissociation of object and spatial processing domains in primate prefrontal cortex. *Science*. 1993;260:1955–1957.

89. Ungerleider LG, Courtney SM, Haxby JV. A neural system for human visual working memory. *Proc Natl Acad Sci USA*. 1998;95:883–890.

90. Kosslyn SM. Seeing and imaging in the cerebral hemispheres: a computational approach. *Psychol Rev*. 1987;94:148–175.

91. Mishkin M, Appenzeller T. The anatomy of memory. *Sci Am*. 1987;256:80–89.

92. Stryker M. Is grandmother an oscillation? *Nature*. 1989;338:297–298.

93. DeSimone R, Albright TD, Gross CG, Bruce C. Stimulus selective properties of inferior temporal neurons in the macaque. *J Neurosci*. 1984;4:2051–2062.

94. Perrett DI, Mistlin AJ, Chitty AJ. Visual neurones responsive to faces. *Trends Neurosci*. 1987;10:358–364.

95. Kanwisher N, McDermott J, Chun MM. The fusiform face area: a module in human extrastriate cortex specialized for face perception. *J Neurosci*. 1997;17:4303–4311.

96. Lu ST, Hamalainen MS, Hari R, et al. Seeing faces activates three separate areas outside the occipital visual cortex in man. *Neuroscience*. 1991;43:287–290.

97. Seeck M, Mainwaring N, Ives J, et al. Differential neural activity in the human temporal lobe evoked by faces of family members and friends. *Ann Neurol*. 1993;34:369–372.

98. Ishai A, Ungerleider LG, Martin A, Schouten JL, Haxby JV. Distributed representation of objects in the human ventral visual pathway. *Proc Nat Acad Sci USA*. 1999;96:9379–9384.

99. Coull JT. Neural correlates of attention and arousal: insights from electrophysiology, functional neuroimaging, and psychopharmacology. *Prog Neurobiol*. 1998;55:343–361.

100. Kastner S, DeWeerd P, Desimone R, Ungerleider LG. Mechanisms of directed attention in the human extrastriate cortex as revealed by functional MRI. *Science*. 1998;282:108–111.

101. Treisman A. Features and objects in visual processing. *Sci Am*. 1986;255:114B–125.

102. Haenny PE, Maunsell JHR, Schiller PH. State dependent activity in monkey visual cortex: II. Retinal and extraretinal factors in V4. *Exp Brain Res*. 1988;30:245–249.

103. Richmond BJ, Sato. Enhancement of inferior temporal neurons during visual discrimination. *J Neurophysiol*. 1987;56:1292–1306.

104. Robinson DL, Petersen SE. The pulvinar and visual salience. *Trends Neurosci*. 1992;15:127–132.

105. Van Essen DC, Anderson CH, Felleman DJ. Information processing in the primate visual system: an integrated systems perspective. *Science*. 1992;255:419–423.

106. Silverman SE, Trick GL, Hart WM. Motion perception is abnormal in primary open angle glaucoma and ocular hypertension. *Invest Ophthalmol Vis Sci*. 1990;31:722–729.

107. Giaschi DE, Regan D, Kraft SP, Hong XH. Defective processing of motion-defined form in the fellow eye of patients with unilateral amblyopia. *Invest Ophthalmol Vis Sci*. 1992;33:2483–2489.

108. Galaburda A, Livingstone M. Evidence for a magnocellular defect in developmental dyslexia. *Ann NY Acad Sci*. 1993;682:70–82.

109. Sadun AA, Bassi CJ. Optic nerve damage in Alzheimer's disease. *Ophthalmology*. 1990;97:9–17.

Part II

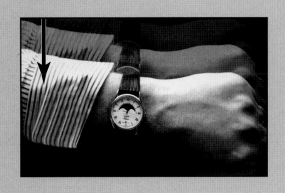

Symptoms of a Failing Visual System

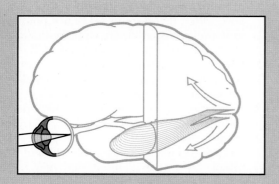

Chapter 2

SYMPTOMS OF OPTICAL DISORDERS

WHAT ARE OPTICAL SYMPTOMS?

VISION WORSE FOR FAR THAN NEAR OBJECTS

VISION WORSE FOR NEAR THAN FAR OBJECTS

FLUCTUATIONS IN IMAGE CLARITY
Variations in the Water Content of Lens or Cornea

Shifts in Lens Position
Changes in Ciliary Muscle Tone

DAZZLE

GLASSES-INDUCED IMAGE DISTORTION

DISCOLORED IMAGE

GHOST IMAGE

SUMMARY

The optical component is the least complex portion of the visual pathway, but its breakdown is the source of most visual symptoms.

WHAT ARE OPTICAL SYMPTOMS?

Optical symptoms derive from uncorrected refractive errors (myopia, hyperopia, astigmatism), failure of accommodation, and imperfections of ocular media (Chapter 1). Identifying optical abnormalities as the cause of the patient's complaints is critical in avoiding unnecessary, uncomfortable, and dangerous neurodiagnostic studies.

Most patients with optical abnormalities report "blurred vision," a nonspecific description that does not identify the disorder as optical, retinocortical, or integrative. Even patients with well-demarcated corneal scars or lens opacities say that their vision is indistinct rather than disturbed in a discrete area of the visual field. This is because corneal and lenticular opacities do not actually impede the flow of light; they scatter it incoherently and degrade its focus on the retina.

The only optical cause of discrete visual loss is a vitreous floater (Box 2-1). Because floaters are compact and lie close to the retina, they cast shadows on the retina (Fig.

VITREOUS FLOATERS

- Are particulate condensates suspended in the vitreous gel.
- Move after the eye starts moving and stop after it comes to rest.
- Occur at all ages, but a sudden increase in number or size is common after age 60 as the vitreous detaches.
- Occur prematurely in patients with high myopia, vitreous inflammation (including primary central nervous system lymphoma), vitreous hemorrhage, or after ocular trauma and surgery.
- Signal traction or holes in the retina if accompanied by flashes of light. Retinal detachment could follow.
- Indicate the need for urgent ophthalmologic examination if they suddenly increase in number or are accompanied by flashes of light or visual loss.

1. Swelling of the lens, usually from poorly controlled diabetes (Fig. 2-1*a*). By uncertain mechanisms, elevated blood sugar promotes osmotic fluid entry into the lens, which increases its refractive power as it swells. Visual clarity typically fluctuates as blood sugar levels rise and fall.
2. Forward displacement of the lens from ocular trauma or medications, principally sulfa-containing agents (Fig. 2-1*b*).[2]
3. Elongation of the globe from retinal detachment surgery or repaired scleral laceration. Retinal detachment surgery often involves placement on the sclera of a plastic encircling element that may increase the axial length of the globe (Fig. 2-1*c*). Following repair of scleral laceration, the globe may be permanently deformed.
4. Excessive accommodation (Fig. 2-1*d*), most commonly occurring in a condition known as *accommodative spasm*. Because convergence, accommodation, and pupil constriction (synkinetic near triad) are centrally linked, the patient may also experience diplopia, as convergence increases along with the excess accommodation.[3,4] Anxiety and malingering are the most common causes, but traumatic brainstem injury and topical parasympathomimetic medications may also evoke this phenomenon.[5]

Myopia that develops after the sixth decade is usually caused by an increase in the refractive index of the lens due to aging degeneration of lens protein (Fig. 2-1*d*). Because the increase in the lens's index of refraction precedes its opacification, there may be no structural changes visible with the slit lamp biomicroscope.

1-6*c*) that the patient interprets as black flecks or cobwebs. These flecks are often called "positive scotomas" to distinguish them from the visual voids, blank areas, or "negative scotomas," which are the typical symptoms of retinocortical pathway lesions (Chapter 3).

Whereas a report of visual blur may not be specific to the optical component of the visual pathway, the symptoms discussed in this chapter are much more specific (Table 2-1).

VISION WORSE FOR FAR THAN NEAR OBJECTS

When vision is less distinct for far than near objects, uncorrected myopia should be the first consideration (Fig. 1-3; Table 2-2). Most myopia either is congenital or develops within the first two decades.[1] Myopia that develops between the third and the sixth decade suggests the following conditions:

VISION WORSE FOR NEAR THAN FAR OBJECTS

This symptom is usually the result of hyperopia, accommodative weakness, or a combination of the two.

Hyperopia (Fig. 1-2; Table 2-3), in which the eye's refractive power is relatively weak, may not be symptomatic during the first three to four decades because the eye's accommodative reserve is able to compensate

Table 2–1. **Symptoms of Optical Disorders**

Symptom	Optical Cause	Nonoptical Cause
Vision worse for far than near objects	Myopia	None
Vision worse for near than far objects	Hyperopia Presbyopia Anticholinergics Ciliary body/nerve lesion Mesencephalic lesion	Impaired downgaze Impaired convergence
Fluctuations in image clarity	Variations in lens or corneal water content Shifts in lens position Changes in ciliary body (accommodative) tone	Demyelinating optic neuropathy
Dazzle	Bright light Corneal lesion Cataract Dilated pupil Reduced ocular pigment Anterior ocular inflammation	Meningeal inflammation Optic neuropathy Cone dystrophy
Glasses-induced image distortion	Differential magnification	
Discolored image	Cataract removal Intraocular hemorrhage Corneal edema	Medication toxicity
Ghost image	Refractive error Presbyopia Corneal lesion Cataract	Retinal lesion Posterior cerebral lesion

Table 2–2. **Causes of Myopia**

Type	Mechanism	Time Course
Congenital	Excessive ocular length	Static
Developmental (genetic)	Excessive ocular length	Progressive over first two decades
Senescent	Increase in lens index of refraction*	Onset after fifth decade, progressive
Metabolic (elevated blood sugar in diabetes mellitus)	Osmotic lens swelling	Fluctuating
Accommodative	Excess accommodation	Fluctuating
Pharmacologic	Forward displacement of lens	Fluctuating
Surgical/traumatic	Elongation of the eye Forward displacement of lens	Acute, persistent

*Premature lens protein degeneration may also occur as the result of ocular inflammation, trauma, surgery, systemic metabolic abnormalities, or familial predisposition.

47

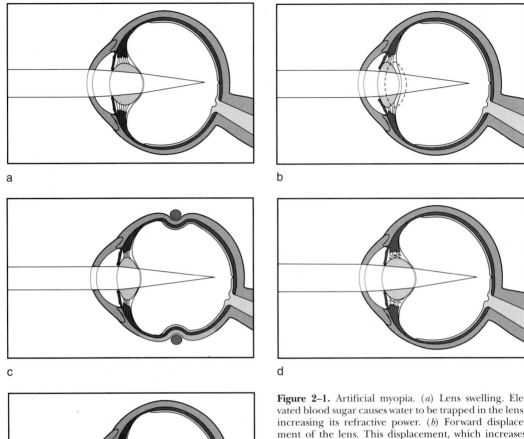

a

b

c

d

e

Figure 2–1. Artificial myopia. (*a*) Lens swelling. Elevated blood sugar causes water to be trapped in the lens, increasing its refractive power. (*b*) Forward displacement of the lens. This displacement, which increases lens refractive power, may be caused by trauma or sulfa-containing medications. (*c*) Elongation of the globe. The plastic encircling element placed outside the sclera in retinal detachment surgery increases the eye's axial length. (*d*) Excess accommodation. When accommodation is employed for viewing a distant object, the eye's refractive power is excessive. Usually a psychogenic phenomenon, it may also result from cholinergic medication or a mesencephalic lesion. (*e*) Increased lens refractive index. This is usually due to degeneration of lens protein during aging.

for it (latent hyperopia). As accommodative power declines physiologically with age, latent hyperopia becomes manifest, typically in early middle age. At first, vision is indistinct only for near objects, but eventually even remote objects become hard to discern.

Hyperopia may also develop acutely from a traumatic backward shift of the crystalline lens (Fig. 2-2*a*) or a shortening of the globe's axial length owing to thickening of the retina by inflammation or indentation by an extrinsic mass (Fig. 2-2*b*). Removal of the lens

in cataract surgery would create hyperopia if the lens power were not replaced. In the past, patients wore thick "Coke-bottle spectacles" or contact lenses to replace missing lens power. An artificial lens is now implanted in the eye following cataract extraction.

An important cause of relatively poor near vision is accommodative paresis (Table 2-4). By far the most common cause is presbyopia, or physiologic decline in accommodative power in the aging eye (Fig. 1-5). But in children and young adults who have not reached

Table 2–3. **Causes of Hyperopia**

Type	Mechanism	Time Course
Congenital	Deficient ocular length	Static
Traumatic/ surgical	Backward displacement of lens Removal of lens	Acute, persistent
Retinal	Forward displacement of retinal surface	Acute, persistent

the stage of presbyopia, insufficient accommodative power can result acutely from topically or systemically administered agents with anticholinergic properties, which weaken the contractility of the ciliary muscle. Trauma or inflammation of the ciliary nerves or ciliary body may also impair accommodative power. Surgical removal of the crystalline lens leads, of course, to loss of accommodation because the plastic implants lack the flexibility of the crystalline lens. Mesencephalic lesions may also impair accommodative ability prematurely.

Optical abnormalities are not the only explanation for the complaint of relatively poor vision for near objects. Here are three nonoptical reasons:

- **High expectations.** Patient expectations of image clarity are higher for near than far-away objects. Most individuals, particularly the elderly and infirm, are willing to accept lesser image clarity for distance viewing than for reading, sewing, cooking, or handicrafts. They may actually have subnormal visual acuity for distance objects as well, but they have not noticed it.

- **Impaired downgaze.** If presbyopic patients cannot look down, they will not be able to use the lower segment of their bifocals to obtain clear near vision. This is a common problem for patients with progressive supranuclear palsy or compressive or infarctive lesions of the midbrain that impair downgaze.[6] Single-vision reading glasses allow clear near vision without having to look down.

- **Impaired convergence.** Patients who have weak convergence develop ocular misalignment (exotropia) in viewing near objects. They are inclined to misinterpret the resultant double vision as blurred vision (Box 2-2). The most common organic causes are Parkinson's disease, progressive supranuclear palsy,[7] and traumatic brain injury. Because convergence is highly effort-dependent, however, it is likely to be judged insufficient unless the patient is cooperating. Convergence insufficiency should not be glibly invoked to explain blurred vision, diplopia, or headache in patients who are otherwise neurologically intact.[8]

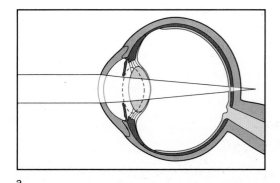
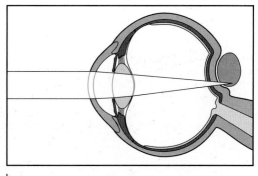

a   b

Figure 2–2. Artificial hyperopia. (*a*) Backward displacement of the lens. This displacement, usually due to trauma, reduces the eye's refractive power. (*b*) Forward displacement of the retina. This displacement, caused by an extrinsic mass (as shown here) or retinal swelling, shortens the eye's axial length.

Table 2–4. **Causes of Impaired Accommodation**

Type	Mechanism	Time Course
Presbyopic	Sclerosis of its protein makes lens inflexible	Onset in middle age, progressive to age 60
Pharmacologic (anticholinergic medication)	Denervation of ciliary muscle	Depends on dose and route of administration
Inflammatory	Ciliary nerve or muscle damage	Subacute
Traumatic	Ciliary nerve or muscle damage	Acute
Surgical	Ciliary nerve or muscle damage; lens extraction	Acute

FLUCTUATIONS IN IMAGE CLARITY

Fluctuations in image clarity *that do not have an abrupt onset* signal variations in water content of the lens or cornea, shifts in lens position, or changes in ciliary muscle tone.

Variations in the Water Content of Lens or Cornea

Changes in serum oncotic pressure give rise to shifts in the refractive power of the lens by altering its shape. As blood sugar rises, myopia becomes prominent, but vision often fluctuates over hours (see above, "Vision Worse for Far than Near Objects," and Fig. 2-1*a*). The most common clinical example is poorly controlled diabetes. Stabilization of blood sugar quickly remedies this symptom.

Changes in corneal water content also may cause fluctuating image clarity. The fault lies in a corneal endothelium damaged by intraocular surgery, trauma, inflammation, or idiopathic degeneration. The cornea maintains its transparency by excluding aqueous fluid by means of an active corneal endothelial metabolic pump. During the

---

Box 2–2

BLURRED VISION, DIPLOPIA, OR OSCILLOPSIA?

When patients report blurred vision, they may not have a visual pathway disturbance, but rather:

1. Ocular misalignment. When the eyes are very slightly misaligned, the diplopic images will appear so close together that the patient may perceive them as one smeared image.

2. Vestibulo-ocular reflex deficiency. To provide clear vision during head motion, the eyes must move in an equal and opposite direction. A malfunctioning vestibulo-ocular reflex (VOR) causes this stabilization to fail. Vision blurs even when the head or body moves slightly, as in driving or walking on uneven surfaces. Viewed objects appear to jiggle or oscillate (oscillopsia).[31,32]

   Failure of the VOR is most commonly found in patients with severe bilateral vestibular damage. A simple way to identify a deficient VOR is to have the patient read a Snellen near card while moving the head rapidly from side to side. Normal VOR compensation permits clear vision to be maintained. If the VOR is defective, acuity will drop by at least two Snellen lines.[33]

3. Ocular oscillation. If the patient develops an acquired, very fine (low-amplitude) ocular oscillation (nystagmus), objects will appear blurred. Only if the oscillation has high amplitude will the patient report that the objects appear to be moving.

waking period, when the eyes are open, evaporation of epithelial edema compensates for a marginal endothelial pump. During sleep, the closed eyes do not permit water evaporation from the water-filled cornea, which now loses its transparency. The patient wakes up with blurred vision that improves as the day goes on. Treatment involves the use of topically applied dehydrating agents. If the corneal endothelium is severely damaged, transplantation may be necessary.

Shifts in Lens Position

When the crystalline lens moves within the eye, its refractive power changes (Fig. 2-1b). The two major causes are traumatic loosening of the lens attachments and a systemically administered agent that produces ciliary body swelling. The ciliary body swelling displaces the lens forward in the eye, thereby increasing its power. Thiazide diuretics and sulfa-containing agents are most commonly implicated in this idiosyncratic and reversible effect.[9,10]

Changes in Ciliary Muscle Tone

Medications with parasympatholytic or parasympathomimetic effects can alter accommodation by affecting ciliary muscle contraction (Chapter 1). Parasympatholytics weaken accommodation and cause blurred vision for near objects that fluctuates with the dose of the medication. Parasympathomimetics enhance ciliary muscle contraction, loosening the lenticular zonules and freeing the lens to assume a more convex shape. This mechanism will cause too much accommodation and create artificial myopia. The patient sees near objects clearly but distant objects as blurred. Effects on the ciliary muscle will not, of course, be apparent in patients aged over 50 years, because they have already lost their ability to accommodate through natural aging and are depending on optical corrections for close viewing.

Fluctuations in visual clarity may be unrelated to accommodative shifts. In patients with multiple sclerosis, they occur because of intermittent conduction block.[11]

DAZZLE

"Dazzle" refers to a light-flooded sensation that includes periocular pain and impaired vision. It is usually provoked by glare, or excessive light reaching the fovea from sources other than the viewed target. The most frequent cause of glare is bright ambient light. But even under normal light conditions, glare may result from an abnormal scatter of light within the eye, as occurs with corneal erosions, scars, and edema, cataract, a widely dilated pupil, or reduced ocular pigment.

The painful component of dazzle cannot be distinguished from photophobia, a ticlike sudden eye pain provoked by normal light levels and associated with inflammation of the anterior ocular structures and cranial base meninges, which receive ample first-division trigeminal innervation. Photophobic patients often squint, close their eyes, or avert their faces to direct light. These gestures can also occur as primitive protective responses in newborns and in those with severe congenital or degenerative brain disorders. The pathways that mediate this protective behavior are unknown.

Dazzle is not always an *optical* symptom. It is reported by patients with optic neuropathy or cone dystrophy. Those with optic neuropathy do not describe pain (Chapter 3). They say that bright light cuts down their visual ability. By contrast, those with cone dystrophy report both pain and loss of vision in ordinary daylight conditions. Normal light levels overwhelm their debilitated cones and create an unpleasant glare (Chapter 3).

GLASSES-INDUCED IMAGE DISTORTION

Patients who are not used to wearing glasses will, upon putting them on for the first time, find that objects look warped along their edges, a sensation called *optical metamorphopsia*. The same sensation will occur if a substantial change in refractive power or base curve is prescribed to long-term wearers of glasses. Convex lenses induce a pincushion distortion, concave lenses a barrel distortion, and cylindrical lenses an elongation along one axis.[12] As edges of objects appear tilted or bowed, the patient often gets nauseated and dizzy from dismaying visual–vestibular interactions[13,14] and develops a periocular pulling sensation and ache as the eyes accommodate in vain to overcome the distortion.

Image distortion can also be generated by *neural visual pathway disorders*. For example, monocular distortion should suggest foveal edema or scarring (retinal metamorphopsia; Chapter 4).[15] As cone photoreceptors are separated by edema, fewer of them are stimulated by the viewed object, which is perceived as smaller than normal (micropsia). Scarring may bring the photoreceptors closer together to cause macropsia. When the macular edema or scarring affects both eyes, retinal metamorphopsia will be binocular, but the image distortion is never completely symmetrical in the two eyes.

Metamorphopsia may rarely be caused by occipital lobe lesions. The distinctive features of this "cerebral metamorphopsia"[16,17] are that the *distortions are always binocular, emanate from partially sighted hemifields and are often accompanied by visual hallucinations* (Chapter 4). Unlike the visual distortion induced by glasses, that which is associated with retinal and cerebral lesions is never accompanied by brow ache or disequilibrium.

DISCOLORED IMAGE

A variety of optical and neural mechanisms can be responsible for the illusion of a discolored image (chromatopsia). For example, before a cataract matures enough to degrade image focus, it absorbs certain photopigments and lends a mild brown discoloration to the appearance of objects. If the cataractous lens is surgically removed, the loss of its color-modulating effects conveys a blue tint (cyanopsia) in normal light conditions[17] and a red tint (erythropsia) in bright sun or snow.[18] The same red glow discolors the vision of patients who have had anterior chamber or vitreous hemorrhages.

Seeing large colored haloes around bright lights is a symptom of corneal edema. Although it is normal to see a small, faint halo with an outer red and an inner violet ring, the appearance of an abnormally large halo is an indication that water droplets have accumulated in the cornea and are producing prismatic color effects.[19] The source of the edema is corneal endothelial injury from acute glaucoma, dystrophy, trauma, or intraocular surgery.

A nonoptical cause of altered image color is medication toxicity. Most medications with neurotropic properties can cause this illusion.[10] Whether the principal site of damage is the retina or the visual cortex is not always known. Digitalis, a cardiac medication, produces a well-documented yellow, orange, or green tint (xanthopsia) or the perception that objects are covered with frost. The damage lies in the retinal photoreceptors, principally cones.[20–22]

GHOST IMAGE

When a patient sees one reasonably clear image overlapped by one or more fuzzy ghost images (optical diplopia; Fig. 2-3), the cause is nearly always an uncorrected refractive error (including presbyopia), early cataract, or a corneal surface lesion.[23,24] Such aberrations cause light to be focused on more than one point on the retina. Because images overlap one another, the patient often reports the experience as blurred rather than multiple vision. Optical disorders may cause ghost images to be seen by both eyes, but the images viewed by each eye are never identical in position and shape.

To determine that the multiple images are of optical origin, instruct the patient to cover each eye separately. If covering *either eye* eliminates the accessory image, presume that ocular misalignment accounts for the symptom. If the extra image persists after occluding one eye, its source is optical. The pinhole test (Chapters 1, 6) can confirm the optical nature of the disorder by screening out peripheral rays of light and eliminating the extra images.[25]

A rare nonoptical cause of a ghost image is retinal (foveal) surface wrinkling.[26] As light rays from the viewed object strike the uneven retinal surface, they evoke a duplicated image. This ghost image will not be as readily eliminated by the pinhole, but the retinal abnormality will be visible on careful ophthalmoscopic examination. Retinal surface-wrinkling lesions are much more likely

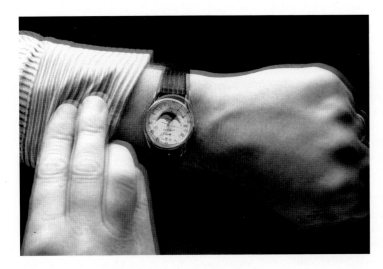

Figure 2–3. Ghost image. Seeing a second fuzzy image near the clear image is usually a manifestation of an uncorrected refractive error, corneal surface abnormality, or cataract. Therefore, it is called "optical diplopia." (Reprinted with permission from Burde RM, Savino PJ, Trobe JD. Clinical Decisions in Neuro-opthalmology, 2nd Ed. Mosby-Yearbook, St. Louis, 1992.)

to cause *binocular* diplopia than *monocular* diplopia, as the disparate images seen by each eye interfere with the fusional forces necessary to maintain bifoveal fixation.[27] The eyes slip very slightly out of alignment and no combination of prisms placed before them will bring about single binocular vision.[27]

Another rare but intriguing nonoptical cause of accessory images is an occipital lobe lesion.[29–33] The multiple images seen by patients with "cerebral polyopia" seem to come and go. When they are visible, they trail off into a homonymous hemianopia (Fig. 4-5 and Chapter 4). The secondary images do not disappear with covering either eye.

SUMMARY

Optical disorders, including refractive errors, accommodative failure, and ocular media imperfections, are responsible for most visual symptoms. They prevent the formation of a clear or faithful image on the retina.

"Blurred vision," the patient's usual complaint, is not localizing to the optical component. Retinocortical and integrative component disorders also evoke this symptom. Symptoms more specific to optical disorders are vision selectively poorer for distant or near objects, fluctuations in image clarity, dazzle, glasses-induced image distortion, discolored image, and ghost image.

Vision worse for far objects is usually due to myopia. Vision worse for near objects usually results from hyperopia or loss of accommodation. After the fourth decade of life, the most frequent cause of accommodative failure is presbyopia, or senescent stiffening of the lens. Earlier in life, accommodative failure may result from parasympatholytic medications and lesions of the ciliary body or mesencephalon.

Fluctuations in image clarity without abrupt onset result from variations in the water content of cornea or lens, shifts in lens position within the eye, and changes in ciliary muscle (accommodative) tone.

Dazzle is a light-flooded sensation that induces periocular pain and decreased vision. Most commonly the result of excessive ambient light, it can also result from ocular media abnormalities, a widely dilated pupil, or reduced ocular pigment. It is closely related to photophobia, a light-induced, ticlike periocular pain associated with inflammation of the anterior globe or meninges. Patients with optic neuropathy and cone dystrophy also complain that they see poorly in daylight; those with cone dystrophy also report that light is painful.

Glasses-induced image distortion results from differential magnification by the glasses; it is always associated with a pulling sensation about the eyes and nausea or disequilibrium from visual–vestibular interactions.

A discolored image can result from cataract, cataract removal, or blood filling the ocular cavities. An nonoptical cause of image discoloration is toxicity due to medication, especially digitalis. The report of seeing large colored haloes around lights signals corneal edema.

The complaint of seeing one or more ghost images is usually the result of an uncorrected refractive error (including presbyopia), early cataract, or a corneal surface lesion. Posterior hemispheric lesions causing homonymous hemianopias may rarely cause the illusion of seeing secondary images.

The report of seeing black spots or cobwebs is likely to be associated with vitreous floaters—solid condensates within the vitreous gel. Floaters may be caused by vitreous detachment from the retina, a common aging condition that is sometimes followed by retinal detachment requiring urgent surgery. Other causes of floaters are vitreous inflammation, bleeding from retinal vessels, ocular surgery or trauma, and myopia.

REFERENCES

1. Whitmore WG. Congenital and developmental myopia. *Eye* 1992;6:361–365.
2. Grinbaum A, Ashkenazi I, Avni I. Drug induced myopia associated with treatment for gynecological problems. *Eur J Ophthalmol.* 1995;5:136–138.
3. Tijssen CC, Goor C, Van Woerkom TCAM. Spasm of the near reflex: functional or organic disorder? *Neuro-ophthalmology.* 1983;3:59–64.
4. Sarkies NJC, Sanders MD. Convergence spasm. *Trans Ophthalmol Soc UK.* 1985;104:782–786.
5. Goldstein JH, Schneekloth BB. Spasm of the near reflex: a spectrum of anomalies. *Surv Ophthalmol.* 1996;40:269–278.
6. Leigh RJ, Zee DS. *The Neurology of Eye Movements.* 3rd ed. Philadelphia: FA Davis; 1999:519.
7. Leigh RJ, Zee DS. *The Neurology of Eye Movements.* 3rd ed. Philadelphia: FA Davis; 1999:307.
8. Krohel GB, Kristan RW, Simon JW, Barrows NA. Posttraumatic convergence insufficiency. *Ann Ophthalmol.* 1986;18:101–104.
9. Bovino JA, Marcus DF. The mechanism of transient myopia induced by sulfonamide therapy. *Am J Ophthalmol.* 1982;94:99–102.
10. Grant WM, Schumann JS. *Toxicology of the Eye.* 4th ed. Springfield, Ill: Charles C Thomas; 1993.
11. McDonald WI, Sears TA. The effects of experimental demyelination on conduction in the central nervous system. *Brain.* 1970;93:583–598.
12. Milder B, Rubin ML. *The Fine Art of Prescribing Glasses without Making a Spectacle of Yourself.* Gainesville, Fla: Triad; 1984:404–408.
13. Brandt T, Daroff RB. The multisensory physiological and pathological vertigo syndromes. *Ann Neurol.* 1980;7:195–203.
14. Demer JL, Oas JG, Baloh RW. Visual-vestibular interaction in humans during active and passive vertical head movement. *J Vestib Res.* 1993;3:101–114.
15. Fine AM, Elman MJ, Murphy RP, Patz A, Aver C. Earliest symptoms caused by neovascular membranes of the macula. *Arch Ophthalmol.* 1986;104:513–514.
16. Critchley M. Types of visual perseveration: "paliopsia" and "illusory visual spread." *Brain.* 1951;74:267–299.
17. Lepore FE. Visual obscurations: evanescent and elementary. *Sem Neurol.* 1986;6:167–175.
18. Sternberg P, Fagadau WR, Massof RW, Stark WJ. Blizzard of '83 erythropsia. *N Engl J Med.* 1983;308:1482–1483.
19. Trick GL. Entoptic imagery and after images. In: Tasman W, Jaeger EA, eds. *Foundations of Clinical Ophthalmology.* Vol 2. Philadelphia: Lippincott; 1995: pp 1–13.
20. Robertson DM, Hollenhorst RW, Callahan JA. Ocular manifestations of digitalis toxicity. *Arch Ophthalmol.* 1966;76:640–645.
21. Weleber RG, Shults WT. Digoxin retinal toxicity: clinical and electrophysiologic evaluation of a cone dysfunction syndrome. *Arch Ophthalmol.* 1981;99:1568–1572.
22. Schneider T, Dahlheim P, Zrenner E. Experimental investigations of the ocular toxicity of cardiac glycosides in animals. *Fortschr Ophthalmol.* 1989;86:751–755.
23. Hirst LW, Miller NR, Johnson RT. Monocular polyopia. *Arch Neurol.* 1983;40:756–757.
24. Records RE. Monocular diplopia. *Surv Ophthalmol.* 1980;24:303–306.
25. Smith JL. Monocular diplopia. *J Clin Neuro-ophthalmol.* 1986;6:184–185.
26. Lepore FE, Yarian DL. Monocular diplopia of retinal origin. *J Clin Neuro-ophthalmol.* 1986;6:181–183.
27. Benegas NM, Egbert J, Engel WK, Kushner BJ. Diplopia secondary to aniseikonia associated with macular disease. *Arch Ophthalmol.* 1999;117:896–899.
28. Burgess D, Roper-Hall G, Burde RM. Binocular diplopia associated with subretinal neovascular membranes. *Arch Ophthalmol.* 1980;98:311–317.
29. Bender MD. Polyopia and monocular diplopia of cerebral origin. *Arch Neurol Psychiatry.* 1945;54:323–338.
30. Kinsbourne M, Warrington EK. A study of visual perseveration. *J Neurol Neurosurg Psychiatry.* 1963;26:468–475.
31. Meadows JC. Observations on a case of monocular diplopia of cerebral origin. *J Neurol Sci.* 1973;18:249–253.
32. Safran AB, Kline LB, Glaser JS, Daroff RB. Television-induced formed visual hallucinations and cerebral diplopia. *Br J Ophthalmol.* 1981;65:707–711.
33. Lessell S. Higher disorders of visual function: positive phenomena. In: Glaser JS, Smith JL, eds. *Neuro-ophthalmology.* Vol 8. St. Louis: Mosby; 1975:27–44.

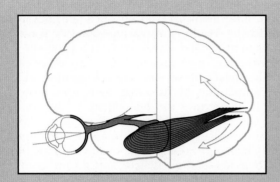

Chapter 3

NEGATIVE SYMPTOMS OF RETINOCORTICAL DISORDERS

NEGATIVE AND POSITIVE SYMPTOMS

PERSISTENT VISUAL DEFICITS
  Impediments to Localization
  Clues to Localization

UNPROVOKED TRANSIENT VISUAL
    DEFICITS
  Monocular
  Binocular

PROVOKED TRANSIENT VISUAL DEFICITS
  Posture Change
  Bright Flash
  Sustained Bright Light
  Sustained Dim Light
  Exercise or Heat
  Eccentric Gaze
  Mild Head Trauma
  Cerebral Angiography
  Rapid Rise in Blood Pressure

SUMMARY

NEGATIVE AND POSITIVE SYMPTOMS

Lesions of the retinocortical component of the visual pathway cause negative and positive symptoms. Negative symptoms are reported as blurred (unclear) vision or scotomas—dim, cloudy, gray, or blank areas within the visual field. They reflect blocked or degraded signal processing. (The word "scotoma" is Greek for dark spot, but patients with retinocortical lesions rarely report scotomas as dark spots. Such a description suggests a vitreous or retinal surface opacity; see Chapter 2.) Positive symptoms are visual illusions and hallucinations. They reflect aberrant signal processing or inappropriate activation of visual circuitry.

Negative and positive symptoms often occur together, yet their phenomenology is sufficiently distinct to deserve separate analysis. Negative symptoms are discussed in this chapter. Positive symptoms are addressed in the next (Chapter 4).

For proper diagnosis, one must determine whether a negative symptom is persistent or transient (lasting 24 hours or less). If the deficit is transient, does it occur spontaneously or is it provoked by specific factors? This chapter is organized according to these principles.

PERSISTENT VISUAL DEFICITS

Impediments to Localization

It is often difficult to surmise from the patient's description that a persisting visual deficit derives from the retinocortical component. First of all, lesions often produce diffuse deficits that the patient simply interprets as "blurred vision," a symptom that does not exclude a disorder of the optical or integrative components. Even when the deficits are exquisitely focal, patients may be largely oblivious of them, for two reasons:

- **The visual fields of each eye overlap.** The visual fields of the two eyes cover a common space in all but the peripheral 30 degrees of visual field on the temporal sides, portions of relatively little functional importance. Therefore, a visual defect limited to one eye is easily ignored, unless the other eye happens to get covered or has a preexisting visual impairment.
- **Defects are perceptually bridged.** Missing parts of the visual field can be perceptually completed, or "filled in."[1,2] In a telling experiment, 40 normal subjects viewed a uniform twinkling background on which a blank spot was suddenly made to appear.[3] The subjects reported that the blank spot had melded into the twinkling background within an average of 5 seconds.

Perceptual completion is more common with pathologic scotomas of retrochiasmal origin than with those of retinal or optic nerve origin.[4,5] Why should this be? One possibility is that retrochiasmal visual pathway defects have borders along the vertical fixational meridian; the missing halves of symmetrical objects can then be readily extrapolated.[6] Perceptual completion occurs even when entire homonymous hemifields are blind. For example, patients who report that they can see the physician's whole face are unable to tell that the physician's eye in their blind hemifield is winking at them! Only when critical images keep disappearing into a blind hemispace during such activities as driving, reading, or playing sports do some patients finally realize there is a problem.[7] However, once they have become aware of the defect, those with intact cognition will compensate by directing their eyes more efficiently into the blind field.[6,8,9] By contrast, those who have enduring global cognitive impairment or hemispatial inattention (Chapter 16) remain perpetually unaware of their hemianopic deficits and do not compensate with eye movements.[8,10]

Even patients who are aware of their focal visual deficits may not recognize them as focal, for two reasons:

- **Defects often lack steep boundaries.** Most visual field defects have sloping boundaries that allow perceptual melding into the intact surrounding field. Patients perceive them not as holes, but vaguely as a loss of clear vision.
- **The peripheral field has low visual discrimination.** The visual field defects most likely to be noticed—those closest to fixation—will be compared to an intact surrounding peripheral field, which normally provides relatively poor resolution of details. Thus a central scotoma would have to be extremely dense and discrete before it would be recognized as a hole.

Clues to Localization

In spite of the foregoing obstacles to localization, it is possible to gain a strong presumption that the lesion lies within the retinocortical component from the following historical features:

- **Acute onset** of persistent visual loss is likely to derive from the retinocortical component, especially if there is no history of trauma to the globe, evidence of a red eye, or opacification of the ocular media. In the case of monocular visual loss, the physician must be sure that patients are reporting *abrupt onset* rather than *abrupt awareness,* which occurs when they happen to occlude the unaffected eye.

- **Visual hallucinations** are consistently of retinocortical origin, provided that the patient has normal cognition and a normal sensorium (Chapter 4).
- **Dim vision** is generally caused by a lesion of the optic nerve or retinal nerve fiber layer, which blocks or temporally disperses axonal conduction. The same complaint may, however, arise if the eye's anterior chamber or vitreous cavity fills with blood.
- **Concurrent neurologic deficits** would usually implicate a retinocortical lesion, although involvement of the integrative component remains a consideration (Chapters 16, 17).

Finally, there are exceptional patients who simplify the physician's task of localization to the retinocortical component by describing the focality of their visual deficits with ringing clarity. When they report binocular defects affecting the same side of visual space in both eyes (homonymous), they are forecasting a lesion in the retrochiasmal pathway. Deficits that involve the temporal fields in both eyes (bitemporal) localize to the optic chiasm. Binocular deficits confined to the upper or lower fields (altitudinal) localize to the optic nerve, retinal nerve fiber layer, or less commonly to both occipital lobes. Monocular altitudinal deficits come exclusively from lesions of the optic nerve or retinal nerve fiber layer. Central scotomas derive from retinal or optic nerve disease.

UNPROVOKED TRANSIENT VISUAL DEFICITS

Most episodes of transient visual deficit have no precipitating circumstances. Diagnosis is especially challenging because examination generally yields no contributory findings.

The first step is to try to determine whether the event involved one eye or both. Unfortunately, patients are egregiously unreliable in making this distinction, for they are likely to attribute homonymous hemifield loss to the eye with the temporal defect. (Apparently they never learned that vision is represented in hemifields.) Certain historical clues help in differentiating between monocular and homonymous visual loss (Box 3-1).

Box 3–1

WAS TRANSIENT VISUAL LOSS MONOCULAR OR BINOCULAR?

Patients do a poor job of distinguishing between transient monocular vision loss and binocular hemifield vision loss. They blame the hemifield loss on the eye with the temporal defect. Here are four clues suggesting that a prior episode of vision loss affected a hemifield rather than an eye:

- Objects disappeared on one side of visual space.
- Reading vision was impaired even with both eyes open.
- Zigzag scintillations were present.
- Headache occurred during or after the visual symptoms.

Monocular Deficits

Transient monocular visual loss (amaurosis fugax, transient monocular blindness) is generally caused by ocular ischemia.[11] As with hemispheric transient ischemic attacks (TIAs), conventional mechanisms include thromboembolism from the heart or anterior circulation as well as low perfusion caused by anterior circulation stenosis superimposed on transient hypotension.

CONVENTIONAL MECHANISMS

As seen in Table 3-1, the eye, just like the cerebral hemisphere, is the target of emboli from the heart, aortic arch, cervical carotid artery, and the systemic veins via a heart wall patency (paradoxical embolism).[12] In addition, Doppler orbital imaging has disclosed that the ophthalmic artery is a source of emboli.[13]

The large arteries of the anterior circulation may produce ocular ischemia by becoming occluded. In the presence of high-grade stenosis, even a brief drop in systemic blood pressure may drop perfusion to the eye enough to induce transient monocular

Table 3–1. **Transient Monocular Visual Loss: Conventional Mechanisms**

Embolism
Aortic arch
Heart valves or wall
Cervical carotid artery
Systemic veins (paradoxical embolism)

Impending Occlusion
Carotid artery

Episodic Systemic Hypotension*
Cardiac arrhythmia
Aortic stenosis
Pulmonary embolus
Congestive heart failure
Hypotensive medication
Dehydration

Increased Viscosity and/or Hypercoagulability
Clotting factor disorder
Blood dyscrasia
Antiphospholipid antibody syndrome
Puerperium
Early postoperative period
Metastatic cancer
Serious systemic infection
Serious trauma
Serious burn
Dehydration
Cigarette smoking
Oral contraceptive use

*Usually causes binocular visual deficits.

(or binocular) visual loss. Hyperviscous or hypercoagulable states have also been associated with transient monocular (and binocular) visual loss.

In the past, reduced ophthalmic or retinal artery pressure was measured by *ophthalmodynamometry,* putting a graded amount of pressure on the sclera by means of a standardized probe and observing the pressure level at which retinal artery pulsations were first noted ophthalmoscopically.[13] Abandoned for lack of precision, ophthalmodynamometry has been supplanted by Doppler orbital imaging, a test that is not in standard clinical use because it requires expertise and expensive equipment.

UNCONVENTIONAL MECHANISMS

In addition to the conventional mechanisms that cause TIAs, Table 3-2 lists six "unconventional mechanisms" that cause transient monocular visual loss: optic disk edema, retinal arterial vasospasm, intermittent angle closure glaucoma, orbital or retro-orbital arteriovenous fistula, recurrent bleeding in the anterior chamber of the eye, and impending optic nerve or retinal vascular occlusion.[12,14]

Optic Disk Edema

Any condition that produces optic disk swelling may give rise to *transient obscurations,* blackouts of vision lasting seconds.[15] The most common cause is elevation of intracranial pressure (ICP) above 200 mg H_2O, which leads to axoplasmic stasis within the optic disk and impaired signal transmission.[16] The special vulnerability of the optic disk to raised ICP may be due to tight tissue packing in the scleral lamina cribrosa and a tenuous ciliary arterial supply (Chapters 1, 12). Although elevated ICP typically causes

Table 3–2. **Transient Monocular Visual Loss: Unconventional Mechanisms**

Optic Disk Swelling
Papilledema
Other causes of optic disk edema

Vasospasm
Idiopathic
Associated with migraine

Episodic Increase in Intraocular Pressure
Intermittent angle closure glaucoma

Ocular Steal
Orbital or cavernous sinus arteriovenous fistula

Recurrent Intraocular Hemorrhage
Leaking iris root vessel after anterior ocular
   segment surgery

Impending Occlusion
Impending ciliary artery occlusion
Impending retinal artery occlusion
Impending retinal vein occlusion

bilateral optic disk edema (papilledema), the degree of swelling may not be equal in the two eyes. Obscurations of vision are often restricted to one eye—the eye with the more swollen disk. Assumption of the upright posture sometimes aggravates the visual symptoms by causing a critical drop in ocular perfusion (see below, "Provoked Transient Visual Deficit").

Vasospasm

Spasm of retinal vessels has become the accepted explanation for episodes of transient monocular visual loss in patients aged under 40 years[17,18] and in older patients whose conventional studies are negative.[19,20] A minority of patients have a history of migraine or Raynaud's phenomenon. Ophthalmoscopic examination is usually negative.[21] Occasionally, however, transient narrowing of retinal arteriolar[19] or veins[22] appears during attacks; these attacks are reported to subside under treatment with nimodipine.[20]

Intermittent Angle Closure Glaucoma

Anatomic anterior chamber abnormalities may lead to episodic plugging of the aqueous drainage channels by the iris. Intraocular pressure climbs rapidly and causes optic nerve ischemia. The patient usually experiences acute periocular and brow pain that may be incorrectly attributed to migraine.[14,23] If the high intraocular pressure (IOP) is sustained, the conjunctiva becomes engorged and the cornea becomes cloudy. If the high IOP has dissipated by the time of examination, the diagnosis must be inferred from history and from examination of the anterior chamber angle with special optical devices.

Retro-ocular Arteriovenous Fistula

Intermittent monocular vision loss may rarely be caused by an orbital or cavernous sinus arteriovenous fistula that diverts arterial blood intended for the eye into orbital or cavernous sinus veins.[24] The diagnosis can usually be made by observing dilated conjunctival or retinal veins and proptosis, which result from high pressure in the venous outflow system within the orbit.

Intermittent Intraocular Hemorrhage

An unusual cause of monocular vision loss is episodic bleeding into the anterior chamber from a traumatized or inflamed vessel in the iris root or within a corneal wound.[25,26] There may be no pain. Patients often describe a reddish turbidity to their vision. Using the slit-lamp biomicroscope, the physician may see a stream of blood coming from the anterior chamber angle into the aqueous. Unless the bleeding is heavy, it will be quickly diluted by the flow of aqueous and clear vision will be restored. This condition can often be corrected surgically.

Impending Optic Nerve or Retinal Vascular Occlusion

Incomplete occlusion of the ciliary supply to the optic nerve or the retinal arteries or veins will often produce transient ischemia exacerbated by standing up (Chapter 10).[27] The patient may also report seeing sparkling lights (photopsias, scintillations; see Chapter 4). In most cases of impending arterial occlusions, ophthalmoscopy is normal. However, in cases of impending ciliary occlusion, especially in association with giant cell arteritis, the optic disk may be slightly swollen, reflecting ischemic axoplasmic stasis. There may be chronically reduced perfusion to the eye(s), as evidenced by retinal cotton wool spots, hemorrhages, dilated veins, and neovascularization, as well as aqueous flare and cells (ischemic oculopathy, ischemic ocular syndrome, chronic ocular ischemia).[27] Even when ophthalmoscopy is normal, fluorescein angiography and Doppler sonography may reveal slow flow across the ocular circulatory bed. In most patients with impending retinal vein occlusion, ophthalmoscopy will disclose distended retinal veins with perivenous hemorrhages concentrated in the retinal periphery.

EVALUATION

The evaluation of patients with spontaneous transient monocular visual loss consists of four components: history, ophthalmic examination, blood studies, and echography of the carotid artery and heart (Fig. 3-1). The

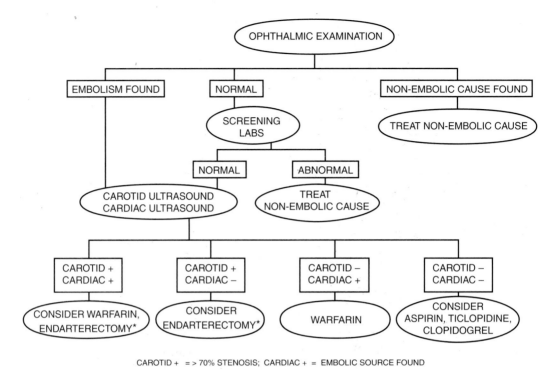

CAROTID + = > 70% STENOSIS; CARDIAC + = EMBOLIC SOURCE FOUND

Figure 3–1. Management of unprovoked monocular transient visual loss. *Risks of endarterectomy may not be justified in patients with transient monocular visual loss alone (see text).

degree to which ancillary studies are used depends on the results of history and ophthalmic examination, the age of the patient, and the presence of arteriosclerotic risk factors.

History

The patient's description of the visual characteristics of an attack *seldom allows the physician to determine its cause.*[28,29] The duration of visual loss can vary from seconds to hours for any cause other than papilledema, where attacks never last more than seconds.[15] Nor does the location of the scotoma within the visual field specify a particular mechanism. For example, an ascending or descending ("curtainlike") spread of blindness, commonly held as specific for embolism, can occur in patients with hypotension and vasospasm.[30] Accompanying monocular sparkles are also nonspecific, merely signaling a lower degree of ischemia than is necessary to produce visual deficits. However, the following accompany-

ing manifestations are helpful in determining a mechanism:

- Zigzag (fortification) scintillations: characteristic of visual cortex migrane, thus incompatible with an ocular origin.
- Headache, scalp tenderness, jaw claudication: impending ciliary occlusion in association with giant cell arteritis.
- Eye or brow pain: intermittent angle closure glaucoma or ciliary ischemia in association with giant cell arteritis.
- Neck pain: cervical carotid dissection.
- Presyncope: hypotension or hyperviscosity syndrome.
- Simultaneous contralateral hemisensory or motor findings: acute cervical carotid or carotid siphon occlusion.[31–33]

Ophthalmic Examination

This is a critical step, both in identifying ocular signs of systemic embolism (retinal intra-arteriolar plaques, branch artery occlusions, cotton wool spots, Roth spots) and in identifying signs of nonembolic causes (optic disk edema, impending retinal vascular occlusion, chronic ocular ischemia, arteriovenous fistula, angle closure, hyphema).

Ancillary Studies

Common hypercoagulable states can be ruled out with conventional screening laboratory studies (CBC, platelet count, sedimentation rate, protein electrophoresis, prothrombin and partial thromboplastin times, connective tissue panel, urinalysis, and standard chemistries). Specialized tests such as protein S and C, antithrombin III, factor V Leiden, and homocysteine are reserved for patients who lack conventional arteriosclerotic risk factors or who have indicators of systemic ischemia.[34]

Carotid and cardiac sources of emboli can be ruled out by ultrasonic examination. But the yield of these echographic studies depends on the age of the patient and the presence of pertinent risk factors. Most individuals who suffer transient monocular visual loss in youth (age <40) will have no ophthalmologic or blood laboratory abnormalities, constitutional manifestations, or important arteriosclerotic risk factors.[34,35] Their chance of future stroke is low.[17,36,37] Should they undergo ultrasonic evaluation of the cervical carotid arteries (atheroma, dissection, dysplasia) or heart (septal, valvular defects)? Considering the low yield of these studies in young people without risk factors, some physicians do not order them at all. Other physicians order them only if ocular TIA episodes are repeated. Still other physicians, pointing out that the studies are risk-free, prescribe them following a single episode if vasospasm cannot be confidently invoked because the patient lacks a history of other forms of migraine.[34]

In older patients, the yield of echographic studies is higher, but the lesions they disclose may have no role in the pathogenesis of ocular TIA. A cardiac embolic source is unlikely to show up under echography in a patient without manifestations of a cardiac disorder. The physician can justify ordering carotid artery echography as a means of detecting carotid disorders that may require treatment. However, carotid artery echography should not be an automatic prelude to carotid endarterectomy, for reasons discussed in the next section.

CAROTID ENDARTERECTOMY

Should patients with transient monocular visual loss and high-grade (>70%) cervical carotid stenosis undergo carotid endarterectomy? Consider the following evidence.

Two large collaborative trials comparing medical therapy to carotid endarterectomy, one conducted in North America,[38–40] the other in Europe,[41] found that endarterectomy significantly reduced the future risk of stroke in symptomatic patients if cross-sectional carotid stenosis was greater than 70%. However, in neither report were the data for ocular TIAs singled out. In 1995, the North American trial compared the results in 70 patients with first-ever hemispheric TIAs to those of 59 patients with first-ever ocular TIAs occurring within 120 days of entry.[42] The estimated 2 year ipsilateral stroke incidence was 43.5% for patients with hemispheric TIAs but *only 16.6% for those with ocular TIAs.* Moreover, patients with ocular TIAs *did not suffer a single major stroke,* defined as a functional deficit persisting beyond 90 days. The lower stroke rate among the medically treated ocular TIA patients could not be attributed to a difference in the frequency of high-grade stenosis, as each group had a mean of 82.9% stenosis.

Why should the future risk of major stroke be so much lower in ocular than hemispheric TIA? There are two possible explanations: (*1*) it takes a much smaller embolus to impair vision than other brain functions, and (*2*) ocular TIA is frequently caused by vasospasm, a mechanism that does not lead to hemispheric stroke as often as do other mechanisms.

The relatively low risk of major stroke after ocular TIA nullifies the benefit of endarterectomy even with a surgical risk of stroke and/or death as low as 4%, well below the levels reported in the two major trials.[35,43,44] There is evidence that the current 30 day perioperative stroke/death rate following endarterectomy performed in community hospitals is not as low as that in the large trials.[45]

Therefore, patients who are considering carotid endarterectomy for transient monocular visual loss should be made aware of the gamble they are taking: an upfront 4% or greater risk of perioperative stroke/death versus a chance of cutting in half a future 4%–8% per year risk of strokes that may not be debilitating.[44] With this information in mind, *knowledgeable observers have favored antiplatelet agents* over endarterectomy in treating ocular TIA alone.[46] Therapy with aspirin, ticlopidine, clopidogrel, and warfarin is a safe alternative to endarterectomy for ocular TIA.

Binocular Deficits

In the absence of papilledema, transient binocular visual loss reflects dysfunction of the visual cortex caused by migraine,[47] vertebrobasilar transient ischemia (TIA),[48–53] or seizure[54–62] (Table 3-3). In differentiating between these three causes of transient binocular sight loss, the visual characteristics of the attack and its accompanying manifestations are the principal clues.

MIGRAINE

Although the visual disturbance of migraine is usually characterized by *scintillations* (Chapter 4), migraine can occur without such positive phenomena.[63,64] In one series involving 70 adults aged 40 years and above, 37% of cases lacked scintillations.[63] A pure visual deficit is especially common in children. In the largest series reported to date, 77 (77%) of 100 children described no scintillations during their visual loss.[65] Rather, they described their vision as indistinct, dim, or empty and did not mention hemianopias. The purely negative visual phenomena of migraine usually disappear within 20 to 30 minutes, but unlike the scintillations, they do not march (expand, spread, build up) across the visual field.

The relationship between headache and migraine is complex. In youth, headache typically follows migrainous visual loss but gradually lessens in severity with advancing age, and it may disappear altogether after age 50 (acephalgic migraine, migraine equivalent, dissociated migraine).[47,63] In children, the headache often precedes or occurs during the visual symptoms.[65]

Migraine is probably the cause of a transient binocular visual deficit if it is followed by numbness or dysphasia. The numbness spreads from the hand to the face over several minutes, beginning 5 and 30 minutes after the visual loss. Dysphasia has a comparable latency of onset after the visual symptoms. In vertebrobasilar TIA, by contrast, *all neurologic manifestations occur at once.*[63] Partial occipital seizures may also be accompanied by numbness, but their spread is typically much faster, and generalized seizures usually follow.

VERTEBROBASILAR TRANSIENT ISCHEMIC ATTACK

Visual impairment is reported in 40%[51] to 50%[50] of patients with vertebrobasilar TIAs.

Table 3–3. **Transient Binocular Visual Loss without Scintillations and with Normal Ophthalmic Examination**

Manifestation	Migraine	Vertebrobasilar TIA	Seizure
Duration	20–30 minutes	Seconds	Variable
Headache frequency	Common	Rare	Uncommon
Headache timing	After visual loss	During or after visual loss	During or after visual loss
Other	Dysphoria, nausea, sleepiness, paresthesias, dysphasia	Dysequilibrium, diplopia, vertigo, amnesia, weakness, numbness	Homonymous hemoanopia, eye deviation, automatisms, clonic movements, depressed consciousness

Visual loss was the only symptom in 2%,[63] 7%,[51,66] and 16%[50] of attacks. Accompanying headache favors migraine but has been reported in 10% of vertebrobasilar TIAs.[50]

To identify vertebrobasilar TIA as the cause of transient binocular visual loss, it is helpful to elicit other symptoms of brainstem ischemia, such as dysequilibrium, diplopia, dysarthria, dysphagia, drop attacks, and dread (the "six D's"), as well as vertigo, nausea, amnesia, facial (especially circumoral) and extremity numbness, extremity weakness, tinnitus, and hearing loss.[50]

Although vertebrobasilar TIA is often attributed to artery-to-artery or cardiogenic embolism,[67] an alternative mechanism is episodic hypotension superimposed on proximal vertebral artery stenosis.

SEIZURE

Binocular visual loss *without positive visual phenomena* is a rare manifestation of seizure. However, purely inhibitory visual phenomena have been described in up to 15% of patients with occipital lobe seizures[54,68] in the three following settings.

- **Occipital absence spells:** episodes of a few minutes' duration occurring only in neurologically intact children, in which binocular blurring or complete blindness may be an isolated manifestation or accompanied by automatisms, especially eye blinking, and slight alterations in consciousness. Occipital spike and wave discharges are recorded during the attacks. Brain imaging is normal, and the episodes disappear by adolescence.
- **Focal occipital discharges:** range in duration from minutes to days, during which a unilateral occipital lobe lesion gives rise to a focal discharge that spreads across to the opposite occipital lobe to cause binocular blindness. In some cases, the persistent seizure discharge remains confined to the occipital lobes, producing a blind nonconvulsive state known as "status epilepticus amauroticus." In other cases, nonvisual focal manifestations, including conjugate eye deviation and loss of consciousness, may follow as the seizure spreads forward or generalizes. These patients usually have an occipital imaging abnormality caused by infarct, trauma, or

tumor, although imaging-negative processes such as hypoglycemia, hyperglycemia, hypoxia–ischemia, meningitis, and encephalitis may be responsible (Chapter 15). In the interictal period, a corresponding homonymous hemianopic visual field defect is usually present.
- **Postictal effects of prolonged generalized seizures:** occur in patients recovering from generalized status epilepticus. They may have delayed recovery of vision or even permanent blindness. These phenomena are attributed to the relative vulnerability of the occipital cortex to hypoxia associated with status epilepticus.

PROVOKED TRANSIENT VISUAL DEFICITS

In a minority of patients who report transient visual loss, the attack is precipitated by a particular circumstance. Recognizing the connection leads to a firmer diagnosis and very different management than when the visual loss is unprovoked (Table 3-4).

Posture Change

Visual loss precipitated by assuming the upright posture (orthostatic visual loss) occurs in patients who have marginal ocular perfusion. This is typically the result of flow-limiting anterior circulation (aortic arch, carotid, ophthalmic artery) stenosis[69] or optic disk edema.

The visual loss probably reflects reduced ciliary blood flow, which nourishes both the outer retina and optic nerve head. The optic nerve circulation is vulnerable to postural change because its small vessels are poorly collateralized, packed in a tight space, exposed to intraocular and intracranial pressures, and in competition with the well-collateralized choroidal circulation, which has the body's highest flow rate.[13,70]

FLOW-LIMITING ANTERIOR CIRCULATION STENOSIS

In the presence of flow-limiting anterior circulation stenosis, vision dims, blurs, or dis-

Table 3–4. **Provoked Transient Visual Loss**

Provoker	Underlying Condition	Mechanism
Posture change	Carotid, ophthalmic artery stenosis Optic disk edema	Impaired perfusion of eye
Bright flash	Carotid, ophthalmic artery stenosis	Impaired regeneration of photopigments after bleaching
	Choroidal or outer retinal lesion	
Sustained bright light	Optic neuropathy Cone dystrophy	Uncertain Impaired regeneration of photopigments after bleaching
Sustained dim light	Rod dystrophy	Impaired dark adadtation
Exercise or heat	Optic neuropathy	Marginal axonal conduction
Eccentric gaze	Orbital mass	Compression of optic nerve
Mild head trauma	None	Postexcitation neuronal exhaustion?
Cerebral angiography	None	Breakdown in blood–brain barrier
Rapid rise in blood pressure	None	Breakthrough in auto-regulation

appears abruptly with upright posture and recovers slowly over minutes to hours.[71] Visual loss, usually binocular, can occur without any other symptoms of global cerebral hypoperfusion (lightheadedness, confusion, diaphoresis, alarm) if the circulation to the eye is already compromised by narrowed vascular caliber. Evidence of chronically low ophthalmic perfusion appears in the optic fundus as retinal microaneurysms, hemorrhages, dilated veins, and neovascularization, on the iris as neovascularization, and in the anterior chamber as flare and cells (ischemic oculopathy).[72,73]

OPTIC DISK EDEMA

Because the optic nerves must pass through a narrow hole in the sclera, pathologic swelling makes them particularly susceptible to ischemia from a posturally mediated drop in blood pressure. When optic disk edema is severe, black-outs of vision may occur without a posture change (see above, "Unprovoked Transient Visual Deficit").

Bright Flash

This symptom represents delayed visual recovery after abrupt exposure to bright sunlight or car headlights.[74,75] As with orthostatic visual loss, it implies flow-limiting atherostenosis of the anterior circulation, causing chronic ocular ischemia. *It can also occur in association with hereditary and inflammatory outer retinal and choroidal diseases.*[76] The mechanism is impaired regeneration of photopigments after bleaching by strong light (Chapter 1).[77–79]

THE PHOTOSTRESS TEST

Delayed regeneration of photopigments in a malfunctioning outer retina is the basis for the photostress test.[80] After baseline visual acuity has been measured, a bright light is shined into the symptomatic eye for 10 seconds. The examiner then measures the delay in the patient's ability to correctly identify the letters on the next larger line on the acuity chart. Following a similar measurement on the asymptomatic eye, the latencies are compared. Full recovery normally occurs within 50 seconds. A doubling of the latency in the affected eye is considered positive for outer retinal dysfunction.

Sustained Bright Light

When patients complain that vision remains relatively poor as long as they are exposed to sunshine or fluorescent lights, they may harbor an optic neuropathy or a cone dystrophy.

OPTIC NEUROPATHY

Patients with any type of optic neuropathy report poor vision during exposure to bright light, but its mechanism is unknown.[81] Because these patients state that their vision also worsens in low light levels (see below), there must be a mesopic, or intermediate, luminance level at which vision is optimal.

CONE DYSTROPHY

Patients with cone receptor dysfunction report markedly impaired vision even in ordinary daylight, a symptom called *day blindness* or *hemeralopia*. The mechanism is presumed to be similar to that which causes impaired vision after bright flash, namely, impaired regeneration of photopigment by damaged cone receptors.

Unfortunately, this symptom carries low specificity because it is so often described both by individuals with normal vision who are abnormally sensitive to glare and by those with refractive abnormalities (Chapters 1, 2).

Sustained Dim Light

Patients who report visual incapacitation in darkness may have rod photoreceptor malfunction. When rods fail, vision does not undergo adaptation to darkness, the physiologic increase in light sense after a 30 minute sustained exposure to low-light stimuli (Chapter 1). Patients stumble into nightclub or cinema seats because they cannot get used to the darkness.

This failure to adapt to low luminance, called *night blindness* or *nyctalopia,* is usually caused by hereditary retinal rod photoreceptor degenerations (retinitis pigmentosa). True nyctalopia is hard to separate from the far more common optical problem of physiologically poorer visual acuity during nighttime than daytime driving, particularly for reading highway signs. Low light levels induce the pupil to dilate, so that the retina is receiving a larger contribution of light refracted by the peripheral portions of the cornea and lens. Because these peripheral light rays are not as accurately refracted, the retinal image becomes blurred even in individuals whose refractive errors are properly corrected for daylight. Moreover, the youthful ciliary muscle does not fully relax in very dim illumination, giving rise to an artificial myopia (night myopia) that keeps highway signs out of focus. Although it may be difficult to separate optical from retinal causes of night vision difficulty based purely on the patient's history, a useful clue is that the retinally night-blind can usually see bright highway signs; it is the objects in the surrounding darkness that they cannot make out.

Patients afflicted with optic neuropathy report that their visual acuity declines on cloudy days or at dusk, as dim light exposes the vulnerability of pathways conveying low-contrast visual information.[82]

Exercise or Heat

Patients with demyelinating optic neuropathy develop blurred vision 5 to 20 minutes after physical exercise, a hot bath or shower, and exposure to ambient heat that elevates body temperature. This phenomenon is attributed to the detrimental effect of heat on axonal conduction.[83,84] When the provoking factor is removed, recovery begins within minutes to hours.

Originally described in 1889 by Uhthoff,[85] and since called "Uhthoff's symptom," exercise-induced or heat-induced visual dimming or blurring has since been reported most often in patients with optic neuritis, where it has been documented in 33%[84] to 50%[83] of cases. It has also been reported uncommonly in patients with compressive optic neuropathies[86] and Leber's hereditary optic neuropathy.[87] There is no correlation between the degree of visual loss and the likelihood of Uhthoff's symptom.[86] But in one study,[83] those with Uhthoff's symptom were more likely to have recurrent attacks of optic neuritis, an abnormal MRI, and later multiple sclerosis than those who did not report this symptom.

ECCENTRIC GAZE

This *monocular* symptom results from compression of the optic nerve by an orbital tumor situated within the extraocular muscle cone.[88,89] Vision is lost in the affected eye 10 to 20 seconds after gaze is directed to one side. It recovers quickly after the eyes return to the straight-ahead position. Orbital imaging shows that in side gaze there is marked deformation of the optic nerve by the intraconal mass, usually a hemangioma or sheath meningioma. Eye movement–induced visual loss may rarely occur without an orbital mass, when the optic nerve is under diffuse pressure from pseudotumor cerebri.[90] The common mechanism is presumed to be marginal blood flow, which is shut off by kinking the optic nerve. A similar symptom is described in patients whose optic nerves are partially demyelinated but under no pressure, presumably because kinking further impairs faulty signal transmission over demyelinated segments.[81]

Eye movement–induced visual loss is actually much less common than head movement–induced visual loss, a *symptom that does not derive from a disorder of the visual pathway, but rather from bilateral lesions of the vestibular pathway*. In order to provide clear vision during head motion, the eyes must move in an equal and opposite direction. A malfunctioning vestibulo-ocular reflex (VOR) causes this stabilization to fail. Vision blurs even when the head or body moves slightly, as in driving or walking on uneven surfaces. Viewed objects appear to jiggle or oscillate (oscillopsia).[91,92] (See Box 2-2.)

A simple way to verify that the VOR is the cause of the symptom is to have a patient read the Snellen near card while moving his or her head rapidly from side to side. Normal VOR compensation permits clear vision to be maintained. If the VOR is defective, acuity will drop by at least two Snellen lines.[93]

Mild Head Trauma

Children and young adults who sustain trivial closed head injury, usually from a fall, may develop transient blindness in a setting of relatively intact neurologic function.[94–96] They can be irritable and confused, but their visual loss is disproportionately severe. Ophthalmic examination is normal, including fully reactive pupils, so that the blindness is presumed to be cortical. Brain imaging is typically normal, but electroencephalography may show bihemispheric posterior slow waves. Within hours, the blindness spontaneously clears. This mystifying posttraumatic transient cortical blindness has been linked to a predisposition to migraine and seizures,[95] reflecting a nonspecific vulnerability of visual cortex. It may represent a postexcitation neuronal "exhaustion," as may be seen after seizure or migraine. In fact, in Britain this phenomenon is called "footballer's migraine," because soccer players develop it after vigorously heading the ball.[97]

Cerebral Angiography

Transient cortical blindness following cerebral angiography has an incidence of 1%–4%.[98,99] Brain imaging usually shows enhancement of posterior occipital regions, reflecting disruption of the blood–brain barrier (BBB) in the posterior cerebral artery domain. The BBB is easily damaged in this region by hyperosmolar contrast agents.[99] Reversibility of the visual loss distinguishes this condition from postangiographic visual cortex infarction.

Rapid Rise in Blood Pressure

A rapid rise in systolic blood pressure above 150 mm Hg can bring on the syndrome of *hypertensive encephalopathy*, consisting of headache, alterations in consciousness, seizures, binocular visual deficits, illusions, or hallucinations.[100] Visual alterations may be the first, the most prominent, or the only manifestation. The eyes sometimes show vaso-occlusive retinopathy, optic neuropathy, or choroidopathy, but the symptoms originate in the white matter adjacent to the visual cortex, which appears edematous on brain imaging.[101] The transudate only temporarily interrupts neurologic function. If blood pressure is not normalized, brain arterioles may develop fibrinoid necrosis and become occluded, infarcting the tissue they serve (Chapter 15). This selective failure in the domain of the posterior cerebral artery could stem from its relatively poor sympathetic innervation.[104] It probably results from a premature failure of cerebrovascular autoregulation, leading to vasodilatation and leakage.[102,103]

SUMMARY

The negative symptoms of retinocortical pathway disease are reported as blurred vision or scotomas—dim, gray, cloudy, or blank areas within the visual field.

Even when visual defects are exquisitely focal, patients are frustratingly vague in describing the nature of their visual deficits, for a variety of reasons. First, monocular deficits may go unnoticed because the visual fields of the two eyes largely overlap. Second, deficits may be ignored because of perceptual "filling in." Third, focal defects often lack distinct boundaries. Fourth, peripheral visual field defects are not well perceived by the patient.

Historical clues to a retinocortical localization are abrupt onset, presence of hallucinations, dimness of vision, and other concurrent neurologic deficits. Confronted with monocular visual symptoms, the physician must differentiate between abrupt onset and abrupt awareness.

When patients are able to describe the focality of their visual deficits, the following information is localizing: homonymous hemianopia—retrochiasmal pathway; bitemporal hemianopia—optic chiasm; altitudinal defect—optic nerve, retinal nerve fiber layer, or, if binocular, rarely visual cortex; central scotoma—retina or optic nerve.

Patients often mislead physicians by attributing transient homonymous defects to the eye with the temporal defect. The deficit is likely to have been homonymous rather than monocular if objects seemed to disappear on one side of visual space, reading vision was impaired even with both eyes open, and the episode included zigzag scintillations and headache.

Transient monocular visual loss is caused by reduced blood flow to the eye. Although the conventional mechanisms used to explain other TIAs apply here (Table 3-1), six mechanisms are unique to monocular transient visual loss: papilledema, vasospasm, intermittent angle closure glaucoma, ocular steal by an orbital or cavernous sinus fistula, recurrent anterior chamber bleeding, and impending ciliary or retinal vascular occlusion (Table 3-2). The patient's description of the visual characteristics of the attack seldom identifies the mechanism, the exception being the ultrabrief obscurations of vision associated with papilledema.

The ophthalmic examination often provides important clues to the cause of transient monocular visual loss. If the ophthalmic examination is unrevealing, however, the physician is left wondering whether the attack was caused by embolism, cervical carotid stenosis with intermittent low perfusion, hyperviscosity or hypercoagulability, or vasospasm. A small battery of blood tests, together with ultrasound of the carotid artery and heart, may suggest a mechanism.

Carotid endarterectomy significantly reduces future stroke risk in patients with hemispheric TIA or mild stroke who have ≥70% cervical carotid stenosis. But it may not be beneficial in patients with ocular TIA alone. This is because the future risk of stroke in patients treated with platelet antiaggregants or warfarin is too low to justify the perioperative risk of endarterectomy.

In the absence of papilledema, the three principal causes of unprovoked binocular transient visual loss are migraine, vertebrobasilar TIA, and occipital lobe seizure. These three causes are best differentiated on the basis of accompanying neurologic manifestations.

In a minority of cases, transient visual loss is provoked by particular circumstances, such as assumption of the upright posture, exposure to a brief bright flash, sustained bright light, sustained dim light, exercise or heat, eccentric gaze, mild head trauma, cerebral angiography, and rapid rise in blood pressure. Pathogenesis is varied and depends on the precipitating condition.

REFERENCES

1. Safran AB, Landis T. Plasticity in the adult visual cortex: implications for the diagnosis of visual field defects and visual rehabilitation. *Curr Opin Ophthalmol.* 1996;7:53–64.

2. Ramachandran VS, Blakeslee S. *Phantoms in the Brain: Probing the Mysteries of the Human Mind.* New York: William Morrow; 1998.

3. Ramachandran VS, Gregory RL. Perceptual filling in of artificially induced scotomas in human vision. *Nature.* 1991;350:699–702.

4. Ramachandran VS. Filling in gaps in perception: Part II. Scotomas and phantom limbs. *Curr Dir Psychol Sci.* 1992;1:56–65.

5. Aulhorn E, Kost G. White noise field campimetry: a new form of perimetric examination. *Klin Monatsbl Augenheilkd.* 1988;192:284–288.

6. Sergent J. An investigation into perceptual completion in blind areas of the visual field. *Brain.* 1988;111:347–373.

7. Trobe JD, Lorber MI, Schlezinger NS. Isolated homonymous hemianopia. *Arch Ophthalmol.* 1973;89:377–381.

8. Gassel MM Williams D. Visual function in patients with homonymous hemianopia: III. The completion phenomenon; insight and attitude to the defect; and visual function efficiency. *Brain.* 1963;86:229–260.

9. Torjussen T. Visual processing in cortically blind hemifields. *Neuropsychologia.* 1978;16:15–21.

10. Warrington EK. The completion of visual forms across hemianopic field defects. *J Neurol Neurosurg Psychiatry.* 1962;25:208–217.

11. Hoyt WF. Transient monocular vision loss: a historical perspective. *Ophthalmol Clin North Am.* 1996;9(3):323–326.

12. Bernstein EF. *Amaurosis Fugax.* New York: Springer-Verlag; 1987:286–303.

13. Alm A. Retinal blood flow and different diagnostic procedures. *Ophthalmol Clin North Am.* 1998;11(40):491–503.

14. Shults WT. Ocular causes of transient monocular visual loss other than emboli. *Ophthalmol Clin North Am.* 1996;9(3):381–391.

15. Hedges TR. The terminology of transient visual loss due to vascular insufficiency. *Stroke.* 1984;15:907–908.

16. Sanders MD. The Bowman Lecture. Papilledema: "the pendulum of progress." *Eye.* 1997;11:267–294.

17. Tippin J, Corbett JJ, Kerber RE, Schroeder E, Thompson HS. Amaurosis fugax and ocular infarction in adolescents and young adults. *Ann Neurol.* 1989;26:69–77.

18. Coppeto JR. Migraine and other head pains. In: Albert DM, Jakobiec FA, eds. *Principles and Practice of Ophthalmology.* Vol 4. Philadelphia: WB Saunders; 1994:2691–2692.

19. Burger SK, Saul RF, Selhorst JB, Thurston SE. Transient monocular blindness caused by vasospasm. *N Engl J Med.* 1991;325:870–873.

20. Winterkorn JMS, Kupersmith MJ, Wirtschafter JD, Forman S. Brief report: treatment of vasospastic amaurosis fugax with calcium-channel blockers. *N Engl J Med.* 1993;329:396–398.

21. Winterkorn JM, Burde RM. Vasospasm—not migraine—in the anterior visual pathway. *Ophthalmol Clin North Am.* 1996;9(3):393–405.

22. Kline LB, Kelly CL. Ocular migraine in a patient with cluster headaches. *Headache.* 1980;20:253–257.

23. Ravits J, Seybold M. Transient monocular visual loss from narrow-angle glaucoma. *Arch Neurol.* 1984;41:991–994.

24. Kupersmith MJ, Berenstein A, Flamm E, Ransohoff J. Neuro-ophthalmologic abnormalities and intravascular therapy of traumatic carotid cavernous fistulas. *Ophthalmology.* 1986;93:906–912.

25. Kosmorsky G, Rosenfeld S, Burde R. Transient monocular obscuration—amaurosis fugax: a case report. *Br J Ophthalmol.* 1985;69:688–692.

26. Cates CA, Newman DK. Transient monocular visual loss due to uveitis-glaucoma-hyphaema (UGH) syndrome. *J Neurol Neurosurg Psychiatry.* 1998;65:131–132.

27. Sharma S, Brown M, Brown GC. Retinal artery occlusions. *Ophthalmol Clin North Am.* 1998;11(4):591–600.

28. Goodwin JA, Gorelick PB, Helgason CM. Symptoms of amaurosis fugax in atherosclerotic carotid artery disease. *Neurology.* 1987;37:829–833.

29. Hedges TR, Lackman RD. Isolated opthalmic migraine in the differential diagnosis of cerebroocular ischemia. *Stroke.* 1976;7:379–381.

30. Gautier J-C. Clinical presentation and differential diagnosis of amaurosis fugax. In: Bernstein EF, ed. *Amaurosis fugax.* New York: Springer-Verlag; 1987: pp 24–42.

31. Bogousslavsky J, Regli F, Zografos L, Uske A. Opticocerebral syndrome: simultaneous hemodynamic infarction of optic nerve and brain. *Neurology.* 1987;37:263–268.

32. Rivkin MJ, Hedges TR, Logigian E. Carotid dissection presenting as posterior ischemic optic neuropathy. *Neurology.* 1990;40:1469.

33. Caplan LR. Transient ischemia and brain and ocular infarction. In: Albert DM, Jakobiec FA, eds. *Principles and Practice of Ophthalmology.* Vol 4. Philadelphia: WB Saunders; 1994:2653–2655.

34. Newman NJ. Evaluating the patient with transient monocular vision loss: the young versus the elderly. *Ophthalmol Clin North Am.* 1996;9(3):455–466.

35. Kline LB. The natural history of patients with amaurosis fugax. *Ophthalmol Clin North Am.* 1996; 9(3):351–357.

36. O'Sullivan FO, Rossor M, Elsten JS. Amaurosis fugax in young people. *Br J Ophthalmol.* 1992;76: 660–662.

37. Poole CMJ, Ross-Russell RW, Harrison P. Amaurosis fugax under the age of 40 years. *J Neurol Neurosurg Psychiatry.* 1987;50:81–84.

38. North American Symptomatic Carotid Endarterectomy Trial Collaborators. Beneficial effect

of carotid endarterectomy in symptomatic patients with high-grade carotid stenosis. *N Engl J Med.* 1991;325:445–453.

39. Haynes RB, Taylor DW, Sackett DI, Thorpe K, Ferguson GG, Barnett HJ. Prevention of functional impairment by endarterectomy for symptomatic high-grade carotid stenosis. *JAMA.* 1994;271:1256–1259.

40. Barnett HJ, Taylor DW, Eliasziw M, Fox AJ, Ferguson GG, Haynes RB. Benefit of carotid endarterectomy in patients with symptomatic moderate or severe stenosis. *N Engl J Med.* 1998;339: 1415–1425.

41. European Carotid Surgery Trialists Collaborative Group. European Carotid Surgery Trial: interim results for symptomatic patients with severe (70–99%) or with mild (0–29%) carotid stenosis. *Lancet.* 1991;337:1235–1243.

42. Streifler JY, Eliasziw M, Benavente OR, et al. The risk of stroke in patients with first-ever retinal vs hemispheric transient ischemic attacks and high-grade carotid stenosis. *Arch Neurol.* 1995;52:246–249.

43. Trobe JD. Carotid endarterectomy: who needs it? *Ophthalmology.* 1987;94:725–730.

44. Trobe JD. Who needs carotid endarterectomy (circa 1996)? *Ophthalmol Clin North Am.* 1996;9(3): 513–519.

45. Tu JV, Hannan EL, Anderson GM, et al. The fall and rise of carotid endarterectomy in the United States and Canada. *N Engl J Med.* 1998;339:1441–1447.

46. Easton JD, Wilterdink JL. Carotid endarterectomy: trials and tribulations. *Ann Neurol.* 1994;35:5–17.

47. Hupp SL, Kline LB, Corbett JJ. Visual disturbances of migraine. *Surv Ophthalmol.* 1989;33:221–236.

48. Hoyt WF. Some neuro-ophthalmic considerations in cerebral vascular insufficiency. *Arch Ophthalmol.* 1959;62:260–272.

49. Hoyt WF. Transient bilateral blurring of vision: considerations of an episodic ischemic symptom of vertebro-basilar insufficiency. *Arch Ophthalmol.* 1963;70:746–751.

50. Williams D, Wilson TG. The diagnosis of the major and minor syndromes of basilar insufficiency. *Brain.* 1962;85:741–774.

51. Minor RH, Kearns TP, Millikan CH, Siekert RG, Sayre GP. Ocular manifestations of occlusive disease of the vertebro-basilar arterial system. *Arch Ophthalmol.* 1959;62:112–124.

52. Fisher CM. The posterior cerebral artery syndrome. *Can J Neurol Sci.* 1986;13:232–239.

53. Fisher CM. Concerning recurrent transient cerebral ischemic attacks. *Can Med Ass J.* 1962;86: 1091–1099.

54. Joseph JM, Louis S. Transient ictal cortical blindness during middle age: a case report and review of the literature. *J Neuro-ophthalmol.* 1995;15:39–42.

55. Engel JL. *Seizures and Epilepsy.* Philadelphia: FA Davis; 1989:146.

56. Kosnik E, Paulson GW, Laguna JF. Post-ictal blindness. *Neurology.* 1976;26:248–250.

57. Jaffe SJ, Roach ES. Transient cortical blindness with occipital lobe epilepsy. *J Clin Neuro-ophthalmol.* 1988;8:221–224.

58. Zung A, Margalith D. Ictal cortical blindness: a case report and review of the literature. *Dev Med Child Neurol.* 1993;35:921–926.

59. Sadeh M, Goldhammer Y, Kuritsky A. Postictal blindness in adults. *J Neurol Neurosurg Psychiatry.* 1983;46:566–569.

60. Barry E, Sussman NM, Bosley TM, Harner RN. Ictal blindness and status epilepticus amauroticus. *Epilepsia.* 1985;26:577–584.

61. Barnet AB, Manson JI, Wilner E. Acute cerebral blindness in childhood. *Neurology.* 1970;20:1147–1156.

62. Roos KL, Tuite PJ, Below ME, Pascuzzi RM. Reversible cortical blindness associated with bilateral occipital EEG abnormalities. *Clin Electroencephalogr.* 1990;21:104–109.

63. Fisher CM. Late-life migraine accompaniments as a cause of unexplained transient ischemic attacks. *Can J Neurol Sci.* 1980;7:9–17.

64. O'Connor PJ. Acephalgic migraine. *Ophthalmology.* 1981;88:999–1003.

65. Hachinski VC, Porchawka J, Steele JC. Visual symptoms in the migraine syndrome. *Neurology.* 1973; 23:570–579.

66. Dennis MS, Sandercock PAG, Bamford JM, Warlow CP. Lone bilateral blindness: a transient ischaemic attack. *Lancet.* 1989;1:185–189.

67. Pessin MS, Lathi ES, Cohen MB, Kwan ES, Hedges TR, Caplan LR. Clinical features and mechanism of occipital infarction. *Ann Neurol.* 1987;21:290–299.

68. Russell WR, Whitty WM. Studies in traumatic epilepsy: 3. Visual fits. *J Neurol Neurosurg Psychiatry.* 1955;18:79–96.

69. Ross-Russell RW, Page NGR. Critical perfusion of brain and retina. *Brain.* 1983;106:419–434.

70. Ernest JT. Choroidal circulation. In: Ryan SJ, ed. *Retina.* Vol 1. St. Louis: Mosby; 1994.

71. Burde RM. Amaurosis fugax: an overview. *J Clin Neuro-ophthalmol.*

72. Young LH, Appen RE. Ischemic oculopathy: a manifestation of carotid artery disease. *Arch Neurol.* 1981;38:358–360.

73. Carter JE. Chronic ocular ischemia and carotid vascular disease. *Stroke.* 1985;16:721–728.

74. Furlan AJ, Whisnant JP, Kearns TP. Unilateral visual loss in bright light: an unusual symptom of carotid artery occlusive disease. *Arch Neurol.* 1979; 36:675–676.

75. Wiebers DO, Swanson JW, Cascino TL, Whisnant JP. Bilateral loss of vision in bright light. *Stroke.* 1989;20:554–558.

76. Glaser JS, Savino PJ, Sumers KD, McDonald SA, Knighton RW. The photostress recovery test: a practical adjunct in the clinical assessment of visual function. *Am J Ophthalmol.* 1977;83:255–260.

77. Heckenlively JR, Arden GB. *Principles and Practice of Clinical Electrophysiology of Vision.* St. Louis: Mosby-Yearbook; 1991.

78. Krill AE, Deutman AF, Fishman G. The cone degenerations. *Doc Ophthalmol.* 1973;35:1–80.

79. Rowe SE, Trobe JD, Sieving PA. Idiopathic photoreceptor dysfunction causes unexplained visual acuity loss in later adulthood. *Ophthalmology.* 1990; 97:1632–1637.

80. Glaser JS. *Neuro-ophthalmology.* 2nd ed. Philadelphia: Lippincott; 1990:18–20.
81. Wray SH. Optic neuritis. In: Albert DM, Jakobiec FA, eds. *Principles and Practice of Ophthalmology.* Vol 4. Philadelphia: WB Saunders; 1994:2541.
82. Fleishman JA, Beck RW, Linares OA, Klein JW. Deficits in visual function after resolution of optic neuritis. *Ophthalmology.* 1987;94:1029–1035.
83. Scholl GB, Song H-S, Wray SH. Uhthoff's symptom in optic neuritis: relationship to magnetic resonance imaging and development of multiple sclerosis. *Ann Neurol.* 1991;30:180–184.
84. Perkin GD, Rose FC. Uhthoff's syndrome. *Br J Ophthalmol.* 1976;60:60–63.
85. McAlpine D, Compston ND, Lumsden CE. *Multiple Sclerosis.* Edinburgh: Churchill Livingstone; 1955.
86. Lepore FE. Uhthoff's symptom in disorders of the anterior visual pathways. *Neurology.* 1994;44:1036–1038.
87. Newman NJ. Leber's hereditary optic neuropathy: new genetic considerations. *Arch Neurol.* 1993;50:540–548.
88. Orcutt JC, Tucker WM, Mills RP, Smith CH. Gaze-evoked amaurosis. *Ophthalmology.* 1987;94:213–218.
89. Manor RS, Ben Sira I. Amaurosis fugax at downward gaze. *Surv Ophthalmol.* 1987;31:411–416.
90. Pascual J, Combarros O, Berciano J. Gaze-evoked amaurosis in pseudotumor cerebri. *Neurology.* 1988;38:1654–1655.
91. Leigh RJ. Management of oscillopsia. In: Barber HO, Sharpe JA, eds. *Vestibular Disorders.* Chicago: Yearbook Medical Publishers; 1988:201–212.
92. JC. Living without a balancing mechanism. *N Engl J Med.* 1952;246:246–247.
93. Demer JL, Honrubia V, Baloh RW. Dynamic visual acuity: a test for oscillopsia and vestibulo-ocular reflex function. *Am J Otol.* 1994;15:340–342.
94. Griffith JF, Dodge PR. Transient blindness following head injury in children. *N Engl J Med.* 1968;278:648–651.
95. Greenblatt SH. Posttraumatic transient cerebral blindness: association with migraine and seizure diatheses. *JAMA.* 1973;225:1073–1076.
96. Hochstetler K, Beals RD. Transient cortical blindness in a child. *Ann Emerg Med.* 1987;16:218–219.
97. Matthews WB. Footballer's migraine. *Br Med J.* 1972;2:326–327.
98. Stoddard WE, Davis DO, Young SW. Cortical blindness after cerebral angiography: case report. *J Neurosurg.* 1981;54:240–244.
99. Lantos G. Cortical blindness due to osmotic disruption of the blood-brain barrier by angiographic contrast material: CT and MRI studies. *Neurology.* 1989;39:567–571.
100. Dinsdale HB. Hypertensive encephalopathy. In: Barnett HJM, Mohr JP, Stein BM, Yatsu FM, eds. *Stroke. Pathophysiology, Diagnosis, and Management.* Vol 2. New York: Churchill Livingstone; 1986:869–874.
101. Schwartz RB, Jones KM, Kalina P, et al. Hypertensive encephalopathy: findings on CT, MR imaging, and SPECT imaging in 14 cases. *Am J Roentgenol.* 1992;159:379–383.
102. Nag S, Robertson DM, Dinsdale HB. Cerebral cortical changes in acute experimental hypertension: an ultrastructural study. *Lab Invest.* 1977;36:150–161.
103. Beausanglinder M, Bill A. Cerebral circulation in acute arterial hypertension—protective effects of sympathetic nervous activity. *Acta Physiol Scand.* 1981;111:193–199.
104. Edvinsson L, Owman C, Sjoberg N. Autonomic nerves, mast cells, and amine receptors in human brain vessel: a histochemical and pharmacological study. *Brain Res.* 1976;115:377–393.

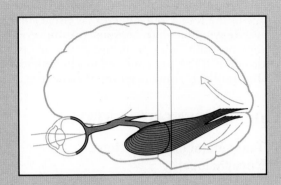

Chapter 4

POSITIVE SYMPTOMS OF RETINOCORTICAL DISORDERS

Positive visual phenomena—illusions and hallucinations—arise from deafferentation states or direct damage to the retinocortical pathway.

ILLUSIONS AND HALLUCINATIONS

The positive symptoms of retinocortical visual pathway disorders are vivid and often frightening illusions and hallucinations. Visual *illusions* are distortions of objects in current view. By contrast, visual *hallucinations* are images generated by endogenous neural activity unrelated to external stimuli. Hallucinations may be unformed, consisting of flashes, flickers (phosphenes) and geometric figures (photopsias, scintillations); or formed, consisting of animate figures and scenes.[1] These positive visual phenomena are generated by conditions which inhibit signal transmission to vision-related cortex (see "Deafferentation States," below)[2] or by direct damage to the visual pathway.

Deafferentation states include toxic-metabolic-infectious encephalopathy, psychosis, dementia, sleep disorders, trancelike states, and blindness, which interfere with signals destined for the visual cortex and allow the emergence into consciousness of endogenous visual activity resulting in hallucinations.[2] Visual hallucinations in these states may have a common pathogenesis: a relative excess of serotonergic input or a relative deficiency of cholinergic input to the lateral geniculate body, which inhibits its ability to transmit visual information to parietal and temporal vision-related cortex.[3] This leads to a release of stored visual memories from those cortical regions (release hallucinations or deafferentation hallucinations).

Positive visual phenomena may also arise from direct damage to the retina, optic nerve, primary visual cortex, or parietal and temporal vision-related cortex. Damage to the middle portions of the visual pathway—the optic chiasm, tracts, and radiations—tends not to create positive visual phenomena unless the patient becomes blind (see "Blindness," below).

The first step in evaluating patients who report visual illusions or hallucinations, then, is to determine if the visual symptoms involve the entire visual field, or if they are confined to the field of one eye or to one hemifield (Fig. 4-1). If visual symptoms involve the entire visual field of both eyes, one should rule out a deafferentation state. If no deafferentation state is present, binocular visual symptoms could arise from direct damage to the retina, optic nerves, or visual cortex. If symptoms are confined to one eye, they probably come from the retina or optic nerve. If they are confined to a hemifield, they probably come from the visual cortex.

DEAFFERENTATION STATES

Toxic-Metabolic-Infectious Encephalopathy

Visual illusions or hallucinations may be a leading or isolated manifestation of a metabolically or pharmacologically induced disorder of consciousness, a delirium.[4] Medications most often implicated are those with anticholinergic, serotonergic, and dopaminergic properties (Table 4-1). Among hallucinogenic street drugs, mescaline, psilocybin, lysergic acid, and amphetamines are most frequently implicated. Withdrawal from habitual use of some of these agents,

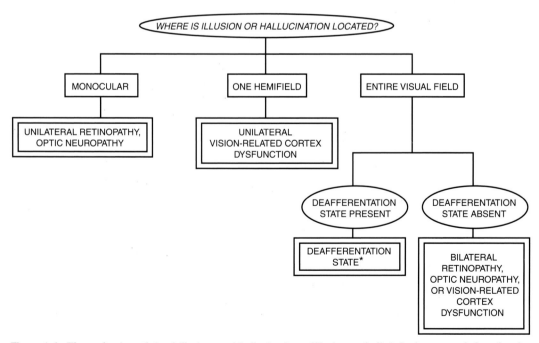

Figure 4–1. The evaluation of visual illusions and hallucinations. *Toxic-metabolic-infectious encephalopathy, dementia, psychosis, sleep disorder, trance-like state, blindness.

Table 4–1. **Psychoactive Agents That Cause Visual Illusions and Hallucinations**

Dopaminergics	*Miscellaneous*
Levodopa	Histamine H_2 receptor antagonists
Selegiline	Narcotic analgesics
Bromocriptine	Antineoplastic agents
Methyldopa	**Cyclosporine**
	Nonsteroidal anti-inflammatory agents
	Calcium channel blockers
	Antifungal agents
	Antiarrhythmics
	Salicylates
Serotonergics	**Intrathecal contrast agents**
Amitriptyline	Benzodiazepines
Nortriptyline	**Anticonvulsants**
Doxepin	**Corticosteroids**
Imipramine	Antibacterial agents
Trazodone	Antiviral agents
Fluoxetine	Nitrates
Sertraline	Methysergide
Beta-Adrenergic Blockers	*Illicit Drugs*
Propranolol	**Amphetamines**
Betaxolol	**Lysergic acid**
Atenolol	**Cocaine**
Timolol	**Mescaline**
	Psilocybin
Adrenergics	
Phenylephrine	
Theophylline	
Pseudoephedrine	
Albuterol	

Common offenders are in boldface type.

Source: Adapted from *The Medical Letter on Drugs and Therapeutics*, Vol. 31, Issue 808, 1989; and Cummings, 1985.[5]

and alcohol, may cause prominent visual hallucinations, often of animals (zoopsia).[5,6]

Dementia

Visual illusions and hallucinations are a common feature of advanced dementia, together with verbal outbursts and paranoid ideation.[7] The hallucinations are usually formed, often reminiscent of earlier life experiences, and sometimes paranoid. They are exacerbated when patients are left alone in darkened rooms, or treated with psychoactive medications ("sundowning"). Visual hallucinations are particularly prominent in patients with diffuse Lewy body dementia[8] and in patients

with Parkinson's disease treated with dopaminergic agents.[9]

Psychosis

The visual hallucinations of psychosis are distinctive in being complex, delusional, and paranoid. They are often integrated with auditory hallucinations.[4,10]

Sleep Disorders

Visual hallucinations occur commonly just before sleep (hypnagogic hallucinations) or upon emergence from sleep (hypnopompic hallucinations). They are also a prominent feature of narcolepsy. Vivid animate hallucinations associated with a sleeplike state may also arise from lesions of the midbrain (peduncular hallucinosis).[11–13] Inasmuch as sleep–wake cycle disturbances are always present, the supposition is that these hallucinations represent dream intrusions generated by a damaged reticular activating system.

Trance-like States

Visual illusions and hallucinations are often reported during hypnosis, intense emotional stress, and religious ritual.[14] The fertile imagination of children quite normally gives rise to fantasies of imaginary playmates they regard as real.

Blindness

Blindness creates a global deafferentation state that generates florid visual hallucinations. It typically occurs in patients aged over 60 years who have 20/200 or worse visual acuity in the better eye. They describe detailed and graphic figments that are usually pleasant ("Charles Bonnet syndrome").[15–18] This phenomenon is more likely to occur against a background of dementia, *but can also occur in patients who have normal cognition.* Patients are usually aware that their "visions" are not real, but if the hallucinations are

bothersome, dopamine antagonists (haloperidol, clozapine, risperidone) may be effective in reducing their frequency.

VISUAL PATHWAY LESIONS

Retina

Visual illusions of retinal origin typically derive from deformation of photoreceptors in the fovea. Hallucinations are caused by lesions of photoreceptors, and, less often, of retinal ganglion cells (Table 4-2).

FOVEAL EDEMA OR SCARRING

When one eye sees an object as warped or distorted (metamorphopsia), the cause is likely to be deformation of foveal retinal photoreceptors by edema or scarring (Fig. 4-2). Foveal edema typically also causes micropsia because cones are spread apart by the fluid. A retina image therefore activates fewer cones than it would if the cones were arrayed normally. Foveal scarring or tugging by an epiretinal membrane usually causes macropsia because cones are dragged into a tighter array (Chapter 11).

VITREORETINAL TUG

Episodic white lightning bolts in the peripheral temporal field are caused by a degenerating vitreous that tugs on retinal photoreceptors. As the vitreous ages, it develops

Table 4–2. **Monocular Visual Illusions and Hallucinations**

Symptom	Causes
Warped vision (metamorphopsia), minified or magnified image	Foveal edema or scarring
Episodic flashes in peripheral field	Vitreous tug on retina
Episodic full-field flickers induced by assuming upright posture	Reduced ocular perfusion
Persistent full-field flickers	Photoreceptor degeneration, inflammation, or infarction
Episodic burst of light induced by loud sound or eye movement	Optic nerve demyelination
Illusion that object swinging in a linear trajectory is moving in an oval trajectory (Pulfrich stereo-illusion)	Optic nerve demyelination

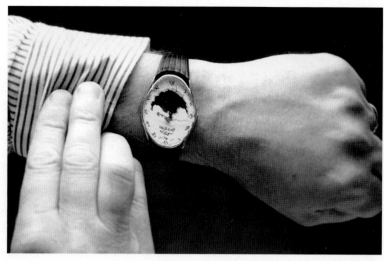

Figure 4–2. Retinal metamorphopsia. The image at fixation appears distorted, sometimes smaller. It is due to edema or scarring of foveal photoreceptors. (Reprinted with permission from Burde RM, Savino PJ, Trobe JD. Clinical Decisions in Neuro-ophthalmology, 2nd Ed. Mosby-Yearbook, St. Louis, 1992.)

pockets of fluid that render it unstable (Chapter 11). Its peripheral attachments to the retinal surface come under increased tension. With quick eye movements, the vitreous sloshes about, pulls at the peripheral retina, and discharges a colony of photoreceptors. If the contracting vitreous severs its circular attachment to the optic disk, the patient will see a black ring or a weblike floater, which is a vitreous condensate that blocks light transmission to the retina. Vitreous detachment occurs most commonly after age 60, but it may also happen earlier as a consequence of myopia, intraocular inflammation, trauma, surgery, or bleeding. In the process of detaching, the vitreous can tear a piece of retina and generate a full-blown retinal detachment—a surgical emergency.

OCULAR HYPOPERFUSION

Episodic flickering lights evoked or exacerbated by assuming the upright posture suggests widespread ischemic irritation of the photoreceptors or retinal ganglion cells caused by severe ipsilateral anterior circulation hypoperfusion.[19] Impending or subtotal retinal arterial and venous infarction may cause transient flickering in one eye that reflects ischemic damage to retinal ganglion cells. If ophthalmoscopy is unrevealing in these cases, orbital Doppler imaging is likely to reveal low ophthalmic artery flow.[19a]

DIFFUSE PHOTORECEPTOR DYSFUNCTION

Persistent binocular flickers that fill the visual field "like snow on a television screen" are usually caused by aberrant firing of sick photoreceptors. Advanced heredodegenerative disorders (retinitis pigmentosa) are usually responsible for this hallucination, but it may also occur in inflammatory, infarctive, and paraneoplastic chorioretinopathies[20,21] and in digitalis[22–25] and clomiphene[26] toxicity (Chapter 11). Among toxic agents, digitalis is distinctive in causing a yellowish green tinge (xanthopsia) or frosting of vision, a reflection of retinal photoreceptor damage.[22–25] Visual acuity and color vision may be impaired as well, but deficits tend to be mild in relation to complaints, which usually rapidly disappear upon normalization of digitalis blood levels. Clomiphene citrate, an ovulatory agent, causes shimmery vision with prolonged afterimages.[26] Persistent monocular full-field flickering is predictive of photoreceptor degeneration, inflammation, or infarction (Chapters 10, 11).[20]

Optic Nerve

Damage to the optic nerve usually causes a visual deficit, but hallucinations may also occur (Table 4-2).

SPONTANEOUS, SOUND-INDUCED, AND EYE MOVEMENT–INDUCED PHOTOPSIAS

A demyelinated optic nerve can set off brief flashes spontaneously, after a loud sound, or with an eye movement. A sudden unanticipated loud sound (cough, dog barking, car door closing) may induce a burst of light (visual-auditory synesthesia).[27–29] This hallucination appears most often when sound breaks a tranquil state such as reading or falling asleep.

The same hallucination can be triggered by rapid horizontal eye motion in a dark room or with eyes closed.[30] This symptom has been likened to Lhermitte's phenomenon of lightning paresthesias evoked by neck flexion. The mechanism is probably a lowered threshold for the development of action potentials in demyelinated optic nerve segments.

PULFRICH STEREO-ILLUSION

Any optic neuropathy that affects the two nerves asymmetrically may create an intriguing illusion in which patients complain that they cannot accurate judge the position of moving objects. Called the "Pulfrich stereo-illusion",[31] it results from unequal conduction rates in the two optic nerves. If shown a pendulum swinging in a plane, patients will incorrectly describe its arc as an ellipse (counterclockwise rotation if the right optic nerve is lesioned, clockwise rotation if the left optic nerve is lesioned) (Fig. 4-3). A neutral density filter placed in front of the unaffected eye may dramatically relieve this symptom.[32]

Visual Cortex

Lesions in primary or vision-related cortex are the source of most binocular visual illusions and hallucinations in patients who do not have deafferentation states (Tables 4-3, 4-4). Illusions are believed to derive from aberrant visual processing. Hallucinations have two pathogenetic mechanisms: (*1*) migrainous or epileptic cortical activation, or (*2*) disinhibition of vision-related parietal and temporal visual cortex by primary visual cortex injury.[3]

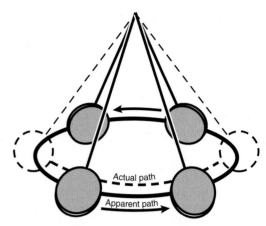

Figure 4–3. The Pulfrich stereo-illusion. Shown a pendulum swinging in a plane, patients will incorrectly describe its arc as an ellipse (counterclockwise rotation if the right optic nerve is lesioned, clockwise rotation if the left optic nerve is lesioned). Any optic neuropathy that affects the two nerves asymmetrically may create this illusion, which results from unequal conduction rates in the two optic nerves. Patients complain that they cannot accurately judge the position of moving objects. (Reprinted with permission from Burde RM, Savino PJ, Trobe JD. Clinical Decisions in Neuro-ophthalmology, 2nd Ed. Mosby-Yearbook, St. Louis, 1992.)

The following binocular illusions are most frequently reported (Table 4-3).

ALTERED SIZE AND SHAPE

Objects appear larger (macropsia) or smaller (micropsia), closer (pelopsia) or farther away (teleopsia) than they really are. In other cases, they seem elongated and warped (cerebral metamorphopsia) (Fig. 4-4). Prominent elongation in a single plane has been called "illusory spread,"[33] a type of visual perseveration in space.[34] Illusory spread produces grotesque images of heads growing from shoulders and gigantic fingers arising from elbows.

INAPPROPRIATE MOTION

Stationary objects may appear to be moving and moving objects to be stationary. Stationary objects seem to oscillate or jump from one place to another. Moving objects seem to have a luminous trail as they trace a path,[35] or to be made up of a sequence of snapshots ("cerebral polyopia for moving objects") (Fig. 4-5).[36] They may strike the viewer as moving too quickly or too slowly, or even to be frozen in space.[37]

Table 4–3. **Binocular Visual Illusions**

Type of Illusion	Features
Size and shape	Objects appear larger, smaller, closer, farther away Objects appear warped, elongated (illusory spread) (Fig. 4-3)
Motion	Stationary objects appear to be moving, shimmering, jumping, oscillating, moving too quickly or too slowly Moving objects appear broken up into snapshots (polyopia for moving objects) (Fig. 4-4)
Position	Objects appear displaced into opposite hemifield (visual allesthesia) Objects appear reduplicated (polyopia for stationary objects) (Fig. 4-5)
Perseveration	Recently viewed objects are superimposed on currently viewed objects (palinopsia) (Fig. 4-6)

DISPLACEMENT

An object in one hemifield may appear at times to be in the opposite hemifield, a phenomenon called *visual allesthesia*.[38] This displacement can occur from a partially defective hemifield into an intact field, or vice versa. The experience lasts from seconds to hours. Right-sided lesions predominate.

If the inciting visual stimulus is still within view in the intact hemifield, patients will see the same image at two different points in space—straight ahead and on the side of the hemianopia (Fig. 4-6). This symptom, called "cerebral polyopia for stationary objects," must be differentiated from the far more common cause of diplopia, namely misalignment of the eyes. The distinguishing features of cerebral diplopia are the presence of hemianopia and the fact that the double vision does not disappear if either eye is closed.

Sometimes cerebral polyopia for stationary objects occurs within an episode of reduced awareness and tonic-clonic movements. In such cases, a focal discharge on the electroencephalogram often signifies partial seizures, for which antiepileptic medications may be effective.[38]

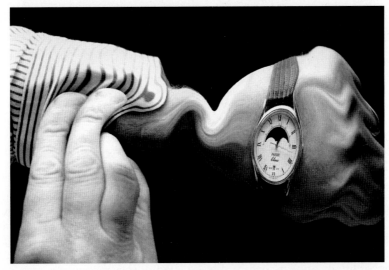

Figure 4–4. Cerebral metamorphopsia. Unlike retinal metamorphopsia, the distortion is not confined to fixation and may be grotesque. (Reprinted with permission from Burde RM, Savino PJ, Trobe JD. Clinical Decisions in Neuro-ophthalmology, 2nd Ed. Mosby-Yearbook, St. Louis, 1992.)

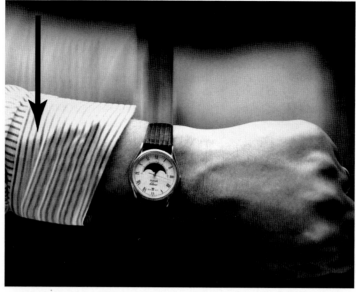

a

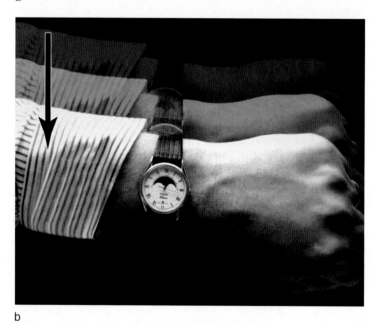

b

Figure 4–5. Cerebral polyopia for moving objects. The viewer sees a faint trail like a comet tail in the wake a moving object (*a*) or a series of faint snapshots of the object (*b*).

PERSEVERATION

An object that was recently seen—usually within the past few minutes—but is no longer in view suddenly appears before the patient (visual perseveration, palinopsia, palinopia, paliopia) (Fig. 4-7).[34,39–43] The palinopsic image is often curiously appro-

priate to the currently viewed scene, an example being a recently seen beard or hat that becomes affixed to the heads of persons now in front of the patient.

Palinopsia symbolizes the crossover between a visual illusion and a hallucination. By definition, it is a hallucination because the stimulus is no longer in view. But it re-

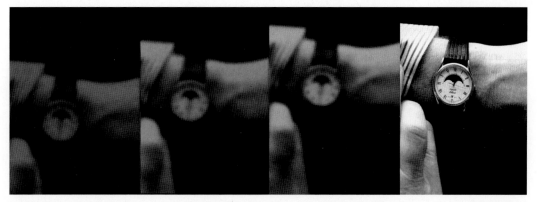

Figure 4–6. Cerebral polyopia for stationary objects. The viewer sees a faint duplicate image in, or on the edge of, a defective hemifield.

sembles an illusion in being based on an exogenous stimulus. Localization is primarily to the right inferior occipitotemporal cortex.[39]

Cortical visual hallucinations are divided into those that are unformed and those that are formed.

UNFORMED HALLUCINATIONS

These consist of stationary or moving, flickering or still, colored or white, linear, circular, or zigzag images. They consistently originate in primary visual cortex and are often confined to a hemifield. There are four common causes: migraine, vertebrobasilar TIAs, seizures, and occipital lobe lesions causing local deafferentation (Table 4-4).

Migraine

The visual aura of migraine accounts for most episodes of binocular unformed visual hallucinations, not only in youth but also in the elderly.[44] The pathogenesis of migraine auras is unknown, but they are nonepileptic excitations of cortex. Among the estimated 20% of migraineurs who have auras, the most common is visual.[45] Nearly every conceivable pattern has been described, but the

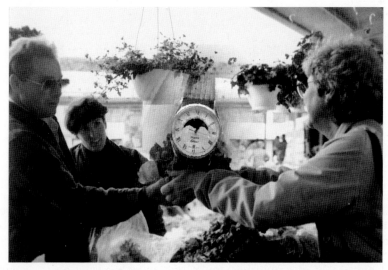

Figure 4–7. Palinopsia. The recently viewed watch becomes superimposed on the currently viewed market scene. This is a visual perseveration. (Reprinted with permission from Burde RM, Savino PJ, Trobe JD. Clinical Decisions in Neuro-ophthalmology, 2nd Ed. Mosby-Yearbook, St. Louis, 1992.)

Table 4–4. **Binocular Visual Hallucinations: Differential Diagnosis**

Manifestation	Migraine	Vertebrobasilar TIA	Seizure	Occipital Lobe Lesion
20–30 minute duration of visual symptoms	Common	Uncommon (usually last only seconds)	Uncommon	Uncommon (may last seconds to hours)
Migration (march) of visual symptoms	Common	Never	Uncommon	Uncommon
Fortification scotoma	Common	Rare	Rare	Uncommon
Formed images	Uncommon	Uncommon	Common	Common*
Headache	Common (but may be absents)	Uncommon	Uncommon	Uncommon
Paresthesias follow visual symptoms	Common	Rare	Uncommon	Rare
Nonvisual symptoms of brainstem dysfunction	Rare	Common	Never	Never
Persistent homonymous hemianopia	Never	Never*	Common	Common
Automatisms	Never	Never	Common	Never
Eye deviation	Never	Never	Common	Never
Loss of consciousness	Never	Uncommon	Common	Uncommon

*Unless infarct has occurred.

"scintillating scotoma," a twinkling zigzag pattern, accounts for about 30%.[44] Likened to the outline of a medieval fortress, the zigzag pattern has also been called a "fortification" or a "teichopsia," from the Greek word teichos, meaning city wall.[46] Its evanescent quality has given rise to the term "fortification spectrum," as in spectral, or ghostlike (Fig. 4-8).

The scintillating scotoma (zigzag, fortification spectrum) is reported very rarely in patients with vertebrobasilar TIA,[47] and uncommonly during posterior hemispheric surface electrode stimulation[48] or electrographically documented spontaneous seizures.[49,50]

Another feature that distinguishes migraine from vertebrobasilar TIA and seizure is a scotoma that traverses the hemifield.

Among patients who have visual auras, an estimated 25% report a 20–40 minute march (migration, expansion, spread, buildup) across the hemifield.[44] This march has never been documented during an electrographic partial seizure. However, it has been documented in single case reports of patients who have occipital lobe lesions, particularly arteriovenous malformations (AVMs).[51–54] Among 70 patients with occipital lobe AVMs, "migrainelike visual phenomena" occurred in 15 (21%).[55] In two occipital AVM cases,[51,53] the migrainelike episodes disappeared after the AVM was excised. *The marching scotoma should be regarded a reaction pattern that occurs mostly as an idiopathic phenomenon in healthy brain and rarely in injured primary visual cortex.*

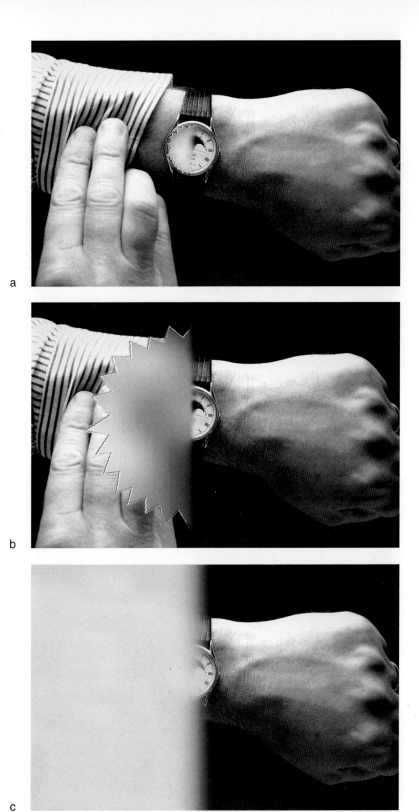

Figure 4–8. The scintillating scotoma of migraine. A small bright light germinates to one side of fixation (*a*) and enlarges (*b*) to occupy the entire hemifield in 20–30 minutes (*c*). Its leading edge has a zigzag ("fortification") pattern. This is the most common positive visual phenomenon in migraine, occurring in an estimated 30% of those who have visual auras. (Reprinted with permission from Burde RM, Savino PJ, Trobe JD. Clinical Decisions in Neuro-ophthalmology, 2nd Ed. Mosby-Yearbook, St. Louis, 1992.)

A less common feature that distinguishes migraine from vertebrobasilar TIA and seizure is the marching paresthesia. It has a time course similar to that of the marching scotoma and begins 5 to 30 minutes after the scotoma. Aphasia may follow. In vertebrobasilar TIA, by contrast, multiple neurologic manifestations typically occur at once; in patients with seizures, the manifestations generally follow each other with a much briefer latency.[44]

Vertebrobasilar Transient Ischemic Attacks

Visual hallucinations are an uncommon manifestation of vertebrobasilar TIAs.[47] In one series, they occurred in only 3%;[56] in another, they were the presenting symptoms in 10% of cases.[57] The hallucinations look like tadpoles, soapflakes, snowflakes, sparklers, pinwheels, or glowing lights. As in migraine, they may occupy the whole visual field or be restricted to a hemifield, depending on whether the hypoperfusion affects one or both posterior cerebral arteries.[47,58]

Although TIAs occasionally produce zigzag shapes, the visual disturbance does not traverse the visual field in the 20 to 30 minutes typical of migraine.[56] It usually lasts only seconds, but it may persist for hours if ischemia is intense. If it lingers beyond a few hours, one should expect to find a persistent homonymous visual field defect, imaging evidence of occipital infarction,[59,60] and sometimes electrographic seizures. After occipital infarction, the hallucinations usually regress within weeks, even as the field defect remains forever.

Distinguishing vertebrobasilar TIA from other causes of binocular positive visual phenomena depends largely on accompanying nonvisual features such as vertigo, disequilibrium, drop attack, diplopia, altered consciousness, nausea, and extremity weakness and numbness.[57] These symptoms are infrequent in patients with seizure and migraine, although there is a rare form of migraine primarily affecting adolescents that may also produce many of them.[61]

Seizures

The hallucinations of primary visual cortex seizures typically begin in one hemifield, but they may spread quickly into the entire field. Anatomic abnormalities are usually evident on brain imaging, and a homonymous hemianopia is nearly always present. The exception is benign childhood epilepsy with occipital paroxysms (CEOP), a self-limited condition affecting mostly preadolescent girls.[62,63]

The nature of visual hallucinations associated with epileptic excitation of primary visual cortex has been discovered by correlating patient descriptions with surface electrode stimulation[64–66] and EEGs recorded during seizures.[49,50,67] They consist of stationary lines, squares, stars, circles, disks, sparkling dots, and zigzags,[49] usually lasting longer than those caused by vertebrobasilar TIA. In contrast to migraine, there is no march and usually no zigzag scintillations. In a series of 20 patients with occipital epilepsy, no one described zigzags.[50]

Identifying seizures as a cause of visual hallucinations is strongly based on finding one or more nonvisual manifestations—nystagmus, frequent blinking or eyelid fluttering, staring or other automatisms, tonic-clonic movements, and eventual loss of consciousness. In one series of 25 patients with occipital lobe partial seizures,[68] eye deviation was present in 16 (64%) and repetitive blinking in 14 (56%).

Occipital Lobe Lesions

Visual hallucinations emanating from occipital lobe lesions (infarcts, dysplasias, inflammations, tumors) are not always manifestations of focal seizures. These lesions may block input to vision-related cortex (local deafferentation) and allow the emergence of endogenous visual activity as release phenomena (Table 4-5). In one large series of patients with occipital infarctions, EEGs failed to document any seizures.[1] But in other instances, seizures have been recorded during the visual spells.[50,69]

FORMED HALLUCINATIONS

These consist of images of animate objects or scenes. In the absence of deafferentation states (see above), they always originate in vision-related cortex. They may be manifes-

Table 4–5. Binocular Visual Hallucinations: Epileptic or Not?

Manifestation	Nonepileptic	Epileptic
Abrupt onset	No	Yes
Same type of hallucination in successive episodes	No	Yes
Eye deviation	No	Yes
Nystagmus	No	Yes
Automatisms	No	Yes
Clonic movements	No	Yes
Loss of consciousness	No	Yes
Reduced by anticonvulsants	No	Yes

tations of a partial seizure originating in temporal or parietal cortex, or of a lesion in primary visual cortex that cuts off input to temporal or parietal cortex and allows release of its endogenous visual activity.[70] *Migraine and vertebrobasilar TIA are so rarely the cause of formed hallucinations that they should not be seriously considered.*

Surface electrode stimulation of the cerebral cortex[64] shows that partial seizures originating in temporal cortex often cause a dreamlike (oneiric) state. The hallucinations evoke feelings of fear, pleasure, strangeness, or familiarity.[64,71] By comparison, partial seizures of parietal origin create formed hallucinations whose details are so vivid and realistic that patients temporarily believe that they are actually seeing them.[71,72] Seizure-associated formed hallucinations have an abrupt onset and generally do not remain confined to a single hemifield.

Supporting a nonepileptic mechanism for some formed visual hallucinations is a study of 13 posterior cerebral artery stroke patients.[1] It disclosed that visual hallucinations were consistently unassociated with electrographic seizures and developed only in those patients whose posterior hemispheric lesions spared vision-related parietal and temporal cortex. The inference is that these regions must be intact in order for patients to experience visual hallucinations. In general, there is a greater tendency for right than left posterior hemisphere lesions to evoke formed hallucinations.[73]

OCULAR MOTOR AND VESTIBULAR LESIONS

Visual illusions are not always the result of visual pathway dysfunction (Box 4-1). For example, the illusion of seeing a stationary object as moving or oscillating can result from either an ocular motor or a vestibular disorder.[74] If the illusion of movement occurs

---

Box 4–1

WHERE ARE THESE VISUAL ILLUSIONS COMING FROM?

Not all illusions come from lesions of the visual pathway. Here are three that result from vestibular or ocular motor system dysfunction.

1. Images oscillate with head still:

   Nystagmus

2. Images oscillate only with head or body movement:

   Vestibulo-ocular reflex (VOR) dysfunction*

3. One of two diplopic images appears tilted:

   Superior oblique palsy

4. Entire visual environment appears shifted 180 degrees—that is, upside down.

   Medullary ischemia[75–77]

*See Box 2-2.

with the head still, the patient should be investigated for nystagmus (oscillation of the eyes). If the sensation occurs only when the head is moving, one must consider failure of both vestibular end organs to provide stabilization of the eyes in space. Medullary ischemia of the vestibular pathway may create an illusion of rotation in which the patient reports that objects are turned 90 degrees or flipped 180 degrees (upside down).[75–77]

SUMMARY

The positive manifestations of retinocortical visual pathway disorders are illusions and hallucinations. Illusions are distortions of objects in current view; hallucinations are images generated by endogenous neural activity unrelated to external stimuli.

Positive visual phenomena arise out of deafferentation states or direct damage to the retinocortical pathway. The deafferentation states include toxic-metabolic-infectious encephalopathy, psychosis, dementia, sleep disorders or trancelike states, and blindness. They cause impairment in the processing of external stimuli that may give rise to distorted imagery or allow the emergence into consciousness of endogenous visual activity that results in hallucinations (release phenomena).

Monocular positive visual symptoms are generated in the retina or optic nerve. In the retina, they include the metamorphopsia of foveal photoreceptor deformation, peripheral flashes of vitreoretinal tug, orthostatic flickering of ocular hypoperfusion, and the twinkling of widespread photoreceptor dysfunction. In the optic nerve, they consist of spontaneous, sound- or eye movement–induced flashes, and the Pulfrich stereoillusion associated with demyelinization.

In the absence of deafferentation states, most binocular positive visual phenomena emanate from primary visual cortex or vision-related parietal or temporal cortex. Illusions are believed to derive from aberrant visual processing. Hallucinations have two pathogenetic mechanisms: (1) migrainous or epileptic cortical activation, or (2) disinhibition of vision-related parietal and temporal visual cortex by primary visual cortex injury. The four common causes are migraine, vertebrobasilar TIA, seizure, and posterior cerebral hemispheric lesion.

The common visual illusions are of altered size, shape, position, and motion of objects. Hallucinations may be unformed (flashes, sparkles, and geometric patterns) or formed (animate objects and scenes).

Two important visual illusions do not emanate from visual pathway lesions. The illusion of environmental tilt derives from medullary ischemia. The illusion of oscillating images derives from damage to either the ocular motor or vestibular system.

REFERENCES

1. Vaphiades MS, Celesia GG, Brigell MG. Positive spontaneous visual phenomena limited to the hemianopic field in lesions of central visual pathways. *Neurology.* 1996;47:408–417.
2. Cogan DG. Visual hallucinations as release phenomena. *Albrecht von Graefes Arch Klin Ophthalmol.* 1973;188:139–151.
3. Manford M, Andermann F. Complex visual hallucinations: clinical and neurobiological insights. *Brain.* 1998;121:1819–1840.
4. Asaad G, Shapiro B. Hallucinations: theoretical and clinical overview. *Am J Psychiatry.* 1986;43:1088–1097.
5. Cummings JL. *Clinical Neuropsychiatry.* Orlando, Fla: Grune & Stratton; 1985:221–233.
6. Critchley M. Neurological aspects of visual and auditory hallucinations. *Br Med J.* 1939;2:634–639.
7. Lerner AJ, Koss E, Patterson MB, et al. Concomitants of visual hallucinations in Alzheimer's disease. *Neurology.* 1994;44:523–527.
8. McShane R, Gedling K, Reading M, McDonald B, Esiri MM, Hope T. Prospective study of relations between cortical Lewy bodies, poor eyesight, and hallucinations in Alzheimer's disease. *J Neurol Neurosurg Psychiatry.* 1995;59:185–188.
9. Rondot R, deRecondo J, Coignet A, Ziegler M. Mental disorders in Parkinson's disease after treatment with L-DOPA. *Adv Neurol.* 1984;40:259–269.
10. Goodwin DW, Alderson P, Rosenthal R. Clinical significance of hallucinations in psychiatric disorders: a study of 116 hallucinatory patients. *Arch Gen Psychiatry.* 1971;24:76–80.
11. Dunn DW, Weisberg LA, Nadell J. Peduncular hallucinations caused by brainstem compression. *Neurology.* 1983;33:1360–1361.
12. McKee AC, Levine DN, Kowall NW, Richardson EP. Peduncular hallucinosis associated with isolated infarction of the substantia nigra pars reticulata. *Ann Neurol.* 1990;27:500–504.
13. Kolmel HW. Peduncular hallucinations. *J Neurol.* 1991;238:457–459.
14. Sarbin TR, Juhasz JB. The social context of hallucinations. In: Siegel RK, West LJ, eds. *Hallucinations: Behavior, Experience, and Theory.* New York: John Wiley & Sons; 1975.

15. Teunisse RJ, Zitman FG, Raes DC. Clinical evaluation of 14 patients with the Charles Bonnet syndrome (isolated visual hallucinations). *Compr Psychiatry*. 1994;35:70–75.
16. Schultz G, Melzack R. Visual hallucinations and mental state: a study of 14 Charles Bonnet syndrome hallucinators. *J Nerv Ment Dis*. 1993;181:639–643.
17. Damos J, Skelton M, Jenner FA. The Charles Bonnet syndrome in perspective. *Psychol Med*. 1982;12:251–257.
18. Teunisse RJ, Cruysberg JR, Hoefnagels WH, Verbeek AL, Zitman FG. Visual hallucinations in psychologically normal people: Charles Bonnet's syndrome. *Lancet*. 1996;347:794–797.
19. Hollenhorst RW. Effect of posture on retinal ischemia from temporal arteritis. *Trans Am Ophthalmol Soc*. 1967;65:94–104.
19a. Alm A. Retinal blood flow and different diagnostic procedures. *Ophthalmol Clin N Am*. 1998;11:491–503.
20. Volpe NJ, Rizzo JF III. Retinal disease in neuro-ophthalmology: paraneoplastic retinopathy and the big blind spot syndrome. *Sem Ophthalmol*. 1995;10:234–241.
21. Jacobson DM, Thirkill CE, Tipping SJ. A clinical triad to diagnose paraneoplastic retinopathy. *Ann Neurol*. 1990;28:162–165.
22. Weleber RG, Shults WT. Digoxin retinal toxicity; clinical and electrophysiologic evaluation of a cone dysfunction syndrome. *Arch Ophthalmol*. 1981;99:1568–1572.
23. Robertson DM, Hollenhorst RW, Callahan JA. Ocular manifestations of digitalis toxicity. *Arch Ophthalmol*. 1966;76:640–645.
24. Schneider T, Dahlheim P, Zrenner E. Experimental investigations of the ocular toxicity of cardiac glycosides in animals. *Fortschr Ophthalmol*. 1989;86:751–755.
25. Piltz JR, Wertenbaker C, Lance SE, et al. Digoxin toxicity: recognizing the varied visual presentations. *J Clin Neuro-ophthalmol*. 1993;13:275–280.
26. Purvin VA. Visual disturbance secondary to clomiphene citrate. *Arch Ophthalmol*. 1995;113:482–484.
27. Jacobs L, Karpik A, Bozian D, et al. Auditory-visual synesthesia: sound-induced photisms. *Arch Neurol*. 1981;38:211–216.
28. Lessell S, Cohen MM. Phosphenes induced by sound. *Neurology*. 1979;29:1524–1526.
29. Page NGR, Bolger JP, Sanders MD. Auditory evoked phosphenes in optic nerve disease. *J Neurol Neurosurg Psychiatry*. 1982;45:7–12.
30. Davis FA, Bergen D, Schauf C, McDonald I, Deutsch W. Movement phosphenes in optic neuritis: a new clinical sign. *Neurology*. 1976;26:1100–1104.
31. Sokol S. The Pulfrich stereo-illusion as an index of optic nerve dysfunction. *Surv Ophthalmol*. 1976;20:432–434.
32. Heron G, Dutton GN. The Pulfrich phenomenon and its alleviation with a neutral density filter. *Br J Ophthalmol*. 1989;73:1004–1008.
33. Critchley M. Types of visual perseveration: "paliopsia" and "illusory visual spread." *Brain*. 1951;74:267–299.
34. Meadows JC, Munro SSF. Palinopsia. *J Neurol Neurosurg Psychiatry*. 1977;40:5–8.
35. Critchley M. *The Parietal Lobes*. New York: Hafner; 1953.
36. Bender MD. Polyopia and monocular diplopia of cerebral origin. *Arch Neurol Psychiatry*. 1945;54:323–338.
37. Zihl J, Von Cramon D, Mai N. Selective disturbance of movement vision after bilateral brain damage. *Brain*. 1983;106:313–340.
38. Jacobs L. Visual allesthesia. *Neurology*. 1980;30:1059–1063.
39. Cummings JL, Syndulko K, Goldberg Z, Treiman DM. Palinopsia reconsidered. *Neurology*. 1982;32:444–447.
40. Michel EM, Troost BT. Palinopsia: cerebral localization with computed tomography. *Neurology*. 1980;30:887–889.
41. Kinsbourne M, Warrington EK. A study of visual perseveration. *J Neurol Neurosurg Psychiatry*. 1963;26:468–475.
42. Bender MB, Feldman M, Sobin AJ. Palinopsia. *Brain*. 1968;91:321–338.
43. Lessell S, Higher disorders of visual function: positive phenomena. Glaser JS, Smith JL, eds. *Neuro-ophthalmology*. Vol 8. St. Louis: Mosby; 1975:27–44.
44. Fisher CM. Late-life migraine accompaniments as a cause of unexplained transient ischemic attacks. *Can J Neurol Sci*. 1980;7:9–17.
45. Davidoff RA. *Migraine: Manifestations, Pathogenesis, and Management*. Philadelphia: FA Davis; 1995.
46. Plant GT. The fortification spectra of migraine. *Br Med J*. 1986;293:1613–1617.
47. Hoyt WF. Transient bilateral blurring of vision: considerations of an episodic ischemic symptom of vertebro-basilar insufficiency. *Arch Ophthalmol*. 1963;70:746–751.
48. Penfield W, Jasper H. *Epilepsy and the Functional Anatomy of the Human Brain*. Boston: Little Brown; 1954.
49. Ludwig BI, Ajmone-Marsan C. Clinical ictal patterns in epileptic patients with occipital electroencephalographic foci. *Neurology*. 1975;25:463–471.
50. Panayiotopoulos CP. Elementary visual hallucinations in migraine and epilepsy. *J Neurol Neurosurg Psychiatry*. 1994;57:1371–1374.
51. Troost BT, Mark LE, Maroon JC. Resolution of classic migraine after removal of an occipital lobe AVM. *Ann Neurol*. 1979;5:199–201.
52. Riaz G, Hennessey JJ. Meningeal lesions mimicking migraine. *Neuro-ophthalmology*. 1991;11:41–48.
53. Kattah JC, Luessenhop AJ. Resolution of classic migraine after removal of an occipital lobe AVM. *Ann Neurol*. 1980;7:93.
54. Weiskrantz L, Warrington EK, Sanders MD, Marshall J. Visual capacity in the hemianopic field following a restricted occipital ablation. *Brain*. 1974;97:709–728.
55. Kupersmith MJ, Vargas ME, Yashar A, et al. Occipital arteriovenous malformations: visual disturbances and presentation. *Neurology*. 1996;46:953–957.
56. Fisher CM. The posterior cerebral artery syndrome. *Can J Neurol Sci*. 1986;13:232–239.
57. Williams D, Wilson TG. The diagnosis of the major and minor syndromes of basilar insufficiency. *Brain*. 1962;85:741–774.
58. Minor RH, Kearns TP, Millikan CH, Siekert RG,

Sayre GP. Ocular manifestations of occlusive disease of the vertebro-basilar arterial system. *Arch Ophthalmol.* 1959;62:112–124.

59. Monteiro LR, Hoyt WF, Imes RK. Puerperal cerebral blindness. *Arch Neurol.* 1984;41:1300–1301.

60. Newman DS, Levine SR, Curtis VL, Welch KM. Migraine-like visual phenomena associated with cerebral venous thrombosis. *Headache.* 1989;29:82–85.

61. Bickerstaff ER. The basilar artery and the migraine-epilepsy syndrome. *Proc R Soc Med.* 1962;55:167–169.

62. Panayiotopoulos CP. Benign childhood epilepsy with occipital paroxysms: a 15-year prospective study. *Ann Neurol.* 1989;26:51–56.

63. Gastaut H, Zifkin BG. Benign epilepsy of childhood with occipital spike and wave complexes. In: Andermann F, Lugaresi E, eds. *Migraine and Epilepsy: An Overview.* Boston: Butterworths; 1987.

64. Penfield W, Perot P. The brain's record of auditory and visual experience. *Brain.* 1963;86:595–696.

65. Dobelle WH, Mladejorsky MG, Garvin JP. Artificial vision for the blind: electrical stimulation of visual cortex offers hope for functional prosthesis. *Science.* 1974;183:440–444.

66. Brindley GS, Lewin WS. The sensations produced by electrical stimulation of the visual cortex. *J Physiol.* 1968;196:479–493.

67. Engel JL. *Seizures and Epilepsy.* Philadelphia: FA Davis; 1989:146.

68. Williamson PD, Thadani VM, Darcey TM, Spencer DD, Spencer SS, Mattson RH. Occipital lobe epilepsy: clinical characteristics, seizure spread patterns, and results of surgery. *Ann Neurol.* 1992;31:3–13.

69. Lance JW, Smee RI. Partial seizures with visual disturbance treated by radiotherapy of cavernous hemangioma. *Ann Neurol.* 1989;26:782–785.

70. Anderson SW, Rizzo M. Hallucinations following occipital lobe damage: the pathological activation of visual representations. *J Clin Exp Neuropsychol.* 1994;16:651–663.

71. Hecaen H, Albert ML. *Human Neuropsychology.* New York: John Wiley & Sons; 1978:215–227.

72. Russell WR, Whitty WM. Studies in traumatic epilepsy: 3. Visual fits. *J Neurol Neurosurg Psychiatry.* 1955;18:79–96.

73. Kolmel HW. Complex visual hallucinations in the hemianopic field. *J Neurol Neurosurg Psychiatry.* 1985;48:29–38.

74. Leigh RJ. Management of oscillopsia. In: Barber HO, Sharpe JA, eds. *Vestibular Disorders.* Chicago: Yearbook Medical Publishers; 1988:201–212.

75. Steiner I, Shahin R, Melamed E. Acute "upside down" reversal of vision in transient vertebrobasilar ischemia. *Neurology.* 1987;37:1685–1686.

76. Charles N, Froment C, Rode G, et al. Vertigo and upside down vision due to an infarct in the territory of the medial branch of the posterior inferior cerebellar artery caused by dissection of a vertebral artery. *J Neurol Neurosurg Psychiatry.* 1992;55:188–189.

77. Horsten G. Wallenberg's syndrome. Part I. General symptomatology, with special reference to visual disturbances and imbalance. *Acta Neurol Scand.* 1974;50:434–446.

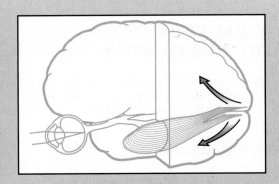

SYMPTOMS OF INTEGRATIVE VISUAL DISORDERS

Once the primary visual cortex has encoded visual signals into luminance, wavelength, and spatial features, this information must be converted into recognizable, meaningful percepts by means of two "extrastriate" integrative pathways (see Figs. 1-29 and 1-30).[1]

THE "WHERE" AND "WHAT" VISUAL INTEGRATIVE PATHWAYS

- The **occipitoparietal "where" pathway,** involving superior visual association, super-olateral temporal and inferior parietal cortex (Brodmann areas 19, 39, and 7), mediates *space* and *motion* perception.

- The **occipitotemporal "what" pathway,** involving inferior visual association (Brodmann area 19) and temporal cortex (Brodmann areas 20 and 37), mediates *form* and *color* perception.

As they exit the primary visual cortex, these two pathways are so close to one another that human lesions—even discrete ones—tend to cause a combination of deficits related to both pathways. In fact, lesions usu-

87

ally damage the primary visual cortex and posterior optic radiations as well, so that elementary (visual acuity and visual field) deficits are often mixed with integrative deficits. *Integrative visual deficits should never be blamed on elementary visual deficits unless the elementary deficits are very severe.* Thus a visual acuity as poor as 20/100 in the better eye and visual fields limited to a maximum diameter of 5 degrees are still compatible with normal scores on integrative vision tests, although patients may take slightly longer than those with normal elementary vision to complete the tests.[2–4] On the other hand, even the mildest integrative dysfunction may interfere with performance on visual acuity and visual field tests.

As the occipitoparietal and occipitotemporal pathways become more remote from primary visual cortex, they are sufficiently segregated so that lesions confined to either pathway generate distinctive constellations of symptoms and signs (Table 5-1). Visual acuity and visual field may well be intact. If so, patients may be misdiagnosed as having nonorganic causes for their visual integrative symptoms.

Visual integrative symptoms consist of difficulty judging distances, orientation, motion, reading, and identifying objects, faces, places, and colors (Chapters 16 and 17). Because memory and attentional deficits often cloud recall, patients may be unable to give a clear accounting of these complex symptoms. If the examiner is not skilled enough to elicit them, assessment will be flawed, since tests of integrative vision are not part of the standard examination repertoire of neurologists or ophthalmologists.

FAILED VISUAL SPATIAL AND ATTENTIONAL SKILLS

Symptoms linked to lesions of the occipitoparietal integrative pathway relate to spatial properties of viewed objects.

Spatial Attention

Patients with unilateral parietal (usually right-sided) lesions behave as if the contralateral half of their surroundings did not exist. They do not respond to visual, tactile, or auditory cues in that hemispace, and they may ignore that half of their body. Testing will disclose elements of hemispatial neglect.[5]

By contrast, patients with bilateral parietal lesions reach inaccurately for objects and have difficulty using kitchen and work implements, setting a table, putting on clothing, walking down stairs, or driving a car. Testing will indicate visual spatial deficits.[6,7]

Patients with these lesions may also state that objects pop in and out of sight and that they cannot interpret simple photographs in the newspaper or follow the story line on television.[8] Caregivers report that patients never seem to see more than one thing at a time. For example, if they are concentrating

Table 5–1. **Symptoms Associated with Integrative Pathway Lesions**

Occipitotemporal "What" Pathway	Occipitoparietal "Where" Pathway
Cannot recognize familiar faces*	Ignores stimuli from left hemispace and hemibody*
Cannot find way in familiar locales*	Cannot dress*
Cannot read[†]	Misreaches for objects[‡]
Cannot recognize objects by sight[†]	Cannot judge distances[‡]
Cannot name or recognize colors[†]	Cannot set table[‡]
	Cannot use household implements[‡]
	Cannot interpret pictures[‡]
	Objects disappear from view[‡]

*Unilateral (usually right-sided) hemispheric lesions.
[†]Unilateral (usually left-sided) or bilateral hemispheric lesions.
[‡]Bilateral hemispheric lesions.

on the meat on their plate, they do not see the potatoes nearby. Rather than being distractible, they seem "fixated" on one item at a time.

When multiple targets are displayed simultaneously before their eyes, these patients do not detect more than one at a time (Chapter 17). Asked to interpret scenes, they identify components but not how they relate to one another. This type of "spotlight" vision, called *simultanagnosia,* represents a failure to spread attention across an array of objects.[9]

Motion

Patients report that flowing water looks frozen and moving objects appear as snapshots at different points in space.[10,11] These spatial illusions are caused by bilateral damage to temporo–parieto–occipital junction.

FAILED RECOGNITION

Symptoms linked to lesions of the occipitotemporal "what" pathway are based on a failure to identify familiar items *by sight.* Lesions of the left hemisphere cause difficulty recognizing items strongly associated with language (words, objects), whereas lesions of the right hemisphere cause difficulty recognizing items weakly associated with language (faces, places).

Letters, Words, and Other Verbal Symbols

Patients complain of an acquired inability to read letters and words. If examination confirms an isolated reading disorder, it will be *pure alexia* (alexia without agraphia).[12–17] A complete right homonymous hemianopia is often present, but patients are rarely aware of it. There may be no other neurologic abnormalities.

The causative lesion, usually a posterior cerebral artery infarct, affects left optic radiations or primary visual cortex and left posterior corpus callosum (splenium) fibers. The alexia often lessens remarkably within weeks to months and may disappear completely; the field defect persists.

Objects

Patients report that they are unable to recognize common objects.[18] If they cannot name or describe the use of objects by sight, but can do so by touch, the diagnosis is visual object agnosia. This disorder results from extensive damage to posterior portions of both cerebral hemispheres, usually in hypoxic-ischemic events, but is rarely caused by tumors or demyelination.[8] Face agnosia (prosopagnosia, see below) and pure alexia often coexist.

Visual object agnosia is often incorrectly diagnosed when patients actually have an aphasia with prominent anomia. Anomia differs from agnosia in that patients can describe the use of viewed objects that they cannot name.

Faces

Patients report that they cannot recognize close friends and relatives. Those who suffer from this face agnosia (prosopagnosia) cannot even recognize themselves in a mirror and will get lost in familiar surroundings.[8,19–25]

On testing, they fail to recognize photographs of friends, relatives, and celebrities, provided they bear no facial characteristics that can be readily expressed in words, such as an unusual hair style, beard, mustache, blemish, or distinctive clothing. The deficit turns out to extend beyond faces to difficulty recognizing members of any subclass. For example, if shown a key and then an array of different types of keys containing the previously viewed key, patients will be unable to identify the previously viewed key. Many patients will be unable to find their way back to the examining room if stranded in the waiting room ("loss of topographic familiarity," see below).[26] These deficits cannot be attributed to elementary visual dysfunction. Visual acuity is typically completely normal. Visual fields may show superior altitudinal defects, but these defects are insufficient to account for the recognition problem.

Places

Patients find themselves unable to navigate in unfamiliar surroundings.[26,27] This symptom is usually associated with loss of recent memory for all visual items, not merely places. In some cases, prosopagnosia and loss of route-finding in familiar locales are present. Lesions, usually posterior cerebral artery infarcts, typically affect inferotemporal white matter on the right side.

Colors

Patients report that objects appear washed out into shades of gray, that their whole environment has turned into an old "black and white" movie. Difficulty reading and recognizing faces and other objects may be other complaints.

On testing, patients will fail to name colors or match those of a similar hue. This combination of deficits suggests an acquired hue discrimination deficit called *cerebral achromatopsia.*[28,29] Preserved visual acuity excludes a binocular retinal or optic nerve cause. Other recognition problems may coexist. The causative lesion lies in the posterior inferior occipitotemporal regions that specialize in the cortical processing of color.

A far more common deficit associated with lesions in this region is *color anomia,* an acquired inability to name colors. Unlike patients who have cerebral achromatopsia, color anomics have no difficulty discriminating hues on informal testing or on standardized tests such as the Farnsworth-Munsell 100-Hue test.

FAILED MENTAL IMAGERY AND DREAMING

The ability to call up mental images and to dream is closely associated with the visual integrative pathway. In most cases, both capacities are lost when patients have object recognition and spatial attentional deficits.[30] A detailed comparison study of two patients and a review of previously published cases disclosed that this type of mental imagery deficit is related to other integrative deficits.[31] For example, a patient with bilateral occipitotemporal damage could neither draw nor describe the features of familiar objects, but could remember the location of fa-miliar landmarks and the furniture in his house. Another patient, who had occipitoparietal (rather than occipitotemporal) damage, could describe object features in detail but could neither place cities on a map nor describe landmarks in his neighborhood.

There are rare patients who have lost mental imagery but no other visual integrative capacities; they are posited to have a deficit in image generation.[32,33] Lesions in these patients are consistently found at the *left* temporo–occipital interface.[30,32] By contrast, spatial tasks requiring mental rotation of images cannot be performed by patients with *right* parieto-occipital lesions.[30,34]

FAILED AWARENESS OF VISION AND ITS LOSS

The relationship between visual deficits and awareness of them has implications for the study of conscious awareness.[35,36] Patients who have intact vision may report that they *cannot* see (denial of sight), and patients who are blind may report that they *can* see (denial of blindness).

Denial of Sight

Patients with hemispatial neglect resulting from lesions of the right parietal regions may not acknowledge seeing targets in the left hemispace even when visual evoked potentials disclose that elementary visual processing in the primary visual cortex is probably normal.[37] This phenomenon demonstrates that an intact visual cortex alone is insufficient for visual awareness.

Some patients with unilateral occipital lobe destruction and homonymous hemianopias will be able, under a forced-choice paradigm, to localize forms, discriminate their orientation, and identify their color in the blind hemifield. Yet these patients insist that they are completely blind in that hemifield![38–40] In the past, this phenomenon of "blindsight" was dismissed as the result of stray light falling on the intact visual field. That objection has been overcome by demonstrating that blindsight does not occur when stimuli are confined to the physiologic blind spot. The argument that conventional visual field techniques conceal tiny islands of intact visual cortex has been dispelled by evidence that blindsight occurs even after hemispherectomy.[41] Now acknowledged as a real phenomenon, blindsight is attributed to visual pathways that bypass primary visual cortex (retina to mesencephalon or retina to pulvinar, and thence to extrastriate cortex). In humans, these detours are able to provide rudimentary sight but do not allow the viewer to be aware of its existence. Evidently, direct passage of visual information from primary visual cortex to integrative centers is a prerequisite for awareness of sight.

Denial of Blindness

Lack of awareness of blindness, called Anton's syndrome,[42] ranges from emphatic denial, to minimization of the deficit, to acknowledgment without concern.

Anton's syndrome is typically found in a small minority of patients with bilateral primary visual cortex damage following posterior cerebral artery occlusion.[43,44] Earlier authors had attributed this phenomenon to an attentional deficit for vision based on a disconnection between occipital and parietal lobes.[45] However, it also occurs when damage appears to be clinically and structurally confined to occipitotemporal regions,[46] wherein profound recent memory loss rather than attention loss is the most characteristic accompanying feature. Denial of blindness can also occur following prechiasmal lesions—even those causing monocular blindness. But in such cases, diffuse encephalopathy, dementia, or bifrontal damage must be present as well.[47] Based on the foregoing evidence, three mechanisms appear to underlie denial of blindness:

- Disruption of occipital–parietal connections (being unaware of one's blindness).
- Disruption of occipital–temporal–limbic connections (forgetting or not caring about one's blindness).
- Disruption of occipital-frontal connections (not keeping track of one's blindness).

SUMMARY

Symptoms of integrative vision disorders are based on deficits arising from lesions of the two "extrastriate" pathways that convey visual information to temporal and parietal lobe vision-related areas.

Lesions of the occipitoparietal "where" pathway give rise to difficulty with spatial attention and motion. Unilateral parietal disorders cause sensory and motor inattention for contralateral hemispace (neglect). Bilateral parietal disorders cause difficulty reaching accurately for objects, setting a table, using household implements, dressing, driving, keeping track of more than one object at a time, or interpreting action pictures. Motion deficits manifest themselves as a misperception of the speed of moving objects.

Lesions of the occipitotemporal "what" pathway give rise to a failure to recognize letters, words and other symbols, objects, faces, places, and colors. Lesions in the left hemisphere cause defects in recognizing verbally based information—words and objects. Lesions in the right hemisphere cause defects in recognizing nonverbally based information—faces and places. Lesions in either hemisphere may give rise to hemifield color loss.

The capacity to call up mental images of features and locations of objects, as well as to dream, is impaired by the same lesions that impair recognition.

Some patients with complete destruction of one occipital lobe appear to have rudimentary vision within the corresponding hemifield, yet lack conscious awareness of sight ("blindsight"). This phenomenon is attributed to intact retinomesencephalic or retinopulvinoextrastriate cortical pathways. In humans, these detours are able to provide rudimentary sight that does not enter consciousness. Apparently an intact pathway from primary visual cortex to extrastriate visual cortex is a prerequisite for awareness of sight.

Lack of awareness (denial) of cortical blindness may result from disconnection of visual from parietal centers for attention, temporal centers for memory, limbic centers for motivation, or frontal centers for monitoring of self. Denial of blindness associated with pregeniculate lesions is always accompanied by dementia, delirium, or bifrontal lesions.

REFERENCES

1. Felleman DJ, Van Essen DC. Distributed hierarchical processing in the primate cerebral cortex. *Cereb Cortex.* 1991;1:1–47.
2. Trobe JD, Butter CM. A screening test for integrative visual dysfunction in Alzheimer's disease. *Arch Ophthalmol.* 1993;111:815–818.
3. Kempen JH, Kritchevsky M, Feldman ST. Effect of visual impairment on neuropsychological test performance. *J Clin Exp Neuropsychol.* 1994;16:223–231.
4. Ettlinger G. Sensory defects in visual agnosia. *J Neurol Neurosurg Psychiatry.* 1956;19:297–307.
5. Weintraub S, Mesulam MM. Neglect: hemispheric specialization, behavioral components and antomical correlates. In: Boller F, Grafman J, eds. *Handbook of Neuropsychology.* Vol 2. Amsterdam: Elsevier Science Publishers; 1989:357–374.
6. Balint R. Seelenlahmung des "Schauens," optische Ataxie, raumliche Storung der Aufmerksamkeit. *Monatschr Psychiatr Neurol.* 1909;25:51–81.
7. Holmes G. Disturbances of visual orientation. *Br J Ophthalmol.* 1918;2:449–468, 506–518.
8. Bauer RM. Agnosia. In: Heilman KM, Valenstein E, eds. *Clinical Neuropsychology.* 3rd ed. New York: Oxford University Press; 1993:215–278.
9. Rizzo M, Robin DA. Simultanagnosia: a defect of sustained attention yields insights on visual information processing. *Neurology.* 1990;40:447–455.
10. Zihl J, Von Cramon D, Mai N. Selective disturbance of movement vision after bilateral brain damage. *Brain.* 1983;106:313–340.
11. Marcar VL, Zihl J, Cowey A. Comparing the visual deficits of a motion blind patient with the visual deficits of monkeys with area MT removed. *Neuropsychologia.* 1997;35:1459–1465.
12. Dejerine J. Contribution à l'étude anatomopathologique et clinique des différentes variétés de cécité verbaie. *Mem Soc Biol.* 1892;4:61–90.
13. Geschwind N, Fusillo M. Color-naming defects in association with alexia. *Arch Neurol.* 1966;15:137–145.
14. Damasio AR, Damasio H. The anatomic basis of pure alexia. *Neurology.* 1983;33:1573–1583.
15. Henderson VW. Anatomy of posterior pathways in reading: a reassessment. *Brain Lang.* 1986;29:119–133.
16. DeRenzi E, Zambolin A, Crisi G. The pattern of neuropsychological impairment associated with left posterior cerebral artery infarcts. *Brain.* 1987;110:1099–1116.
17. Greenblatt SH. Alexia without agraphia or hemianopia: anatomical analysis of an autopsied case. *Brain.* 1973;96:307–316.
18. Farah MJ. *Visual Agnosia: Disorders of Object Vision and What They Tell Us about Normal Vision.* Cambridge, Mass: MIT Press/Bradford; 1990.
19. Meadows JC. The anatomical basis of prosopagnosia. *J Neurol Neurosurg Psychiatry.* 1974;37:489–501.
20. DeRenzi E, Scotti G, Spinnler H. Perceptual and associative disorders of visual recognition. *Neurology.* 1969;19:634–642.
21. Benton AL, Van Allen MW. Prosopagnosia and facial discrimination. *J Neurol Sci.* 1972;15:167–172.
22. Hecaen H, Angelergues R. Agnosia for faces (prosopagnosia). *Arch Neurol.* 1962;7:92–100.
23. Damasio AR, Damasio H, Van Hoesen GW, Cornell S. Prosopagnosia: anatomic basis and behavioral mechanisms. *Neurology.* 1982;32:331–341.
24. Levine DN. Prosopagnosia and visual object agnosia: a behavioral study. *Brain Lang.* 1978;5:341–365.
25. Bauer RM, Trobe JD. Visual memory and perceptual impairments in prosopagnosia. *J Clin Neuroophthalmol.* 1984;4:39–46.
26. Landis T, Cummings JL, Benson DF, Palmer EP. Loss of topographic familiarity: An environmental agnosia. *Arch Neurol.* 1986;43:132–136.
27. Hecaen H, Albert ML. *Human Neuropsychology.* New York: John Wiley & Sons; 1978:215–227.
28. Damasio AR. Disorders of complex visual processing: agnosias, achromatopsia, Balint's syndrome, and related difficulties of orientation and construction. In: Mesulam M-M, ed. *Principles of Behavioral Neurology.* Philadelphia: FA Davis; 1985:259–288.
29. Zeki S, Watson JDG, Lueck CJ, Friston KJ, Kennard C, Frackowiak RSJ. A direct demonstration of functional specialization in human visual cortex. *J Neurosci.* 1991;11:641–649.
30. Farah MJ. The neural basis of mental imagery. *Trends Neurosci.* 1989;12:395–399.
31. Levine DN, Warach J, Farah MJ. Two visual systems in mental imagery: dissociation of "What" and "Where" in imagery disorders due to bilateral posterior cerebral lesions. *Neurology.* 1985;35:1010–1018.
32. Farah MJ. The neurological basis of mental imagery: a componential analysis. *Cognition.* 1984;18:245–272.
33. Kosslyn SM. *Image and Mind.* Cambridge, Mass: Harvard University Press; 1980.
34. Goldenberg G. The ability of patients with brain damage to generate mental images. *Brain.* 1989;112:305–325.
35. Crick F, Koch C. Are we aware of neural activity in primary visual cortex? *Nature.* 1995;375:121–122.
36. Farah MJ, Feinberg TE. Consciousness of perception after brain damage. *Sem Neurol.* 1997;17:145–152.
37. Vallar G, Sandroni P, Rusconi ML, Barbieri S. Hemianopia, hemianesthesia, and spatial neglect: a study with evoked potentials. *Neurology.* 1991;41:1918–1922.
38. Weiskrantz L. Blindsight. In: Boller F, Grafman J, eds. *Handbook of Neuropsychology.* Vol 2. Amsterdam: Elsevier Science; 1989:375–385.
39. Barton JJS. Higher cortical visual function. *Curr Opin Ophthalmol.* 1998;9(VI):40–45.
40. Stoerig P, Cowey A. Blindsight in man and monkey. *Brain.* 1997;120:535–559.
41. Ptito A, Lassonde M, Lepore F, Ptito M. Visual discrimination in hemispherectomized patients. *Neuropsychologia.* 1987;25:869–879.

42. Anton G. Ueber die Selbstwahrnehmung der Herderkränkungen des Gehirns durch den Kranken bei Rindenblindheit und Rindentaubheit. *Arch Psychiatr.* 1898;32:86–127.

43. Gloning I, Gloning K, Hoff H. *Neuropsychological Symptoms and Syndromes in Lesions of the Occipital Lobe and the Adjacent Areas.* Paris: Gauthier-Villars; 1968.

44. Aldrich MS, Alessi AG, Beck RW, Gilman S. Cortical blindness: etiology, diagnosis and prognosis. *Ann Neurol.* 1987;21:149–158.

45. Potzl O. *Die optisch-agnostichen Störungen.* Leipzig: F Deuticke; 1928.

46. Fisher CM. Neurologic fragments: II. Remarks on anosognosia, confabulation, memory, and other topics; and an appendix on self-observation. *Neurology.* 1989;39:127–132.

47. McDaniel KD, McDaniel LD. Anton's syndrome in a patient with posttraumatic optic neuropathy and bifrontal contusions. *Arch Neurol.* 1991;48:101–105.

Part III

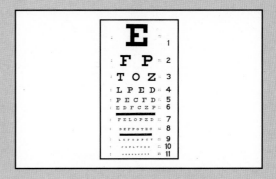

Measures of a Failing Visual System

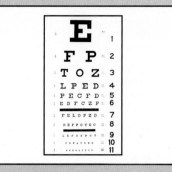

Chapter 6

VISUAL ACUITY, CONTRAST SENSITIVITY, BRIGHTNESS SENSE, AND COLOR VISION

The basic psychophysical tests used to assess elementary visual function are visual acuity, contrast sensitivity, brightness sense, color vision, and visual fields. Visual field testing is complicated enough to merit its own chapter (Chapter 7). The tests described in this chapter require no elaborate or expensive equipment, but they demand cooperation from the patient and expertise from the examiner. Part of this expertise is an appreciation of the limitations of each test (Table 6-1).

VISUAL ACUITY

Rationale

Visual acuity is the most valuable test of high-contrast achromatic vision, notwithstanding its four important limitations:

- **Impracticality.** It requires a well-illuminated Snellen chart located at a 20 foot viewing distance; anything less compromises the accuracy of measurement.

Table 6–1. **Limitations of Basic Visual Function Tests**

Test	Purpose	Limitation
Visual acuity	Measures high-contrast foveal vision	Impractical Subjective Insensitive Nonlocalizing
Contrast sensitivity	Measures low-contrast foveal vision	Subjective Nonlocalizing Degraded by optical abnormalities
Brightness sense	Measures retinal axonal traffic	Subjective
Color vision	Measures cone function	Subjective Screening tests do not differentiate congenital from acquired color loss or optic neuropathy from cone dysfunction Definitive tests are time-consuming and require skill

- **Subjectivity.** It requires patient cooperation. Although visual acuity can be assessed objectively with visual evoked potentials, this test is complicated and is not standardized.[1,2]
- **Insensitivity.** Normal visual acuity (20/15) does not rule out retinocortical disease, which may damage only low-contrast (see "Contrast Sensitivity," below) or nonfixational vision (see Chapter 7).
- **Lack of specificity.** Subnormal visual acuity does not differentiate between lesions of the optical and retinocortical components.

These drawbacks can be minimized by adhering to proper technique and by acknowledging that visual acuity must be used diagnostically in combination with other types of tests.

Testing Methods

Visual acuity tests are summarized in Table 6-2[3] and Fig. 6-1. Of the many ways to assess visual acuity subjectively,[4] use of the Snellen chart is most practical for literate patients.[5] It has endured because the examiner can instantly spot correct and incorrect answers and response inconsistencies. Owing to their special shapes, some smaller Snellen letters are easier to identify than larger ones. This feature offers a built-in trap for patients with nonorganic visual loss. Unaware of this trap, they will correctly identify all letters on a particular line, yet claim that all the letters on the next (smaller) line are beyond their resolution (Chapter 18).

SNELLEN DISTANCE TEST

The Snellen distance chart (Fig. 6-1a) displays high-contrast block print letters ("optotypes") in lines of diminishing size. Each line is defined according to the distance at which the letters can be read by a person with normal acuity (Box 6-1). Results are expressed by a numerator and a denominator, but the notation is not a fraction. The numerator is the testing distance (20 feet or 6 meters); the denominator is the smallest line of letters the patient can identify at that testing distance.

SNELLEN NEAR TEST

The Snellen near vision card (Fig. 6-1b) is a scaled-down version of the Snellen distance

Table 6–2. Visual Acuity Tests: Advantages and Disadvantages

Method	Advantages	Disadvantages
Snellen distance acuity test	Standardized Easy to interpret	Requires special chart
Snellen near acuity test	Standardized Practical	Inaccurate
Tumbling E's	Useful in preliterate or illiterate patients	Inaccurate
Picture cards	Useful in preliterate or illiterate patients	Inaccurate
Preferential looking	Useful in infants	Requires special equipment, expertise, time
Fixation and pursuit eye movements	Useful in those who cannot do E's or pictures	Very inaccurate
Blink to threat or bright light	Useful in those who cannot do any other tests	Very inaccurate

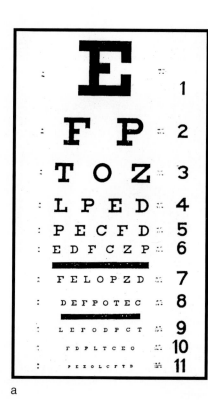

a

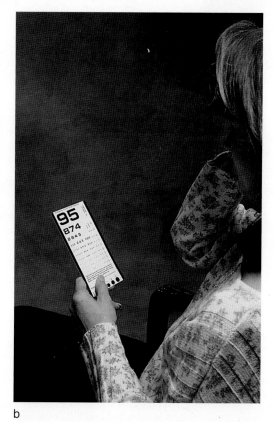

b

Figure 6–1. Visual acuity tests. (*a*) Snellen Distance Acuity. Visual acuity is expressed with a numerator designating testing distance (usually 20 feet or 6 meters) and a denominator designating optotype size. For example, the optotypes on the 20/50 line can just be identified at a distance of 50 feet by a person with normal acuity. (*b*) Snellen Near Acuity. This is a scaled down Snellen Distance Acuity Chart, meant to be held at 14 inches from the eye. (*continued*)

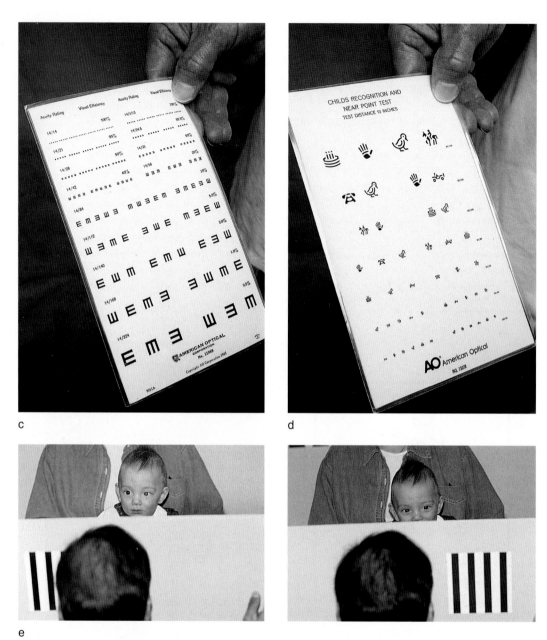

c

d

e

Figure 6–1. (*continued*) (*c*) Tumbling E's. Used for preliterate or illiterate patients, the symbols are E's arrayed in one of four orientations. The patient is instructed to indicate by hand gesture or verbal response the direction of the open end of the three prongs. Scored just like Snellen acuity. (*d*) Allen Pictures. Used for preliterate or illiterate patients, these are standard icons of familiar items (horse, birthday cake, duck, telephone, wagon). The patient is instructed to identify them either by verbal response or by matching to symbols held in the lap. (*e*) Preferential Looking. Used for testing infants, this consists of two panels of black and white stripes displayed side by side. As different spatial frequency patterns are displayed, the examiner observes the direction of the baby's gaze. The baby will consistently gaze in the direction of panels where stripes can be discerned. The highest spatial frequency that evokes consistent gaze is converted into a measure of visual acuity.

Box 6–1

SNELLEN DISTANCE VISUAL ACUITY TESTING

- Test each eye separately with the customary refractive correction in place.
- Instruct patients to read the line containing the smallest letters legible to them. If they identify more than half of the letters on a line, give full credit.
- If acuity is poorer than the largest Snellen letter (either 20/200 or 20/400), instruct patients to approach the Snellen chart as close as necessary to correctly read the largest symbol. If the viewing distance is 5 feet, record the acuity as 5/200 or 5/400, depending on the size of the largest letter correctly identified.
- If patients still cannot see the largest Snellen letter, record acuity as:

  Counting fingers (CF): counts stationary fingers displayed at a distance of 1 foot.

  Hand movements (HM): distinguishes horizontal from vertical hand motions at 1 foot.

  Light perception (LP): sees a bright light shined directly into the eyes.

  No light perception (NLP): does not see a bright light shined directly into the eyes.

chart. It serves as a practical but inaccurate substitute when Snellen distance testing is not available. The patient should be wearing the customary reading correction and holding the card 14 inches from the eye. Because even the slightest misestimate of testing distance will result in an incorrect measurement, this test is most valuable in disclosing a *difference in the visual acuities between the two eyes.* The difference should not normally be greater than one Snellen line.

TUMBLING E'S

This test (Fig. 6-1*c*) is used to assess acuity in children aged 3 to 5 years and in mildly demented, uncooperative, illiterate, or mute adults. Instruct the patient to indicate, by

means of hand gestures, the direction of the open portion of the letter E, which appears in diminishing sizes and various orientations. The E's are displayed on a Snellen chart at a distance of 20 feet or on a standard near vision card held 14 inches from the eye. Measurement is carried out as with Snellen testing.

PICTURE CARDS

This test (Fig. 6-1*d*) should be used when patients are unable to perform the Tumbling E's test. They should identify standard pictures of diminishing size displayed at a distance of 20 feet or on a card held at the standard 14 inch lap distance. Measurement is identical to that used in Snellen testing.

PREFERENTIAL LOOKING

Used primarily in babies, this test (Fig. 6-1*e*) is based on the fact that the eyes will be more attracted to a grating pattern of alternating dark and white stripes than to a featureless target.[6] As subjects are exposed to gratings of different spatial frequencies, their eyes are watched for movement. A semiquantitative acuity can be measured by determining a spatial frequency threshold that no longer attracts attention. This method has limited practical value because it requires special equipment, skill of administration, cooperation from the subject, and time to allow enough responses.

When patients are unable to cooperate with these semiquantitative tests of visual acuity, the examiner is forced to drop down to a cruder level of assessment.

FIXATION AND PURSUIT EYE MOVEMENTS

This maneuver should be used with children aged 6 months to 2 years and with severely demented or otherwise uncooperative adults. Occluding one eye at a time, observe if the patient will fixate a stationary target (face, toy, or light) or pursue a moving target at arm's length. In infants, marked resistance to covering an eye is indirect evidence that the uncovered eye sees poorly.

BLINK TO THREAT OR BRIGHT LIGHT

These tests are used when there are no fixation or pursuit eye movements because of severely depressed vision or consciousness. Wave a closed fist toward the patient's face and briskly open it with a fanning movement of the fingers. Do not get so close that you generate an air current on the cornea, which will induce a tactile blink reflex. To rule out a homonymous hemianopia, approach first the right eye from the extreme right side and then the left eye from the extreme left side. However, the lack of a blink to threat is not necessarily an indication of blindness; a severe attentional deficit, as in a persistent vegetative state, will preclude it. The blink response to a bright light is reliable only at light intensities beyond those of the standard flashlights (the indirect ophthalmoscope is most commonly used). At that high intensity, even patients who have hemispheric blindness will produce an aversive response, presumably mediated by retinotectal pathways.

Interpretation

Normal visual acuity does not exclude visual pathway disease. Abnormal visual acuity does not, of course, differentiate between optical and neural defects.

NORMAL VISUAL ACUITY

Although 20/20 acuity is traditionally considered "normal," 80% of patients who are properly refracted and have clear ocular media have an acuity of 20/16 or better.[7,8] Even a visual acuity of 20/16 does not rule out a retinocortical lesion, because the lesion may spare high-contrast achromatic fixational vision.

For example, optic neuritis tends to spare visual acuity relative to contrast sensitivity and color vision.[9,10] Retinal infarcts, glaucoma, chronic papilledema, and dysplastic optic neuropathies often spare visual acuity altogether.

Lesions involving the optic chiasm, particularly those that compress it from outside, leave visual acuity unaffected unless they are very advanced. In their early stages, these lesions typically damage only the crossing fibers that emanate from the nasal half of the retina; preservation of the temporal (noncrossing) fibers is enough to maintain normal visual acuity.[11]

Unilateral retrochiasmal lesions *never depress visual acuity*. In other words, damage to one optic tract, lateral geniculate body, optic radiations, or visual cortex leaves visual acuity unimpaired—*even if the visual field defect involves the central 5 degrees in both hemifields*. The patient may struggle to place the Snellen letters onto the intact half of the fixational area, but once the letters are found, they will be correctly identified. Bihemispheric retrochiasmal lesions depress visual acuity only if fibers coming from both halves of the foveal area are affected.

ABNORMAL VISUAL ACUITY

Abnormal visual acuity does not differentiate between optical and retinocortical disorders. However, a retinocortical abnormality is likely under one or more of the following conditions:

1. An optimal refraction does not normalize visual acuity and careful slit-lamp biomicroscopic examination fails to disclose ocular media imperfections.
2. The pinhole test (Box 6-2; Fig. 6-2) fails to improve visual acuity.
3. Visual fields disclose a focal defect (Chapter 7).
4. An ipsilateral relative afferent pupillary defect is present (Chapter 8).

CONTRAST SENSITIVITY

Rationale

Contrast sensitivity complements visual acuity as a test of foveal achromatic vision *at low contrast*. It increases the sensitivity of detecting optical and retinocortical lesions, which may spare high-contrast vision. Unfortunately, its localizing value is minimal because lesions in all three components of the visual pathway can impair it.[4,12,13]

USING THE PINHOLE

- The pinhole is an occluder perforated with multiple holes of 2.5 mm diameter. It limits light entry to a narrow beam that bypasses the eye's optical aberrations—refractive errors and media imperfections.

- Measures "potential visual acuity"—the maximum visual acuity that the neural pathway could provide if optical disorders were eliminated.

- If the pinhole improves visual acuity by two or more Snellen lines, a refractive cause of subnormal vision is likely.

- Unfortunately, children under age 6 and mentally impaired adults typically have difficulty locating a hole to look through. Therefore, *failure of visual acuity to improve with the pinhole does not entirely exclude a refractive cause.*

- There are more sophisticated optical devices than the pinhole for assessing potential acuity;[37] sometimes they improve visual acuity when the pinhole fails.

Testing Methods

Two types of stimulus presentation are used (Fig. 6-3).

SINE-WAVE GRATINGS

These tests (Arden Plates,[14] Vistech Vision Contrast Test System[15]) consist of alternating black and white bars of varying width (spatial frequency) and contrast. The minimum contrast that permits the patient to identify the orientation of the bars at various spatial frequencies is called the *contrast sensitivity threshold*. The line that joins the contrast sensitivity thresholds at each tested spatial frequency generates a curve called the *contrast sensitivity function*. Grating acuity is favored by those who consider it necessary to test the full range of spatial frequencies in order to detect abnormalities in restricted regions (notch defects).[16,17] But this method

is time-consuming and subject to false positive results.

LOW-CONTRAST OPTOTYPES

The Regan Low Contrast Letter Chart[18,19] uses two letter charts at 95% contrast and 9% contrast. An even simpler design, the Pelli-Robson Chart,[20] uses letters of a single spatial frequency but declining contrast. Proponents of the optotype method argue that the entire spatial frequency range tends to be equally affected by visual pathway disease, so that measurement of contrast sensitivity at multiple spatial frequencies is unnecessary and time-consuming.[13] This method is faster and easier to interpret than the grating method.

Interpretation

Both types of contrast sensitivity test are highly sensitive but nonspecific indicators of

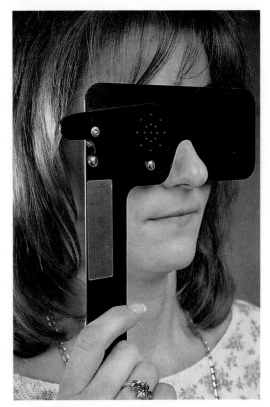

Figure 6–2. The pinhole. See Box 6-2.

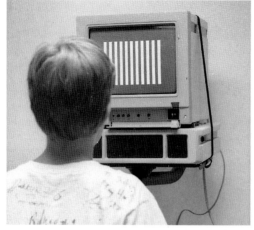

a

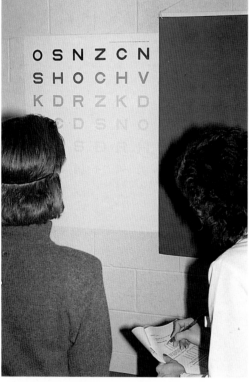

b

Figure 6–3. Contrast sensitivity charts. (*a*) Gratings (Vistech). This popular method requires patients to identify the orientation of lines at various spatial frequencies. At each spatial frequency tested, the contrast sensitivity threshold is the minimum contrast needed to identify orientation. (*b*) Low-contrast optotypes (Pelli-Robson). With this method, only one spatial frequency is used. The threshold is the minimum contrast at that spatial frequency. The low-contrast optotypes test is faster to administer than the gratings and probably equally sensitive.

visual dysfunction.[9,21] Lesions in all components of the visual system will depress this function, and the pattern of contrast sensitivity loss bears no relationship to lesion location.[22] Abnormalities should therefore be interpreted cautiously, and only in the context of other persuasive evidence.

BRIGHTNESS SENSE

Rationale

The brightness of a viewed object is based on the ratio of its light reflectance to that of surrounding elements.[23] This test subjectively measures the volume of retinal ganglion axon traffic exiting from each eye, the same component that is objectively assessed by pupillary light reactions (Chapter 9). It is a sensitive screener for asymmetric optic nerve disease.

Testing Methods

Brightness sense is assessed qualitatively by asking the patient if a light shined consecutively in the two eyes appears brighter in one eye than the other. A quantitative measure may be obtained by means of light-polarizing filters.[24] Two such filters with their gratings in parallel are placed in spectacle-carriers in front of each eye. The patient is asked to equalize the brightness of a white piece of paper in the two eyes by rotating the front filter before the eye that sees the brighter image. In this process, the light transmission is progressively reduced until the brightness is perceived as equal. The percentage of full light transmission is calculated from the final orientation of the front filter.

Interpretation

Brightness sense may be abnormal even when visual acuity and color vision are normal; it correlates best with the afferent pupillary defect (Chapter 9). It is reduced to a slight degree in patients with maculopathies but only if the maculopathies cause severe loss of visual acuity. *Patients with dense cata-*

racts do not manifest brightness sense loss. Test–retest constancy tends to be high for patients with organic causes of visual loss and low for patients with nonorganic causes.[24] Thus brightness sense loss serves as a psychophysical backup of the afferent pupillary defect. It is particularly valuable when the iris sphincter muscle is damaged in both eyes, such that the presence of an afferent pupil defect cannot be determined.

COLOR VISION

Rationale

Color vision tests are used predominantly to test for congenital color vision disturbances. But they occupy a neurodiagnostic niche for two reasons:

1. Color vision loss may be greater than achromatic vision loss in damage to the retinocortical pathway. The explanation for this consistent observation is not known.
2. Color vision may be entirely absent in all field quadrants while achromatic vision is intact in inferior field quadrants. This combination of findings can occur in lesions of V4, in the inferior occipitotemporal region, where color vision may be separately processed (cerebral achromatopsia; Chapter 17).[25] Lesions typically also extend into inferior primary visual cortex to impair achromatic vision in superior field quadrants, but inferior quadrant achromatic vision is spared unless lesions are very large.

Regrettably, the rapid color vision screening batteries in common clinical use were designed to detect *congenital* color vision disturbances and are relatively insensitive to acquired color vision loss. In using these tests to diagnose acquired neurovisual disorders, the examiner must have a passing knowledge of congenital color abnormalities in order to avoid being confounded (Box 6–3).

Testing Methods

Several color vision tests are used in clinical practice (Fig. 6-4).[5,25–29]

Box 6–3

CONGENITAL COLOR VISION DISTURBANCES

- Genetic cone receptor abnormalities.
- Binocularly symmetrical, nonprogressive, and rarely a cause of depression in achromatic visual function.
- Most common condition is an x-linked disorder affecting 8% of males and 0.5% of females with a "red-green" deficiency, a confusion of reds and browns, purples and blues.
- Only 0.0001% of males suffer from congenital achromatopsia, an autosomal recessive disorder resulting from the absence of cones (rod monochromatism). Such patients typically have photophobia, nystagmus, and approximately 20/200 acuity in each eye.
- Except for patients with congenital achromatopsia, those with congenital color deficiencies are not functionally impaired by their deficits and notice them only when fine distinctions are required.

COLOR CONFUSION TESTS

These tests (Ishihara, Hardy-Rand-Rittler) consist of a series of plates formed by closely spaced colored dots. The patient is instructed to identify numbers, letters, or a path made up of dots of equal hue. Although brief, simple to administer, and easy to interpret, they are insensitive to acquired color vision disorders. False positive results occur if patients have a visual spatial disorder.[30,31] Those with alexia or aphasia must be instructed to trace the symbols or paths.

COLOR DISCRIMINATION TESTS

In taking the Farnsworth-Munsell or Lanthony tests, the patient is given a series of colored chips, each of different hue, and instructed to assemble them in the correct sequence based on their hue. Although more quantitative and sensitive to acquired color vision deficits than color confusion tests, they are time-consuming. The Farnsworth

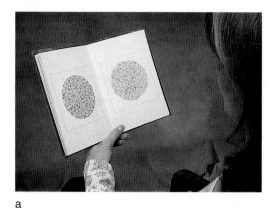
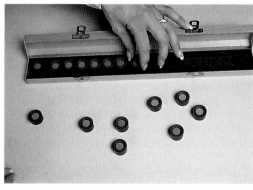

a   b

Figure 6–4. Color vision tests. (*a*) Ishihara Plates. Color plates are made of closely spaced colored balls. The patient is instructed to identify numbers or paths formed by balls of equal hue. (*b*) Farnsworth D-15. In this test, an abbreviated version of the Farnsworth-Munsell 100 Hue, patients must sort 15 colored chips by hue. They are given a starter chip and asked to choose the chip whose color is closest to the "starter," and then one whose color is closest to the last chip selected, and so on.

D-15 is most widely used, as its testing time is relatively brief.

COLOR VISUAL FIELD TESTS

In these tests, chromatic targets (matchsticks, swizzle sticks, eyedropper bottle caps, colored paper squares) are displayed statically or kinetically in the field of vision and the patient is asked to identify their color or compare their saturation (color intensity) to identical targets displayed elsewhere in the visual field (Chapter 8). This technique is valuable in disclosing loss of color vision in regions where achromatic vision is grossly intact.

Interpretation

Color vision tests are clinically useful in four settings.

SUSPECTED CONE PHOTORECEPTOR DYSFUNCTION OR TOXIC-NUTRITIONAL OPTIC NEUROPATHY

The patient complains of slowly progressive visual loss, visual acuity is slightly subnormal in both eyes, visual fields show central scotomas bilaterally, and ophthalmoscopic examination is normal. Color confusion tests are reasonably sensitive, but color discrimination tests are better.[32,33] The distinction between optic neuropathy and cone dysfunction depends on the results of electroretinography (Chapter 9).

SUSPECTED CHIASMAL DISEASE

The patient reports slowly progressive visual loss and has slightly depressed visual acuity in one eye, normal pupillary reactions, and confrontation visual field testing that is equivocally abnormal. Confrontation visual field testing with chromatic (especially red) targets may reveal a bitemporal hemianopia, because chiasmal lesions typically affect chromatic more than achromatic peripheral vision. The other color vision tests would not be helpful.

SUSPECTED CEREBRAL ACHROMATOPSIA

The patient complains that colors suddenly appear gray but has no other neurologic symptoms. If visual acuity is normal, the diagnosis to rule out is cerebral achromatopsia, acquired color vision loss owing to inferior occipitotemporal lesions, usually caused by infarction (Chapter 17).[25,34–36]

In using color visual fields, the first step is to perform finger confrontation (Chapter 8). In patients with cerebral achromatopsia, there should be a dense loss of *achromatic vision* involving the superior visual field quadrants but sparing the inferior quadrants. If such a pattern of field loss is found, test all field quadrants with red targets. If color vision is lost everywhere, the patient probably has bilateral lesions of inferior temporal cortex, the region putatively responsible for color processing and designated as V4.[25] If color confrontation loss is subtotal, confirm cerebral achromatopsia by looking for a failure score on the Farnsworth-Munsell D-15 or 100-Hue test. Although alexia, prosopagnosia, and visual object agnosia defects are often present, cerebral achromatopsia may exist in isolation.

Cerebral achromatopsia can also be confined to one hemifield, but patients with this limited affliction tend to complain more of an associated pure alexia (Chapters 5, 17).

COLOR MISNAMING

If the patient misnames the color of common objects, the differential diagnosis includes a hue discrimination (achromatopsic) disorder and a color naming (anomic) disorder (Chapter 17). The definitive way to distinguish anomia from achromatopsia is with the color confusion and sorting tests. Properly instructed, anomic patients have normal scores on these tests, provided they do not have congenital color vision loss, which usually gives typical fault patterns.

SUMMARY

Visual acuity is the simplest test of high-contrast, achromatic vision, but it is subjective and insensitive to retinocortical dysfunction.

Abnormal visual acuity does not distinguish between optical and retinocortical abnormalities. The pinhole acuity test is helpful in identifying an optical cause, but many patients have difficulty performing this test properly, so that lack of visual acuity improvement is not diagnostic of a retinocortical disorder.

Contrast sensitivity measures low-contrast foveal achromatic vision. It is sensitive to visual pathway disorders but not helpful in their localization.

Brightness sense assesses whether a target appears relatively dim to the viewer. It is a psychophysical measure of retinal axonal traffic, which also mediates the afferent limb of the pupillary reflex arc. This test serves as a psychophysical backup of the afferent pupil defect. It is especially useful in diagnosing patients with asymmetric optic nerve disorders when pupillary reactions are uninterpretable.

Color vision tests are most useful in identifying cone receptor disorders, subtle chiasmal lesions, and cerebral achromatopsia. They are also used in differentiating color anomia from cerebral achromatopsia in patients with color naming abnormalities.

REFERENCES

1. Towle VL, Harter MR. Objective determination of human visual acuity: pattern evoked potentials. *Invest Ophthalmol Vis Sci.* 1977;16:1073–1078.
2. Norcia AM, Tyler CW. Spatial frequency sweep VEP: visual acuity during the first year of life. *Vision Res.* 1985;25:1399–1408.
3. Trobe JD. *The Physician's Guide to Eye Care.* San Francisco: American Academy of Ophthalmology; 1993: 1–7.
4. Johnson CA. Evaluation of visual function. In: Tasman W, Jaeger EA, eds. *Foundations of Clinical Ophthalmology.* Vol 2. Philadelphia: Lippincott; 1999: Chapter 17.
5. Frisen L. *Clinical Tests of Vision.* New York: Raven Press; 1990.
6. McDonald MA, Dobson V, Sebris SL, Baitch L, Varner D, Teller DY. The acuity card procedure: a rapid test of infant acuity. *Invest Ophthalmol Vis Sci.* 1985;26:1158–1162.
7. Beck RW, Diehl L, Cleary PA, Optic Neuritis Study Group. The Pelli-Robson letter chart: normative data for young adults. *Clin Vis Sci.* 1993;8:207–210.
8. Frisen L, Frisen M. How good is normal visual acuity? A study of letter acuity thresholds as a function of age. *Albrecht von Graefes Arch Klin Exp Ophthalmol.* 1981;215:149–157.
9. Trobe JD, Beck RW, Moke PS, Cleary PA. Contrast sensitivity and other vision tests in The Optic Neuritis Treatment Trial. *Am J Ophthalmol.* 1996;121: 547–553.
10. Grigsby S, Vingrys A, Benes S, King-Smith PE. Correlation of chromatic, spatial, and temporal sensitivity in optic nerve disease. *Invest Ophthalmol Vis Sci.* 1991;32:3252–3262.
11. Frisen L. The neurology of visual acuity. *Brain.* 1980;103:639–670.
12. Kupersmith MJ, Holopigian K, Seiple WH. Contrast sensitivity testing. In: Wall M, Sadun AA, eds. *New Methods of Sensory Testing.* New York: Springer-Verlag; 1989:53–67.
13. Rubin GS. Reliability and sensitivity of clinical contrast sensitivity function. *Clin Vis Sci.* 1988;2:169–177.
14. Arden GB, Jacobson JJ. A simple grating test for contrast sensitivity: preliminary results indicate value in screening for glaucoma. *Invest Ophthalmol Vis Sci.* 1978;17:23–32.

15. Ginsburg AP. A new contrast sensitivity vision test chart. *Am J Optom Physiol Opt.* 1984;61:403–407.

16. Bodis I. Visual acuity and contrast sensitivity in patients with cerebral lesions. *Science.* 1972;178:769–771.

17. Bodis I, Diamond SP. The measurement of spatial contrast sensitivity in cases of blurred vision associated with cerebral lesions. *Brain.* 1976;99:695–710.

18. Regan D, Neima D. Low-contrast letter charts in early diabetic retinopathy, ocular hypertension, glaucoma, and Parkinson's disease. *Br J Ophthalmol.* 1984;68:885–889.

19. Drucker MD, Savino PJ, Sergott RC, Bosley TM, Schatz NJ, Kubilis PS. Low-contrast letter charts to detect subtle neuropathies. *Am J Ophthalmol.* 1988; 105:141–145.

20. Pelli DG, Robson JG, Wilkins AJ. The design of a new letter chart for measuring contrast sensitivity. *Clin Vis Sci.* 1988;2:187–199.

21. Kupersmith MJ, Siegel IM, Carr RE. Subtle disturbances of vision with compressive lesions of the anterior visual pathway measured by contrast sensitivity. *Ophthalmology.* 1982;89:68–72.

22. Hess RF, Zihl J, Pointer JS, Schmid C. The contrast sensitivity in cases with cerebral lesions. *Clin Vis Sci.* 1990;5:203–215.

23. Sadun AA. Brightness sense testing. In: Wall M, Sadun AA, eds. *New Methods of Sensory Testing.* New York: Springer Verlag; 1989: Chapter 2.

24. Sadun AA, Lessell S. Brightness sense and optic nerve disease. *Arch Ophthalmol.* 1985;103:39–43.

25. Zeki S. A century of cerebral achromatopsia. *Brain.* 1990;113:1721–1777.

26. Hart WM. Acquired dyschromatopsias. *Surv Ophthalmol.* 1987;32:10–31.

27. Pokorny J, Smith VC, Verriest G, Pinckers AJLG. *Congenital and Acquired Color Vision Defects.* New York: Grune & Stratton; 1979.

28. Birch J. *Diagnosis of Defective Colour Vision.* Oxford: Oxford University Press; 1993.

29. Lanthony PH. Clinical examination of the chromatic saturation. *Neuro-ophthalmology.* 1990;10:119–128.

30. Trobe JD, Butter CM. A screening test for integrative visual dysfunction in Alzheimer's disease. *Arch Ophthalmol.* 1993;111:815–818.

31. Brazis PW, Graff-Radford NR, Newman NJ, Lee AG. Ishihara color plates as a test for simultanagnosia. *Am J Ophthalmol.* 1998;126:850–851.

32. Krill AE, Deutman AF, Fishman G. The cone degenerations. *Doc Ophthalmol.* 1973;35:1–80.

33. Rowe SE, Trobe JD, Sieving PA. Idiopathic photoreceptor dysfunction causes unexplained visual acuity loss in later adulthood. *Ophthalmology.* 1990; 97:1632–1637.

34. Pearlman AL, Birch J, Meadows JC. Cerebral color blindness: an acquired defect in hue discrimination. *Ann Neurol.* 1979;5:253–261.

35. Damasio AR, Yamada T, Damasio H, Corbett J, McKee J. Central achromatopsia: behavioral, anatomic, and physiologic aspects. *Neurology.* 1980;30: 1064–1071.

36. Green GL, Lessell S. Acquired cerebral dyschromatopsia. *Arch Ophthalmol.* 1977;95:121–128.

37. Spurny RC, Zaldivar R, Belcher CD, Simmons RJ. Instruments for predicting visual acuity: a clinical comparison. *Arch Ophthalmol.* 1986;104:196–200.

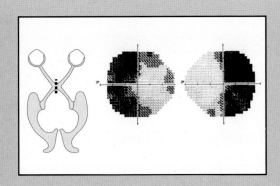

VISUAL FIELDS

Visual field testing ought to be the most powerful tool in localizing disease within the visual pathway. Despite major improvements in testing methods, however, it remains deeply flawed, and is rarely used properly.

RATIONALE AND OBSTACLES

The diagnostic power of visual field testing is based on the topographic organization of the retinocortical pathway, and the fact that the topography changes from the retina to the visual cortex. Lesions of each segment of the pathway produce visual field defects with specific configurations. But mapping and interpreting them appropriately is impeded by the following problems:

- Testing is long and boring. Patients must keep their eyes on a fixation target displayed in a white bowl for 10 to 20 minutes as they wait to signal awareness of momentarily displayed spots of light only slightly brighter than the background. As they gaze at this featureless canopy, their attention soon begins to flag.
- Testing requires special equipment. Perimetric devices are well-standardized and relatively trouble-free, but they are costly to buy and maintain.

109

- Testing requires examiner supervision and skill. Unless the examiner is very skilled, manual perimetry gives misleading information. Automated devices have obviated the need for skill in presenting stimuli, but they provide misleading information unless the proper protocols are selected and patient compliance is monitored.
- Results vary from one test session to another. Intrasubject consistency of responses is low when visual field abnormalities are present,[3–5] making this test unreliable as a measure of the clinical course of visual pathway disease.
- Results are difficult to interpret. The data generated by the automated devices, which now dominate visual field testing, are full of psychophysical "noise." This is because the computer accepts all responses, even those that a human perimetrist, operating a manual device, would reject as accidental or inappropriate. These extraneous responses often obscure clinically meaningful defect patterns.

TESTING METHODS

Visual field testing is divided into informal techniques (identifying face components, patient drawing, and confrontation), which require no elaborate equipment, and formal techniques (bowl perimetry), which require carefully calibrated instruments and either a skilled perimetrist or a computer (Table 7-1).

Identifying Face Components

In this method, the patient is asked to stare at the examiner's nose and declare whether all parts of the face are seen equally well. If the patient replies that all parts are well-visualized, the examiner should confirm this by asking if each eye and each cheek is seen equally well, and if the eyes are seen as well as the chin. The limitation of this simple test is that patients will perceptually "fill in" the missing parts of their visual fields (Chapter 3).

Table 7–1. **Visual Field Tests**

Method	Advantages	Disadvantages
Identifying face components	Simple and quick screen for hemianopic and altitudinal defects	Nonquantitative Insensitive
Patient drawing	Quick screen for small paracentral defects	Nonquantitative Insensitive Samples only the central 10 degrees
Confrontation	Quick screen for hemianopic and altitudinal defects	Nonquantitative Insensitive Requires skill
Kinetic bowl perimetry	Examiner can guide the testing, prodding the patient and rejecting spurious responses Surveys the entire field More sensitive and quantitative than confrontation	Requires testing skill Requires special equipment Boring and time-consuming Subject to examiner bias Relatively insensitive compared to static perimetry
Static bowl perimetry	Very sensitive Quantitative Reproducible	Requires special equipment Boring, impersonal, and time-consuming Samples limited area Difficult for inattentive patients Examiner cannot guide the testing Overly sensitive Results difficult to interpret

Patient Drawing

This is the fastest, simplest way to uncover small but discrete scotomas close to the point of fixation. It is also useful for detecting metamorphopsia (altered image size or shape), an illusion that is nearly always caused by edema or scarring of foveal photoreceptors (Chapter 4) (Fig. 7-1; Box 7-1).

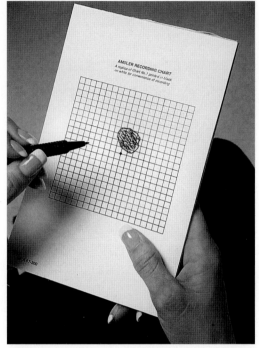

a

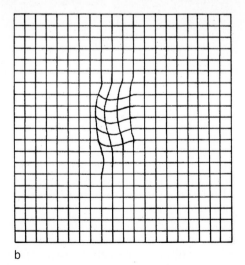

b

Figure 7–1. Patient drawing (Amsler grid). (*a*) Scotoma. (*b*) Metamorphopsia.

However, this method suffers the same limitation as the previous test: patients will "fill in" their tiny defects. Another drawback of this method is that it samples only a limited region of the central visual field, thereby forfeiting the ability to detect peripheral defects.

Finger Confrontation

This method is useful in screening for two types of defects: (*1*) constriction, and (*2*) hemianopic and altitudinal defects.[6] Constriction is detected by advancing one's finger from the periphery toward the center. By performing this maneuver at two testing distances, one can effectively screen for nonorganic (tubular) field constriction (Fig. 18-6). Hemianopic and altitudinal defects are best screened by displaying stationary fingers in two field quadrants simultaneously, thereby comparing visual sensitivity across the vertical or horizontal meridians passing through visual fixation (Fig. 7-2; Box 7-2). Finger confrontation testing has also been used to screen for central scotomas, but technique and interpretation are so difficult that reliability is poor.

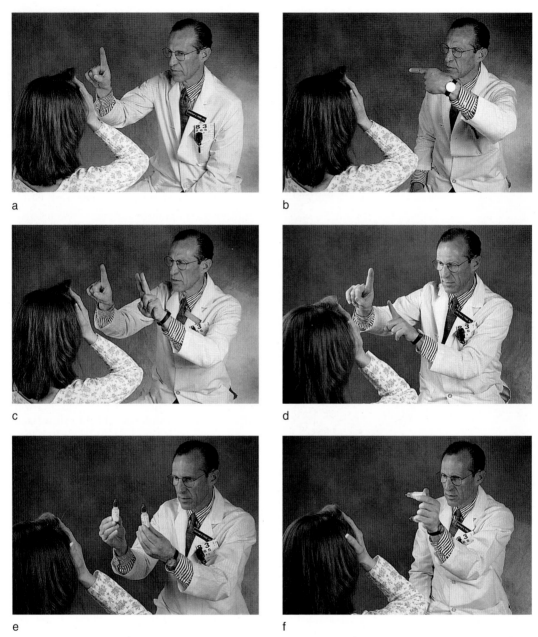

Figure 7–2. Confrontation visual field testing. (See Box 7-2 for explanation.)

Bowl Perimetry

Although informal techniques are helpful screening tests for visual field loss, they are not sufficiently standardized, quantitative, or sensitive to stand alone. Definitive diagnosis usually depends on bowl perimetry, which tests the patient's ability to identify a round, white light slightly brighter than the background of a white cupola. The stimulus can be displayed either as a moving (kinetic) or stationary (static) target.

Bowl perimetry replaced tangent screen testing, which is now a relic. Adherents still use it to magnify very small scotomas and to trap suspected malingerers, but other meth-

Box 7–2

CONFRONTATION FIELD TESTING FOR
HEMIANOPIC AND ALTITUDINAL DEFECTS

- Position yourself so that your head is 2 feet from the patient's head.
- Cover the patient's left eye and instruct her to fixate your nose.
- Inquire if a part of your face appears missing or blurred. If so, use this information to guide finger confrontation.
- Present one or two stationary fingers (more than two fingers takes up too much space) sequentially in each visual field quadrant of the right eye, well within 30 degrees of fixation, midway between you and the patient (Fig. 7-2*a*).
- Instruct the patient to count the displayed finger(s). Instruct those unable to verbalize this response (children, illiterate, demented, or very poorly sighted adults) to mimic the number of fingers presented. If that fails, watch for an eye movement directed at the stimulus.
- If fingers are consistently not seen in one or more quadrants, move the fingers toward the horizontal and vertical meridians, asking the patient to identify the number of fingers as soon as they become visible. Note whether the defect border is aligned to the meridians (Fig. 7-2*b*).
- If all the fingers are counted correctly after each quadrant has been tested twice, present one or two fingers from each hand in two quadrants *simultaneously,* asking the patient to total the number of fingers seen. Always present one finger in one hand and two in the other hand, so you will know in which quadrant the error is made (Fig. 7-2*c*).
- If you suspect a chiasmal or retrochiasmal lesion, or hemispatial neglect, test across the vertical meridian (one nasal and one temporal quadrant at a time) (Fig. 7-2*c*); if you suspect a prechiasmal lesion, test across the horizontal meridian, particularly on the nasal side (Fig. 7-2*d*).
- If all fingers are counted correctly and yet your index of suspicion is high, instruct the patient to compare the *brightness* of single fingers presented simultaneously on each side of the relevant fixation meridian.
- To increase sensitivity further, present red stimuli (bottlecaps, matchsticks, swizzle sticks) instead of fingers and ask the patient to compare the "brightness" of the colors (Fig. 7-2*e*).
- If the patient reports consistent brightness differences, move the color-deficient target toward the fixational meridian and ask the patient if there is an abrupt increase in brightness as the target crosses the meridian (Fig. 7-2*f*).

ods are just as good at these tasks and more versatile (Chapter 18).

The visual field map generated by bowl perimetry consists of two sets of coordinates related to the fixation point, the radial meridians (Fig. 7-3*a*) and the circles of eccentricity (Fig. 7-3*b*). All abnormalities are sited by means of these coordinates.

KINETIC TECHNIQUE

The patient's head is positioned inside a hemispheric bowl. The examiner projects a stimulus on the cupola and moves it from a position outside the normal perimeter of

the patient's visual field to a point where the patient signals awareness of the target (kinetic threshold) (Fig. 7-4). The examiner then removes the stimulus beyond the patient's visual field to another eccentric position and begins moving it inward until threshold is reached. After moving the target inward from many different eccentric positions and mapping a locus of kinetic threshold points, the examiner connects them by an oval line, or isopter, that approximates the perimeter of the field for that stimulus. The examiner can present targets of different size and/or brightness to generate a series of isopters, or concentric

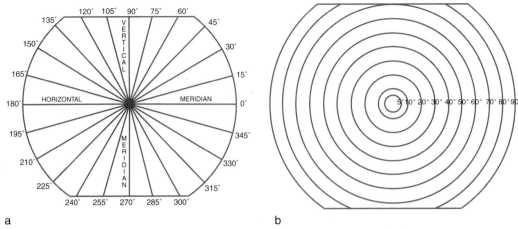

Figure 7–3. The coordinates of the visual field map. (*a*) The radial meridians. (*b*) The circles of eccentricity.

ovals that provide a reasonable sampling of the contour of the visual field. The greater the number of threshold points produced by various targets, the more accurate is the contour estimate. If the isopters are in the expected position and there are no scotomas, the kinetic field is considered normal (Fig. 7-5). If the isopters are evenly displaced inward, the patient has a diffuse deficit (Fig. 7-6). And if the isopters are locally displaced inward or there are scotomas within the field, the patient has a focal deficit (Fig. 7-7).

The advantage of kinetic perimetry is that it allows the examiner the flexibility to cover large areas of the visual field quickly, hone in on expected vulnerable areas of the visual field, reject responses that may be based on poor attention or anticipation, and modify the strategy as the examination evolves.

There are also many disadvantages.[1,7] The results depend on examiner skill and are confounded by examiner bias. Reproducibility is poor because it is difficult to maintain a constant speed of stimulus presentation. Finally, this technique is relatively insensitive to retinocortical dysfunction because moving stimuli are spatially summated by retinal receptors as the stimulus crosses receptive fields. These disadvantages of kinetic perimetry have led to its replacement by static perimetry, as microprocessor technology has become capable of sophisticated manipulation of stimulus luminance and field position.

STATIC TECHNIQUE

As with kinetic perimetry, the patient's head is positioned inside a cupola (Fig. 7-8). Instead of a moving target, the subject sees a static target of standard size and varying luminance presented at different places on the cupola. Over the course of the examination, the computer presents targets enough times at each test point to determine a threshold, or a luminance that permits detection on 50% of exposures. Thus the automated perimeter does not measure borders between seeing and nonseeing as the kinetic perimeter does. Rather, it measures visual thresholds at spatial intervals determined by the testing protocol.[7] The selection of a particular array of test points depends on the anticipated location of the defects within the visual field.

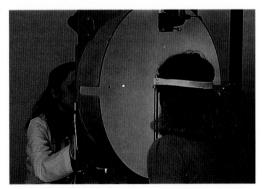

Figure 7–4. Kinetic bowl perimetry. The patient maintains fixation on a central spot in the white cupola while the examiner manually displays a moving stimulus.

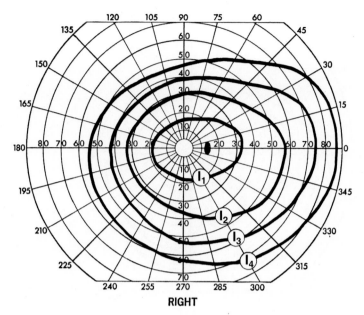

Figure 7–5. The normal kinetic visual field. Four isopters are shown in their normal position. An isopter is formed by connecting kinetic thresholds determined by the points at which the patient first signaled awareness of an inwardly moving target. Each isopter represents the locus of kinetic thresholds for a target of given size and brightness. The label on each isopter contains a Roman numeral indicating size and an Arabic numeral indicating brightness. The outermost target is the largest and/or brightest; the innermost target is the smallest and/or dimmest. The black dot 15 degrees temporal to fixation is the physiologic blind spot due to the optic disk.

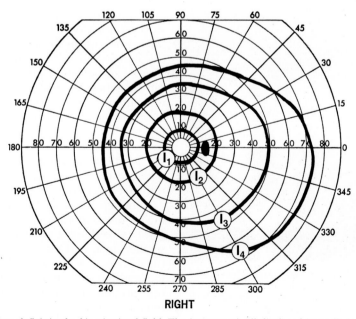

Figure 7–6. Diffuse deficit in the kinetic visual field. The isopters are all displaced inwardly in an even fashion.

115

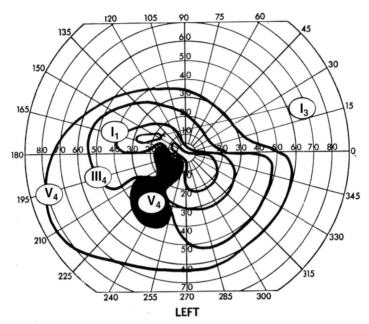

Figure 7–7. Focal deficit in the kinetic visual field. Isopters are locally deviated (warped) and there are scotomas within the field.

Computer-driven static perimeters generate a bewildering amount of data (Fig. 7-9). The nucleus is a set of thresholds determined at the various loci tested. These data

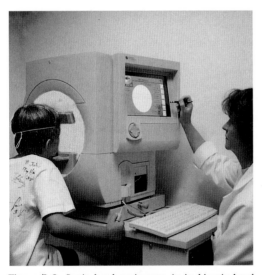

Figure 7–8. Static bowl perimetry. As in kinetic bowl perimetry, the patient maintains fixation on a central spot in the white cupola, but a microprocessor selects the intensity and position of static stimuli.

are presented as raw decibel numbers (raw threshold data), compared to age-matched normals (total deviation), and mathematically manipulated to tease out areas of particularly low sensitivity (pattern deviation). The patient's overall performance is mathematically summarized with an average sensitivity (mean deviation) and a measure of unevenness of the field terrain caused by focal deficits (pattern standard deviation). The mean deviation gives an indication of diffuse deficit; the pattern deviation gives an indication of focal deficit. Finally, an attempt is made to monitor patient compliance with test directions through a series of catch trials (reliability indices). Unfortunately, these catch trials are an imperfect measure of how the patient follows directions (see below).

Although automated static visual field testing produces more sensitive and quantitative results than kinetic perimetry,[8] it samples a smaller area, and the interpreter must sort through a vast amount of irrelevant data ("psychophysical noise"). To be successful in interpreting the results, one must have a systematic approach.[2,5]

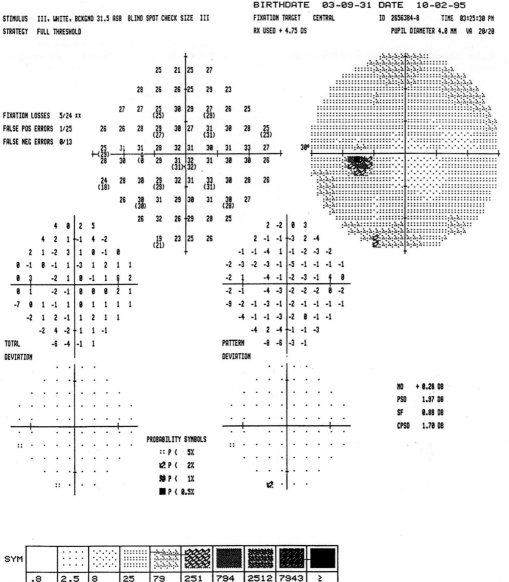

NAME SMITH, JOHN   LEFT EYE

BIRTHDATE 03-09-31 DATE 10-02-95

STIMULUS III, WHITE, BCKGND 31.5 ASB BLIND SPOT CHECK SIZE III
STRATEGY FULL THRESHOLD

FIXATION TARGET   CENTRAL   ID 2656384-8   TIME 03:25:30 PM
RX USED + 4.75 DS   PUPIL DIAMETER 4.0 MM   VA 20/20

FIXATION LOSSES   5/24 xx
FALSE POS ERRORS 1/25
FALSE NEG ERRORS 0/13

TOTAL
DEVIATION

PATTERN
DEVIATION

MD   + 0.28 DB
PSD   1.97 DB
SF   0.88 DB
CPSD   1.70 DB

PROBABILITY SYMBOLS
:: P < 5%
⚇ P < 2%
▓ P < 1%
■ P < 0.5%

SYM									
ASB	.8 / .1	2.5 / 1	8 / 3.2	25 / 10	79 / 32	251 / 100	794 / 316	2512 / 1000	7943 / 3162	≥ 10000
DB	41 / 50	36 / 40	31 / 35	26 / 30	21 / 25	16 / 20	11 / 15	6 / 10	1 / 5	≤0

a

Figure 7–9. The normal static visual field (Humphrey Field Analyzer, San Leandro, Calif.). (*a*) Complete printout. (*continued*, *pp. 118–120*)

General Information

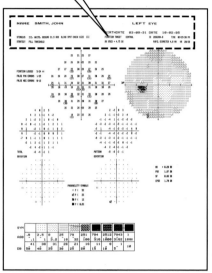

NAME   SMITH, JOHN   **LEFT EYE**

BIRTHDATE   03-09-31 DATE   10-02-95

STIMULUS   III, WHITE, BCKGND 31.5 ASB BLIND SPOT CHECK SIZE III   FIXATION TARGET   CENTRAL   ID 2656384-8   TIME 03:25:30 PM

STRATEGY   FULL THRESHOLD   RX USED + 4.75 DS   PUPIL DIAMETER 4.0 MM   VA 20/20

b

Reliability Indices

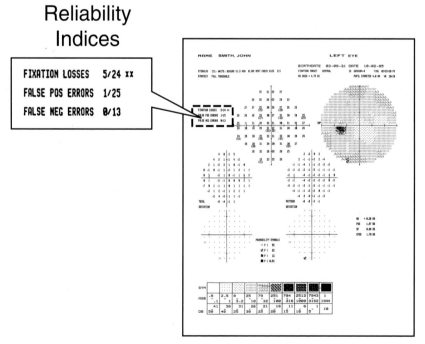

FIXATION LOSSES   5/24 xx

FALSE POS ERRORS 1/25

FALSE NEG ERRORS 0/13

c

Figure 7–9. (*continued*) The normal static visual field (Humphrey Field Analyzer, San Leandro, Calif.). (*b*) General information. (*c*) Reliability indices. These are measures of how well the patient complied with directions. (*continued*)

Raw Threshold Data

Gray Scale Interpolation

Gray Scale Index

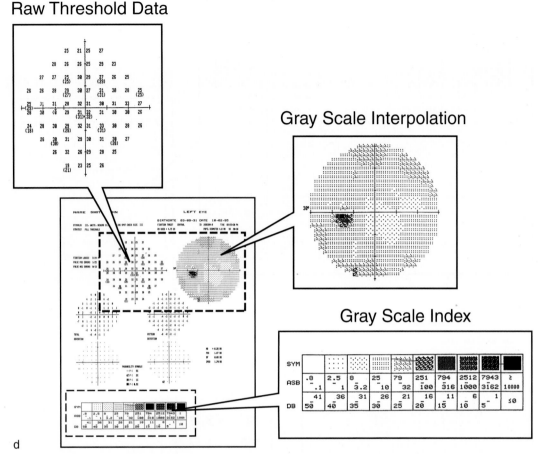

d

Figure 7–9. (*continued*) The normal static visual field (Humphrey Field Analyzer, San Leandro, Calif.). (*d*) Raw threshold data, gray scale interpolation, and gray scale index. The raw threshold data plot contains an array of threshold sensitivities in decibels (dB) corresponding to points tested. Numbers in parentheses are thresholds established on retesting the same points. The gray scale interpolation of these data points is based on the gray scale index. The gray scale index converts decibel values from the raw threshold data plot into shades of gray according to the symbol guide. In the gray scale interpolation, areas between the tested points are assigned an interpolated gray scale value. The gray scale interpolation allows the examiner to get a pictorial overview of the configuration of defects. But it is deceptive in that only a small fraction of the plot comes from points actually tested; the rest is interpolated. (*continued*)

INTERPRETATION

The results of formal perimetry should be analyzed according to a four-step plan (Table 7-2; Fig. 7-10).

Step 1: Is the field normal or abnormal?

KINETIC PERIMETRY

Check if the isopters are in the expected contour and position (by comparison to age-expected norms) and if there are any scotomas, or regions within the field where some stimuli are not seen (Figs. 7-5 to 7-7).

STATIC PERIMETRY

Check the global indices, which summarize performance (Fig. 7-9*f*). A normal mean deviation indicates that there is no diffuse defect in the visual field. A normal pattern deviation indicates that there are no focal defects.

Before dismissing a field as normal, one must heed some nuances. As with any psy-

Threshold Deviations from Normal

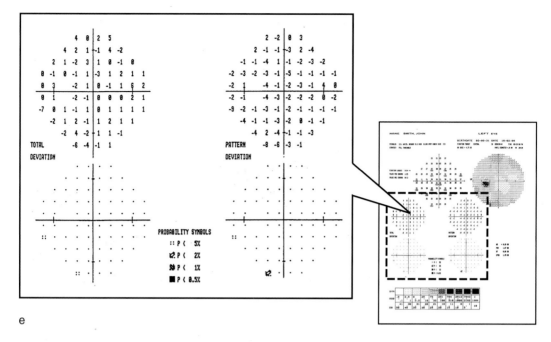

e

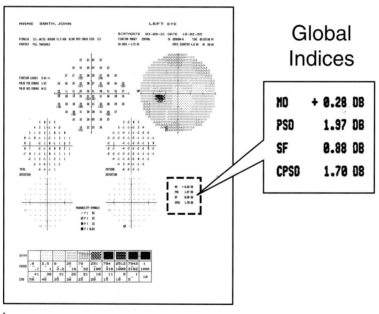

f

Global Indices

MD	+ 0.28 DB
PSD	1.97 DB
SF	0.88 DB
CPSD	1.70 DB

Figure 7–9. (*continued*) The normal static visual field (Humphrey Field Analyzer, San Leandro, Calif.). (*e*) Threshold deviations from normal. On the upper left is an array of data points representing deviations from normal (total deviation). These values are derived by comparing the values in the raw threshold data plot to those of age-matched normals, and they are converted into probability symbols (*lower left*). On the upper right is an array of data points that are mathematically adjusted to eliminate threshold losses reflecting diffuse depression of the visual field (*lower right*). This plot accentuates focal defects (pattern deviation). (*f*) Global indices. These give a mathematical summary of the patient's overall performance. MD = mean deviation, a weighted mean (peripheral points are discounted because of greater test–retest variance) of the total deviation plot. It is the best single measure of extent of field loss, but it does not differentiate between diffuse and focal loss. PSD = standard deviation of the difference of each sensitivity value from an expected value. It measures focal field loss. SF = short-term fluctuation, or a weighted standard deviation of repeated threshold measurements of the same points. It represents a measure of patient reliability but may also be high if the visual field is badly damaged. CPSD = the PSD adjusted for a high SF. The CPSD is therefore a more reliable index than the PSD.

Table 7–2. **Visual Field Signs**

Perimetric Method	Signs of Global Defect	Signs of Focal Defect	Measures of Poor Compliance
Kinetic	Isopters displaced inward symmetrically	Isopters displaced inward asymmetrically One or more scotomas	Inconsistent responses Poor fixation
Static	Abnormal mean deviation	Abnormal pattern deviation	>20% fixation losses >33 1/3% false positive responses >33 1/3% false negative responses >2 dB short-term fluctuation

chophysical study, results are considered normal in terms of probabilities. Although deviations that have a greater than 10% chance of being normal are probably non-pathologic, that determination depends on the physician's index of suspicion. With this caveat, normal global indices indicate a normal test result, and there is no need to examine the rest of the printout.

If the mean or the pattern deviation is abnormal, the interpreter must go on to Step 2 and determine whether the abnormality reflects poor cooperation or a true defect in vision.

Step 2: Is the abnormal field the result of poor cooperation?

KINETIC PERIMETRY

Check the information provided by the perimetrist about the patient's ability to maintain fixation and consistent responses. If either is poor, the test result is of questionable value.

STATIC PERIMETRY

Check the four reliability indices, the built-in catch trials that assess patient compliance (Fig. 7-9c).[7]

1. *Fixation losses:* the fraction of instances that the patient signaled awareness of a target displayed within the physiologic "blind spot," the region corresponding to the optic disk, where there is normally no sight. Early in the test, the instrument es-

tablishes the region of the blind spot for that individual. As the test proceeds, 5% of stimulus presentations fall within that region. If the patient signals awareness of the stimulus, fixation must have been wandering. If fixation losses exceed 20%, fixation is unreliable.

2. *False positive responses:* the instrument records the number of times the patient signaled awareness of a stimulus when none was shown, indicating how "trigger-happy" the patient was. If false positives exceed $33\frac{1}{3}\%$, the patient's responses must be considered untrustworthy.

3. *False negative responses:* the instrument records the number of times the patient failed to signal awareness of a stimulus when he had previously seen a target of higher luminance displayed in that spot. This index tends to reflect inattentiveness or fatigue. If the false negative responses exceed $33\frac{1}{3}\%$, the result is not reliable.

4. *Short-term fluctuation:* although not conventionally included among the reliability indices, this global index measure displays the standard deviation of test–retest thresholds at certain designated points in the visual field. Therefore, it is the best measure of the consistency of the patient's responses. Short-term fluctuation should not exceed 2 decibels.

Unfortunately, the reliability indices themselves are not always reliable indicators of poor cooperation! For example, an excessive number of fixation losses and false negative responses and a wide short-term fluctuation may occur in the presence of large organic defects. Such defects can impair fixation and,

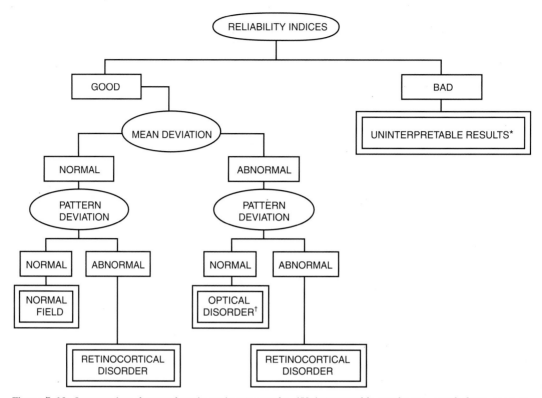

Figure 7–10. Interpreting abnormal static perimetry results. *Uninterpretable results may result from poor patient compliance or large visual field defects. Before rejecting the results entirely, consider whether large defects could account for the results and examine the global indices. †Optic neuropathy may also rarely cause this deficit pattern.

because of moment-to-moment changes in axonal conduction, cause major shifts in thresholds at the same point in visual space. Furthermore, these indices do not detect a consistent but deliberate response pattern perpetrated by a faker (Chapter 18). Thus these indices may be completely normal as a malingerer goes about fashioning a complete homonymous hemianopia out of whole cloth.[9–11]

If the reliability indices are acceptable, the interpreter must go on to Step 3 and determine if the defects are caused by a lesion in the optical or retinocortical component.

Step 3: Is the abnormal field the result of an optical or retinocortical abnormality?

To answer this question, the examiner must determine if the field shows global defects alone, focal defects alone, or a combination of global and focal defects (Table 7-2). Global defects alone, which indicate that the sensitivity of the visual pathway is diffusely reduced, usually signify that an optical disorder exists. Focal defects, alone or in combination with global defects, are always a sign of a retinocortical disorder. How do you recognize global and focal defects?

KINETIC PERIMETRY

Global defects appear as symmetrical inward displacement of isopters as compared to age-expected norms (Figs. 7-5, 7-6). Focal defects appear as asymmetrical inward displacement (warping) of isopters or as scotomas (Fig. 7-7).

STATIC PERIMETRY

Global defects are represented by widespread equal elevation of thresholds as compared to age-expected norms (Fig. 7-11), and they are summarized numerically in an elevated mean deviation. Focal defects are clusters of two or more adjacent test points that have elevated thresholds (Fig. 7-12).

If the field shows focal defects, go on to Step 4 to decide where they originate in the retinocortical pathway.

Step 4: Can the retinocortical abnormality be localized?

Localization depends on the shape and location of the focal defects. There are three types of focal defects: nerve fiber bundle defects, hemianopic defects, and nonlocalizing defects (Table 7-3).

Nerve Fiber Bundle Defects

These defects are named for the three anatomically separate bundles of axons of retinal ganglion cells that make up the retinal nerve fiber layer (Fig. 1-12).[1]

PAPILLOMACULAR BUNDLES

Axons emanating from the ganglion cells of the macula and the area between the macula and the optic disk make up the papillomacular bundle ("papilla" = optic nerve head) (Figs. 1-12, 1-13). Damage to this bundle produces *central scotomas*, round defects centered at fixation (Fig. 7-13*a*), and *cecocentral scotomas*, oval or cigar-shaped defects linking fixation to the physiologic blind spot (Fig. 7-13*b*). Injury to this bundle is caused most commonly by optic nerve or retinal ganglion cell disorders: compression, inflammation, nutritional deprivation, hereditary disorders, or toxins. The reason for the susceptibility of the papillomacular axons in these conditions is unknown.

ARCUATE BUNDLES

Axons that arc above and below the papillomacular bundle make up the arcuate bundles. The scimitar shape of arcuate scotomas comes from the fact that these fibers fan out toward the retinal periphery (Fig. 7-13*c*; Fig. 1-14*b*). When scotomas are very small, their arcuate nature may not be evident unless they have a border along the nasal horizontal meridian, called a *nasal step* (Fig. 1-14*a*). When the entire arcuate compartment above or below the horizontal meridian is destroyed, the defect is called *altitudinal* (Figs. 1-14*c*). Injury to the arcuate bundles is most frequently found in patients with glaucoma and in those with ischemic and inflammatory optic neuropathies. There is no consistent explanation for the vulnerability of arcuate bundles in these disorders.

NASAL RADIAL BUNDLES

Axons take a converging radial course from the nasal retina toward the optic disk. In the visual field, damage to these fibers appears as a temporal wedge scotoma that usually emerges from the physiologic blind spot (Figs. 1-15, 7-13*d*). Relatively uncommon, this scotoma occurs in conjunction with dysplastic and inflammatory optic neuropathies. Why this bundle is selectively affected by these conditions remains a mystery.

Hemianopic Defects

Caused by lesions of the optic chiasm and retrochiasmal pathways, these defects are defined by the fact that one border is aligned to the vertical fixational meridian.

CHIASMAL LESIONS

As the optic nerve axons approach the optic chiasm, those that emanate from the nasal side of the retina (with the fovea as reference point) begin to segregate from the temporal fibers (Fig. 1-8). The nasal fibers then cross in the chiasm to enter the opposite optic tract. All lesions of the chiasm—no matter whether they are extrinsic or intrinsic, compressive or inflammatory—selectively damage the median bar of the chiasm where these fibers cross. The vulnerability of this region derives from its relatively weak arterial supply.[12] The result is a temporal visual field defect whose border occurs at the vertical meridian—a *temporal hemianopia* (Fig.

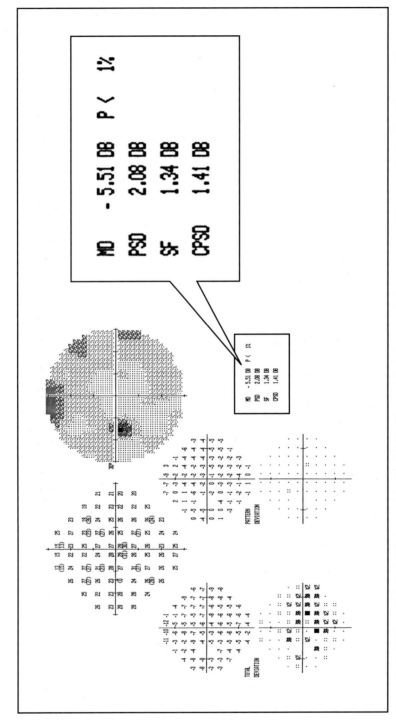

Figure 7–11. Diffuse (global) deficit in the static visual field. The total deviation plot shows many points falling outside the $P < 5\%$ range. The pattern deviation plot is much less abnormal. The global indices show an abnormal MD but a normal CPSD. (The high thresholds on the upper and nasal edges of the field are discounted because of the wide range of normal at these points.)

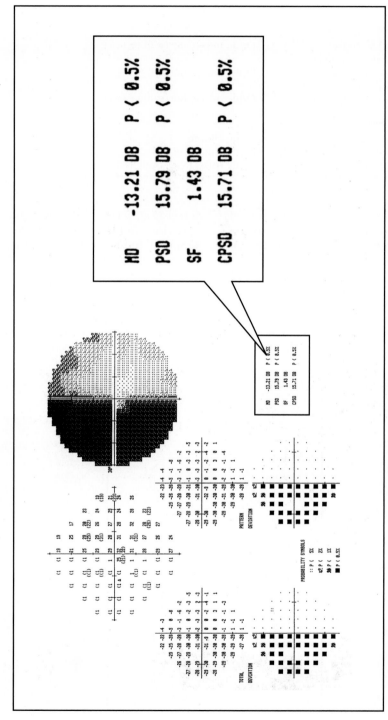

Figure 7–12. Focal deficit in the static visual field. The total and pattern deviation plots both show many points falling outside the $P < 5\%$ range in the temporal field. The global indices show an abnormal MD and an abnormal CPSD.

Table 7–3. **Localizing Visual Field Defects**

Defect Type	Localization
Nerve Fiber Bundle	
Central scotoma	Optic nerve, nerve fiber layer
Cecocentral scotoma	
Arcuate, altitudinal, nasal step	Optic nerve, nerve fiber layer
Temporal wedge	Optic nerve, nerve fiber layer
Hemianopic	
Bitemporal	Optic chiasm
Junctional	Optic chiasm
Homonymous	Optic tract, LGB, optic radiations, visual cortex

7-14*a*). Unless the chiasm is deeply lesioned, only a portion of the temporal field will be damaged. Indeed, the mildest lesions produce only subtle elevation of static or kinetic thresholds—but always on the temporal side of fixation.

Bitemporal hemianopia is the dominant pattern. However, a lesion located in the optic nerve near the chiasm may produce an ipsilateral monocular temporal hemianopic defect (Fig. 7-14*b*).[13] It reflects the fact that posteriorly in the optic nerve, the nasal and temporal retinal axons are already segregated, and that the nasal fibers are particularly vulnerable. A slightly more posterior optic nerve lesion may produce a pattern consisting of a nerve fiber bundle defect in the field of the ipsilateral eye and a temporal hemianopia in the field of the contralateral eye (Fig. 7-14*c*). This pattern is found in

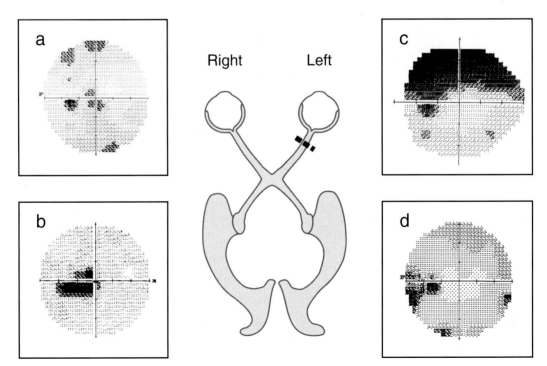

Figure 7–13. Optic nerve lesions: nerve fiber bundle defects. (*a*) Central scotoma. (*b*) Cecocentral scotoma. (*c*) Arcuate defect. (*d*) Temporal wedge defect.

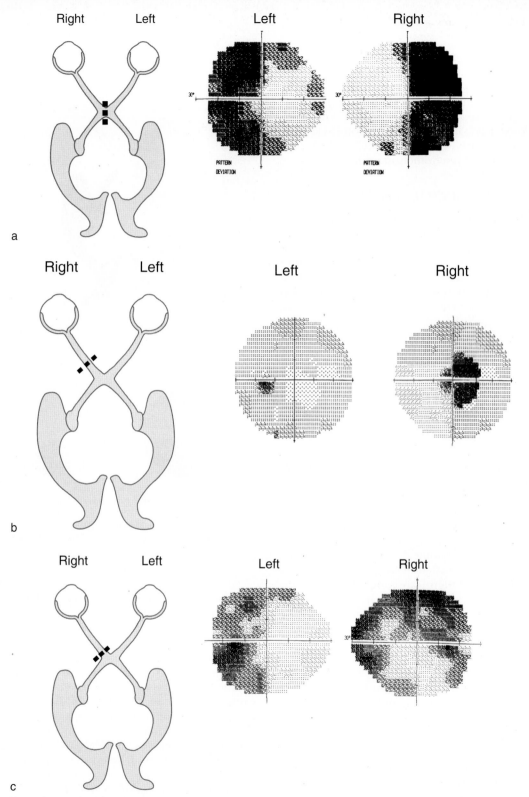

Figure 7–14. Chiasmal lesions: bitemporal and junctional defects. (*a*) Chiasmal lesion (left), causing bitemporal hemianopia (right). (*b*) Anterior lesion of optic nerve-chiasm junction (left), causing ipsilateral temporal hemianopic defect (right). (*c*) Posterior lesion of optic nerve-chiasm junction (left), causing ipsilateral nerve fiber bundle defect and contralateral temporal hemianopic defect.

up to 50% of patients with perichiasmal tumors.[14] It is believed to arise because lesions injure nasal crossing fibers from the contralateral inferior retina which loop forward into the ipsilateral optic nerve ("Wilbrand's knee") (Chapter 1). This anatomic explanation has been challenged[15] (Chapter 1), but the clinical phenomenon endures.

RETROCHIASMAL LESIONS

As they course through the optic chiasm, retinal axons undergo a spatial realignment. Once they enter the optic tract, adjacent fibers represent a spatial hemifield rather than a monocular field. Reflecting that transformation, all visual field defects caused by retrochiasmal lesions are *homonymous,* that is, on the same side of visual space. A complete lesion interrupting the retrochiasmal pathway anywhere from optic tract to visual cortex will cause a complete homonymous hemianopia (Fig. 7-15).

As the retrochiasmal visual pathway fibers proceed toward visual cortex, those that subserve retinotopically corresponding points in hemifields will come to lie closer together. Within the optic tract, these fibers have not yet approximated each other. As a result, incomplete optic tract lesions will produce homonymous hemianopias that are not identical in size, shape, or depth (incongruous) (Fig. 7-16a). It is not until the midportion of the optic radiations that retinotopically corresponding fibers have come to lie side by side, so that incomplete lesions here will produce identical (congruous) homonymous defects in fields of the two eyes (see Fig. 16b). A point to emphasize is that the concept of congruity applies only to *incomplete* homonymous hemianopias; once the defect is complete, the concept of congruity becomes meaningless.

There are other important configurational features of incomplete retrochiasmal field defects that allow localization *within* the retrochiasmal pathway (Table 7-4).

Homonymous Sector Defects (Fig. 7-17)

Homonymous hemianopic defects that selectively spare or obliterate a sector along

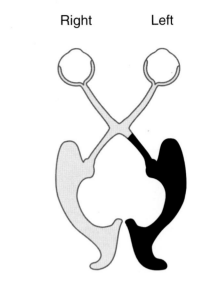

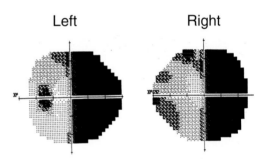

Figure 7–15. Complete retrochiasmal lesion: complete homonymous hemianopia. A complete lesion located anywhere in the retrochiasmal visual pathway (indicated in black) would produce a complete homonymous hemianopia.

the horizontal meridian are associated with lesions of the lateral geniculate body (LGB). These visual field patterns are based on the LGB's dual blood supply from anterior and posterior choroidal arteries, which nourish separate domains. Infarction in the domain of the lateral posterior choroidal artery causes a wedge defect that straddles the horizontal meridional region (sectoranopia) (Fig. 7-17a),[16] while infarction in the territory of the anterior choroidal artery spares that sector of the visual field (sector-sparing) (Fig. 7-17b).[17] However, *homonymous sector defects are probably not specific to LGB damage.* Defects preferentially involving the horizontal meridian sector have also been reported in

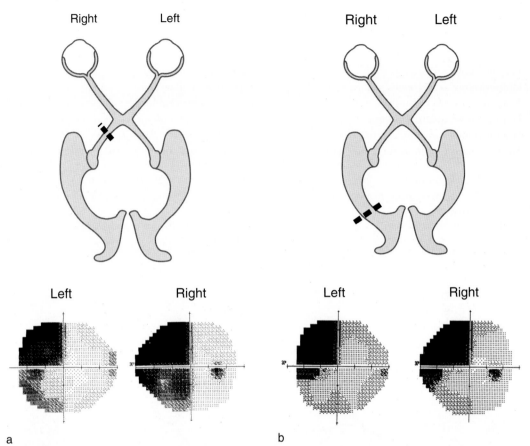

Figure 7–16. (*a*) Incomplete optic tract lesion: incongruous homonymous hemianopia. (*b*) Incomplete optic radiation lesion: congruous homonymous hemianopia.

lesions affecting the optic radiations[18] and visual cortex.[19]

Homonymous Pie-in-the-Sky Defects (Fig. 7-18)

After they exit from LGB, optic radiation fibers conveying contralateral superior visual field information sweep forward around the anterior temporal horn (Meyer's loop; Chapter 1). Damage to this portion of the optic radiations, often the result of amputation of the anterior temporal pole during epilepsy surgery, produces wedge-shaped defects in the superior visual field.[20,21] The defect generally has linear margins, with one border aligned to the vertical meridian and the other extending radially toward fixation. Its wedge shape and superior quadrant location give rise to its descriptive name: the "pie-in-the-sky" defect.

Homonymous Quadrantanopia (Figs. 7-19a,b)

As the optic radiations approach the visual cortex, they split into superior and inferior fascicles. Lesions, especially infarcts, can selectively damage either of these fascicles or their terminations in cortical gray matter to produce homonymous hemianopic defects that have borders *aligned to the horizontal as well the vertical fixational meridian*. Retrochiasmal lesions located elsewhere would be un-

Table 7–4. Localizing Retrochiasmal Visual Field Defects

Defect	Localization
Homonymous sectoranopia	Lateral geniculate body
Homonymous sector-sparing	Lateral geniculate body
Homonymous pie-in-the-sky	Anterior temporal lobe
Homonymous quadrantanopia	Posterior optic radiations, visual cortex
Homonymous paracentral scotomas	Posterior primary visual cortex
Macular-sparing homonymous hemianopia	Primary visual cortex (sparing posterior portion)
Temporal crescent only	Far anterior primary visual cortex
Temporal crescent-sparing homonymous hemianopia	Primary visual cortex (sparing far anterior portion)
Bilateral homonymous hemianopia	Bilateral posterior optic radiations or primary visual cortex

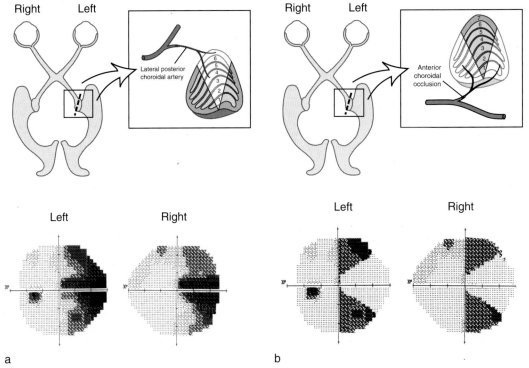

Figure 7–17. Incomplete lateral geniculate body lesions: sector defects. (*a*) Central wedge-shaped homonymous sectoranopia (*bottom*) caused by lateral posterior choroidal artery occlusion (*top*). (*b*) Central sector-sparing homonymous hemianopia (*bottom*) caused by anterior choroidal artery occlusion (*top*).

Right   Left

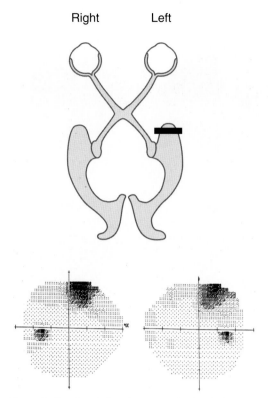

Figure 7–18. Meyer's loop lesion: pie-in-the-sky homonymous hemianopia.

Homonymous Paracentral Scotomas (Fig. 7-19c)

These are homonymous visual field defects confined to the central 10 degrees. Their cause is occipital tip injury (stroke, trauma). The importance of foveal vision in primates is exemplified by the fact that foveal fibers, which occupy less than 1% of retinal area, project to the posterior 50% of the primary visual cortex (magnification factor) (Chapter 1).[22] Thus lesions that destroy this large region cause field defects confined to the central 10 degrees of the visual field! Yet these tiny paracentral defects devastate the patient's ability to read because only half of a given word can be seen at a time. With extreme effort, visual acuity will be normal, inasmuch as half of the macular projections are spared by unilateral lesions. Standard static perimetry testing protocols often miss these defects because test points are spaced every 6 degrees. A special program designed to test intensively (every 2 degrees) within the central 10 degrees is necessary to detect these small scotomas. Patients can often draw them on the (Amsler) grid, providing a valuable diagnostic clue that a high-intensity central static testing program should be used.

Macular-Sparing Homonymous Hemianopia (Fig. 7-19d)

Homonymous hemianopias that spare at least 5 degrees of the central visual field are called *macular-sparing*. They are the mirror images of homonymous paracentral scotomas. In these cases, the posterior half of the occipital region has been at least partially spared by the lesion. Such sparing is very common,[23,24] owing to the relatively large domain of the central projections and the dual blood supply of the occipital pole in many individuals.[25] The principal blood supply of the visual cortex comes from calcarine branches of the posterior cerebral artery, but in about 50% of individuals, the occipital tip receives a collateral supply either from branches of middle cerebral artery or from occipitotemporal or parieto-occipital branches of posterior cerebral artery. Thus macular-sparing defects are more likely to occur with stroke than with

likely to produce a defect border aligned to the horizontal meridian, because only in the primary visual cortex are the upper and lower field quadrants anatomically divided. (In temporal lobe lesions, the lower bound of the defect usually radiates above the horizontal meridian; in parietal lobe lesions, the optic radiations are tightly packed, and the defect edge rarely bears any relation to the horizontal meridian.) Homonymous quadrantanopias are therefore specific to occipital lobe lesions. Inasmuch as the cortical regions immediately surrounding primary visual cortex, known as V2 and V3, replicate the retinotopic arrangement of V1, it is conceivable that lesions confined to these areas could cause visual field defects identical to those caused by lesions confined to V1. In fact, cases of homonymous quadrantanopias have been documented by imaging or necropsy[22] where lesions were limited to extrastriate regions.

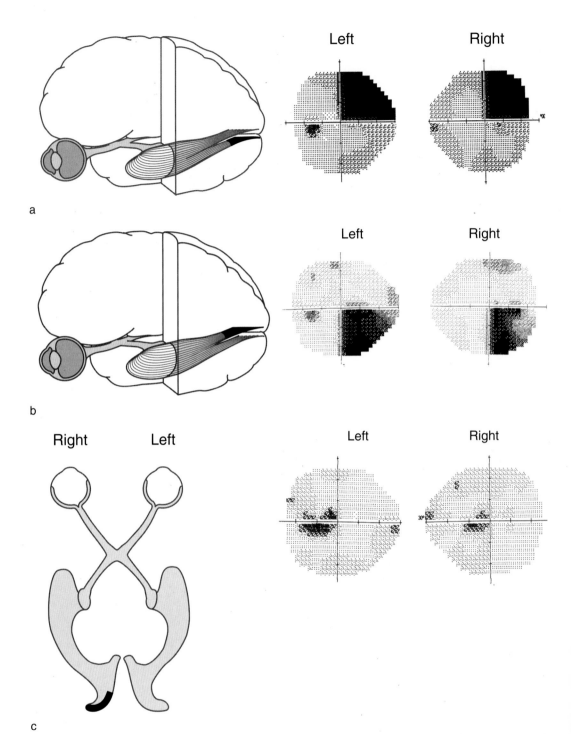

Figure 7–19. Visual field defects associated with primary visual cortex lesions. (*a*) Right superior homonymous quadrantanopia (*right*), caused by damage to left inferior cortex (*left*). (*b*) Right inferior homonymous quadrantanopia (*right*), caused by damage to left superior visual cortex (*left*). (*c*) Left homonymous paracentral scotomas (*right*), caused by damage to the posterior half of right visual cortex (*left*). (*continued, pp. 133–134*)

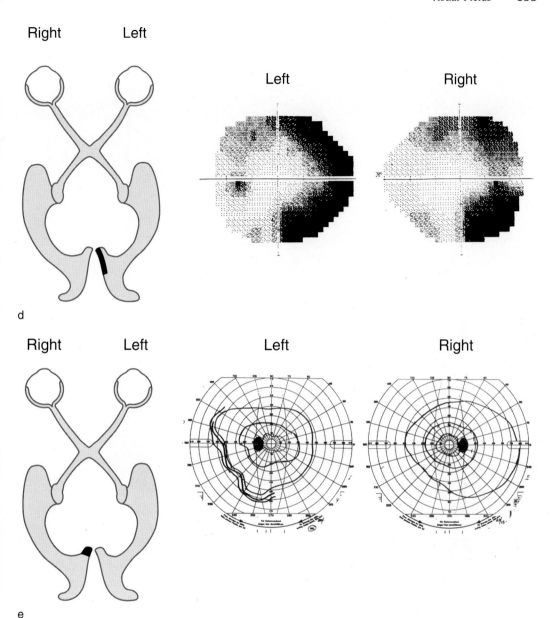

Figure 7–19. (*continued*) Visual field defects associated with primary visual cortex lesions. (*d*) Right macular-sparing homonymous hemianopia (*right*), caused by damage to the anterior half of left visual cortex (*left*). (*e*) Left monocular temporal crescent defect (*right*), caused by damage limited to the anterior 10% of right visual cortex (*left*). Such a peripheral defect, shown here in kinetic perimetry, is not captured by standard threshold static automated perimetry because the peripheral field is not tested. (*continued*)

other occipital lesions such as tumor, vascular malformation, or trauma, which tend to involve the occipital pole as well. These defects are specific to primary visual cortex lesions. That is, lesions in any other portion of the retrochiasmal pathway typically cause macular-splitting, perhaps because the macular region axons have not yet had the chance to fan out over their expanse in posterior cortex. *Caution:* macular sparing of 3 degrees or less is not clinically meaningful; it may be the result of wandering fixation.[26]

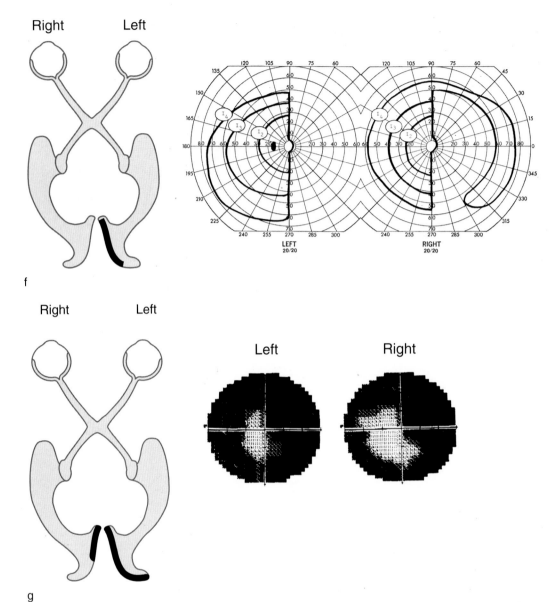

Figure 7–19. (*continued*) Visual field defects associated with primary visual cortex lesions. (*f*) Right temporal crescent-sparing, macular-sparing homonymous hemianopia (*right*), caused by damage sparing the anterior 10% and posterior 20% of left visual cortex (*left*). The crescent-sparing, shown here in kinetic perimetry, would be missed in standard threshold static automated perimetry because the peripheral field is not tested. (*g*) Bilateral homonymous hemianopia with macular-sparing on the left side (*right*), caused by bilateral damage to visual cortex, but sparing the posterior 50% on the right (*left*). The localizing features are alignment of defect borders to the vertical meridian. This defect is often misdiagnosed as the field constriction of a malingerer (Chapter 18).

Temporal Crescent Loss (Fig. 7-19e)
In these extremely rare cases, the lesion is confined to the anterior 10% of primary visual cortex, skimming off the outermost crescent in the temporal field of the eye contralateral to the involved hemisphere. The

lesion is usually an infarct.[27,28] The missing sliver of field is likely to go unnoticed by the patient and may easily be overlooked by examiners because current static techniques tend to concentrate stimuli in the central 30 degrees of the field. *Temporal crescent loss is the only example of a monocular visual field defect caused by a retrochiasmal lesion.* (All other defects are binocular and homonymous.)

Temporal Crescent-Sparing Homonymous Hemianopia (Fig 7-19f)

The most peripheral 30 degrees of the temporal field viewed by each eye is not overlapped by a corresponding nasal field in the other eye. Called the *temporal crescent,* this portion of the field has monocular representation in the anteriormost 10% of the contralateral visual cortex located near the parieto-occipital fissure.[22,29] Primary visual cortex lesions often spare this region.[30,31] The resulting homonymous hemianopia may, upon first analysis, appear incongruous because the temporal crescent of field viewed by one eye remains intact. Upon careful scrutiny, however, the examiner realizes that the defects are perfectly congruous if the unpaired temporal crescent is subtracted. Current static visual field testing often misses the spared area because stimuli are not displayed beyond 30 degrees eccentricity, but this corridor of sight is critical to patients—it preserves their mobility by orienting them to moving targets on their blind side.[31]

Bilateral Homonymous Hemianopias (Fig. 7-19g)

Bilateral homonymous defects are nearly always a reflection of bilateral visual cortex lesions, although bilateral optic radiation lesions do rarely occur. Because these defects involve both halves of the visual field, they are generally misinterpreted as reflecting binocular retinal or optic nerve damage. If macular sparing is a feature, the examiner may wrongly assume they are the "tunnel fields" of a malingerer (Chapter 18). Correct localization depends on formal perimetry, which discloses defect borders *aligned to the vertical meridian on both sides of fixation.*

Bilateral homonymous hemianopia may rarely be restricted to the inferior or superior halves of the visual field. In such a case, it would be called homonymous altitudinal hemianopia. It usually results from concomitant or consecutive selective occlusion of the calcarine, occipitotemporal (inferior altitudinal defects), or occipitoparietal (inferior altitudinal defects) branches of both posterior cerebral arteries.[32]

Nonlocalizing Focal Defects

Focal defects that do have the configurational features of nerve fiber bundle or hemianopic defects are nonlocalizing. Three interpretations of these defects are possible:

1. The outer retina is damaged. The retinal photoreceptors and their polysynaptic connections to retinal ganglion cells lack the architecture that gives rise to nerve fiber bundle visual field defects. Damage to this "preganglionic" retinal region produces visual field defects that correspond to the boundaries of the injury, often visible on ophthalmoscopic examination. Some outer retinal disorders characteristically affect certain portions of the visual field. The best example is the midperipheral ring visual field defect (Fig. 7-20) caused by photoreceptor dystrophies. It coincides with a band of excess or deficient retinal pigmentation observed through the ophthalmoscope in that region (Chapter 11; Plate 1).

2. The defects are too small to show nerve fiber bundle or hemianopic features. In such cases, applying a more sensitive perimetric protocol might bring out the localizing features. In other cases, time and the evolution of the disease process may eventually reveal their localizing features.

3. The nerve fiber bundle or hemianopic features are buried by noise or extensive loss. The patient's responses are so abnormal, because of either disease or poor compliance, that localizing features are hidden. In such cases, applying a less sensitive, shorter duration perimetric protocol (or informal techniques) may bring out more useful information.

To recapitulate, focal visual field defects should be divided into those that are nonhemianopic and those that are hemianopic (Fig. 7-21). Of those that are nonhemianopic, some will have nerve fiber bundle features that permit localization predominantly to the optic nerve. Others will have no nerve fiber bundle features and must be

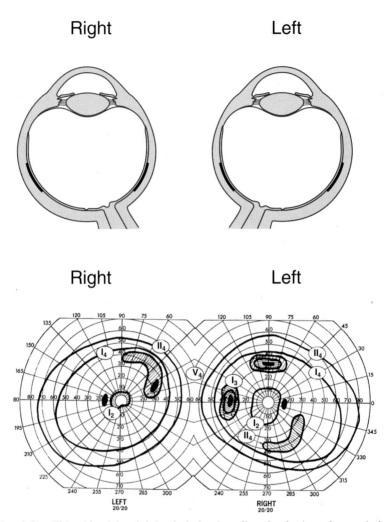

Figure 7–20. Ring defect. This midperipheral defect lacks borders aligned to horizontal or vertical meridians. It is nonlocalizing until correlated with typical ophthalmoscopic or electroretinographic features of retinitis pigmentosa. This hereditary photoreceptor degeneration initially damages photoreceptors in the equatorial region of the retina corresponding to the defect.

considered nonlocalizing. Among those with hemianopic features, recognition of special characteristics will allow localization within the chiasmal and retrochiasmal portions of the retinocortical component.

Sadly, the results of static perimetry often do not allow even the most astute interpreter to find localizing information. This is not necessarily the fault of the testing procedure. Some retinocortical lesions do not produce discrete defects. In other cases, patient cooperation is limited. Alternative perimetric testing methods[33–40,40a] appear to be less variable, more sensitive, and more patient-friendly, but none has gained wide clinical

acceptance. Stimulating the retina with a small focal light stimulus[41] or measuring pupil constriction in response to stimuli projected onto the cupola[42] may eventually solve current perimetry's inherent problems of subjectivity, but these novel techniques remain experimental.[40a]

SUMMARY

Visual field testing offers the most powerful clinical means of localizing lesions because it directly accesses the retinocortical pathway's topographical arrangement. But as a

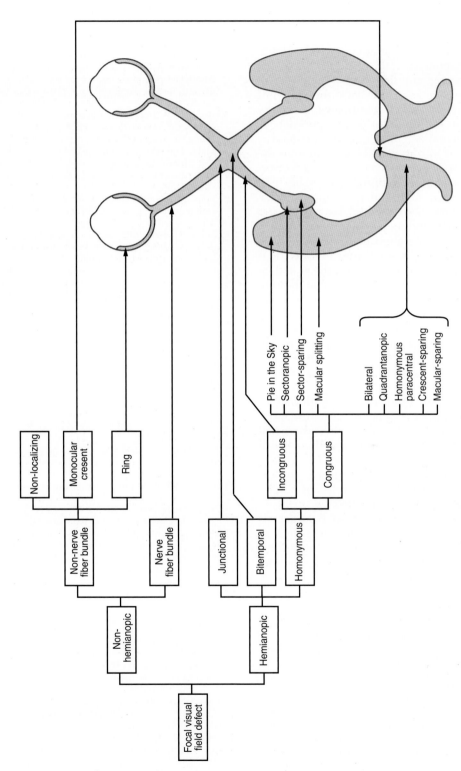

Figure 7–21. Retinocortical visual field defects—at a glance.

diagnostic tool, it is constrained by the need for long testing times, patient cooperation, special equipment, and interpretive skill.

Informal testing methods include identifying components of the examiner's face, patient drawing, and finger confrontation. Although valuable as previews, they are not sufficiently sensitive, quantitative, or reproducible to substitute for formal perimetry.

Formal perimetry was, until the last decade, performed with manual kinetic stimulus delivery. It is now performed almost exclusively with automated microprocessors. The new, computerized method may be a more sensitive and quantitative method, but it generates a lot of confounding psychophysical "noise."

In interpreting abnormal results of static perimetry, the examiner must first decide if there are any defects, based on the global indices (mean and pattern deviations). If there are defects, the next step is to decide if the study is reliable. This is done by scanning the reliability indices. If they are very poor, the results may have to be rejected as evidence of poor compliance with the test.

If the reliability indices are acceptable, the examiner should scan the mean and pattern deviations. An abnormal mean deviation, together with a normal pattern deviation, suggests an optical disorder. An abnormal pattern deviation suggests a retinocortical disorder.

To localize retinocortical defects, the examiner must then hunt for relevant configurational features of focal defects.

The three types of focal visual field defects are (*1*) nerve fiber bundle defects, reflecting retinal fiber layer and optic nerve lesions; (*2*) hemianopic defects, reflecting chiasmal and retrochiasmal lesions; and (*3*) nonlocalizing focal defects, reflecting outer retinal lesions or nerve fiber bundle defects that are not diagnosable because they are too small or buried by global defects.

REFERENCES

1. Trobe JD, Glaser JS. *The Visual Fields Manual: A Practical Guide to Testing and Interpretation.* Gainesville, Fla: Triad; 1983.
2. Walsh TJ. *Visual Fields: Examination and Interpretation.* San Francisco: American Academy of Ophthalmology; 1996.
3. Wall M, Kutzko KE, Chauhan BC. Variability in patients with flaucomatous visual field damage is reduced using size V stimuli. *Invest Ophthalmol Vis Sci.* 1997;38:426–435.
4. Wall M, Johnson CA, Kutzko KE, Nguyen R, Brito C, Keltner JL. Long- and short-term variability of automated perimetry in patients with optic neuritis and healthy subjects. *Arch Ophthalmol.* 1998; 116:53–61.
5. Werner EB. Interpreting automated visual fields. *Ophthalmol Clin North Am.* 1995;8(2):229–257.
6. Trobe JD, Acosta PC, Krischer JP. Confrontation visual field techniques in the detection of anterior visual pathway lesions. *Ann Neurol.* 1981;10:28–34.
7. Anderson DA. *Automated Static Perimetry.* St. Louis: Mosby; 1992.
8. Keltner JL, Johnson CA. Current status of automated perimetry. *Arch Ophthalmol.* 1986;104:347–349.
9. Smith TJ, Baker RS. Perimetric findings in functional disorders using automated techniques. *Ophthalmology.* 1987;94:1562–1566.
10. Glovinsky Y, Quigley HA, Bisset RA, Miller NR. Artificially produced quadrantanopsia in computed visual field testing. *Am J Ophthalmol.* 1990;110:90–91.
11. Thompson JC, Kosmorsky GS, Ellis BD. Fields of dreamers and dreamed-up fields. *Ophthalmology.* 1996;103:117–125.
12. Bergland RM, Ray BS. The arterial blood supply of the human optic chiasm. *J Neurosurg.* 1969;31:327–334.
13. Miller NR, Newman NJ. Topical diagnosis of lesions in the visual sensory pathway. In: Miller NR, Newman NJ, eds. *Walsh & Hoyt's Clinical Neuro-ophthalmology.* 5th ed. Vol 1. Baltimore: Williams & Wilkins; 1998: pp 307–309.
14. Trobe JD, Tao AH, Shuster JJ. Perichiasmal tumors: diagnostic and prognostic features. *Neurosurgery.* 1984;15:391–399.
15. Horton JC. Wilbrand's knee of the primate optic chiasm is an artifact of monocular enucleation. *Trans Am Ophthalmol Soc.* 1997;95:579–609.
16. Frisen L, Holmegaard L, Rosencrantz M. Sectorial optic atrophy and homonymous horizontal sectoranopia: a lateral choroidal artery syndrome? *J Neurol Neurosurg Psychiatry.* 1978;41:374–380.
17. Frisen L. Quadruple sectoranopia and sectorial optic atrophy—a syndrome of the distal anterior choroidal artery. *J Neurol Neurosurg Psychiatry.* 1979; 42:590–594.
18. Carter JE, O'Connor P, Schacklett D, Rosenberg M. Lesions of the optic radiations mimicking lateral geniculate nucleus visual field defects. *J Neurol Neurosurg Psychiatry.* 1985;48:982–988.
19. Grossman M, Galetta SL, Nichols CW, Grossman RI. Horizontal homonymous sectoral field defect after ischemia infarction of the occipital cortex. *Am J Ophthalmol.* 1990;109:234–236.
20. Cogan DG. *Neurology of the Visual System.* Springfield, Ill: Charles C Thomas; 1966:263.
21. Miller NR. *Walsh & Hoyt's Clinical Neuro-ophthalmology.* 4th ed. Vol 1. Baltimore: Williams & Wilkins; 1982:134–136.
22. Horton JC, Hoyt WF. The representation of the vi-

sual field in human striate cortex: a revision of the classic Holmes map. *Arch Ophthalmol.* 1991;109:816–824.

23. McFadzean R, Brosnahan D, Hadley D, Mutlukan E. Representation of the visual field in the occipital striate cortex. *Br J Ophthalmol.* 1994;78:185–190.

24. Gray LG, Galetta SL, Siegal T, Schatz NJ. The central visual field in homonymous hemianopia: evidence for unilateral foveal representation. *Arch Neurol.* 1997;54:312–317.

25. Smith CG, Richardson WFG. The course and distribution of the arteries supplying the visual (striate) cortex. *Am J Ophthalmol.* 1966;61:1391–1396.

26. Leventhal AG, Ault SJ, Vitek DJ. The nasotemporal division in primate retina: the neural bases of macular sparing and splitting. *Science.* 1988;240:66–67.

27. Landau K, Wichmann W, Valavanis A. The missing temporal crescent. *Am J Ophthalmol.* 1995;119:345–349.

28. Chavis PS, Alhazmi A, Clunie D, Hoyt WF. Temporal crescent syndrome with magnetic resonance imaging. *J Neuro-ophthalmol.* 1997;17:151–155.

29. Horton JC, Dagi LR, McCrane EP, de Monasterio FM. Arrangement of ocular dominance columns in human visual cortex. *Arch Ophthalmol.* 1990;108:1025–1031.

30. Benton S, Levy I, Swash M. Vision in the temporal crescent in occipital infarction. *Brain.* 1980;103:83–97.

31. Meienberg O. Sparing of the temporal crescent in homonymous hemianopia and its significance for visual orientation. *Neuro-ophthalmology.* 1981;2:129–134.

32. Newman RP, Kinkel WR, Jacobs L. Altitudinal hemianopia caused by occipital infarctions: clinical and computerized tomographic correlations. *Arch Neurol.* 1984;41:413–418.

33. Frisen L. High-pass resolution targets in peripheral vision. *Ophthalmology.* 1987;94:1104–1108.

34. Wall M. High-pass resolution perimetry in optic neuritis. *Invest Ophthalmol Vis Sci.* 1991;32:2525–2529.

35. Wall M, Ketoff KM. Random dot motion perimetry in patients with glaucoma and in normal subjects. *Am J Ophthalmol.* 1995;120:587–596.

36. Sample PA, Taylor JDN, Martinex G, Lusky M, Weinreb RN. Short-wavelength color visual fields in glaucoma suspects at risk. *Am J Ophthalmol.* 1993;115:225–228.

37. Stewart WC, Chauhan BC. Newer visual function tests in the evaluation of glaucoma. *Surv Ophthalmol.* 1995;40:119–135.

38. Chauhan BC, Johnson CA. Test–retest variability of frequency-doubling perimetry and conventional perimetry in gaucoma patients and normal subjects. *Invest Ophthalmol Vis Sci.* 1999;40:648–656.

39. Chauhan BC, House PH, McCormick TA, LeBlanc RP. Comparison of conventional and high-pass resolution perimetry in a prospective study of patients with glaucoma and healthy controls. *Arch Ophthalmol.* 1999;117:24–33.

40. Polo V, Abecia E, Pablo LE, Pinilla I, Larrosa JM, Honrubia FM. Short-wavelength automated perimetry and retinal nerve fiber layer evaluation in suspected cases of glaucoma. *Arch Ophthalmol.* 1998;116:1295–1298.

40a. Donahue SP. Perimetry techniques in neuro-ophthalmology. *Curr Opin Ophthalmol.* 1999;10:420–428.

41. Varano M, Scassa C. Scanning laser ophthalmoscope microperimetry. *Sem Ophthalmol.* 1998;13:203–209.

42. Kardon RH, Kirkali PA, Thompson HS. Automated pupil perimetry: pupil field mapping in patients and normal subjects. *Ophthalmology.* 1991;98:485–496.

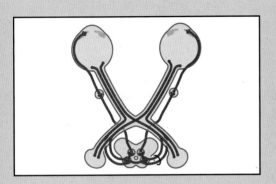

Chapter 8

PUPILLARY REACTIONS

THE PUPILLARY REFLEX ARC

TESTING AND INTERPRETATION
  Pupil Reactions to Direct Light
  Swinging-Light Test

SUMMARY

The pupillary reactions are an indirect but objective measure of visual function. The swinging light test for an afferent pupil defect is an efficient way to detect asymmetric optic nerve disease, but its accuracy depends on proper technique.

THE PUPILLARY REFLEX ARC

The anterior neural circuits that mediate visual processing are closely associated with pupillary reactions to light (Fig. 8-1).[1] This linkage offers an objective means to identify unilateral or bilaterally asymmetric optic nerve disease and to separate pregeniculate from geniculate or retrogeniculate blindness.

The pupillary reflex pathway (Fig. 8-1; Box 8-1) consists of an afferent (input) loop and an efferent (output) loop. In the afferent loop, neural signals are conveyed by the very same retinal ganglion cell axons that convey visual information. Because of a lack of perfect concordance between anterior visual pathway visual loss and pupillary reactions, some investigators believe that these two functions are subserved by separate populations of ganglion cells.[1] The pupillary reflex fibers branch off rostral to the lateral geniculate body and synapse in pretectal nuclei. Signals are then distributed to pretectal nuclei on the opposite side and to the Edinger-Westphal subnuclei of the third cranial nerve. The efferent loop is a two-neuron pathway extending from the Edinger-Westphal subnucleus to the iris sphincter. Axons travel with other components of the third cranial nerve to synapse in the ciliary ganglion on the long posterior ciliary nerves which carry the signal to the iris.

THE PUPILLARY REFLEX ARC

- Light on the retina generates a smooth muscle response in the iris sphincter in order to refine focus and optimize light levels.[1]

- The afferent loop uses foveal axons that pass through the optic nerve, chiasm, and tract and then split off as collateral fibers destined for the pretectal nuclei rostral to the superior colliculus.

- Pretectal nuclear output goes to the autonomic (Edinger-Westphal) portion of the third (oculomotor) nerve nuclei in the midbrain tegmentum.

- Edinger-Westphal output is conveyed through the oculomotor nerve in its parasympathetic division to synapse in the ciliary ganglion located in the midorbit.

- Ciliary ganglion outflow is to the iris and ciliary muscle via short ciliary nerves that pierce the back of the eyeball and travel within the sclera to the front of the eye.

- Light input facilitates pupil constriction; suprasegmental influences on the pupillary reflex arc from limbic, neocortical, and brainstem reticular formations are both inhibitory and excitatory.[1]

Four features of the reflex arc must be borne in mind in testing and interpreting the pupillary reactions:

1. Light-evoked neural impulses are distributed equally to both iris sphincters. Before they reach the efferent loop, the neural impulses delivered by the optic nerves undergo hemidecussation, so that each third cranial nerve parasympathetic nucleus receives identical innervation from both eyes (Fig. 8-1). Thus *an afferent loop lesion never produces a difference in pupil size (anisocoria)*. Only an efferent loop (parasympathetic or muscular) lesion will do so.

2. Focusing on a near target induces pupil constriction. The mere intention to see a near target induces pupil constriction via input from both cerebral hemispheres onto the pupillary reflex arc (the near response).[2] Therefore, when pupil reactions are tested, *the patient must maintain fixation on a distant target*, or else the pupils will constrict without relation to the light stimulus.

3. Pupil size fluctuates physiologically. The pupils fluctuate rapidly on the basis of momentary changes in alertness (physiologic pupillary unrest, or hippus).[3] To avoid being confounded by hippus, one must introduce a *strong light in a dark setting in repeated brisk rhythmic trials*.

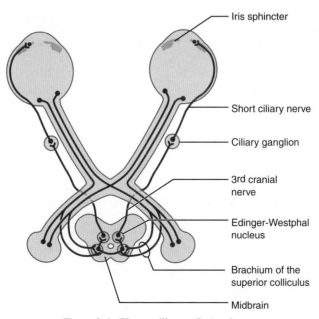

Figure 8–1. The pupillary reflex pathway.

4. The intensity of pupil constriction to light varies from one individual to another. Many factors reduce pupil constriction, including infancy, late adulthood, anxiety, diabetes, previous eye surgery or trauma, systemic narcotics, or anticholinergic agents. Therefore, judging whether a pupillary response to light is "normal" may be difficult. The swinging-light test is designed to bypass this problem by directly *comparing the pupillary responses to light between the two eyes.*

TESTING AND INTERPRETATION

After observing the size of the pupils in dim illumination, the pupillary responses to light are tested in a two-step sequence: (*1*) pupil reactions to direct light; and (*2*) swinging light-test.

Pupil Reactions to Direct Light

In a dimly lit setting, instruct the patient to fixate on a distant target. Shine a bright light directly at the right eye from about 10 inches below the inferior orbital rim, noting that the patient does not shift fixation onto the light and create a pupillary near response. Observe the amplitude of the first response and score it on a qualitative scale from 1 (least) to 4 (normal). Remove the light and introduce it below the left eye, as before. In this way, the responses of each pupil are observed and scored separately.

A reduced constriction to light may be caused by a lesion in either the afferent or efferent loop of the pupillary reflex arc. A distinction can be made by hunting for other evidence of an efferent loop disorder (anisocoria, somatic oculomotor deficits) and by performing the swinging-light test (see below) in search of an afferent loop disorder.

A normal response to light shined in each eye is compatible with a bilateral retrogeniculate cause of visual loss because the afferent loop pupillary reflex fibers exit the retinocortical pathway anterior to the lateral geniculate body. However, some pregeniculate lesions impair pupillary responses so

minimally that the responses may appear normal. The swinging-light test links the responses of the two eyes sequentially in time, in order to bring out a subtle difference in afferent function.

Swinging-Light Test

This maneuver differs from the pupil reaction to direct light test in that the light is shifted back and forth between the eyes in a rhythmic pattern in order to compare the direct reactions to light in the two eyes (Box 8-2; Fig. 8-2). If technique is suboptimal, the results will be meaningless (Box 8-3).[4,5]

In the swinging-light test, the pupil size should not normally change as the light is swung back and forth. If one pupil consistently dilates as the light is shined on the eye, or if it shows relatively more rapid escape dilation as the light remains on the eye, the response is abnormal and the patient is con-

---

Box 8–2

THE SWINGING-LIGHT TEST: PROPER TECHNIQUE

- Instruct the patient to fixate a distant target in a dark room.

- Direct a bright light at the pupil of the right eye for a count of "one-one thousand" (1 second). Aim from below the eye, so that the patient will not be tempted to fixate it (and evoke pupillary constriction to a near target).

- Shift the light briskly across the nose to the pupil of the left eye, noting whether the pupil constricts, remains the same size, or dilates.

- Shift the light back to the pupil of right eye, noting again whether the right pupil constricts, remains the same size, or dilates.

- An afferent defect is present when the pupil of one eye consistently dilates faster and more widely than that of the fellow eye after three to five repetitions of light movement across the nose.[5]

Normal   Left Afferent Pupil Defect

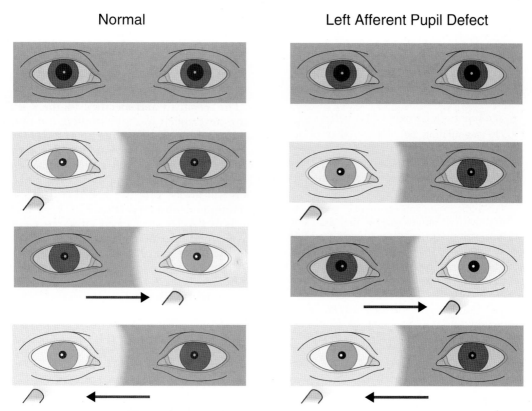

Figure 8–2. The swinging-light test. Normal result (*left column*). Patient stares at distant target in a dimly illuminated room (*top frame*). Bright light is directed at right eye from below; both pupils constrict amply and equally. Light is swung past nose and directed at left eye; both pupils remain constricted. Light is swung past nose and redirected at right eye; both pupils remain constricted. Left afferent pupil defect (*right column*). Patient stares at distant target in a dimly illuminated room (*top frame*). Bright light is directed at right eye from below and both pupils constrict amply and equally. Light is swung past nose and directed at left eye and both pupils dilate. Light is swung past nose and redirected at right eye; both pupils constrict amply.

sidered to have a relative afferent pupillary defect (RAPD) on the abnormal side.[6] Pupillometry has disclosed that a minimal RAPD may be observed as a normal finding, but its magnitude (≤ 0.3 neutral density filter log units) is so low that it is barely clinically observable.[7]

The intensity of the RAPD depends on the ratio of the volume of impulses transmitted through the two optic nerves. As a consequence, six axioms hold true.

OCULAR MEDIA OPACITIES DO NOT GENERALLY CAUSE A RAPD

Most cornea, lens, and vitreous opacities do not block light transmission, they scatter it.

In fact, mature cataracts may, by excessive light scatter, actually cause a small RAPD *in the contralateral eye.*[8] Only a dense vitreous or anterior chamber hemorrhage reduces the volume of light-induced impulses in the optic nerves.[9]

OUTER AND MIDDLE LAYER RETINAL LESIONS DO NOT CAUSE LARGE RAPDS

Damage to photoreceptors, retinal pigment epithelium, bipolar cells, and Mueller cells must be widespread or produce major structural alteration in the macular region in order to give rise to a RAPD.[10,11] For an obvious RAPD to be seen, at least half of the

Box 8–3

THE SWINGING-LIGHT TEST: ERRORS IN TECHNIQUE

- The room is too bright.
- The stimulating light is too dim or too bright.
- The light is held in front of the eye, evoking pupillary constriction as the patient fixates it.
- The light is not moved quickly and rhythmically from side to side, so that the examiner cannot differentiate an afferent pupillary defect from hippus.[3]
- The light is not swung back and forth enough times to allow a consistent pattern to emerge.
- The light is shined too long into one pupil, creating asymmetric retinal bleaching and an artificial afferent pupil defect in that eye.

retina must be detached and macular disease must cause visual acuity of 20/200 or worse.[5,12] The explanation for this phenomenon is uncertain. However, it may be that subtotal lesions in this region disturb the orderliness rather than the volume of conducted impulses. Disordered or degraded impulses impair vision but do not cause a RAPD so long as the volume of axonal traffic is maintained.

ASYMMETRIC OPTIC NERVE OR RETINAL NERVE FIBER LAYER LESIONS CAUSE MOST RAPDS

A lesion asymmetry between the two optic nerves that may barely be measurable with visual function tests can account for a RAPD. For example, in association with a variety of optic neuropathies, visual acuity[13,14] and static perimetry[15] may be completely normal, and yet the eye has a reproducible RAPD! In cases of optic neuropathy, the intensity of the RAPD, as measured with neutral density filters (Box 8-4), is correlated

with the interocular difference in central (within 30 degrees) visual field—not visual acuity.[15–18] The correlation is not perfect; that is, there is considerable variation in the intensity of RAPD associated with a given interocular difference in visual field loss.

The sensitivity and specificity of the RAPD have never been formally studied, but optic neuropathies causing more than 2 decibels of interocular difference in static mean deviation (Chapter 9) will generally cause a RAPD, and those causing more than 6 decibels will always produce a RAPD if proper technique is observed (Box 8-2).[15,16] Falsely positive RAPDs are caused either by errors in technique, a dense monocular cataract (in the other eye),[8] or anisocoria of 2 mm or greater (the eye with the smaller pupil will be relatively dark-adapted and more sensitive to light)[5] (Box 8-3).

THE RAPD PRODUCED BY ASYMMETRIC INNER RETINAL (NERVE FIBER LAYER) LESIONS IS OF MUCH LOWER INTENSITY THAN THAT PRODUCED BY ASYMMETRIC OPTIC NEUROPATHIES

The explanation probably lies in the fact that nerve fiber layer lesions, which are usually caused by retinal arterial or venous infarcts, are usually less pervasive than those caused by optic nerve disorders.

OPTIC TRACT LESIONS PRODUCE SMALL RAPDS

Because more than half the optic nerve axons cross in the chiasm, optic tract lesions cause contralateral low-intensity ($\leq$0.6 log unit) afferent pupillary defects.[19–21,25] The best explanation for this phenomenon is that the crossing fibers outnumber the noncrossing fibers in the optic chiasm. Therefore, input to the iris sphincters from the eye contralateral to the tract lesion will be reduced relative to that from the ipsilateral eye. The homonymous hemianopic visual field defects that produce afferent pupil defects are complete or nearly complete.[22]

Box 8–4

THE SWINGING-LIGHT TEST: QUANTIFYING THE RESULTS[25]

- Place a 0.3 log unit neutral density filter in front of the eye that does not appear to have an afferent pupil defect.
- Perform the swinging-light test as before, increasing the filters by 0.3 log unit steps until there is no longer any afferent pupil defect. Bracket the defect by adding an additional 0.3 log unit to see if you induce an afferent pupil defect in the other eye. The density of the filter that neutralizes the afferent pupil defect is entered on the record as the intensity of the defect.
- If you are not certain if an afferent pupil defect is present, place the 0.3 filter over each eye and compare the pupillary responses. If you see a consistent difference in pupillary dynamics, you have unmasked a small defect by enhancement.

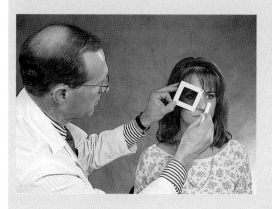
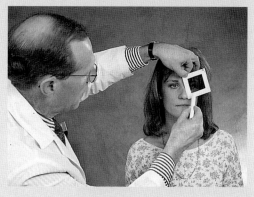

PRETECTAL LESIONS MAY RARELY PRODUCE RAPDS

An asymmetric pretectal lesion, such as a small glioma, can cause a RAPD by interrupting incoming impulses to the dorsal midbrain on one side.[23] The RAPD produced by a unilateral pretectal lesion is based on the same mechanism as that governing the RAPD associated with a unilateral optic tract RAPD (see above). Unlike optic tract lesions, however, tectal lesions do not damage the optic pathway, and therefore visual function is normal.

The RAPD is a more sensitive means of detecting asymmetric optic neuropathy or retinal nerve fiber layer lesions than visual evoked potentials (Chapter 9), the other objective test used in this setting.[14,24]

SUMMARY

Pupillary reactions to light are valuable in identifying monocular or asymmetric binocular optic nerve lesions and in differentiating pregeniculate from postgeniculate lesions.

The swinging-light test is designed to bring out subtle differences in pupil reactions to light between the two eyes. A relative afferent pupil defect (RAPD) is an objective and sensitive indicator of asymmetric optic nerve lesions, but the test fails if technique is flawed.

Low-intensity RAPDs may also be found in optic tract and pretectal lesions. They are never caused by ipsilateral lens or corneal opacities, but a dense intraocular hemorrhage may cause them.

REFERENCES

1. Kardon RH. Anatomy and physiology of the pupil. In: Miller NR, Newman NJ, eds. *Walsh & Hoyt's Clinical Neuro-ophthalmology.* 5th ed. Vol 1. Baltimore: Williams & Wilkins; 1998:847–897.
2. Weinstein JM. Anatomy and physiology of accommodation. In: Miller NR, Newman NJ, eds. *Walsh & Hoyt's Clinical Neuro-ophthalmology.* 5th ed. Vol 1. Baltimore: Williams & Wilkins; 1998:899–915.
3. Kawasaki A, Moore P, Kardon RH. Variability of the relative afferent pupillary defect. *Am J Ophthalmol.* 1995;120:622–633.
4. Thompson JS, Corbett JJ, Cox TA. How to measure the relative afferent pupillary defect. *Surv Ophthalmol.* 1981;26:39–43.
5. Thompson HS, Corbett JJ. Asymmetry of pupillomotor input. *Eye.* 1991;5:36–39.
6. Bell RA, Waggoner PM, Boyd WM, et al. Clinical grading of relative afferent pupillary defects. *Arch Ophthalmol.* 1993;111:938–942.
7. Kawasaki A, Moore P, Kardon RH. Long-term fluctuation of relative afferent pupillary defect in subjects with normal visual function. *Am J Ophthalmol.* 1996;122:875–882.
8. Lam BL, Thompson HS. A unilateral cataract produces a relative afferent pupillary defect in contralateral eye. *Ophthalmology.* 1990;97:334–338.
9. Abrams GW, Knighton RW. Falsely extinguished bright-flash electroretinogram: its association with dense vitreous hemorrhage. *Arch Ophthalmol.* 1982; 100:1427–1429.
10. Thompson HS, Watsky RC, Weinstein JM. Pupillary dysfunction in macular disease. *Trans Am Ophthalmol Soc.* 1980;78:311–317.
11. Slamovits TL, Glaser JS. The pupils and accommodation. In: Glaser JS, ed. *Neuro-ophthalmology.* 2nd ed. Philadelphia: Lippincott; 1990:459–486.
12. Newsome DA, Milton RC, Gass JDM. Afferent pupillary defect in macular degeneration. *Am J Ophthalmol.* 1981;92:396–402.
13. Burde RM, Gallin PF. Visual parameters associated with recovered retrobulbar optic neuritis. *Am J Ophthalmol.* 1975;79:1034–1037.
14. Han DP, Thompson HS, Folk JC. Differentiation between recently resolved optic neuritis and central serous retinopathy: use of tests of visual function. *Arch Ophthalmol.* 1985;103:394–396.
15. Johnson LN, Hill RA, Bartholomew MJ. Correlation of afferent pupillary defect with visual field loss on automated perimetry. *Ophthalmology.* 1988;95:1649–1655.
16. Kardon RH, Haupert CL, Thompson HS. The relationship between static perimetry and the relative afferent pupillary defect. *Am J Ophthalmol.* 1993; 115:351–356.
17. Thompson HS, Montague P, Cox TA, et al. The relationship between visual acuity, pupillary defect and visual loss. *Am J Ophthalmol.* 1982;93:681–688.
18. Brown RH, Zilis JD, Lynch MG, Sanborn GE. The afferent pupillary defect in asymmetric glaucoma. *Arch Ophthalmol.* 1987;105:1540–1543.
19. Bell RA, Thompson HS. Relative afferent pupillary defect in optic tract hemianopias. *Am J Ophthalmol.* 1978;85:538–540.
20. Newman SA, Miller NR. Optic tract syndrome: neuro-ophthalmologic considerations. *Arch Ophthalmol.* 1983;101:187–193.
21. Anderson DR, Trobe JD, Hood TW, Gebarski SS. Optic tract injury after anterior temporal lobectomy. *Ophthalmology.* 1989;96:1065–1072.
22. Miller NR. *Walsh & Hoyt's Clinical Neuro-ophthalmology.* 4th ed. Vol 1. Baltimore: Williams & Wilkins; 1982:130.
23. Forman L, Behrens MM, Odel JG, Spector RT, Hilal S. Relative afferent pupillary defect with normal visual function. *Arch Ophthalmol.* 1990;108:1074–1075.
24. Cox TA, Thompson HS, Hayreh SS, Snyder JE. Visual evoked potential and pupillary signs: a comparison in optic nerve disease. *Arch Ophthalmol.* 1982;100:1603–1607.
25. Fineberg E, Thompson HS. Quantitation of the afferent pupillary defect. In: Smith JL, ed. *Neuro-ophthalmology Focus 1980.* New York: Masson; 1979: 25–30.

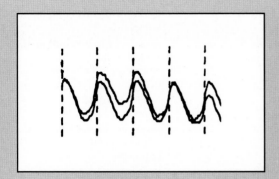

Chapter 9

DARK ADAPTOMETRY, ELECTRORETINOGRAPHY, AND VISUAL EVOKED POTENTIALS

Dark adaptometry, electroretinography, and visual evoked potentials are ancillary studies of the visual system. Available only in referral centers, their indications are limited. Dark adaptometry offers a subjective assessment of rod photoreceptor function. Electroretinography objectively measures the function of rods, cones, Mueller cells, and bipolar cells. Visual evoked potentials document signal transmission from the photoreceptors to visual cortex (Table 9-1).

DARK ADAPTOMETRY

Rationale

Dark adaptometry (DA) measures the eye's ability to detect the dimmest light presented at various points eccentric to fixation. It predicts how visually impaired a patient will be in low light conditions, but it is a subjective measure of rod function. Dark adaptometry complements electroretinography (ERG),

147

Table 9–1. **Ancillary Tests of Vision**

Test	Advantages	Disadvantages
Dark adaptometry	Quantitative measure of rod function	Requires special equipment Subjective
Full-field electroretinography	Objective and quantitative measure of cone and rod function	Requires special equipment Sensitive only to widespread disease
Foveal electroretinography	Objective measure of foveal function	Requires special equipment and expertise Expensive
Multifocal electroretinography	Objective measure of regional retinal function	Requires special equipment and expertise Expensive
Visual evoked potentials	Objective measure of retino-cortical conduction	Requires special expertise Unreliable

an objective test used to assess photoreceptor function (see below).

Testing Methods

After being exposed to a bright light (bleaching stimulus), the patient is seated with her head positioned to view the inside of a white bowl that is similar to that used in perimetry (Fig. 9-1). With one eye occluded, the patient fixes on a light-emitting diode. An eccentric spot of light of varying intensities is shown until the dimmest detectable intensity, the dark adaptation threshold, is determined. Thresholds are sequentially determined for several positions away from the point of fixation. A curve of dark adaptation is computed by measuring thresholds at given time intervals against stimulus intensity (in microapostilbs). An initial increase in dark adaptation is mediated by cones, carrying sensitivity to 10^5 microapostilbs. After 10 minutes, rod adaptation begins and, in normal subjects, sensitivity reaches 10^1 to 10^2 microapostilbs (Fig. 9-2a). The normal latency of rod adaptation creates a kink in the dark adaptation curve known as the *cone–rod break.*

Interpretation

In cases of damage to the rod photoreceptors, the dark adaptation final threshold will be elevated 1 or more log units (Fig. 9-2b).

In cases of preferential damage to the cone photoreceptors (cone dystrophies), the cone–rod break will be elevated by 1 or more log units (Fig. 9-2c). Night blindness (nyctalopia), the complaint of poor vision in low light, emerges only in conditions that elevate the rod final threshold elevation above 3 log

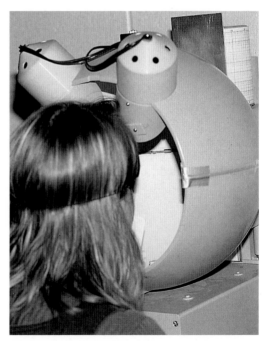

Figure 9–1. Dark adaptation testing. The patient wears occluders on both eyes for 40 minutes, then uncovers one eye and places her head in the bowl. At several points eccentric to fixation, a spot of light is presented monocularly at increasing intensities until a detection threshold is determined.

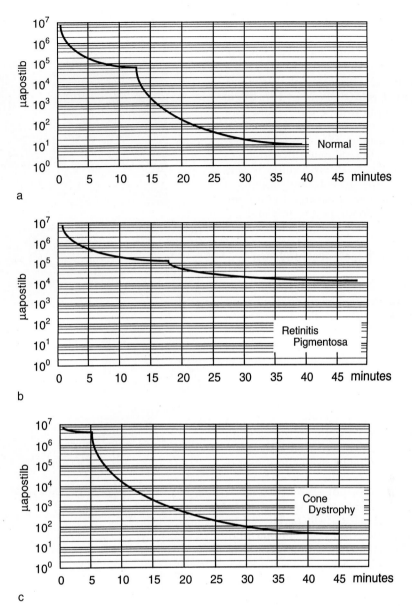

Figure 9–2. Normal and abnormal dark adaptation. (*a*) Normal dark adaptation. (*b*) Abnormal dark adaptation in hereditary rod photoreceptor degeneration (retinitis pigmentosa). (*c*) Abnormal dark adaptation in cone dystrophy.

units (Fig. 9-2). Such elevations occur most commonly in patients with hereditary retinal degeneration (retinitis pigmentosa). Elevations of 1 to 2 log units are found in patients who have a variety of neurodegenerative states, such as multiple system atrophy, spinocerebellar degenerations, mitochondrial encephalomyopathies, and storage disorders.[1] They do not complain of night vision difficulty.

ELECTRORETINOGRAPHY

Rationale

The electroretinogram (ERG) is an objective, sensitive, and specific indicator of outer retinal function.[2] However, the standard full-field ERG is sensitive only to *widespread* outer retinal disorders. *The full-field ERG will be normal in all disorders limited to the inner retina and in regional outer retinal disorders,* including those limited to the critically important foveal region where visual acuity is mediated.

Modifications in the ERG have extended its capability to the measurement of regional, including foveal, retinal disorders (the foveal ERG[3] and the multifocal ERG).[4,5] All forms of the ERG require expensive equipment and scrupulous technique. When properly performed, however, the full-field ERG produces reliable signals whose interpretation is well-standardized.[6] The foveal and multifocal ERGs are not perfected enough to have entered the clinical arena on a wide scale.

The Full-Field Electroretinogram

The eye is fitted with a corneal contact lens containing a recording electrode referenced to another electrode on the conjunctiva, forehead, or earlobe (Fig. 9-3). The patient's head is placed within a white bowl. A diffuse, bright flash of light reflected off the bowl illuminates the entire retina (ganzfeld stimulus). The voltage change in the retina induced by the light flash is recorded by the corneal contact lens electrode.

The full-field ERG waveform consists of an initial cornea-negative potential, called the "a wave," that originates from the photoreceptors. This is followed by a cornea-positive "b wave" generated by potassium currents in the Mueller cells (Fig. 9-4). One or more components of the ERG will be altered by disease of the outer retina, including photoreceptors, Mueller cells, and bipolar cells. Lesions of the photoreceptors will reduce the amplitude of both the a and b waves because photoreceptor transmission is necessary to generate Mueller cell potassium currents. Lesions limited to the Mueller and bipolar cells, but sparing photoreceptors, will depress only the b wave, sparing the a wave. *Lesions of the inner retina—the retinal ganglion cells and their axons—do not affect the full-field ERG.*

By varying the stimulus parameters and the state of the eye's adaptation to light, the full-field ERG can determine whether rods or cones are selectively damaged. When the ERG is recorded under bright (photopic) conditions and after a bright white flash or a 30-hertz flickering white light, the wave is generated principally by cones. When it is

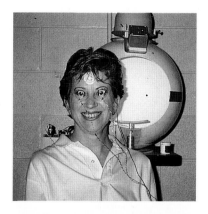

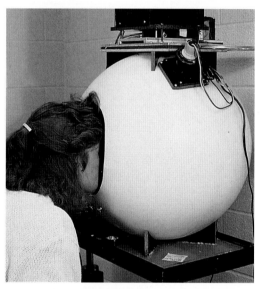

Figure 9–3. Full-field electroretinography testing. A corneal contact lens containing a recording electrode is referenced to another electrode on the conjunctiva, forehead, or earlobe. The patient's head is then placed within a white bowl. A diffuse, bright light is flashed intermittently within the bowl. The voltage change in the retina induced by the light flash is recorded by the corneal contact lens electrode.

recorded under dark (scotopic) conditions, and after a dim white or blue flash, the wave is generated principally by rods (Fig. 9-4).

Because of its sensitivity and objectivity, the full-field ERG is a critical test for evaluating widespread outer retinal disorders, particularly the heritable retinal photoreceptor degenerations that occur as isolated manifestations or as part of neurodegenerative states. In the presence of night vision difficulty or a finding of pigmentary retinopa-

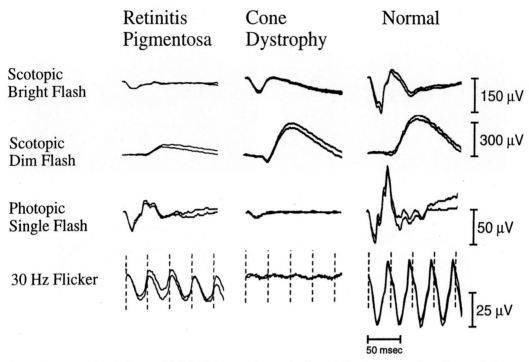

Figure 9–4. Normal and abnormal full-field electroretinography. In retinitis pigmentosa (hereditary rod photoreceptor dystrophy) (*left column*), the wave amplitude is particularly low when the eye is stimulated under scotopic conditions. These stimulus conditions selectively challenge rod function. In patients with cone dystrophy (*middle column*), which primarily damages cones, wave amplitude is normal under scotopic conditions but low in photopic and flicker conditions, which selectively challenge cone function.

thy, a normal full-field ERG excludes a hereditary retinal degeneration.

The full-field ERG is sensitive to minimal photoreceptor damage, but only if a majority of the receptor population is affected. Thus the waveform will generally not be deformed by conditions limited to the macula (such as age-related macular degeneration or some rare heritable photoreceptor disorders), or to other sectors of the outer retina. It is in the diagnosis of these regionally limited conditions that the foveal and multifocal ERG have become especially useful.

The Foveal Electroretinogram

This test differs from the full-field ERG in that the stimulus consists of a sinusoidal red flicker aimed at the fovea from a ganzfeld bowl or hand-held ophthalmoscope. (When the stimulus is delivered from the ganzfeld bowl, the peripheral retina is desensitized by background light in the bowl.) To overcome the low intensity of the evoked potential, it

is summated by signal-averaging, as is customary in performing cortical evoked potentials. Measurements of phase lag of the foveal ERG at several flicker frequencies provide an assessment of foveal (macular) cone function.[3]

The foveal ERG is sensitive enough to foveal disorders (maculopathies) that it becomes abnormal even when structural changes are not evident on ophthalmoscopy.[7,8] It can also be used to determine the source of an abnormal visual evoked potential (VEP; see below). Thus if both the foveal ERG and the VEP are abnormal, damage must lie within the fovea.

The Multifocal Electroretinogram

The multifocal ERG (Fig. 9-5) is recorded in a fashion similar to the full-field ERG, but the patient fixates a cathode ray tube monitor and watches 241 flickering hexagons that stimulate 23 degrees of the visual field. An array of miniature ERG wavelets is produced. The amplitude of the b wave indicates the

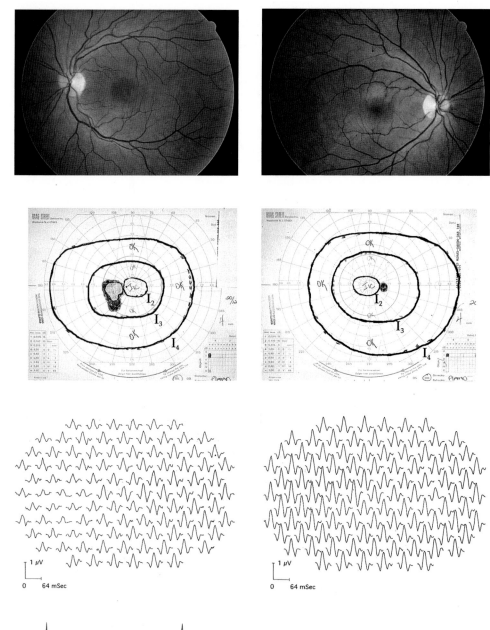

Figure 9–5. Multifocal electroretinography. A 32-year-old woman complained of a flickering scotoma temporal to fixation in her left eye of one month's duration. Ophthalmoscopy showed only mild nasal disk margin blurring in the left eye (a). Visual acuities were 20/15 in each eye, but Goldmann perimetry disclosed enlargement of the physiologic blind spot in the left eye (b). Full-field ERG was normal. Multifocal electroretinography revealed depressed wavelets in the region of the blind spot in the left eye and was normal in the right eye (c). Scalar representation of wavelet amplitude (d) shows depression of perifoveal function in the left eye. (Courtesy of Randy Kardon, M.D.)

integrity of the corresponding region of the outer retina.[4]

The major contribution of the multifocal ERG is the ability to provide objective evidence of regional (multifocal, sectoral) outer retinal dysfunction, that is, disease concentrated in particular areas rather than widely spread. This tool extends the physician's ability to diagnose cases of multifocal retinal pigment epitheliopathies (Fig. 9-5),[5] hereditary retinal photoreceptor degenerations limited to small sectors, and macular dystrophies that produce little or no ophthalmoscopic or angiographic abnormalities. These entities would escape detection on the full-field ERG because they do not cause widespread dysfunction.

VISUAL EVOKED POTENTIALS

Rationale

Visual evoked potentials[9] are the only electrophysiologic means to assess function across the entire retinocortical pathway. Unlike ERGs, VEPs are easily degraded by poor cooperation, defocusing, and nystagmus,[10] and they are further compromised by a lack of sensitivity and specificity (Table 9-1).[11,12]

Testing Methods

Visual evoked potential tests utilize flash stimuli when visual fixation is poor, as it may be with babies, uncooperative adults, and those with very poor vision. Otherwise, the standard stimulus is a checkerboard pattern of black and white squares reversing at 1 or 2 hertz. The sizes of the square or check range from a subtense of 15 to 60 minutes of arc (Fig. 9-6). The VEP response is generally recorded by an occipital scalp electrode attached 5 cm above the inion and referenced to the midfrontal area. Waveforms are produced as an average of 100 to 200 checkerboard reversals.

Interpretation

Almost entirely generated by the central (foveal) 5 degrees of the visual field, the nor-

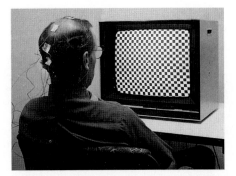

Figure 9–6. Visual evoked potentials testing.

mal signal-averaged VEP wave has an amplitude of 5 to 10 microvolts and a major positive peak at about 100 milliseconds (P100 peak) (Fig. 9-7). The amplitude of the VEP, usually measured from the P100 to the next trough, is too variable between subjects to use as a measure of pathology. Because amplitude is relatively constant between eyes, however, it confirms the presence of unilateral or asymmetric optic nerve disease if there is at least a twofold difference between eyes. The latency of the P100 is the most reliable VEP parameter because its intersubject values fall within a narrow range.

The VEP latency will be prolonged in any disorder affecting signal transmission from the outer retina to the primary visual cortex. Its contribution to medical diagnosis is best considered in the context of the five settings in which it is commonly used (Table 9-2).

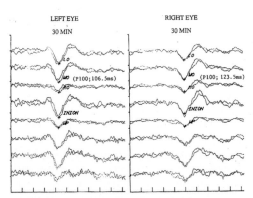

Figure 9–7. Abnormal pattern visual evoked potentials. In a patient with right eye optic neuritis, the tracing from the left eye shows a normal latency, whereas that from the right eye shows a prolongation.

Table 9–2. **Clinical Use of Visual Evoked Potentials**

Clinical Problem	Limitations
Searching for a subclinical "other" lesion in suspected multiple sclerosis	Insensitive relative to MRI
Making a diagnosis of multiple sclerosis in a patient with obvious optic neuritis	Insensitive relative to MRI
Making a diagnosis of optic neuropathy when there are visual complaints but equivocal clinical findings	Useful only if optic neuropathy is symmetrical and there is no afferent pupil defect
Differentiating optic neuritis from other optic neuropathies	Nonspecific
Assessing vision in infants who appear blind	Unreliable
Assessing vision in patients suspected of nonorganic blindness	Unreliable

SEARCHING FOR A SUBCLINICAL "OTHER" LESION IN SUSPECTED MULTIPLE SCLEROSIS

The VEP test is less helpful here than magnetic resonance imaging (MRI). Visual evoked potential latencies are found in 30%–95% of patients with suspected multiple sclerosis, depending on the degree of clinical signs and symptoms.[13] In a study of 200 patients with clinically possible or probable MS, VEPs were abnormal in 46%, approximately as sensitive as somatosensory evoked potentials, spinal fluid oligoclonal bands, and MRI.[14] However, in 25% of the VEP-normal cases, laboratory-supported definite MS could be diagnosed by means of MRI or oligoclonal bands. In only 12 cases (6%) was the VEP the only abnormal paraclinical test. A further drawback in using VEP to support a diagnosis of MS is that its findings are nonspecific. Prolonged latencies have been reported in such conditions as Parkinson's disease, Huntington's disease, Friedreich's ataxia, ataxia telangiectasia, Alzheimer's disease, and hepatic encephalopathy—even without overt signs of visual dysfunction.[15] Therefore, VEP has lost its preeminence within the matrix of tests used to support a clinical diagnosis of MS.

A common misapplication of the VEP is in the evaluation of patients presenting with acute and clinically isolated optic neuropathy. A VEP is typically performed to document abnormal latency in the unaffected eye. (Prolonged latency in the eye with optic neuritis is expected.) A large study found a 27% prevalence of prolonged latency in the unaffected eyes of patients with contralateral optic neuritis.[16] But MRI signal abnormalities highly suggestive of MS have been found in 50%–70% of these patients,[13,17–19] making VEP less sensitive to dissemination than MRI in this setting.

MAKING A DIAGNOSIS OF OPTIC NEUROPATHY WHEN THERE ARE VISUAL COMPLAINTS BUT EQUIVOCAL CLINICAL FINDINGS

A VEP is not necessary in this setting if an afferent pupil defect is found (Chapter 8). With proper technique, the swinging-light test (Chapter 8) offers a more rapid, more sensitive, and less expensive measurement than VEP.[20] On the other hand, VEP is useful as the only objective means of documenting *bilateral, symmetrical* optic neuropathies in association with toxic,[21] nutritional, hereditary, or degenerative conditions where clinical examination is equivocal (Chapter 13).

DIFFERENTIATING OPTIC NEURITIS FROM OTHER OPTIC NEUROPATHIES

If an optic neuropathy is evident but its etiology is unclear, a VEP is of limited value in refining the diagnosis. Although reduced-amplitude VEPs with relatively normal latency are typical of ischemic optic neuropathy (an axonal rather than demyelinating lesion) and greatly prolonged latencies are characteristic of optic neuritis, compressive lesions and even amblyopia may prolong latency.[12,22] History and clinical examination provide more reliable differential diagnostic information.

ASSESSING VISION IN INFANTS WHO APPEAR BLIND

Because of poor fixation, flash VEPs must be used to evaluate babies. They offer only a gross assessment of neurotransmission in the visual pathway. Flash VEPs have been intact in blind babies despite anatomic evidence of destruction of extrastriate visual cortex.[23,24] Even pattern VEPs may be normal in patients with cortical blindness.[25–27] These tests evidently sample only a part of the pathway needed for seeing.[28] *Among infants who appear to have poor vision but no apparent encephalopathy, the first test to perform is not the VEP but the full-field ERG,* which will be abnormal in those with congenital retinal receptor disorders (rod monochromatism, Leber's congenital amaurosis) or synaptic disorders (congenital stationary night blindness). The ERG will, however, be normal in cases of macular and optic nerve hypoplasias. These latter conditions might be diagnosed only if the stimulus were placed on the fovea with an ophthalmoscope.

ASSESSING VISION IN PATIENTS SUSPECTED OF NONORGANIC BLINDNESS

Here the VEP is disappointingly limited as a screening test because it is so dependent on visual fixation. Despite attempts at monitoring fixation, malingerers find a way to defocus or look away from the target often enough to degrade the VEP.[29–31] Moreover, a normal VEP is no guarantee of normal vision.

ELECTROPHYSIOLOGIC EVALUATION OF VISION LOSS: ALL TOOLS CONSIDERED

Combined use of the standard (full-field) and modified (foveal, multifocal) ERGs and VEPs offers the potential of localizing visual pathway disease by electrophysiologic means

alone (Table 9-3). Diffuse damage to the outer retina (photoreceptor, Mueller, and bipolar cells) causes an abnormal full-field ERG. Diffuse disease of cones disturbs the phototopic and flicker ERGs; diffuse disease of rods disturbs the scotopic ERG. Regional (multifocal) damage of the outer retina causes an abnormal multifocal ERG but spares the full-field ERG. Disease limited to the fovea (macula) causes an abnormal multifocal and foveal ERG, but it also spares the full-field ERG. Damage to the inner retina (retinal ganglion cells and axons), the optic nerve, optic chiasm, or retrochiasmal visual pathway disease spares all forms of the ERG but alters the VEP.

SUMMARY

Dark adaptometry is a subjective test of rod function. It measures the rod threshold, the ability of the eye to detect light of low intensity in the dark. Patients with night blindness (nyctalopia), a common complaint among patients with hereditary photoreceptor dystrophies, typically have a 3 or more log unit elevation in rod threshold. Although rod dysfunction is common in many neurodegenerative conditions, the rod threshold elevations are typically too low to cause night blindness.

Full-field electroretinography is a sensitive and objective measure of outer retinal (rod, cone, bipolar cell, Mueller cell) function. It becomes abnormal only if a preponderance of the outer retina is damaged. The foveal ERG is sensitive to dysfunction limited to the fovea. The multifocal ERG detects regional disorders of the retina, including those limited to the fovea.

Visual evoked potentials are used to investigate subclinical optic neuropathy in MS, diagnose subtle optic neuropathy in patients with visual complaints, differentiate demyelinating from other optic neuropathies, and assess vision in babies who appear to be blind and in individuals suspected of having nonorganic (psychogenic) blindness. In most of these tasks, the clinical value of VEPs is compromised either by lack of sensitivity or specificity or by the fact that other tests provide better information. Visual evoked potentials are, however, helpful in investigating bilaterally symmetrical (toxic, nutri-

Table 9–3. Electrophysiologic Evaluation of Vision Loss: All Tools Considered

Test	Diffuse Damage to Outer Retina	Diffuse Damage to Cones	Diffuse Damage to Rods	Regional (Multifocal) Damage to Outer Retina	Damage Limited to the Fovea	Damage from Inner Retina to Primary Visual Cortex
Full-field scotopic ERG	Abnormal	Normal	Abnormal	Normal	Normal	Normal
Full-field photopic ERG	Abnormal	Abnormal	Normal	Normal	Normal	Normal
Full-field flicker ERG	Abnormal	Abnormal	Normal	Normal	Normal	Normal
Foveal ERG	Abnormal	Abnormal	Normal	Normal or abnormal	Abnormal	Normal
Multifocal ERG	Abnormal	Abnormal	Abnormal	Abnormal	Abnormal	Normal
Visual evoked potentials	Abnormal	Abnormal	Abnormal	Normal or abnormal	Abnormal	Abnormal

tional, hereditary) optic neuropathies when clinical signs are equivocal.

Combined use of the full-field ERG, foveal ERG, multifocal ERG, and VEP allows reasonable objective localization of visual pathway disease. Diffuse damage to the photoreceptor, Mueller, and bipolar cells alters the full-field ERG. Damage to cones disturbs the photopic and flicker ERGs, whereas damage to rods disturbs the scotopic ERG. Regional damage of the outer retina causes an abnormal multifocal ERG. Disease limited to the fovea (macula) causes an abnormal multifocal and foveal ERG. Damage to the retinal ganglion cells, their axons, the optic nerve, optic chiasm, or retrochiasmal visual pathway disease spares all forms of the ERG but alters the VEP.

REFERENCES

1. Bateman JB, Lang GE, Maumenee IH. Multisystem genetic disorders associated with retinal dystrophies. In: Ryan SJ, ed. *Retina.* 2nd ed. Vol 1. St. Louis: Mosby; 1994:467–491.
2. Heckenlively JR, Arden GB. *Principles and Practice of Clinical Electrophysiology of Vision.* St. Louis: Mosby-Yearbook; 1991.
3. Carr RE, Siegel IM. *Electrodiagnostic Testing of the Visual System.* Philadelphia: FA Davis; 1990.
4. Sutter EE, Tran D. The field topography of ERG components in man. 1. The photopic luminance response. *Vision Res.* 1992;32:433–446.
5. Kondo M, Miyake Y, Horiguchi M, Suzuki S, Tanikawa A. Clinical evaluation of multifocal electroretinogram. *Invest Ophthalmol Vis Sci.* 1995;36:2146–2150.
6. Marmor MF. An updated standard for clinical electroretinography. *Arch Ophthalmol.* 1995;113:1375–1376.
7. Matthews GP, Sandberg MA, Berson EL. Foveal cone electroretinograms in patients with central visual loss of unexplained etiology. *Arch Ophthalmol.* 1992;110:1568–1570.
8. Miyake Y, Horiguchi M, Tomita N, et al. Occult macular dystrophy. *Am J Ophthalmol.* 1996;122:644–653.
9. Celesia GG, Peachey NS, Brigell M, DeMarco PJ Jr. Visual evoked potentials: recent advances. *Electroenceph Clin Neurophysiol Suppl.* 1996;46:3–14.
10. Smith DN. The clinical usefulness of the visual evoked response. *J Pediatr Ophthalmol Strabismus.* 1984;21:235–236.
11. Eisen A, Cracco RQ. Overuse of evoked potentials: caution. *Neurology.* 1983;33:618–621.
12. Aminoff MJ, Goodin DS. Visual evoked potentials. *J Clin Neurophysiol.* 1994;11:493–499.
13. Chiappa KH. *Evoked Potentials in Clinical Medicine.* New York: Raven Press; 1983.
14. Paty DW, Oger JJF, Kastrukoff LF, et al. MRI in the diagnosis of MS: a prospective study with comparison of clinical evaluation, evoked potentials, oligoclonal banding, and CT. *Neurology.* 1988;38:180–185.
15. Verhagen WIM, Horsten GPM. The visual evoked potential and the electroretinogram in clinical neuro-ophthalmology. In: Lessell S, Van Dalen JTW, eds. *Current Neuro-ophthalmology.* Vol. 1 Chicago: Year Book Medical Publishers; 1988:305–318.
16. Miller DH, Newton MR, Van der Poel EPGH, et al. Magnetic resonance imaging of the optic nerve in optic neuritis. *Neurology.* 1988;38:175–179.
17. Ormerod IE, McDonald WI, DuBoulay GH, et al. Disseminated lesions at presentation in patients with optic neuritis. *J Neurol Neurosurg Psychiatry.* 1986;49:124–127.
18. Jacobs L, Kinkel PR, Kinkel WR. Silent brain lesions in patients with isolated idiopathic optic neuritis: a clinical and nuclear magnetic resonance imaging study. *Arch Neurol.* 1986;43:452–455.
19. Johns K, Lavin P, Elliott JH, Partain CL. Magnetic resonance imaging of the brain in isolated optic neuritis. *Arch Ophthalmol.* 1986;104:1486–1488.
20. Cox TA, Thompson HS, Hayreh SS, Snyder JE. Visual evoked potentials and pupillary signs: a comparison in optic nerve disease. *Arch Ophthalmol.* 1982;100:1603–1607.
21. Yannikas C, Walsh JC, McLeod JG. Visual evoked potentials in the detection of subclinical optic toxic effects secondary to ethambutol. *Arch Neurol.* 1983;40:645–648.
22. Sokol S. Abnormal evoked potential latencies in amblyopia. *Br J Ophthalmol.* 1983;67:310–314.
23. Bodis I, Atkin A, Raab E, Wolkstein M. Visual association cortex and vision in man: pattern-evoked occipital potentials in a blind boy. *Science.* 1977;198:629–631.
24. Spehlmann R, Gross RA, Ho SU, Leetsma JF, Norcross KA. Visual evoked potentials and postmortem findings in a case of cortical blindness. *Ann Neurol.* 1977;2:531–534.
25. Celesia GG, Archer CR, Kurosiwa Y, Brigell MG. Visual function of the extrageniculo-calcarine system in man: relationship to cortical blindness. *Arch Neurol.* 1980;37:704–706.
26. Hess CW, Meienberg O, Ludin HP. Visual evoked potentials in acute occipital blindness: diagnostic and prognostic value. *J Neurol.* 1982;227:193–200.
27. Aldrich MS, Alessi AG, Beck RW, Gilman S. Cortical blindness: etiology, diagnosis and prognosis. *Ann Neurol.* 1987;21:149–158.
28. Celesia GG, Bushnell D, Cone-Toleikis S, Brigell MC. Cortical blindness and residual vision: Is the second visual system in humans capable of more than rudimentary visual perception? *Neurology.* 1991;41:862–869.
29. Bumgartner J, Epstein CM. Voluntary alteration of visual evoked potentials. *Ann Neurol.* 1982;12:475–478.
30. Tan CT, Murray NMF, Sawyers D, Leonard TJK. Deliberate alteration of the visual evoked potential. *J Neurol Neurosurg Psychiatry.* 1984;47:518–523.
31. Morgan RK, Nugent B, Harrison JM, O'Connor PS. Voluntary alteration of pattern visual evoked responses. *Ophthalmology.* 1985;92:1356–1363.

Part IV

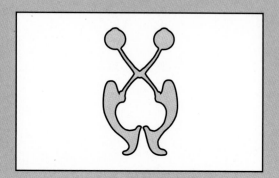

Topographic Disorders

Chapter 10

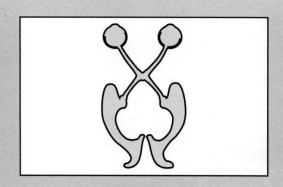

RETINA AND CHOROID I: VASCULAR DISORDERS

RETINAL AND CHOROIDAL ARTERIAL
    CIRCULATIONS
RETINAL VASCULAR REACTION
    PATTERNS
    Arteriolar Wall Changes
    Arterial Occlusion
    Precapillary Arteriolar Occlusion
    Venous Stasis
    Venous Occlusion
    Inner Blood–Retinal Barrier
        Incompetence

    Neovascularization
    Vasculitis
    Vascular Malformation
CHOROIDAL VASCULAR REACTION
    PATTERNS
    Choriocapillaris Occlusion
    Arteriolar Occlusion
    Neovascularization
    Hemangioma
SUMMARY

The retina and its underlying vascular tunic, the choroid, behave as a physiologic unit and are jointly affected by many disorders (Fig. 10-1a and Plate 1). Diagnosis depends on recognizing specific ophthalmoscopic abnormalities (Table 10-1). Dilating the pupils makes this task much easier (Box 10-1; Fig. 10-2), and skilled ophthalmoscopy is critical in obtaining a decent view (Box 10-2; Fig. 10-3).

Even through a widely dilated pupil and clear ocular media, experienced examiners will encounter retinal and choroidal disorders that display only the most subtle findings—or none at all (Table 10-2). A familiarity with these conditions is critical, because *ophthalmoscopic findings are often overlooked by ophthalmologists*. Patients are then referred to neurologists in the mistaken belief that the disease process is retrobulbar. When ophthalmoscopy is unhelpful, localization depends on other clinical features (Table 10-3).

Vascular disease accounts for a large portion of retinochoroidal disorders. This chap-

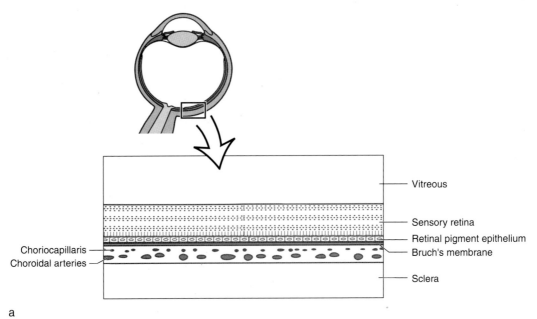

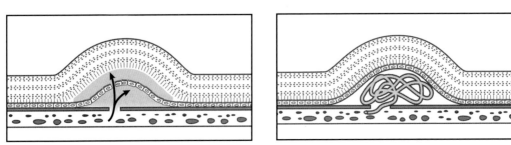

a

b   c

Figure 10–1. (*a*) The normal retina and choroid in cross section. (*b*) Breakdown of the outer blood–retinal barrier. Damage to choroidal vessels and/or overlying retinal pigment epithelium (RPE) produces a hole in the RPE that allows serous fluid to enter the sensory retina and cause a focal detachment. This occurs most commonly in the macular region. (*c*) Choroidal neovascularization. In the macular region, new blood vessels have formed in the choroid and have burrowed through the retina. They bleed easily and cause scarring.

Table 10–1. **Important Ophthalmoscopic Findings**

Abnormality	Interpretation
Optic disk rim pallor	Optic neuropathy
Optic disk cup > 1/2 disk diameter	Glaucoma
Indistinct optic disk margins	Elevated ICP, optic neuropathy, congenital disk anomaly
Retinal yellow area	Hard exudate, drusen, infiltrate
Retinal white area	Retinal microinfarct (cotton-wool spot), infiltrate, chorioretinal atrophy, drusen
Retinal gray area	Subretinal hemorrhage or tumor, gliosis
Retinal red area	Intraretinal, preretinal hemorrhage
Increased retinal arteriolar light reflection ("copper-wiring")	Arteriosclerosis
Arteriovenous nicking	Arteriosclerosis
Arteriolar cuffing	Vasculitis
Arteriolar plaque	Retinal embolus

DILATING THE PUPILS

- The safest mydriatic agent is phenylephrine 2.5%, a sympathomimetic agent that stimulates the iris dilator. It is a weaker pupil dilator than the parasympatholytic drugs (tropicamide, cyclopentolate) that paralyze the iris sphincter, but it is adequate and carries no risk of angle-closure glaucoma. If wider dilatation is necessary, a parasympatholytic agent should be used.
- Instill two drops into each eye. The pupil will dilate about 2–3 mm within 15 minutes and remain dilated for approximately 2 hours.

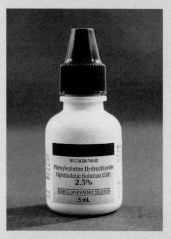

Figure 10–2. Phenylephrine hydrochloride 2.5%.

ter is devoted to that topic. Nonvascular retinochoroidal disorders are presented in the next chapter.

RETINAL AND CHOROIDAL ARTERIAL CIRCULATIONS

The ophthalmic artery divides into retinal and ciliary branches that supply the eye (Fig. 1-16). The central retinal artery nourishes the inner retina, which includes the ganglion cells and their axons. The ciliary arteries nourish the optic nerve and, via the choroidal circulation, the outer retina, including the retinal pigment epithelium (RPE), photoreceptors, Mueller cells, and bipolar cells.

RETINAL VASCULAR REACTION PATTERNS

Retinal vessels are subject to nine principal reaction patterns: wall changes, arterial occlusion, precapillary arteriolar occlusion, venous stasis, venous occlusion, inner blood–retinal barrier incompetence, neovascularization, vasculitis, and congenital malformation (Table 10-4).

Arteriolar Wall Changes

In response to acute and severe elevations in blood pressure, the muscular wall of the retinal arteries and arterioles contracts in segments. Through the ophthalmoscope,

Box 10–2

EXAMINING THE OPTIC FUNDUS

- Use your right eye to examine the patient's right eye, your left eye to examine the patient's left eye.
- Place your free hand on the patient's brow and use your thumb to gently elevate the upper lid. (This precaution is especially useful in "squeezers.")
- Select the smaller direct ophthalmoscope aperture size if the pupils are small and place the ophthalmoscope as close as possible to your eye.
- Approach the patient's eye, aiming the beam at the optic disk (15 degrees medially), so as to cause minimal pupil constriction, stopping when the ophthalmoscope is 1/4 cm from the upper lashes. Adjust the dioptric power until the disk is in focus.
- Evaluate the optic disk for color, cup size, and distinctness of margins and the retina for color changes (Table 10-1). Examine the macular region last because it is most light-sensitive.

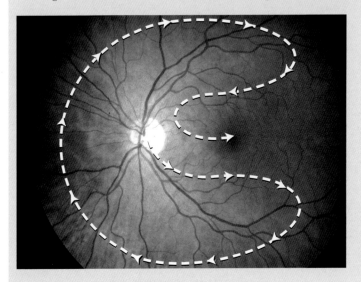

Figure 10–3. Fundus photo showing path of ophthalmoscopy.

the vessels appear focally narrowed, like beads.[1,2] By contrast, chronic (even apparently well-controlled) hypertension causes thickening of retinal arteriolar walls.[1] The basement membrane widens, lipid is deposited in the intima, and collagen forms within the media. These changes produce a brightened light reflection from the vessel wall, which at first has a bronzen sheen ("copper-wiring") and later a grayish glint ("silver-wiring"). At arteriovenous crossing points, the flaccid venous wall is flattened and the vein appears to be deviated in its course (arteriovenous nicking) (Plate 2).

Arterial Occlusion

The central retinal artery or its arteriolar branches may be occluded by local thrombosis or embolism from the heart, aortic arch, carotid artery, or ophthalmic artery (Plates 3, 4, 5).[3] The relative prevalence of thrombosis and embolism is unknown. Through the ophthalmoscope, an embolus appears as a yellow or white plaque embedded at an arterial bifurcation on the optic disk or retinal surface. Even if no embolus is seen, occlusion may still have been embolic. The embolus could be impacted deep

Table 10–2. Easy-to-Overlook Retinal Disorders That Cause Visual Acuity Loss

Category	Disorder
Dystrophy	Cone dystrophy Stargardt's disease X-linked retinoschisis
Inflammation	Choroiditis
Trauma	Contusion (commotio) Photic injury
Paraneoplasia	Cancer-associated Melanoma-associated
Ischemia	Resolved branch retinal arterial occlusion Subtle macular edema Foveal nonperfusion
Toxin	Hydroxychloroquine Deferoxamine Thioridazine
Degeneration	Macular holey Cellophane maculopathy

Table 10–3. Features That Differentiate Retinochoroidal Disorders from Other Visual Pathway Disorders

Clinical Feature	Inner Retinal Disorder	Outer Retinal or Choroidal Disorder	Optic Nerve Disorder	Optic Chiasm or Retrochiasmal Disorder
Metamorphopsia	Common	Common	Never	Rare, always binocular and temporary
Photopsias	Uncommon	Common	Uncommon	Common with visual cortex lesions, but usually temporary
Reduced color vision	Uncommon	Only if diffuse cone disorder	Common	Uncommon
Visual field defects	Often nerve fiber bundle type	Correspond to area of damage	Always nerve fiber bundle type	Hemianopic
Afferent pupil defect	Uncommon and mild	Only if very extensive and uniocular lesion	Always if involvement of two optic nerves is asymmetric	Only with optic tract lesions, and then mild

Table 10–4. **Retinal Vascular Reaction Patterns**

Reaction Pattern	Manifestations	Common Causes
Arteriolar wall changes	Focal narrowing Increased vascular light reflex Arteriovenous nicking	Acute hypertension Chronic hypertension Aging
Artery occlusion	Ischemic whitening Cherry-red spot	Arteriosclerosis Hypertension Hypercoagulable states Emboli
Precapillary arteriolar occlusion	Cotton-wool spot	Diabetes Hypertension Connective tissue disease Severe anemia HIV disease Purtscher's-like
Venous stasis	Dilated, tortuous veins Perivenous hemorrhages Cotton-wool spots Macular edema Hard exudates	Arteriosclerosis Aortic arch/carotid/ophthalmic artery stenosis Hypertension Hyperviscosity Hypercoagulability Retinal venous obstruction
Venous occlusion	Flame-shaped hemorrhages Cotton-wool spots Swollen disk	Arteriosclerosis Aortic arch/carotid/ophthalmic artery stenosis Hypertension Hyperviscosity Hypercoagulability Retinal venous obstruction
Inner blood–retinal barrier incompetence	Hemorrhages Hard exudates Edema	Diabetes Hypertension Uveitis Retinal venous stasis Vascular malformation Intraocular surgery
Neovascularization	Netlike surface vessels Fibroglial fronds Hemorrhage Retinal detachment	Diabetes Aortic arch/carotid/ophthalmic artery stenosis Sickle cell diseases Retinal vein occlusion Prematurity Idiopathic (Eales' disease)
Vasculitis	Waxlike perivascular cuffing Sausagelike vascular narrowing Ischemic whitening Cotton-wool spots Retinal hemorrhages Roth spots Vitreous haze	Sarcoidosis Behcet's disease Syphilis Tuberculosis Whipple's disease Multiple sclerosis Herpesviruses Idiopathic (Eales' disease)
Malformations	Hard exudates Exudative retinal detachment Red-pink masses Tortuous vessels	Coats' disease Von Hippel-Lindau disease Wyburn-Masson disease

within the optic nerve or have broken up and moved out of the ocular circulation. Fortunately, most emboli pass through the retinal vessels without obstructing flow enough to create infarcts. They arrive at the retina from many sources (talc from intravenous drug abusers, air from pump oxygenators, fat from long bone fractures), but there are three main types of endogenous emboli:[4]

- **Cholesterol (Hollenhorst).** Small, yellow, refractile particles derived from the carotid system or aortic arch atheromas can lodge for days to weeks at bifurcations (Plates 4, 6). Because they do not typically impede blood flow completely, they are usually found incidentally. Patients who have incidentally discovered Hollenhorst plaques and who have no history of ocular or hemispheric TIA or stroke have a 50% likelihood of developing myocardial infarction within seven years.[5] The future risk of stroke in these patients has not been prospectively studied. If their risk is akin to that of other asymptomatic patients with high-grade carotid stenosis (2% per year),[6] then the hazards of carotid endarterectomy outweigh its benefits.[7–10]
- **Platelet-fibrin.** Dull white, waferlike particles derived from the cervical carotid atheromas or heart valves mold themselves to the distal retinal vessels and usually break up within hours to days and disappear. Before moving on, they may cause retinal infarcts.
- **Calcium.** Large, white, nonrefractile particles derived from heart valves or calcified atheromas may, due to their stiffness, become impacted in proximal vessels, where they often obstruct flow, cause infarcts, and linger (Plate 7).

If an embolus or thrombus thoroughly plugs a proximal retinal arteriole, the inner retina becomes infarcted because its arterial supply is poorly collateralized. The patient complains of sudden monocular loss of vision, which is painless because the tissue has no nociceptive receptors. An infarcted retina loses its transparency and fails to transmit the red-orange color of the choroid, so it looks cloudy (ischemic whitening). If the infarction involves the macular region, a foveolar "cherry-red spot" will be visible within several hours. The cherry-red spot arises because the foveola contains no ganglion cells or axons.

It transmits the red color of the underlying choroid, surrounded by a halo of cloudy, infarcted perifoveolar retina. If the retina displays perifoveolar whitening but has no cherry-red spot, suspect a combined retinal and choroidal arterial infarction, owing to occlusion of the parent ophthalmic artery. Patients with ophthalmic artery infarcts typically suffer more profound and enduring visual loss than those with retinal artery infarcts. Ophthalmic artery infarcts have four major causes: severe anterior circulation arteriosclerosis, giant cell arteritis, mucormycosis, and orbitocranial trauma (Table 10-5).

Retinal transparency returns within three weeks of the infarct,[4] but death of its inner layers thins out the tissue. Ischemic retinal thinning can be visualized only with great skill and biomicroscopic aids. If the infarct has been extensive, clues include a narrowed retinal arterial tree and a pale optic disk. But if the patient has suffered a less extensive infarct, there may be no obvious ophthalmoscopic evidence for visual loss. Months after the event, occluded retinal arterioles may develop focal whitish yellow sheathing that is often mistakenly diagnosed as a fresh embolic plaque or active vasculitis (Plate 8).

Although central retinal artery occlusion is managed as an ophthalmic emergency, therapies have never been proved to be effective. Efforts are made to quickly lower intraocular pressure by withdrawing aqueous fluid with anterior chamber needle puncture, massaging the globe, and administering intravenous acetazolamide. Another traditional treatment is the breathing of a 95% oxygen/5% carbon dioxide gas mixture in order to produce higher oxygen tension and vasodilatation. Thrombolysis, delivered by catheterization of the ophthalmic artery, has been anecdotally effective and safe.[11,12] However, no large controlled trials have been conducted to verify the efficacy of this intervention.

Even if emergency treatment does not work, some recovery of vision may eventually occur. The patient requires an evaluation for the same conditions that predispose to ischemic stroke elsewhere in the central nervous system: hypertension, atherosclerosis, aortic arch and cervical carotid stenosis, cardiac valvular, mural, or rhythm abnormalities, hypercoagulable states, and connective

Table 10–5. **Causes of Retinal Vascular Occlusions**

Ophthalmic Artery Occlusion	Central Retinal Artery Occlusion	Branch Retinal Artery Occlusion	Retinal Precapillary Arteriole Occlusion (Cotton-Wool Spot)	Central Retinal Vein Occlusion	Branch Retinal Vein Occlusion
Arteriosclerosis	Hypertension	Hypertension	Diabetes	Arteriosclerosis	Arteriosclerosis
Giant cell arteritis	Arteriosclerosis	Heart, aortic arch, carotid system embolism	Hypertension	Hypertension	Hypertension
Mucormycosis	Heart, aortic arch, carotid system embolism		Blood dyscrasia	Hypercoagulable states	
Orbitocranial trauma			HIV	Hyperviscosity states	
	Hypercoagulable state		X-irradiation	Orbital lesion	
	Hypotension		IV drug abuse	Cavernous sinus fistula	
			Chest trauma	Venous obstructive neck or thoracic lesion	
			Pancreatitis		
			Bacteremia		
			Syphilis		
			Rickettsiosis		
			Altitude sickness		

tissue disorders.[3] In young individuals, and those who lack ample arteriosclerotic risk factors, the workup is tilted strongly toward unusual hypercoagulable states and cardiac disorders.

Survival after retinal artery occlusion is relatively reduced. Death is due largely to myocardial infarction.[13] The future risk of hemispheric stroke after ipsilateral retinal artery occlusion in patients with high-grade carotid stenosis who are treated with aspirin alone is believed to be about 2%–3% per year,[7,14,15] much lower than that for hemispheric TIA or minor stroke. Whether this low stroke risk justifies the hazards of carotid endarterectomy is doubtful (Chapter 3).

Precapillary Arteriolar Occlusion

If an occlusion affects a small precapillary arteriole rather than a large arteriole, the infarct will smudge the retinal surface with a tiny patch of gray-white—a "cotton-wool spot" (Plate 9).

Located in the posterior retina within ten disk diameters of the optic disk, cotton-wool spots are clusters of distended and exploded retinal ganglion cell axons. Their axoplasmic flow is halted by hypoxia-ischemia.[16] They are often surrounded by hemorrhage because the ischemic vessel also leaks blood. Such a white-centered hemorrhage is called a *Roth spot.* Incorrectly believed to be pathognomonic for bacterial endocarditis,[17] it is merely a modified cotton-wool spot.

Any condition that causes retinal microvascular occlusion will produce cotton-wool spots.[18] Diabetes, hypertension, connective tissue disorders, and severe anemia (<6 g hemoglobin)[19] lead the list, joined recently by HIV disease. Other considerations are retinal venous obstruction, cardiogenic or arteriogenic embolism, intravenous drug abuse, cranial arteritis, exposure to therapeutic x-irradiation, chest trauma, pancreatitis, bacteremia, spirochetal and rickettsial diseases, blood dyscrasias, and altitude sickness. As with larger retinal infarcts, the pathogenesis may be embolic (cardiogenic or septicemic) or thrombotic (leukemic plug, severe anemia, vasculitis, immune complex deposition, antiphospholipid antibody, malignant hypertensive fibrinoid wall necrosis).

A plethora of cotton-wool spots scattered in a corona around the optic disk is called *Purtscher's retinopathy* (Plate 10). This observation was first made in patients with severe head trauma.[20] Later it was described in those suffering multiple extracranial fractures and attributed to fat emboli from the fractured bones.[21] However, an identical pattern is seen in patients with acute pancreatitis, HIV disease, exacerbations of lupus, malignant hypertension, obstetrical complications, burns, and various other prothrombotic states.[4] Preferably called "Purtscher's-like retinopathy," this phenomenon represents retinal microinfarction caused by a variety of mechanisms: autoregulatory vasoconstriction (malignant hypertension), antiphospholipid antibody or other vascular endothelial injury (connective tissue disorders), and occlusion by leukocyte–fibrin aggregates (pancreatitis).[22]

Cotton-wool spots do not usually interfere with vision unless they are especially numerous or clustered together between the fovea and the optic nerve. They resolve within five to seven weeks. High-resolution perimetry may detect tiny scotomas corresponding to their current or previous location.

If obliteration of precapillary arterioles occurs gradually rather than acutely, then inner retinal tissue becomes ischemic without the appearance of an infarct or a cotton-wool spot. This phenomenon, especially common in diabetic patients, tends to affect the macular region. Careful ophthalmoscopy discloses a thinning of the retinal nerve fiber layer, and fluorescein angiography displays a widening of the foveal capillary-free zone.

Venous Stasis

When the retina is subjected to chronic hypoperfusion owing to stenosis, hyperviscosity, or increased venous back pressure, it will manifest the signs of venous stasis, or "slow-flow" retinopathy. Ophthalmoscopic features are retinal venous distention and tortuosity and perivenous hemorrhages in the retinal periphery (Plate 11). These signs may result from impaired inflow or outflow. The following features signal *impaired inflow:*

1. Symptoms and signs of ischemia of the entire globe and orbit (ocular ischemic

syndrome).[23] The patient reports periocular pain (orbitotrigeminal ischemia), transient (especially orthostatic) monocular blindness, scintillations, and persistent afterimages from bright lights. The eyes may disclose hyperemia of the episcleral vessels, anterior chamber aqueous flare and cells, and low intraocular pressure (ischemia to the ciliary body's secretory apparatus), cataract, pupillary areflexia, and iris neovascularization (Plate 12).

2. Low retinal artery pressure. Applying minimal suction or indentation pressure to the globe evokes retinal arterial pulsations (ophthalmodynamometry).

3. Delayed arm-to-eye circulation time. Fluorescein angiographic dye has a prolonged latency in arriving in the retinal or choroidal arterioles after intravenous injection.

In the absence of these signs, dilated, incompetent retinal veins are probably caused by *impaired outflow,* owing to increased venous back pressure. Retinal veins may be compressed by sclerotic arterioles at arteriovenous crossing points on the retinal surface or within the optic nerve, where the central retinal vein and artery share a common adventitial sheath. The central retinal vein is also subject to chronic increased pressure from elevated intraocular pressure, a crowded orbit, a dural cavernous sinus fistula, or obstructive neck or thoracic pathology.

Venous Occlusion

If venous flow becomes slow enough, blood may clot and obstruct flow. The effects depend on whether the central or branch vein is obstructed and if so, how completely.[24] The ischemic venous wall swells and bursts, casting a swath of flame-shaped hemorrhages across the retinal surface (Plate 13). The degree of retinal ischemia is related to the number of cotton-wool spots and the presence of an afferent pupil defect. Both signify a poor visual prognosis. In the absence of these signs, visual recovery depends chiefly on whether macular edema or neovascularization develops.

There is no acute treatment for retinal vein occlusion. Evaluation is directed at di-agnosis of arteriosclerosis and the three H's: hypertension, hyperviscosity, and hypercoagulability.[25] Orbitocranial mass lesions or fistulas are rarely responsible. Some young adults seem to develop retinal vein occlusion without identifiable cause or arteriosclerotic risk factors.[26] Because the optic disk is often swollen in these patients, some observers have, without foundation, considered the process to be primarily an inflammatory optic neuropathy with secondary vein occlusion (papillophlebitis).[27] Visual prognosis is relatively good.

Approximately two-thirds of patients who sustain ischemic central retinal vein occlusions develop neovascularization of the iris within the following year.[28] New vessels grow into the anterior chamber angle, "zipper" the iris over the aqueous drainage channels, and produce dangerously high intraocular pressure (neovascular glaucoma). Panretinal photocoagulation generally reverses these effects.

A florid but generally benign ophthalmoscopic picture resembling central retinal vein occlusion may arise when intracranial pressure rises suddenly, as from subarachnoid hemorrhage. Blood bursts out of the central retinal vein and into the subhyaloid space between retina and vitreous (Terson's syndrome).[29,30] The patient reports the sudden appearance of a dark spot (positive scotoma) as the layered blood blocks the retina's access to light rays. If the hemorrhage dissects into the vitreous cavity, vision may appear red-orange (erythropsia). Hemorrhages within the substance of the retina and in the subhyaloid space are usually absorbed within months. Those within the vitreous will generally settle out of view toward the bottom of the vitreous cavity, where a yellow-white ropy matrix may sometimes be observed indefinitely with the indirect ophthalmoscope. If the intravitreal hemorrhage is large, it may not be absorbed and will have to be removed surgically.

Inner Blood–Retinal Barrier Incompetence

Retinal arterioles and capillaries resemble cerebral capillaries in having endothelial tight junctions that prevent the escape of macromolecules. This "inner blood–retinal barrier" is akin to the blood–brain barrier of other CNS vessels. But retinal capillaries differ from cerebral capillaries in having mural cells, or pericyctes, which, together with endothelial cells, maintain the integrity of the blood–retina barrier. If either cell type becomes defective, retinal capillaries will leak. Their seepage will be visible as discrete yellow lipoproteinaceous residues called "hard exudates" (Plate 14) and as retina-thickening clear edema, which accumulates in petaloid pockets that radiate outward from the fovea (cystoid macular edema) (Plate 15). Incompetent vessels also leak blood, which appears as small perivascular hemorrhages (Plate 14). These phenomena occur in the following settings.

DIABETES

A loss of pericytes creates tiny outpouchings in the retinal capillaries called *microaneurysms,* barely visible with the direct ophthalmoscope as pinpoint red spots.[31] These microaneurysms are the source of the hard exudates that often collect in ringlike (circinate) patterns around the important leakpoints. Edema also results from diffuse leakage of the ischemic perifoveal capillaries. Collaborative trials have proven that early laser photocoagulation significantly reduces ultimate visual loss from diabetic macular edema.[32]

MALIGNANT HYPERTENSION

Autoregulatory vasoconstriction is believed to result in ischemic damage to vessel walls, making them leak (and, as the walls swell, occlude and infarct tissue).[33–35] Optic disk edema and cotton-wool spots are often present.

UVEITIS

Retinal vessels may appear ophthalmoscopically normal, yet the retina will be wet from their seepage, a phenomenon well highlighted by fluorescein angiography.

BRANCH RETINAL VEIN OCCLUSION

Serum often escapes from ischemic veins, causing macular edema that impairs vision. If fluorescein angiography reveals that there is adequate perfusion of the macula, grid photocoagulation applied to the leaking region significantly improves visual outcome.[36]

INTRAOCULAR SURGERY

Following cataract surgery, and other intraocular procedures, parafoveal capillaries may leak serum into the macular region.[4] This phenomenon occurs in about 2% of patients who undergo standard extracapsular cataract extraction and lens implantation. Prevalence is higher in diabetic and hypertensive patients, and if vitreous loss complicates the surgery.[4] Surgically induced inflammation is the suspected mechanism. Topical ketorolac and other nonsteroidal agents are considered mildly effective in postoperative treatment, but no solid data support their use. When there is vitreous incarceration in the wound, its removal may reverse the leakage.

COAGULOPATHY

Retinal hemorrhages are anecdotally documented in patients with various coagulation disorders,[37] but the most consistent association is with thrombocytopenia in the context of anemia[38] or acute leukemia.[39,40] In one study of patients with anemia of 8 g/100 ml or worse,[38] the presence of a platelet count below 50,000/mm^3 increased the likelihood of retinal hemorrhages from 10% to 70%. In cases of acute leukemia, both the degree of thrombocytopenia[39] and the degree of leukocytosis[41] have been directly related to the prevalence of retinal hemorrhages.

Neovascularization

Another phenomenon that sets retinal vessels apart from other CNS vessels is the development of new vessels under conditions of chronic ischemia. How this happens is unclear, although a humoral vasogenic agent has been identified in chronically ischemic retina.[42,43] Neovascular nets form on the surface of the retina and finally break through into the space between retina and vitreous (Plate 16). The fragile vessels of these nets often bleed into the vitreous cavity. As they proliferate, the new vessels attract a fibroglial scaffold that tugs, distorts, and finally detaches the retina (Plate 17). Three settings give rise to this sequence.

RETINAL VASCULAR OCCLUSION

Diabetes is the most common cause, but a similar phenomenon also occurs in patients with ocular exposure to therapeutic x-irradiation,[44] sickle cell diseases (mostly sickle-C and sickle-Thal, rarely SS, and never SA),[45] branch retinal vein occlusion,[46] and in an idiopathic condition called Eales' disease.[47,48] In diabetic, venous occlusive, and radiation retinopathy, neovascularization predominantly affects the posterior retina; in sickle cell and Eales' disease, the neovascularization lies predominantly in the anterior retina.

Retinal hypoxia is the mechanism common to all these conditions. In cases of diabetes, capillary basement membrane thickening may impede flow. In x-irradiation, intimal hyperplasia obliterates the vascular lumen; in sickle diseases, deformed red blood cells plug the lumen; in retinal vein occlusions, slow flow causes stagnant hypoxia; in Eales' disease, the pathogenesis is unknown.

Retinal neovascularization is the hallmark of proliferative diabetic retinopathy. It develops within 15 years of diagnosis in 25% of insulin-dependent diabetics diagnosed before age 30.[49] Among diabetics diagnosed after age 30, proliferative signs are present 15 years after diagnosis in 15% of insulin users and in only 4% of non-users of insulin.[50] Intensive glucose control reduces by 50% the chances of developing or worsening retinopathy.[51]

The ophthalmic treatment of diabetic neovascularization consists of scattering laser burns across the retina, excluding only the territory around the optic disk and macula. This "panretinal" carpetbombing of the retina often causes the neovascularization to regress, perhaps by reducing the amount of ischemic retinal tissue. Collaborative trials have clearly established the value of panretinal photocoagulation in reducing visual loss.[32] Such a treatment has also proved effective in treating branch vein occlusion in a large controlled trial.[46] A similar scatter approach is used to treat radiation retinopathy

and Eales' disease, but no controlled studies have been done to verify its efficacy. In patients with sickle retinopathy, treatment is applied by scatter technique or directly to feeder vessels.[52]

POOR ARTERIAL FLOW PROXIMAL TO THE EYE

Stenosis of the aortic arch, carotid, or ophthalmic artery may cause chronic hypoperfusion of the eye, giving rise to a constellation of symptoms and signs called the *ischemic ocular syndrome* (see "Venous Stasis," above).[23] Carotid endarterectomy and bypass procedures have been anecdotally considered effective, but data are sparse. Panretinal photocoagulation is sometimes successful.

PREMATURITY

Infants with birth weights of 2 g or less or gestational ages of 36 weeks or less have immature peripheral retinal vasculature, especially in the temporal region. This vasculature fails to develop if exposed to atmospheric oxygen after birth.[53] A distinct ridgelike demarcation develops at the border between vascularized and nonvascularized peripheral retina. In some cases, these signs regress spontaneously; in others, neovascular channels grow behind the ridge, bleed, and cause contraction of the overlying vitreous, leading to retinal detachment. In cases where retinopathy of prematurity (ROP) is proceeding rapidly, retinal veins near the optic disk and macula will become dilated and tortuous, a sign called "plus disease" to emphasize its serious import. The incidence of ROP increases with lower birth weights and gestational ages, as well as intercurrent illness.[54] Infants should undergo ophthalmoscopy of the retinal periphery between 6 and 8 weeks postnatally. Early cryotherapy reduces visual morbidity in high-risk cases.[55]

Vasculitis

Inflammation affects retinal veins more than arterioles. In many cases, it is restricted to the eye. In other cases, it is associated with a systemic infectious or inflammatory disorder.[56]

Direct ophthalmoscopic evidence of vasculitis consists of diffuse or focal (sausage-like) narrowing of vessels together with white waxlike cuffing that reflects mural and perimural leukocytic infiltration (Plate 18). Vasculitis should not be inferred merely on the basis of finding retinal leakage or infarction, because these signs are not specific to vasculitis. They are more often pathologically associated with noninflammatory occlusion, such as venous stasis or vascular malformation. Vasculitis is more likely to be the cause of leakage if the white perivascular cuffs vary in thickness and there is an overlying vitreous haze.

When vascular inflammation subsides, the cuffing goes away, but if the vessel has become permanently occluded, it looks like a white strand, or a pipe cleaner (Plate 8). This vascular appearance is often misinterpreted as a sign of active vasculitis.

Important causes of retinal vascular inflammation are sarcoidosis, Behçet's disease, the herpesviruses, syphilis, tuberculosis, Whipple's disease, and multiple sclerosis. Retinal vasculitis is often described in association with Cogan's syndrome, Susac's syndrome,[57,58] lupus erythematosus, scleroderma, polymyositis, dermatomyositis, polychondritis, Sjogren's syndrome, and inflammatory arthropathies and enteropathies,[59] but pathology rarely shows inflammation. In conjunction with some of these conditions, intravascular immune complex or complement deposition has been found; in others, the pathogenesis of retinal vascular occlusion is uncertain. True retinal vasculitis is most often an isolated finding without systemic association.[4]

SARCOIDOSIS

In patients with sarcoidosis, retinal vasculitis is rare (<10%) compared to anterior uveitis (25%).[59] The characteristic ophthalmoscopic abnormality is a whitish cuffing of the midperipheral venules. The infiltrates may become so large that they appear to be dripping from the vessels. In one series, the axiom that the finding of retinal vasculitis markedly increases the likelihood of intracranial sarcoidosis was not supported.[60]

BEHÇET'S DISEASE, SYPHILIS, TUBERCULOSIS, WHIPPLE'S DISEASE, AND MULTIPLE SCLEROSIS

The retinitis associated with these conditions has few distinguishing features. Behçet's disease tends to affect the peripheral vessels first.[61] The retinal vasculitis of Whipple's disease often has a prominent vitreous haze, aspiration of which may allow for identification of the causative organism, *Tropheryma whippelii*, by polymerase chain reaction.[62] In multiple sclerosis, peripheral venous sheathing has been described in 14 (28%) of 50 cases.[63] Among more than 2000 patients with multiple sclerosis, peripheral vitreous clouding ("snowbanking," "pars planitis") was found in 1%.[64] However, in a cohort of 53 patients with pars planitis, 6 (16%) developed multiple sclerosis.[65] Both studies emphasized that ocular findings may precede CNS findings by months to years.

HERPESVIRUSES

Retinal inflammation caused by the herpesviruses appears to originate within vessels but quickly spreads into adjacent parenchyma to cause a confluent retinitis.

Cytomegalovirus (CMV) retinitis produces a florid hemorrhagic yellow-white necrosis of the retina that spreads flamelike across the fundus ("pizza-pie retinopathy").[66] If untreated, the infection leads within days to weeks to total destruction of the retina (Plate 19). Treatment with intravenous or intraocular implant ganciclovir often arrests its progression,[67] but once the drug is withdrawn, the destruction resumes. These findings are most often encountered in AIDS and organ transplant cases; they generally precede other CNS manifestations of CMV.

Acute retinal necrosis, a retinal vasculitis that advances posteriorly from the retinal periphery, has been described as an isolated phenomenon in otherwise healthy individuals.[68] It is marked by full-thickness retinal and optic nerve necrosis, choroidal granulomas, and retinal vasculitis. Herpesvirus is the suggested pathogen, based on antigens in intravascular immune complexes, intraocular antibody production, and viral particles on electron microscopy. Early treatment with intravenous acyclovir may arrest and even partially reverse this process. Traction retinal detachment is a late threat.

Vascular Malformation

Hamartomas of retinal vessels may leak profusely into the retina and disturb vision, or they may signal the existence of intracranial vascular malformations with equally disastrous consequences.[69]

LEAKY MALFORMATIONS LIMITED TO THE EYE

Retinal telangiectasis (Coats' disease, Leber's miliary aneurysms) is the most common example of a leaky malformation isolated to the retina.[70] An idiopathic monocular affection occurring sporadically and mostly in boys, it is generally discovered within the first two decades of life. The porous walls of dilated retinal vessels leak yellow exudates that are initially confined to the macula (Plate 20). As fluid continues to pour out of these incompetent vessels, the retina balloons forward to cause a white pupil ("cat's-eye reflex," or leukocoria). Pathologic examination discloses a patchy absence of vascular pericytes and endothelium. Photocoagulation treatment can prevent visual loss only if given before massive exudation has occurred.

LEAKY OCULAR MALFORMATIONS ASSOCIATED WITH CNS MALFORMATIONS

Angiomatosis retinae (von Hippel's disease) is the most important example of a leaky retinal vascular malformation (Plate 21) associated with a CNS malformation.[71] In this condition, which is familial and autosomal dominant in about 20% of cases, retinal hemangioblastomas may coexist with similar lesions in the cerebellum and spinal cord. Polycystic lesions may affect the abdominal viscera, and carcinoma may involve the kidney. When extraocular manifestations exist, the disorder is called von Hippel-Lindau disease.

The prevalence of extraocular malformations in patients who are identified by their retinal angiomas is 25%.[72] Cerebellar he-mangioblastomas are the most common extraocular manifestations.[73] From 40% to 60% of patients identified with extraocular manifestations will have retinal hemangioblastomas.[69,71]

The retinal angiomas are red or pink masses that are typically multiple and located beyond the range of the direct ophthalmoscope in the peripheral retina. Occasionally, however, they may appear on the optic disk and create the misimpression of optic disk edema from other causes. The angiomas are fed by large arterioles, drained by large veins, and ringed by yellow exudates. Early photocoagulation or cryotherapy to seal the vessels prevents or reverses vision-threatening leakage.

NONLEAKY OCULAR MALFORMATIONS ASSOCIATED WITH CNS MALFORMATIONS

In this group, the retinal malformations do not leak, but they may slowly enlarge and rarely bleed. Examples are retinal arteriovenous malformation (racemose angioma, Wyburn-Mason syndrome) and cavernous retinal hemangioma.

In patients with retinal AVM, a serpentine tangle of massively enlarged retinal arteries and veins typically emanates from the optic nervehead (Plate 22). Despite this angry appearance, visual function is usually normal unless the central retinal vein becomes occluded or the optic nerve axons become severely compressed. Recognition of this syndrome is important because AVMs of the anterior visual pathway, facial bones, cranial base, and posterior fossa may cause problems.[74,75]

Cavernous retinal hemangiomas are rare, stagnant lesions that appear as clusters of large, dark red grapes on the retinal surface near the optic nervehead.[4,69] Visual symptoms occur only if the lesions bleed, but their discovery is important because of a common association with similar cerebral malformations.[76]

CHOROIDAL VASCULAR REACTION PATTERNS

Choroidal vessels exhibit four pathologic reaction patterns: choriocapillaris occlusion,

Table 10–6. **Choroidal Vascular Reaction Patterns**

Reaction Pattern	Manifestations	Common Causes
Choriocapillaris occlusion	Acute: small, faint milky spots +/− focal retinal detachment Healed: black dots with yellow rims (Elschnig spots)	Acute hypertension ITP, TTP, DIC*
Arteriolar occlusion	Acute: ischemic whitening Healed: pigmentary retinopathy	Atherosclerosis Giant cell arteritis Mucormycosis Orbitocranial trauma
Neovascularization	Acute: submacular hemorrhage Healed: yellow-white glial scar	Age-related macular degeneration Choroiditis Ocular trauma Elastic disorders High myopia Retinal photocoagulation
Hemangioma	Diffusely red fundus Focal yellow submacular lesion, macular detachment	Sturge-Weber syndrome Unknown

*ITP = idiopathic thrombocytopenic purpura; TTP = thrombotic thrombocytopenic purpura; DIC = disseminated intravascular coagulation.

choroid arteriolar occlusion, neovascularization, and hemangioma (Table 10-6).

Choriocapillaris Occlusion

The choriocapillaris is subject to occlusions that may produce small, multifocal infarctions. During sudden extreme blood pressure elevations (acute glomerulonephritis, pregnancy-induced hypertension, scleroderma, pheochromocytoma), strong sympathetic innervation reduces flow enough to cause spot infarctions that injure the overlying RPE and photoreceptors.[77-79] Choriocapillaris occlusions also result from vascular plugging by hematologic or immune aggregates in association with idiopathic thrombocytopenic purpura (ITP) and thrombotic thrombocytopenic purpura (TTP), and in disseminated intravascular coagulopathies in the peripartum state, sepsis, metastatic carcinoma, leukemia, severe burns, drug allergies, trauma, and major surgery.[80]

In the acute phase of choriocapillaris occlusion, the patient complains of sudden, painless monocular or binocular central visual loss. Focal choriocapillaris infarcts appear ophthalmoscopically as faint milky spots deep within the retina. Sometimes there is an overlying bubblelike retinal detachment. This minidetachment arises because of ischemic breakdown of the outer blood–retinal barrier that is maintained by RPE tight junctions. The serum that normally escapes from the choroidal vessels, but is ordinarily shut out of the retina by tight RPE junctions, now enters the retina and lifts the photoreceptors off their moorings to the RPE (Fig. 10-1*b*). This phenomenon is most common in the macular region, but it can affect any area of the retina. Early phases of the fluorescein angiogram reveal underperfusion in affected areas. Later phases show fluorescein dye staining of ischemic RPE cells and seepage into the cleft between the RPE and the photoreceptors (see Fig. 11-2). After several weeks, the focal retinal detachment resolves and leaves behind an "Elschnig spot," a readily overlooked, tiny, round, black dot surrounded by a yellow rim.

Arteriolar Occlusion

Although the choroidal arteriolar walls are affected by arteriosclerosis, their rich anastomoses and high blood flow preclude large infarctions. Occlusion of the ophthalmic artery will, however, cause a combined retinal and choroidal infarction that usually renders the patient completely blind. In the acute phase, the retina displays ischemic whitening without a cherry-red spot (see "Retinal Arterial Occlusion," above). In the healed phase, irritated and metaplastic RPE cells migrate into the inner retina, so that the fundus displays a speckled black pigmentation often mistaken for a heritable pigmentary retinopathy or ocular trauma.

Neovascularization

In several conditions, the submacular choriocapillaris burrows into the overlying retina (Fig. 10-1c). This "choroidal neovascularization" is as visually devastating as retinal neovascularization. Unlike retinal neovascularization, however, which is provoked by chronic hypoxia, choroidal neovascularization appears to develop if there has been any damage to Bruch's membrane, the elastic barrier between the choriocapillaris and the RPE.

Ophthalmoscopically invisible, the choroidal neovascular membrane is readily detected on fluorescein angiography because it stains the overlying retina. Most choroidal neovascular membranes are first recognized when they bleed into the retina and cause blurring and image distortion (Plate 23). The blood triggers a glial reaction that causes the macular region to look like scrambled eggs. Cycles of bleeding and scarring eventually deprive the patient of all central vision. Age-related macular degeneration, choroidal inflammation, systemic disorders of elastin, trauma, and retinal photocoagulation are the common settings. In a small fraction of patients, direct photocoagulation of the membrane improves visual outcome (Chapter 11).[81]

Hemangioma

The most important choroidal vascular hamartoma is the hemangioma.[4] It occurs in two forms.

Diffuse hemangioma is a lesion involving nearly the entire choroid in patients with en-

cephalotrigeminal angiomatosis (Sturge-Weber syndrome), which includes ipsilateral facial and meningeal hemangiomas. The diffuse choroidal hemangioma confers a red color, suggesting velvet, to the fundus, but it does not usually grow or damage the overlying RPE.

Focal hemangioma is a yellow lesion usually lying under the macula. Unlike the hemangioma of Sturge-Weber, this one has no syndromic associations, and it often grows during puberty and depresses visual acuity by injuring the overlying RPE and creating a macular detachment. This lesion is easily mistaken for an amelanotic malignant melanoma or a choroidal metastasis (see "Neoplastic Disorders," Chapter 11). Light surface photocoagulation of the parafoveal portion of the tumor often restores vision.

SUMMARY

The retinal vessels display nine pathologic reaction patterns: wall changes, arterial occlusion, precapillary arteriolar occlusion, inner blood–retinal barrier incompetence, neovascularization, venous stasis, venous occlusion, vasculitis, and congenital malformation.

The choroidal vessels exhibit four pathologic reaction patterns: choriocapillaris occlusion, arteriolar occlusion, neovascularization, and hemangioma.

REFERENCES

1. Klein R, Klein BEK, Moss SE, Wang Q. Hypertension and retinopathy, arteriolar narrowing, and arteriovenous nicking in a population. *Arch Ophthalmol.* 1994;112:92–98.
2. Daniels SR, Lipman MJ, Burke MJ, Loggie JM. The prevalence of retinal vascular abnormalities in children and adolescents with essential hypertension. *Am J Ophthalmol.* 1991;111:205–208.
3. Sharma S, Brown M, Brown GC. Retinal artery occlusions. *Ophthalmol Clin North Am.* 1998;11:591–600.
4. Gass JDM. *Stereoscopic Atlas of Macular Diseases: Diagnosis and Treatment.* 4th ed. St. Louis: Mosby; 1997.
5. Pfaffenbach DD, Hollenhorst RW. Mortality and survivorship of patients with embolic cholesterol crystals in the ocular fundus. *Am J Ophthalmol.* 1973; 75:66–72.
6. Executive Committee for the Asymptomatic Carotid Atherosclerosis Study. Endarterectomy for

asymptomatic carotid artery stenosis. *JAMA*. 1995; 273:1421–1428.

7. Trobe JD. Who needs carotid endarterectomy (circa 1996)? *Ophthalmol Clin North Am*. 1996;9:513–519.

8. Barnett HJM, Eliasziw M, Meldrum HE, Taylor DW. Do the facts and figures warrant a 10-fold increase in the performance of carotid endarterectomy on asymptomatic patients? *Neurology*. 1996;46:603–608.

9. Mayberg MR, Winn HR. Endarterectomy for asymptomatic carotid artery stenosis: resolving the controversy. *JAMA*. 1995;273:1459–1461.

10. European Carotid Surgery Trialists Collaborative Group. Risk of stroke in the distribution of an asymptomatic carotid artery. *Lancet*. 1995;345:209–212.

11. Richard G, Lerche R-C, Knospe V, Zeumer H. Treatment of retinal arterial occlusion with local fibrinolysis using recombinant tissue plasminogen activator. *Ophthalmology*. 1999;106:768–773.

12. Schumacher M, Schmidt D, Wakhloo AK. Intra-arterial fibrinolytic therapy in central retinal artery occlusion. *Neuroradiology*. 1993;355:600–605.

13. Savino PJ, Glaser JS, Cassady J. Retinal stroke: Is the patient at risk? *Arch Ophthalmol*. 1977;95:1185–1189.

14. Trobe JD. Carotid endarterectomy. Who needs it? *Ophthalmology*. 1987;94:725–730.

15. Kline LB. The natural history of patients with amaurosis fugax. *Ophthalmol Clin North Am*. 1996; 9(3):351–357.

16. McLeod D, Marshall J, Kohner EM, Bird AC. The role of axoplasmic transport in the pathogenesis of retinal cotton wool spots. *Br J Ophthalmol*. 1977; 61:177–191.

17. Duane TD, Osher RH, Green WR. White centered hemorrhages: their significance. *Ophthalmology*. 1980;87:66–69.

18. Brown GC, Brown MM, Hiller T, Fischer D, Benson WE, Magargal LE. Cotton wool spots. *Retina*. 1985;5:206–214.

19. Aisen ML, Bacon BR, Goodman AM, Chester EM. Retinal abnormalities associated with anemia. *Arch Ophthalmol*. 1983;101:1049–1052.

20. Purtscher O. Angiopathia retinae traumatica: lymphorrhagien des Augengrundes. *Albrecht von Graefes Arch Ophthalmol*. 1912;82:347–371.

21. Pratt MV, DeVenecia G. Purtscher's retinopathy: a clinicohistopathological correlation. *Surv Ophthalmol*. 1970;14:417–423.

22. Jacob HS, Craddock PR, Hammerschmidt DE, Moldow CF. Complement-induced granulocyte aggregation; an unsuspected mechanism of disease. *N Engl J Med*. 1980;302:789–794.

23. Brown GC. The ocular ischemic syndrome. In: Ryan SJ, ed. *Retina*. 2nd ed. St. Louis: Mosby; 1994: 1515–1527.

24. Hayreh SS. Central retinal vein occlusion. *Ophthalmol Clin North Am*. 1998;11:559–590.

25. Elman MJ, Bhatt A, Quinlan PM, Enger C. The risk of systemic vascular disease and mortality in patients with central retinal vein occlusion. *Ophthalmology*. 1990;97:1543–1548.

26. Walters RF, Spalton DJ. Central retinal vein occlusion in people aged 40 years or less: a review of 17 patients. *Br J Ophthalmol*. 1990;74:30–35.

27. Hart CD, Sanders MD, Miller SJH. Benign retinal vasculitis: clinical and fluorescein angiographic study. *Br J Ophthalmol*. 1971;55:721–733.

28. Central Vein Occlusion Study Group. A randomized clinical trial of early panretinal photocoagulation for ischemic central retinal vein occlusion. The Central Vein Occlusion Study Group N Report. *Ophthalmology*. 1995;102:1434–1444.

29. Terson A. De l'hémorragie dans le corps vitre au cours l'hémorrhagie cérébrale. *Clin Ophtalmol*. 1900;6:309.

30. Garfinkle AM, Danys IR, Nicolle DA, Colohan AR, Brem S. Terson's syndrome: a reversible cause of blindness following subarachnoid hemorrhage. *J Neurosurg*. 1992;76:766–771.

31. Frank RN. On the pathogenesis of diabetic retinopathy: a 1990 update. *Ophthalmology*. 1991;98: 586.

32. Early Treatment Diabetic Retinopathy Study Group. Early photocoagulation for diabetic retinopathy. ETDRS report number 9. *Ophthalmology*. 1991;98:766–785.

33. Hayreh SS, Servais GE, Virdi PS. Hypertensive retinopathy. *Ophthalmologica*. 1989;198:173–177.

34. Tso MOM, Jampol LM. Pathophysiology of hypertensive retinopathy. *Ophthalmology*. 1982;89:1132–1138.

35. Garner A, Ashton N, Tripathi R, Kohner EM, Bulpitt CJ, Dollery CT. Pathogenesis of hypertensive retinopathy: an experimental study in the monkey. *Br J Ophthalmol*. 1975;59:3–12.

36. Branch Retinal Vein Study Group. Argon laser photocoagulation for macular edema in branch vein occlusion. *Am J Ophthalmol*. 1984;98:271–282.

37. Gold DH, Weingeist TA. *The Eye in Systemic Disease*. Philadelphia: Lippincott; 1990.

38. Rubenstein RA, Yanoff M, Albert DM. Thrombocytopenia, anemia, and retinal hemorrhage. *Am J Ophthalmol*. 1968;65:435–439.

39. Schachat AP. The leukemias and lymphomas. In: Ryan SJ, ed. *Retina*. Vol 1. St. Louis: Mosby; 1989: 775–791.

40. Culler AM. Fundus changes in leukemia. *Trans Am Ophthalmol Soc*. 1951;49:445–473.

41. Kincaid MC, Green WR. Ocular and orbital involvement in leukemia. *Surv Ophthalmol*. 1983;27: 211–232.

42. Adamis AP, Miller JW, Bernal MT, et al. Increased vascular endothelial growth factor levels in the vitreous of eyes with proliferative diabetic retinopathy. *Am J Ophthalmol*. 1994;118:445–450.

43. Adamis AP, Shima DT, Tolention MJ, et al. Inhibition of vascular endothelial growth factor prevents retinal ischemia-associated iris neovascularization in a nonhuman primate. *Arch Ophthalmol*. 1996;114: 66–71.

44. Archer DB, Amoaku WMK, Gardiner TA. Radiation retinopathy—clinical, histopathological, ultrastructural and experimental correlations. *Eye*. 1991;5: 239–251.

45. Nagpal KC, Goldberg MF, Rabb MF. Ocular manifestations of sickle hemoglobinopathies. *Surv Ophthalmol*. 1977;21:391–411.

46. Branch Retinal Vein Study Group. Argon laser scatter photocoagulation for prevention of neovascularization and vitreous hemorrhage in branch vein

occlusion; a randomized clinical trial. *Arch Oph-thalmol.* 1986;104:34–41.

47. Eales H. Causes of retinal hemorrhage associated with epistaxis and constipation. *Birm Med Rev.* 1880; 9:262.

48. Gieser SC, Murphy RF. Eales' disease. In: Albert DM, Jakobiec FA, eds. *Principles and Practice of Ophthalmology.* Vol 2. Philadelphia: Saunders; 1994:791–795.

49. Klein R, Klein BEK, Moss SE, Davis MD, De Mets DL. Diabetic retinopathy: II. Prevalence and risk of diabetic retinopathy when age at diagnosis is less than 30 years. *Arch Ophthalmol.* 1984;102:520–525.

50. Klein R, Klein BEK, Moss SE, Davis MD, De Mets DL. Diabetic retinopathy: III. Prevalence and risk of diabetic retinopathy when age at diagnosis is 30 or more years. *Arch Ophthalmol.* 1984;102:527.

51. Diabetes Control and Complications Trial Study Group. The effect of intensive treatment of diabetes on the development and progression of long-term complications of insulin-dependent diabetes mellitus. *N Engl J Med.* 1993;329:977–986.

52. Jacobson MS, Gagliano DA, Cohen SB, et al. A randomized clinical trial of feeder vessel photocoagulation of sickle cell retinopathy. *Ophthalmology.* 1991;98:581–585.

53. Charles S, Devine C. Retinopathy of prematurity. *Ophthalmol Clin North Am.* 1998;11(4):517–524.

54. Palmer EA, Flynn JT, Hardy RJ, et al. Incidence and early course of retinopathy of prematurity. *Ophthalmology.* 1991;98:1628–1640.

55. Cryotherapy for Retinopathy of Prematurity Study Group. Multicenter trial of cryotherapy for retinopathy of prematurity; one-year outcome—structure and function. *Arch Ophthalmol.* 1990;108:1408–1416.

56. Chee SP. Retinal vasculitis associated with systemic disease: Behcet's disease, sarcoidosis, inflammatory bowel disease and others. *Ophthalmol Clin North Am.* 1998;11:655–672.

57. O'Halloran HS, Pearson PA, Lee WB, Susac JO, Berger JR. Microangiopathy of the brain, retina, and cochlea (Susac's syndrome). *Ophthalmology.* 1998;105:1038–1044.

58. Papo T, Biousse V, Lehoang P, et al. Susac syndrome. *Medicine.* 1998;77:3–11.

59. Jabs DA. The rheumatic diseases. In: Ryan SJ, ed. *Retina.* Vol 2. St. Louis: Mosby; 1989:457–480.

60. Spalton DJ, Sanders MD. Fundus changes in histologically confirmed sarcoidosis. *Br J Ophthalmol.* 1981;65:348–358.

61. Michelson JB, Chisari FV. Behcet's disease. *Surv Ophthalmol.* 1982;26:190–203.

62. Rickman LS, Freeman WR, Green WR, et al. Brief report: uveitis caused by *Tropheryma whippelii* (Whipple's bacillus). *N Engl J Med.* 1995;332:363–366.

63. Lightman S, McDonald WI, Bird AC, et al. Retinal venous sheathing in optic neuritis: its significance for the pathogenesis of multiple sclerosis. *Brain.* 1987;110:405–414.

64. Biousse V, Trichet C, Bloch-Michel E, Roullet E. Multiple sclerosis associated with uveitis in two large clinic-based series. *Neurology.* 1999;52:179–181.

65. Raja SC, Jabs DA, Dunn JP, et al. Pars planitis. Clinical features and Class II HLA associations. *Ophthalmology.* 1999;106:594–599.

66. Bloom JN, Palestine AG. The diagnosis of cytomegalovirus retinitis. *Ann Intern Med.* 1988;109:963–969.

67. Musch DC, Martin DF, Gordon JF, Davis MD, Kuppermann BD. Treatment of cytomegalovirus retinitis with a sustained-release ganciclovir implant. *N Engl J Med.* 1997;337:83–90.

68. Culbertson WW, Clarkson JG, Blumenkranz MS, Lewis ML. Acute retinal necrosis. *Am J Ophthalmol.* 1983;106:426–429.

69. Amin HI, Ai E. Retinal vascular malformations. *Ophthalmol Clin North Am.* 1998;11:503–515.

70. Horn G, Rabb MF, Lewicky AO. Retinal telangiectasis of the macula: a review and differential diagnosis. *Int Ophthalmol Clin.* 1981;21:139–155.

71. Hardwig P, Robertson DM. Von Hippel-Lindau disease: a familial, often lethal, multisystem phakomatosis. *Ophthalmology.* 1984;91:263.

72. Ebert EM, Albert DM. The phakomatoses. In: Albert DM, Jakobiec FA, eds. *Principles and Practice of Ophthalmology.* Vol 5. Philadelphia: Saunders; 1994: 3301–3328.

73. Maher ER, Yates JRW, Harris R. Clinical features and natural history of von Hippel-Lindau disease. *Q J Med.* 1990;77:1151–1163.

74. Theron J, Newton TH, Hoyt WF. Unilateral retinocephalic vascular malformations. *Neuroradiology.* 1974;7:185.

75. Bech K, Jenson OA. On the frequency of coexisting racemose haemangiomata of the retina and brain. *Acta Psychiat Neurol Scand.* 1961;36:47.

76. Hassler W, Zentner J, Wilhelm H. Cavernous angiomas of the anterior visual pathways. *J Clin Neuroophthalmol.* 1989;9:160–164.

77. DeVenecia G, Jampol LM. The eye in accelerated hypertension. II. Localized serous detachments of the retina in patients. *Arch Ophthalmol.* 1984;102:68–73.

78. DeVenecia G, Wallow I, Houser D, Wahlstrom M. The eye in accelerated hypertension. I. Elschnig's spots in nonhuman primates. *Arch Ophthalmol.* 1980;98:913–918.

79. Hayreh SS, Servais GE, Virdi PS. Fundus lesions in malignant hypertension. VI. Hypertensive choroidopathy. *Ophthalmology.* 1986;93:1383–1400.

80. Bird AC. Pathogenesis of serous detachment of the retina and pigment epithelium. In: Ryan SJ, ed. *Retina.* Vol 2. St. Louis: Mosby; 1989:99–105.

81. Zimmer-Galler IE, Bressler NM, Bressler SB. Treatment of choroidal neovascularization: updated information from recent Macular Photocoagulation Study Group reports. *Int Ophthalmol Cl.* 1995(4); 35:37–57.

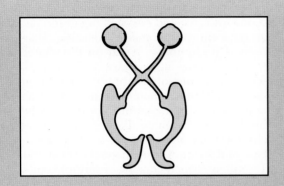

Chapter 11

RETINA AND CHOROID II: INFLAMMATORY, DEGENERATIVE, TOXIC, AND NEOPLASTIC DISORDERS

Retinal and choroidal inflammatory, degenerative, toxic, and neoplastic disorders are the topics of this chapter.

INFLAMMATORY DISORDERS

Retinal and choroidal inflammation may be based in blood vessels (vasculitis) or in extravascular tissues. Retinal vasculitis is dis-

cussed in Chapter 10; extravascular retinal inflammation is reviewed here. Choroidal vasculitis, a poorly defined entity, is discussed under the general topic of choroidal inflammation in this chapter.

Retinal Inflammation

Patients who have retinal inflammation report painless, blurred, or scotomatous visual

179

loss, sometimes accompanied by metamorphopsia and floaters (Chapter 10). The fundus discloses whitish yellow patches with indistinct margins often tinged with hemorrhage. These patches consist of cellular infiltrates and perhaps necrotic retinal tissue. There may be an overlying vitreous haze and swelling of the optic disk. The four principal causes of such inflammations are toxoplasmosis, toxocariasis, bacterial (including luetic) sepsis, and fungal sepsis. (Sarcoidosis, Behcet's disease, the herpesviruses, tuberculosis, Whipple's disease, and multiple sclerosis also cause retinal inflammation, but it originates as a retinal vasculitis and is therefore discussed under that topic in Chapter 10.)

Toxoplasmic retinitis may develop *in utero* in immune-competent hosts or as an acquired infection in immune-compromised hosts.[1] In either case, the retina displays one or more white patches with fuzzy edges and an overlying vitreous haze (Plate 24). An anterior uveitis (Box 11-1; Fig. 11-1) may also be present. The white patches, usually located in or near the macula, contain necrotic retina with free and encysted organisms and an adjacent granulomatous reaction. Diagnosis is presumptive, based on the characteristic fundus appearance. (Toxoplasma serum immunoglobins are not a reliable indicator.) Without treatment, the inflammation subsides over months, but it leaves behind a distinctive craterlike area of complete chorioretinal atrophy with a white scleral base and a rim of black pigment (Plate 25). Treatment, which consists of various combinations of oral pyrimethamine, sulfadiazine, clindamycin, and corticosteroids, limits the area of retinal destruction and hastens inactivation. Recurrence of disease appears as a retinitis adjacent to old toxoplasma retinal scars (Plate 24).

Toxocara retinitis is a disease of children, the

WHAT IS UVEITIS?

- **Uveitis:** inflammation of the uveal tract, the vascular tunic of the eye consisting of the choroid, ciliary body, and iris. Each segment may be separately involved, or they may be involved together as "panuveitis."

- **Choroiditis:** "posterior uveitis," manifests with faint yellow patches behind the retina, exudative detachment of the retina, and vitreous cells (vitritis). Patients complain of blurred or scotomatous vision, floaters, photopsias, and sometimes pain.

- **Cyclitis and pars planitis:** ciliary body–pars plana inflammation, or "intermediate uveitis," manifests with low intraocular pressure (as aqueous secretion shuts down) and vitreous cells. Patients complain of pain, photophobia, floaters, and sometimes blurred vision.

- **Iritis:** "anterior uveitis," manifests as turbidity (flare) and floating cells in the anterior chamber, bloblike cellular deposits on the corneal endothelium (keratic precipitates), and adhesions of the iris margin to the anterior lens capsule. If the anterior chamber aqueous outflow channels become inflamed, the intraocular pressure may rise. The conjunctival and episcleral vessels dilate, particularly at the margin of the cornea (ciliary flush). Patients complain of pain, photophobia, red eye, and sometimes blurred vision.

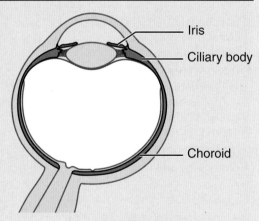

Figure 11–1. The uveal tract.

average age at diagnosis being two years. The causative organism is a roundworm acquired by children who ingest the ova shed in the feces of infected puppies. The larva-filled ova disseminate to viscera, brain, and eye. In the eye, a white granulomatous cocoon forms on the retinal surface and seeds the vitreous. Diagnosis is confirmed by means of an elevated enzyme-linked immunosorbent assay (ELISA) titer (>1:16); treatment consists of periocular corticosteroids.

Bacterial and fungal retinitis are characterized by very similar ophthalmoscopic findings. Candida sepsis and bacterial endocarditis are the most common settings for the infectious retinitis of blood-borne bacterial and fungal organisms. The embolic retinal lesion may begin as a small white retinal patch (cotton-wool spot) or white-centered retinal blot hemorrhage (Roth spot), as detailed in Chapter 10. Within days, it matures into a fluffy infiltrate on the retinal surface and posterior vitreous that will ultimately destroy the eye if not checked with appropriate systemic and intravitreal anti-infective agents.

If retinal inflammation is arrested, and there has been no tissue necrosis, the retina will return to normal appearance and function. Following mild necrosis, the retina will be thinned and dysfunctional, but the structural abnormality may be visible only with specialized techniques. If necrosis has extended into the choroid, the aftermath will be a chorioretinal scar, a yellow-white patch with a distinct border and a rim of black pigment (Plate 25).

Choroidal Inflammation

The choroid may become inflamed in isolation, as part of a contiguous retinitis, or as part of a uveitis that also affects the anterior portion of the uveal tract (Box 10-1; Fig. 10-1).

SYMPTOMS AND SIGNS

As with retinitis, patients complain of blurred vision, scotomas, floaters, photopsias, or metamorphopsia. But *ophthalmoscopic signs are often more subtle than in retinitis* because the choroid hides behind the retina.

Choroidal inflammatory lesions consist of faint whitish yellow or grayish white patches (Plates 27, 28). If the overlying retinal pigment epithelium (RPE) is damaged, it allows entry into the retina of serum that exudes from porous choroidal vessels. Bubblelike elevations appear in the retina, especially in the fovea, as the photoreceptors are lifted off their tenuous moorings to the RPE (Figs. 10-1b, 11-2). Inflammatory cells in the vitreous produce a haze that obscures the view of the retina. Optic disk edema and a relative afferent pupil defect are sometimes present and suggest a coexisting optic neuritis. In chronic choroiditis, choroidal neovascular membranes may develop in the macular region. Patients must be advised to report a sudden drop in vision or metamorphopsia, so that photocoagulation therapy can prevent the disastrous visual consequences of recurrent bleeding into the retina.

CAUSES

The principal systemic causes of choroiditis are tuberculosis, nocardiosis, cryptococcosis, *Pneumocystis carinii*, syphilis, Lyme disease, bacterial sepsis, and Whipple's disease. There are two important noninfectious systemic conditions: sarcoidosis and Vogt-Koyanagi-Harada syndrome (Table 11-1). In cases of sarcoidosis, choroiditis appears as multiple yellow nodules (Plate 27), but it is less common than retinal vasculitis, optic neuritis, and anterior uveitis. The distinctive ophthalmic feature of Vogt-Koyanagi-Harada syndrome is a confluent exudative retinal detachment.[2] Its nonophthalmic components are vitiligo, poliosis, alopecia, hearing loss, and sterile meningitis (uveomeningitis syndrome).[3,4]

In considering the systemic causes of choroiditis, note that *primary CNS lymphoma may look just exactly like a choroidal inflammation.*[5,6] Vitreous aspiration or vitrectomy can be diagnostic (see "Choroidal Malignancies," below).

Choroiditis may be limited to the eye, without an underlying systemic cause. Such an "isolated" choroiditis may involve the entire choroid (full-thickness choroiditis) or merely the choriocapillaris.

Full-thickness choroiditis isolated to the

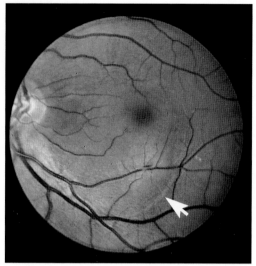
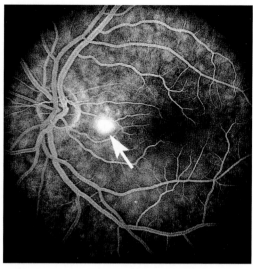

a   b

Figure 11–2. Serious retinal detachment. Focal choroidal infarction or inflammation damages the RPE and impairs the outer blood–retinal barrier, allowing fluid to escape into the retina and elevate the macula (arrow indicates lower margin of detached retina) (*a*); the leak point is visible as a white spot (arrow) on fluorescein angiography (*b*). (Also see Box 11-2.)

eye is believed to be an idiopathic autoimmune vasculopathy that usually leads to destruction of the deep and superficial (choriocapillaris) layers of the choroid (Fig. 10-1).[7] Ocular manifestations are similar to those of choroiditis associated with systemic conditions, but some variants have sufficiently distinctive features to allow a presumptive clinical diagnosis (Table 11-2). Systemic and periocular corticosteroids are used in treatment, but they are often ineffective. The choroid is eventually destroyed, together with the overlying retina, producing profound visual loss. Intriguingly, an unclassi-

fied nematode wandering through the subretinal space can cause this syndrome (diffuse unilateral subacute neuroretinitis).[8] Seeing the worm move through the choroid is a diagnostic coup, for the ocular abnormalities will disappear within months if the nematode is stopped in its tracks by photocoagulation.

Choroiditis restricted to the choriocapillaris (Table 11-3) has a much better prognosis than full-thickness choroiditis. Like full-thickness choroiditis, its pathogenesis is believed to be an immunogenic vasculopathy, but limited to the choriocapillaris.[9–13] *Even if the choriocapillaris is the target, the RPE is always secondarily damaged.* Fortunately, inflammation often resolves spontaneously or following systemic corticosteroid therapy, leaving minimal visual deficit.

In these superficial choroidal inflammations, ophthalmoscopy—even with special instruments—may be completely normal. In other cases, it discloses faint cream-colored deposits under the retina (Plate 28), macular edema, or bubbles of focal retinal detachment elsewhere. Fluorescein angiography may highlight abnormalities invisible or barely visible on ophthalmoscopy. In the initial phase of the angiogram, normal cho-

Table 11–1. **Systemic Causes of Choroidal Inflammation**

Systemic Infections

Tuberculosis	Syphilis
Nocardiosis	Lyme disease
Cryptococcosis	Bacterial sepsis
Pneumocystis carinii	Whipple's disease

Systemic Idiopathic Inflammations

Sarcoidosis
Vogt-Koyanagi-Harada
   (uveomeningitic) syndrome

Table 11–2. Full-Thickness Choroidal Inflammation Unassociated with Systemic Inflammation

Condition	Symptoms	Host	Acute Signs	Healed Signs	Clinical Course	Fluorescein Angiography*	Other DX Tests	Treatment[†]
Multifocal choroiditis	Blurred vision Floaters	Age 20–50 F > M	Gray-white patches Vitritis, + / − anterior uveitis	Large scars of choroid/ RPE, often peripapillary	Recurrent Visual outcome may be poor	Early: hypo Late: hyper	Epstein-Barr titers may be elevated	Cortico-steroids
Birdshot choroiditis	Blurred vision Floaters Photopsias Nyctalopia	Age 40–70 F > M	Small cream-colored spots Vitritis	Small unpig-mented scars of choroid/ RPE	Recurrent Visual outcome may be poor	Early: hypo Late: hyper, disk, macular leakage	ERG: usually depressed Dark adapta-tion thresh-olds elevated HLA A29 + in >80%	Cortico-steroids
Serpiginous choroiditis	Blurred vision Scotomas	Age 30–50 M = F	Gray-white patches at edge of scars centered at disk	Pseudopodlike scars emanating from disk	Recurrent Visual out-come usually poor CNVM[‡] common	Early: hypo Late: hyper	None	Cortico-steroids
Punctate inner choroidopathy	Blurred vision Scotomas Photopsias	Age 20–40 F > M Myopia	Small yellow patches, often around disk Often extensive field loss	Small pigmented scars of choroid/RPE	Resolves 4–6 weeks with minimal/no vision loss, but CNVM[‡] common later	Early: hyper Late: stain	None	None[†]

*hypo = hypofluorescent; hyper = hyperfluorescent.
[†]Apart from photocoagulation of submacular neovascular membranes.
[‡]CNVM = choroidal neovascular membrane.

Table 11–3. Choriocapillaris Inflammation

Condition	Symptoms	Host	Acute Signs	Healed Signs	Clinical Course	Fluorescein Angiography*	Other DX Tests	Treatment
Central serous chorio-retinopathy	Blurred vision Micropsia Metamorphopsia	Age 20–50 M > F	Macular detachment	Macular RPE atrophic spots	Usually spontaneous recovery	Macular leak	None	Photocoagulation if recovery protracted
Acute posterior multifocal placoid pigment epitheliopathy	Blurred vision Photopsias Scotomas	Age 20–40 M = F Flulike illness	Large gray patches +/− vitritis Optic neuritis	Scattered focal RPE atrophic spots	Resolves 1–2 weeks with minimal/no visual loss Rare CNS vasculitis	Early: hypo Late: stain	None	None
Multiple evanescent white dot syndrome	Blurred vision Photopsias Scotomas Floaters	Age 15–50 F > M	Perifoveal white dots Granular macula +/− optic disk edema	None except +/− enlarged blind spot on perimetry	Resolves 6–10 weeks with minimal/no visual loss Lingering photopsias	Early: hyper Late: stain	ERG: reduced A waves	None
Acute retinal pigment epitheliitis	Blurred vision Central scotoma	Age 15–40 M > F	None; two weeks later, dark macular spots with halo	None	Resolves within weeks with no visual loss	Early: hyper in haloes	None	None
Diffuse unilateral subacute neuro-retinopathy	Blurred vision	Age 7–65 M = F	Mild optic disk swelling, vitreous cells; later scattered gray-white RPE-level spots; Motile worm or worm tracks	Patchy chorioretinal atrophy Pale optic disk Narrowed vessels (retinitis pigmentosa–like)	Relentless progression if untreated; proper photocoagulation stops progression	Early: hyper Late: disk staining	Afferent pupil defect ERG: reduced B wave	Photocoagulation of worm

*hypo = hypofluorescence; hyper = hyperfluorescence.

roidal fluorescence is usually blocked; in the late phases, there is staining of damaged RPE and sometimes leakage into the overlying retina (Plate 28). There are no serum markers, but the multifocal ERG may be abnormal (Fig. 9-5). In the healed phase, patients may develop patchy RPE atrophy, especially around the optic disk. A common example of a superficial choroidopathy is central serous chorioretinopathy (Box 11-2; Figs. 10-1b, 11-2).[9]

Because the fundus findings are so subtle in the acute phase of choriocapillaris inflammations, the lesions are often completely overlooked—even by well-trained ophthalmologists. Afflicted patients may then be subjected to unnecessary neurodiagnostic evaluations or dismissed as malingerers. One condition—acute posterior multifocal placoid pigment epitheliopathy (APMPPE)—occasionally violates the rule of having no systemic associations. It has been reported in association with granulomatous CNS angiitis, stroke, and death.[14]

MANAGEMENT

The management of choroiditis depends on its ophthalmic appearance, host characteristics, and clinical course (Fig. 11-3). If the patient is immune-competent, there is no evidence of systemic illness, and the inflammation appears nonprogressive and limited to the choriocapillaris, then only a minimal screening test battery is warranted. Otherwise, a specific infectious or neoplastic diagnosis should be intensively sought.

Treatment of choroiditis associated with systemic conditions is aimed at the underlying condition. For choroiditis limited to the eye, corticosteroids are the mainstay of treatment; they are particularly effective in the superficial choroiditides. In some patients with choriocapillaris inflammation, photocoagulation improves visual outcome (diffuse unilateral subacute neuroretinitis, central serous chorioretinopathy).

DEGENERATIVE DISORDERS

Degenerative retinochoroidal disorders include a wide variety of conditions in which tissues are abnormal or deteriorate over time without a recognized insult such as ischemia, inflammation, toxins, or trauma. There are three groups of disorders, based on the primary site of damage: diffuse photoreceptor–RPE complex disorders, macular disorders, and vitreoretinal interface disorders.

Box 11–2

CENTRAL SEROUS CHORIORETINOPATHY

- Most frequently occurring idiopathic inflammation of the choriocapillaris.
- Affects otherwise healthy individuals (male:female = 8:1) of all ages.
- Subacute onset of blurred and distorted vision in one eye; objects appear smaller (micropsia) and warped (metamorphopsia). Visual acuity is mildly depressed.
- High-magnification ophthalmoscopy discloses elevation of the macula by clear fluid (Fig. 11-2a). The micropsia and metamorphopsia are attributed to uneven separation of photoreceptors by the edema.
- Fluorescein angiography shows a minute hyperfluorescent spot at the level of the RPE where dye appears to leak into the subretinal space between RPE and photoreceptors (Fig. 11-2b).
- Leakage subsides within months and vision usually returns to normal or near normal.
- Laser photocoagulation directed at the hyperfluorescent spot is advocated in cases where vision worsens or fails to recover within four to six months.

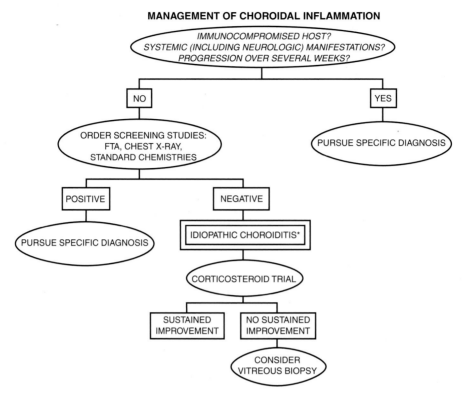

MANAGEMENT OF CHOROIDAL INFLAMMATION

Figure 11–3. Management of choroidal inflammation. *If clinical characteristics suggest acute posterior multifocal placoid epitheliopathy (APMPPE), lumbar puncture and MRA may be indicated to rule out meningitis and CNS vasculitis. In an older patient, also consider primary CNS lymphoma.

Diffuse Photoreceptor–Retinal Pigment Epithelium Disorders

In these conditions, there is diffuse involvement of the photoreceptor–RPE junction throughout the retina. Most cases are caused by heritable genetic abnormalities, but there are some important nongenetic mimickers.

HERITABLE DEGENERATIONS

Retinitis pigmentosa, or pigmentary retinopathy, is a term that encompasses the many heritable diffuse photoreceptor–RPE disorders.[15] For a small number, the genetic mutation is already known; none is treatable at this time.

In most cases of photoreceptor degeneration, rods and cones are damaged, but usually the rods are affected earlier and more profoundly. If so, the patient will suffer slowly progressive binocular loss of dark adaptation (nyctalopia), constriction of the visual field, and depression in the rod-mediated portion of the full-field electroretinogram (ERG) (Chapter 9). Once cone function becomes disturbed, color vision and visual acuity decline, and the cone-mediated ERG becomes abnormal.

Ophthalmoscopy typically reveals a retina speckled with black pigment, especially in the midperiphery (Plate 29). The pigment comes from migrating RPE cells. As the disease progresses, the speckling encroaches on the region of the optic disk and macula. The pigment may be clumped in thick spicules along blood vessels ("bone corpuscular" pattern) or sprinkled about like pepper ("salt and pepper" pattern). There are many instances in which no pigment is seen, forcing the use of the qualifier "retinitis pigmentosa *sine pigmento.*" In cases where cones are affected and rods are relatively spared (cone degeneration, cone dystrophy), the retinal periphery will be normal, but pigment loss will typically occur around the fovea—a so-called bull's-eye maculopathy. An ophthalmoscopic feature common to all heritable retinal degenerations is diffusely narrowed retinal arterioles, due to the relatively increased amounts of oxygen diffusing from the choroid through a damaged outer retina.

An important variant of retinitis pigmentosa known as Leber's congenital amaurosis[16] causes blindness in babies. Diagnosis is often delayed because the fundus lacks pigmentary abnormalities. Clues are the presence of a fine pendular nystagmus, narrowed retinal arterioles, and a lack of other neurologic abnormalities. The diagnosis is secured by finding an extinguished ERG.

Heritable photoreceptor degenerations also occur in conjunction with a vast number of systemic genetically determined disorders (Table 11-4). Visual deficits are relatively minor, except in Usher syndrome, Laurence syndrome, Cockayne syndrome, peroxisomal disorders, ceroid lipofuscinoses, abetalipoproteinemia, and adult Refsum's disease. Ophthalmoscopy may be entirely normal or show mild arteriolar narrowing and a salt-and-pepper retinopathy. Olivopontocerebellar atrophy, ceroid lipofuscinoses, myotonic dystrophy, and Hallervorden-Spatz disease deviate from this pattern. In these conditions, the cones are affected more than the rods, so that the principal fundus sign is a bull's-eye maculopathy (Table 11-7).

MIMICKERS OF HERITABLE DEGENERATIONS

Certain systemic toxins have a proclivity for the RPE and produce ocular manifestations that resemble those of retinitis pigmentosa ("Toxic Disorders," see Table 11-5 below). A coarse pigmentary retinopathy, together with severe visual and electrophysiologic dysfunction, may follow severe ocular trauma or ophthalmic artery occlusion (see "Choroidal arteriolar occlusion," Chapter 10). These conditions may be differentiated from the heritable forms by history and by the fact that they are generally monocular. A fine salt-and-pepper retinopathy resembling the heritable retinopathies also occurs in association with congenital rubella and syphilis. It

Table 11–4. **Heritable Systemic Disorders Associated with Pigmentary Retinopathy**

Lysosomal Disorders
Mucopolysaccharidosis
Oligosaccharidosis
Gangliosidosis*
Mucolipidosis*

Peroxisomal Disorders
Zellweger's syndrome
Neonatal adrenoleukodystrophy
X-linked adrenoleukodystrophy
Infantile Refsum's disease

Ceroid Lipofuscinosis
Haltia-Santavuori
Jansky-Bielschowsky
Spielmeyer-Vogt
Kuf's

Mitochondrial cytopathies
Chronic progressive external ophthalmoplegia
Kearns-Sayre syndrome
Mitochondrial encephalopathy, lactic acidosis, and strokelike episodes (MELAS)
Myoclonic epilepsy and ragged red fiber disease (MERRF)
Leigh's disease

Miscellaneous
Abetalipoproteinemia
Olivopontocerebellar atrophy
Spinocerebellar degeneration
Hereditary sensorimotor neuropathy of Charcot-Marie-Tooth
Adult Refsum's disease
Pelizaeus-Merzbacher disease
Cockayne's syndrome
Marinesco-Sjögren syndrome
Osteopetrosis
Hallervorden-Spatz disease
Incontinentia pigmenti
Idiopathic pallidal degeneration
Laurence-Moon-Bardet-Biedl syndrome
Usher syndrome
Myotonic dystrophy
Cystinosis

*GM$_1$ type 1, GM$_2$ types 1 and 2, Gaucher's type 1, Niemann-Pick disease type A, mucolipidoses types 1 and 2, and multiple sulfatase deficiency produce cherry-red maculas rather than pigmentary retinopathy (see Table 11-8).

is readily distinguished from retinitis pigmentosa by the fact that visual function and the ERG are normal or nearly normal.

Rapidly progressive photoreceptor degeneration manifested by loss of peripheral and

Table 11–5. Nonheritable Causes of Pigmentary Retinopathy

Quinoline toxicity
Thioridazine toxicity
Deferoxamine toxicity
Ophthalmic artery occlusion
Severe ocular trauma
Congenital rubella
Congenital syphilis
Cancer-associated retinopathy
Melanoma-associated retinopathy

night vision, retinal arteriolar narrowing, and a depressed ERG has been attributed to a paraneoplastic disorder ("cancer-associated retinopathy," or CAR) (Plate 30).[17,18] It differs from heritable retinopathies clinically in that it may proceed to complete blindness over months. Pathologic damage is limited to photoreceptors (RPE and choriocapillaris are spared).[19] In CAR, the overwhelming association is with small (oat) cell carcinoma of the lung, although the cancers have also originated from the breast, colon, prostate, and cervix. Current belief is that these cancers and photoreceptors share a 23 kilodalton antigenic protein to which antibodies cross-react.[17,18]

An even rarer retinal paraneoplastic disorder is associated with metastatic skin melanoma (melanoma-associated retinopathy, or MAR).[17,18] Patients with MAR differ from those with CAR in occasionally having relatively preserved visual acuity, prominent photopsias, an ERG resembling congenital stationary night blindness, hearing loss, vitiligo, signs of uveitis, and antibodies to retinal bipolar cells. Unfortunately, there is no effective treatment for either of these paraneoplastic retinopathies.

Macular Disorders

The macular region is the predominant or exclusive site of damage for an important class of retinal degenerative disorders. Patients with macular disorders typically exhibit normal or nearly normal full-field ERGs, so that diagnosis depends on recognizing the abnormal configuration of the macula by inspection and confirming dysfunction with the foveal or multifocal ERG (Chapter 9).

SYMPTOMS AND SIGNS OF ALL MACULAR DISORDERS

The chief complaint of patients with macular disorders is progressive visual acuity loss, sometimes accompanied by metamorphopsia. Loss of visual acuity and steep-margined central scotomas are the principal deficits. Color vision is often preserved by intact perimacular cones. There may be no ophthalmoscopic abnormalities in the earliest stages, and findings may be faint even in advanced stages. One must be adept at looking at the retina with high dioptric, handheld, slit-lamp mounted or corneal surface lenses. Fluorescein angiography may highlight subtle ophthalmoscopic abnormalities (Box 11-3).

Box 11–3

RETINAL FLUORESCEIN ANGIOGRAPHY

- **What?** Intravenous administration of fluorescein dye followed by fundus photography with special camera and film.

- **Why?** Highlights retinal abnormalities that cannot be well seen with ophthalmoscopy alone. Shows abnormal vascular formations, leakage created by defects in the inner and outer blood–retinal barriers, and window transmission defects created by atrophy of the RPE.

- **What do results mean?** Normal retinal vessels are impermeable to fluorescein; damaged vessels leak and stain the adjacent tissue. Normal RPE tight junctions prevent entry of fluorescein into the retina; damaged RPE stains with fluorescein and may allow fluorescein seepage into the retina. Choroidal or retinal tumors or inflammatory masses block the view of the underlying choroidal fluorescence. Abnormal vascular formations become more obvious.

AGE-RELATED MACULAR DEGENERATION

This idiopathic disorder of the elderly is the most common cause of blindness in the developed world.[20] Cigarette smoking is the only established risk factor.[21,22] The fundamental abnormality in this condition lies in the macular RPE,[23] which, for unknown reasons, fails to catabolize expended photoreceptor outer segments. Debris piles up on the inner surface of Bruch's membrane, a five-layered structure interposed between the RPE and the choriocapillaris. The yellow-gray mounds created by these imperfectly catabolized outer segments are called *drusen* (Plate 31). As drusen form, RPE cells and their overlying photoreceptors begin to die off. Visual acuity fails when atrophy of the RPE–photoreceptor unit becomes confluent. (The correlation between ophthalmoscopic signs of RPE atrophy, drusen, and visual acuity loss is not very precise.) This common variant of macular degeneration is called *atrophic*, or *dry*, because, unlike the "wet" form (see below), there is no exudate. Unfortunately, there is no treatment for this dry form of age-related macular degeneration.

Although the other form of macular degeneration, called *disciform*, or *wet*, accounts for only 10% of all cases, it is responsible for most of the severe visual acuity loss associated with this condition. It is caused by choroidal neovascularization that arborizes through cracks in Bruch's membrane, bleeds, and disrupts macular tissues (Fig. 10-1c). The stimulus for the growth of these incompetent new blood vessels is unknown. Subretinal blood and serum may be detected by the experienced examiner and enhanced with fluorescein angiography (Plate 23; Fig. 10-1c).

Collaborative trials have shown that laser photocoagulation may attenuate the progression of visual loss in a small percentage of patients with wet macular degeneration but vision is rarely restored.[24] Given the relatively limited therapeutic impact of photocoagulation, several alternatives are actively being investigated. One of them is low-dose (800–1500 centigray [cGy]) irradiation applied externally or by plaques sutured temporarily to the sclera. Although small clinical studies are promising, no randomized trials have been completed.[25] Also under way are pilot trials with oral antiangiogenesis agents, including interferon alfa, antivascular endothelial growth factor (anti-VEGF), anti–alpha integrins, angiostatin, and thalidomide.[26] Surgical removal of choroidal neovascular membranes, a technical tour-de-force, has thus far failed to improve vision because the adherent macular RPE always gets removed as well. Efforts are now directed at transplanting RPE or inducing adjacent RPE to grow into the space left after submacular surgery.[27]

HIGH MYOPIA

A degenerative maculopathy with many of the features of age-related macular degeneration may also occur in conjunction with pathologic myopia (greater than 10 diopters). Fine yellow-white stretch marks in Bruch's membrane, called "lacquer cracks," forewarn of the later development of choroidal neovascularization.[28]

ANGIOID STREAKS

In patients with pseudoxanthoma elasticum, a heritable disorder of elastic tissue, wide gulfs occur in the elastic portion of Bruch's membrane.[29] These clefts are visible ophthalmoscopically as reddish brown streaks that radiate out from the optic nervehead (Plate 32). Often mistaken for abnormal vessels, they are called *angioid streaks*. Their significance is that in 75% of cases, choroidal neovascularization occurs in these regions and causes problems similar to those of age-related macular degeneration. Angioid streaks occur less commonly in individuals with sickle cell diseases, Paget's disease, and Ehlers-Danlos syndrome.[29]

DYSTROPHIC DISORDERS

The macula can be damaged by a variety of inborn metabolic errors. Some are limited to the eye, and others are systemic. Currently, no treatment is available for these disorders.

Dystrophic Maculopathies without Systemic Associations

These conditions are classified according to the ophthalmoscopic appearance of the macula and on the results of electro-oculography, electroretinography, and fluorescein angiography (Table 11-6). Most are

Table 11–6. **Dystrophic Maculopathies without Systemic Associations**

Dystrophic Maculopathy	Inheritance/Age of Onset/Mechanism	Ophthalmoscopic Features	Special Features
Juvenile retinoschisis	X-linked/first decade/splitting of nerve fiber layer	Stellate foveal cysts; peripheral schisis cavity inferotemporally in 50%	ERG loss of B wave Visual acuity loss (20/50–20/100) Acuity loss may precede ophthalmoscopic changes
Stargardt's (fundus flavimaculatus)	AR*/1st to 3rd decade/accumulation of lipofuscin in RPE	Macular RPE atrophy, +/− fishtail-shaped yellow flecks in macula and elsewhere	Distinctive blockage of choroidal vessel pattern on fluorescein angio because of RPE lipofuscin ("dark choroid") Progressive but variable acuity loss; ERG usually normal
Best's (vitelliform)	AD*/first decade/unknown	First phase: egg yolk Second phase: meniscus Third phase: scrambled egg Fourth phase: atrophy	Ophthalmoscopic features proceed through phases Acuity normal until scrambled-egg phase EOG† often very abnormal
Inherited drusen	Any pedigree/any age/unknown	Yellowish round flecks at RPE level not limited to macular region	Visual acuity usually good unless drusen confluent in fovea
Sorsby's	AD*/midlife/lipid deposit between RPE and Bruch's membrane/abnormal gene codes for tissue inhibitor for metalloproteinase	Drusen, then subfoveal choroidal neovascular choroidal atrophy and scarring	Produces same picture as any condition causing subfoveal neovascularization
Central areolar	AD*/early adulthood/unknown but in one form, gene mapped to chromosome 6	Macular RPE atrophy with discrete border	Often confused with age-related macular degeneration or toxoplasmosis
Pattern	AD*/midlife/peripherin–RDS mutation in some cases	Reticular or butterfly-shaped black pigment	Late onset, generally good visual prognosis

*AR = autosomal recessive; AD = autosomal dominant.

†EOG = electro-oculogram. The test is performed by attaching active electrodes to the medial and lateral canthi and a ground electrode to the forehead. With head positioned in a white bowl, the patient is instructed to make horizontal saccades to targets placed 15 degrees eccentric to fixation on either side. Two trials are conducted, one in darkness, the other in room light. An instrument records the amplitude of the change in potential of the ocular dipole as the eye moves. The relevant EOG measure is the ratio of the highest amplitude in darkness ("dark trough") to the highest amplitude in light ("light peak"). The cutoff is 1.65. A lower value indicates dysfunction of the macular RPE.[64,65] This test is most helpful in diagnosing Best's (vitelliform) maculopathy, because it is abnormal even when ophthalmoscopy is normal or near-normal. In other macular disorders, it is only mildly abnormal and only when ophthalmoscopic features are very evident.

characterized by slowly progressive binocular visual acuity loss and yellow flecks that eventually appear at the level of the RPE, the suspected target tissue.[30]

Given the lack of obvious ophthalmoscopic abnormalities, diagnosis is challenging. Central scotomas detected on high-resolution perimetry are missed with standard protocols. Color vision is relatively preserved by intact perimacular cones. The full-field electroretinogram (ERG), which measures global retinal transmission, is often normal. Visual evoked potentials (VEP), which depend heavily on macular input, are abnormal, but they misdirect attention toward optic nerve and intracranial visual pathway disease. The foveal or multifocal ERGs, which can measure macular function, provide the clue to correct localization (Chapter 9). In Best's vitelliform maculopathy, the electro-oculogram is a critical diagnostic test[64,65] (see Table 11-6).

Two particularly subtle dystrophic maculopathies are juvenile retinoschisis (Plate 33) and Stargardt's disease (Plate 34). Juvenile retinoschisis is an x-linked disorder that becomes symptomatic in the first decade with binocular progressive visual acuity loss. The retinal nerve fiber layer splits, causing a subtle cyst with fine radial folds in the fovea.[31] In 50% of cases, the peripheral retina shows similar splitting. Stargardt's disease is an autosomal recessive disorder that presents in the first to third decades with progressive binocular acuity loss. In the early stages, ophthalmoscopy may be utterly normal, as may be the ERG. In 85% of cases, fluorescein angiography is diagnostic in showing a "dark choroid"; normal fluorescence is blocked by the diffuse accumulation of lipofuscin in the RPE. Eventually, focal RPE atrophy occurs in the perifoveal region to produce a bull's-eye maculopathy; in some cases, fish-shaped (pisciform) yellow-white flecks appear scattered through the posterior fundus.

Dystrophic Maculopathies with Systemic Associations

Several systemic metabolic conditions that affect the nervous sytem may also affect the macula (Table 11-7). Ophthalmoscopy discloses one of two patterns:

- Cherry-red spot: impaired lysosomal catabolism in retinal ganglion cells allows a

Table 11–7. **Heritable Disorders with Cherry-Red Spot or Bull's-Eye Maculopathy**

Cherry-Red Spot

GM 1 gangliosidosis type 1 (generalized)
GM 2 gangliosidosis type 1 (Tay-Sachs)
GM 2 gangliosidosis type 2 (Sandhoff's)
Sialidosis type 1 (Cherry-red spot–myoclonus syndrome)
Sialidosis type 2, juvenile onset (cherry-red spot–dementia syndrome)
Niemann-Pick type A
Multiple sulfatase deficiency
Farber's disease

Bull's-Eye

Gaucher's type 1
Niemann-Pick type B
Metachromatic leukodystrophy
Ceroid lipofuscinosis
Olivopontocerebellar atrophy
Hallervorden-Spatz disease
Cystinosis

buildup of metabolic products that impair retinal transparency. This effect is most noticeable around fovea, where the ganglion cells are most numerous. A gray-white ring, caused by the swollen ganglion cells, contrasts with the red-orange color reflected from the choroid in the foveal region (Plate 35).

- Bull's-eye: catabolic products damage the RPE around the fovea, causing a pale halo, or bull's-eye (Plate 36).

Vitreoretinal Interface Disorders

Degenerations sometimes affect the junction between the vitreous and retina (Fig. 11-4). With advancing age, ocular trauma, intraocular surgery, inflammation, or high myopia. the vitreous gel undergoes liquefaction. The resulting inhomogeneity of the vitreous gel stresses and eventually breaks its firm fibrous attachments to the retinal periphery, fovea, and optic disk. In autopsied eyes of patients aged over 70 years, more than 50% have posterior vitreous detachment.[32]

Vitreous detachment may cause no symptoms, but often the patient reports the sudden appearance of flashes or floaters and, less commonly, turbid vision. The flashes

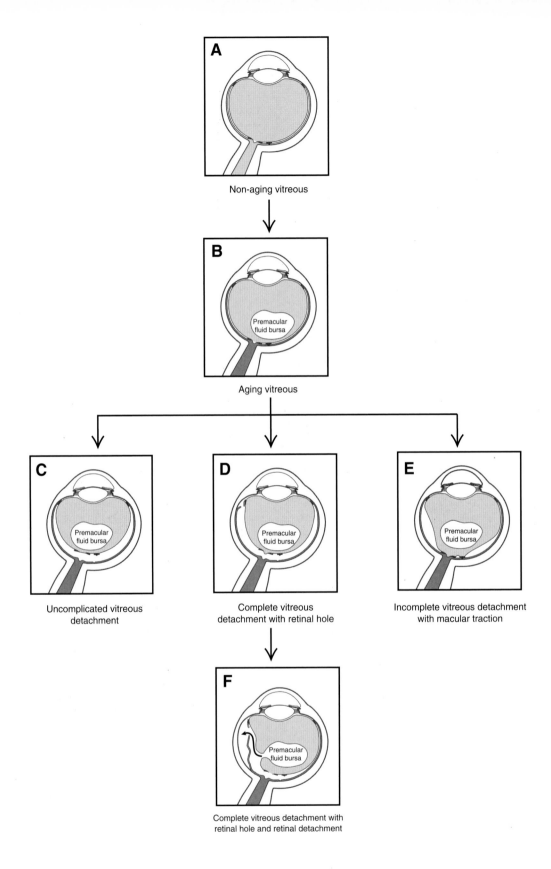

A

Non-aging vitreous

B

Premacular
fluid bursa

Aging vitreous

C

Premacular
fluid bursa

Uncomplicated vitreous
detachment

D

Premacular
fluid bursa

Complete vitreous
detachment with retinal hole

E

Premacular
fluid bursa

Incomplete vitreous detachment
with macular traction

F

Premacular
fluid bursa

Complete vitreous detachment with
retinal hole and retinal detachment

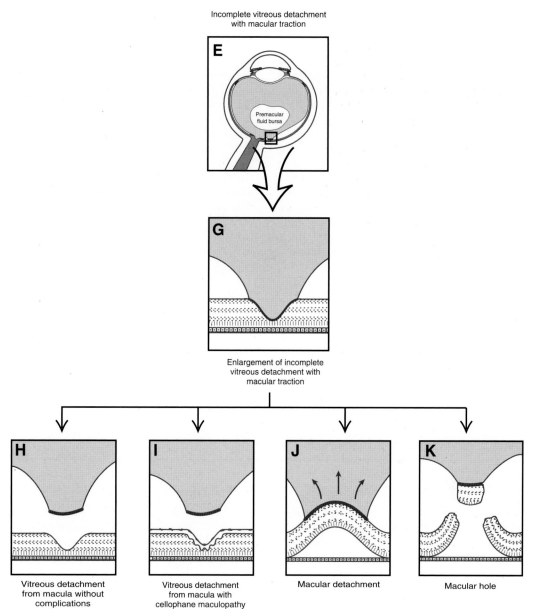

Incomplete vitreous detachment
with macular traction

E

Premacular
fluid bursa

G

Enlargement of incomplete
vitreous detachment with
macular traction

H

Vitreous detachment
from macula without
complications

I

Vitreous detachment
from macula with
cellophane maculopathy

J

Macular detachment

K

Macular hole

Figure 11–4. Vitreoretinal interface disorders. (*A*) The nonaging vitreous has uniform consistency and is attached firmly to the retina at the macula, optic disk, and retinal periphery. (*B*) The aging vitreous has developed a premacular fluid bursa but remains attached to the retina. (*C*, *D*, *E*) Three types of vitreous detachments from the retina. In *C*, the vitreous has successfully detached itself. In *D*, vitreous detachment is complete but has torn a hole in the peripheral retina. In *E*, vitreous detachment has occurred in the retinal periphery, but persisting attachments at the macula and optic disk create traction. (*F*) Retinal detachment. Fluid vitreous has seeped into the retinal hole and separated the neurosensory retina from the RPE. (*G*) Vitreous traction on the macula. (*H*, *I*, *J*, *K*) Four types of vitreous detachment from the macula. In *H*, vitreous detachment from the macula is uncomplicated. In *I*, vitreous detachment from the macula is followed by surface membrane overgrowth (cellophane maculopathy), creating distorted vision. This complication may also follow complete, successful detachment of the vitreous (*C*). In *J*, vitreous traction elevates the macula. In *K*, the vitreous detaches but tears a hole in the macula, degrading visual acuity.

come from photoreceptors deformed by a contracting vitreous that is tugging on the retina. The threadlike or weblike floaters derive from the broken fibrous attachments to the optic disk that become suspended in front of the retina and block its view (Fig. 1-6). Turbid vision is caused by blood escaping from a retinal vessel torn by the detaching vitreous.

The flashes normally cease after a few days. The floaters settle out of view within months, and the turbid vision resolves within months as the blood is absorbed. However, the process of vitreous separation can go awry in three ways that lead to enduring vision loss: retinal detachment, cellophane maculopathy, and vitreomacular traction (Table 11-8).

RETINAL DETACHMENT

In 15% of patients with flashes or floaters, the detaching vitreous tears a hole in the peripheral retina (Fig. 11-4D).[33] If a hemorrhage accompanies the vitreous detachment, the chances of finding a retinal break are much higher.[33] Vitreous fluid may seep through the hole and dissect the photoreceptors from their tenuous attachments to the RPE (Fig. 11-4F). As the retina separates, the patient loses peripheral vision. Because the detachment starts in the retinal periphery, it is visible only with an indirect ophthalmoscope through a widely dilated pupil. In time, the detachment spreads to the posterior retina and interrupts macular function. Treatment consists of sealing the hole, together with procedures aimed at reducing vitreous traction. Unfortunately, once the macula has become detached, the chance that surgical repair of the detachment will restore a visual acuity of 20/50 or better falls from 87% to 37%.[34]

CELLOPHANE MACULOPATHY

Cellophane maculopathy, also known as macular pucker, epiretinal membrane, premacular fibroplasia, or surface-wrinkling maculopathy, is a common cause of disturbed vision in the elderly. Even if the vitreous detaches uneventfully from the retina, a thin layer of fibroblasts, glia, and RPE cells may develop on the retinal surface and form a

Table 11–8. **Vitreoretinal Interface Disorders**

Disorder	Symptoms	Signs	Pathogenesis	Treatment
Retinal detachment	Flashes Floaters Visual loss	Retinal separation	Detaching vitreous tears hole in retina Liquid vitreous seeps in and detaches retina	Surgical retinal reattachment procedures
Cellophane maculopathy (macular pucker, epiretinal, membrane, premacular fibroplasia, surface wrinkling)	Metamorphopsia Visual acuity loss	Wrinkled macular surface Tortuous vessels Crinkled light reflection	Vitreous detaches successfully, but residual membrane on retinal surface contracts	Retinal surface membrane peeling
Vitreomacular traction syndrome	Metamorphopsia Visual acuity loss	Cystoid macular edema Macular hole	Vitreous detaches from retinal periphery but not from macula, leaving a reaction strand	Vitrectomy, gas bubble postoperative prone positioning

contracting (epiretinal) membrane over the macula (Fig. 11-4*I*).[35] As the membrane contracts, it wrinkles and puckers up the retinal tissues, causing metamorphopsia and blurred central vision. The ophthalmoscopic findings are subtle—a translucent covering on the retina, increased tortuosity of macular vessels, and a crinkled, cellophane-like light reflection (Plate 37). This surface-wrinkling process progresses slowly and often arrests; it may rarely reverse spontaneously. But if it persists, and vision is badly degraded, treatment involves peeling the membrane off the retinal surface. Visual improvement may be expected in about 75% of cases.[36]

VITREOMACULAR TRACTION

Sometimes the vitreous successfully separates from its retinal attachments in all but the macular region, leaving behind a taut stalk that causes leakage of perifoveal capillaries and cystoid macular edema (Fig. 11-4*E,G,J*).[37] The remaining attachment may spontaneously break free in time (Fig. 11-4*H*). If not, it can be cut surgically with a 67% chance of improving vision.[38] The same finding may be seen in patients whose vitreous has been injured by intraocular surgery, ocular trauma, or inflammation.

In some patients with vitreomacular traction syndrome, the retina is ripped off in the foveal region (Fig. 11-4*K*) (Plate 38).[39,40] The first sign of a threatened break is a tiny yellow dot within the fovea. As the foveal photoreceptors detach from the underlying RPE, a faint yellow foveal ring appears. Within weeks to months, 50% of cases have spontaneous resolution as the posterior vitreous detaches, and 50% go on to have a foveal dehiscence if the vitreous remains attached. Dehiscence causes a sudden central scotoma and a drop in visual acuity.

Treatment for this type of macular hole consists of vitrectomy, peeling of the posterior vitreous off the retina, injecting a gas bubble into the vitreous, and instructing the patient to lie face down for a period of weeks so that the gas bubble will tamponade the freed edges. If each of these steps is rigorously followed, the margins seem to grow back together and visual acuity improves substantially in 75% of cases with an acceptably low complication rate.[41–43]

TOXIC DISORDERS

Visual disturbance may result from retinal toxicity of quinolines (chloroquine and hydroxychloroquine), thioridazine, deferoxamine, tamoxifen, digitalis, and clomiphene. With the quinolines, thioridazine, deferoxamine, digitalis, and clomiphene, symptoms appear without ophthalmoscopically visible abnormalities. As a result, visual symptoms are often dismissed. By contrast, tamoxifen usually causes more structural than functional alterations. Digitalis and clomiphene produce florid symptoms that disappear without lasting effects once the medication level is normalized (digitalis) or stopped (clomiphene). There are no antidotes for retinal toxicity; the only treatment is discontinuation of the medication.

Chloroquine and Hydroxychloroquine

As a group, the quinolines are fiercely toxic to the retina. They are most avidly taken up by perifoveal RPE cells to cause a bull's-eye maculopathy; in severe cases, the peripheral RPE cells also atrophy. Chloroquine hydrochloride (Aralen), used now primarily in prevention of malaria, is likely to cause retinopathy after daily doses of greater than 250 mg or a cumulative dose of greater than 100 g.[44] Hydroxychloroquine sulfate (Plaquenil), which has largely replaced chloroquine for treatment of connective tissue disorders, is much less toxic, but it may cause retinopathy at daily doses greater than 6.5 mg/kg or in patients with impaired renal function.[45]

The first symptom of quinoline retinal toxicity is the appearance of fuzzy borders on viewed objects. Small paracentral scotomas are noted next, and finally visual acuity falls. At the earliest stage, ophthalmoscopy may be normal. Central visual field testing with grids and stationary red objects is probably the most sensitive diagnostic test. Fluorescein angiography will display subtle perifoveal window defects. Later, a loss of the normal orange color around the fovea will be evident through the ophthalmoscope (Plate 36). Much later, pigmentary changes and atrophy may appear in the peripheral retina and retinal arterioles will narrow, just as they do in heritable and metabolic pigmentary retinopathies. At this stage, the visual fields will be narrowed and the ERG abnormal. Damage is irreversible. Although it often stabilizes once the medication is withdrawn, visual loss may progress.

Thioridazine

Thioridazine (Mellaril), an antipsychotic agent favored for its relatively low parkinsonian side-effects, causes a severe retinopathy at daily doses above 800 mg/day.[46] Symptoms appear soon after treatment is begun—within three to six weeks. The patient complains of blurred or brownish discoloration of day vision and poor night vision. No fundus changes may yet be evident. Soon a uniform salt-and-pepper pattern appears everywhere. If the medication is not stopped, this pattern will evolve into a blotchy loss of RPE and choriocapillaris that resembles the most severe forms of heritable retinochoroidal degeneration, gyrate atrophy and choroideremia. Primary toxicity appears to be to photoreceptors as well as RPE. Damage is typically irreversible.

Deferoxamine

Deferoxamine mesylate (Desferal), used to chelate iron in transfusion-induced hemosiderosis, causes impairments in color vision, visual acuity, night vision, and peripheral visual field.[47] Damage may occur with accepted dose regimens even in patients with normal renal clearance of the drug. Well after initial symptoms have emerged, the macula develops a speckled appearance that eventually appears in the rest of the retina. Eventually, the retinal arterioles narrow. The pathogenesis is unclear, although damage is seated within the RPE. Withdrawing the medication often leads to improvement, unless damage is advanced. Cochlear hearing loss often coexists.

Tamoxifen

Tamoxifen citrate (Nolvadex), an antiestrogenic medication used to treat breast cancer, causes crystalline deposits in the macular nerve fiber layer, macular edema, and a loss of visual acuity. The toxic dose limits are not clear, but one study showed that 4 (6%) of 63 patients treated at standard doses (average 20 mg/day) developed retinopathy within 10 to 35 months after initiation of treatment, at a total mean dose of 14 g.[48] Fortunately, these changes are largely reversible upon discontinuing the drug.

Digitalis

Digitalis toxicity causes a yellowish-green tinge (xanthopsia) or frosting of vision, as well as mild visual acuity and color vision loss, attributed to photoreceptor damage.[49–52] Symptoms and deficits disappear quickly when digitalis blood levels return to normal.

Clomiphene

Clomiphene citrate, an ovulatory agent, causes shimmery vision with prolonged afterimages.[53] Symptoms are fully reversible after drug withdrawal. Damage is presumed to occur at the photoreceptor level, although it could also be at the visual cortex.

High-Intensity Light

Toxicity to the retina may also occur following exposure to high-intensity light. Common settings include sun-gazing, inappropriate use of high-intensity illuminators during eye surgery, and accidental injury from industrial lasers.

NEOPLASTIC DISORDERS

Retinal and choroidal malignancies present a diagnostic challenge because a false-negative diagnosis could lead to a loss of life, and a false-positive diagnosis to unnecessary removal of an eye. Adding to the complexity of the task are two critical factors: (1) the manifestations of these tumors resemble those of nonmalignant processes (Table 11-9), and (2) performing a biopsy carries the danger of destroying vision or spreading the tumor.

Retinal Malignancies

The most important primary retinal malignancy is retinoblastoma,[54] a tumor of infancy

Table 11–9. **Mimickers of Retinal and Choroidal Neoplasms**

Neoplasm	Mimickers
Retinoblastoma	Toxocariasis
	Astrocytic hamartoma
	Retinal telangiectasis
	Retinopathy of prematurity
	Persistent hyperplastic primary vitreous
	Retinal dysplasia
	Traumatic chorioretinopathy
	Familial exudative vitreoretinopathy
Choroidal melanoma	Nevus
	Melanocytoma
	Metastatic carcinoma
	Hemangioma
	Hemorrhagic RPE detachment
	Focal choroiditis
	Primary CNS lymphoma
	Osseous choristoma

and early childhood caused by a mutation in chromosome 13q14. Patients who have multiple tumors in one eye and tumors in both eyes must have germ line mutations. Their offspring have a 50% of being carriers and 45% of having the disease. By contrast, patients who have only a single tumor in one eye have a 12% chance of having germ line mutations. Their offspring have a 6% chance of being carriers and a 5.4% chance of having the disease. However, if an offspring develops retinoblastoma, the mutation must lie within the germ line.

The retinoblastoma tumor usually grows into the vitreous as a tapiocalike white mass (Fig. 11-5). Necrosis causes inflammation within the eye, exhibited by vitreous and anterior chamber cells and perhaps a hyperemic conjunctiva. Sporadic forms of retinoblastoma are detected in one (or more) of four ways:

- **Leukocoria** (white pupil, cat's-eye reflex). The dark pupillary space appears white because the tumor has grown forward to reach the lens. The tumor can be detected before the pupil becomes white by shining the ophthalmoscope light through it and observing that the reflection is gray or black rather than red. Nonmalignant processes may also cause leukocoria.
- **Poor vision.** The the tumor obstructs the visual axis or distorts the retina. The re-

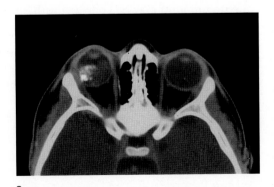
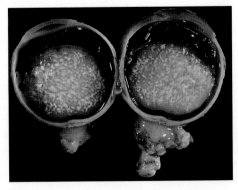

a   b

Figure 11–5. Retinoblastoma. (*a*) CT shows a calcified mass in the posterior vitreous of the right eye. (*b*) Enucleated right eye, cut in half, shows tapiocalike white mass.

sulting poor vision may be detected on routine screening or by finding that an infant resists occlusion of the seeing eye.

- **Ocular misalignment.** The eyes go out of alignment because of loss of binocular vision. The misalignment (strabismus) is usually in the inward direction, that is, esotropia.
- **Chronic uveitis.** Signs of intraocular inflammation together with a retinal or vitreous mass eventually lead to the diagnosis.

Retinoblastoma can usually be separated from its imitators when one or more tapiocalike masses are found in the retina on ophthalmoscopy, which must be performed under general anesthesia to achieve adequate compliance. Computed tomography and ultrasound are helpful diagnostic adjuncts in revealing the presence of intratumoral calcium (Fig. 11-5), which is distinctive for retinoblastoma. Treatment alternatives include enucleation, plaque radiation therapy, photocoagulation, and chemotherapy.

The retina is not a favorite site for metastatic tumors, but one important tumor does settle here: immunoblastic (primary CNS–ocular) lymphoma. Formerly called "reticulum cell sarcoma," it is a non-Hodgkin's lymphoma variant that involves the eye far more commonly than any other type of lymphoma.[5,6] In two-thirds of cases, it is found simultaneously in brain parenchyma. In most other cases, the brain lesions are discovered later, with an average latency of two years. Diagnosis of the isolated ocular form is often delayed because it masquerades as an inflammatory disorder of the retina or choroid (see "Inflammatory Disorders," above).

Adults aged 60–70 years are most at risk. They complain of blurred vision, floaters, and periocular pain. Both eyes are generally affected, the initial site being the space between the choroid and the RPE. There, the lymphoma forms cream-colored mounds (Plate 39) over which the retina develops focal detachments. The vitreous is usually turbid with inflammatory and neoplastic cells. In some cases, the vitreous cells precede the focal sub-RPE lesions. In time, focal white patches of retinal necrosis, branch arteriolar occlusions, optic disk swelling, and anterior uveitis may develop.

Primary CNS lymphoma in the eye is usually suspected when inflammation fails to respond to corticosteroid treatment or if CNS symptoms develop. Definitive diagnosis can often be made by cytologic examination of cells derived from biopsy of the vitreous. This procedure is particularly useful when MRI of the brain fails to disclose distinctive lesions and lumbar puncture is negative. Lymphoma cells may be so scant that inspection of the specimen must be meticulous.[55]

In cases of combined ocular–CNS disease, treatment consists of whole brain and ocular irradiation, together with systemic chemotherapy. If the lymphoma is isolated to the eye, ocular irradiation is the treatment of choice. Vitrectomy is an alternative if the visual loss is largely attributable to vitritis. Although treatment prolongs life, the disease is uniformly fatal within four years once brain lesions appear. Survival is longer with disease limited to the eye.

Choroidal Malignancies

Choroidal malignancies may take the form of malignant melanoma or metastatic carcinoma. (Choroidal involvement by systemic lymphoma is rare;[56] choroidal leukemic infiltration is a common autopsy finding but is not often identified during life.[57,58]

MALIGNANT MELANOMA

The most common primary intraocular tumor, choroidal melanoma usually presents as a single, domelike brown mass that elevates the retina (Plate 40).[59] The darkly pigmented mound may be confused with a nevus, melanocytoma, or RPE hamartoma. When lightly pigmented, this lesion is difficult to distinguish from a choroidal hemangioma, metastasis, inflammation, and other less common lesions (Table 11-9). However, the combination of skilled ocular examination, fluorescein angiography, and ultrasound has allowed experts to make a correct diagnosis with high accuracy.[59,60] The tumor's proclivity to spread hematogenously outside the eye and kill the patient depends on two factors: its size and its proportion of epithelioid cells. If no metastases are found elsewhere, traditional management has been to remove the eye (enucleation). Alternative strategies, including observation of small tumors for growth and radiation by means of plaque sources sown onto the sclera, are undergoing study in a large randomized trial.[60]

METASTASES

Metastatic tumors to the choroid are usually carcinomas.[61–63] Prognosis for survival is poor, averaging seven months from diagnosis.[61] The breast and lung are by far the most prevalent source of primary tumor. Less common origins are kidney and skin (melanoma). Gastrointestinal and urogenital carcinomas hardly ever deposit in the choroid.

The choroid is favored as a destination for metastases because of its lush blood flow. In fact, no primary or other metastatic foci may found at the time of a choroidal metastasis, particularly in the case of lung cancer. The diagnosis depends on the clinical characteristics of the ocular mass, inasmuch as performing a biopsy would be visually disruptive.

Choroidal metastases are often asymptomatic (and are discovered only at autopsy) unless they underlie the macular region (loss of acuity, metamorphopsia), create a vitreous inflammation (floaters, foggy vision), or elevate large areas of nonmacular retina (visual field defects). They appear as yellow, gray, or white plaques with indistinct margins and often minimal mass effect. There may be one or more discrete lesions or a diffuse infiltration. When they affect the submacular region, they often cause considerable vision loss by damaging the outer blood–retinal barrier and producing serous detachment of the overlying retina. Local low-dose (3000 cGy) x-irradiation is dramatically effective in restoring vision and shrinking metastatic deposits.

SUMMARY

The principal causes of extravascular retinal inflammation are toxoplasmosis, toxocariasis, syphilis, candidiasis, and bacterial sepsis.

The principal systemic causes of choroidal inflammation are tuberculosis, nocardiosis, cryptococcosis, *Pneumocystis carinii*, syphilis, Lyme disease, bacterial sepsis, Whipple's disease, sarcoidosis, and Vogt-Koyanagi-Harada syndrome. Primary CNS lymphoma is a neoplastic disorder whose ophthalmic manifestations precisely mimic choroiditis.

Choroiditis unassociated with a systemic process may involve the full-thickness choroid or be restricted to the choriocapillaris. Patients with full-thickness choroidal inflammations have a poor visual prognosis. Those with choriocapillaris inflammations have a better visual prognosis but often go undiagnosed because signs are subtle.

Degenerative retinochoroidal diseases include disorders that affect the photoreceptors and RPE throughout the retina, the macular region only, or the vitreoretinal interface. The most common diffuse photoreceptor-RPE disorder is retinitis pigmentosa. The most common macular disorder is age-related macular degeneration. The most common vitreoretinal interface disorder is senescent vitreous detachment.

Retinal toxicity may result from many medications. Chloroquine, thioridazine, and deferoxamine can cause irreversible visual loss. The principal site of damage is the photoreceptor–RPE unit.

The most important primary retinal malignancy is retinoblastoma, a tumor of infancy and early childhood. Early diagnosis is critical to therapy, which can save vision and even life. Primary ocular–CNS lymphoma is a multicentric tumor that may manifest in the outer retina before it appears in deep brain structures.

The most important primary choroidal tumor is malignant melanoma. Choroidal metastasis may be the first sign of a lung carcinoma.

REFERENCES

1. Tamesis RR, Foster CS. Toxoplasmosis. In: Albert DN, Jakobiec FA, eds. *Principles and Practice of Ophthalmology.* Vol 2. Philadelphia: Saunders; 1994:929–934.
2. Snyder DA, Tessler HH. Vogt-Koyanagi-Harada syndrome. *Am J Ophthalmol.* 1980;90:69.
3. Beniz J, Forster DJ, Lean JS, Smith RE, Rao NA. Variations in clinical features of the Vogt-Koyanagi-Harada syndrome. *Retina.* 1991;11:275–280.
4. Moorthy RS, Inomata H, Rao NA. Vogt-Koyanagi-Harada syndrome. *Surv Ophthalmol.* 1995;39:265–292.

5. Freeman IN, Schachat AP, Knox DL, Michels RG, Green WR. Clinical features, laboratory investigations, and survival in ocular reticulum cell sarcoma. *Ophthalmology.* 1987;94:1631–1639.

6. Ridley ME, McDonald R, Sternberg P, Blumenkranz MS, Zarbin MA, Schachat AP. Retinal manifestations of ocular lymphoma (reticulum cell sarcoma). *Ophthalmology.* 1992;99:1153–1161.

7. Dunlop AAS, Cree IA, Hague S, Luthert PJ, Lightman S. Multifocal choroiditis: clinicopathologic correlation. *Arch Ophthalmol.* 1998;116:801–803.

8. Gass JDM, Gilbert WR, Guerry RK, Scelfo R. Diffuse unilateral subacute neuroretinitis. *Ophthalmology.* 1978;85:521–545.

9. Gass JDM. *Stereoscopic Atlas of Macular Diseases: Diagnosis and Treatment.* 4th ed. St. Louis: Mosby; 1997.

10. Young NJA, Bird AC, Sehmi K. Pigment epithelial diseases with abnormal choroidal patterns. *Am J Ophthalmol.* 1980;90:607–618.

11. Lewis H, Lozano D. Retinal pigment epithelial inflammations. *Ophthalmol Clin North Am.* 1993;6:97–108.

12. Lam S, Tessler HH. "New stuff" in uveitis. *Ophthalmol Clin North Am.* 1993;6(1):81–95.

13. Sheppard JD. Posterior uveitis. *Ophthalmol Clin North Am.* 1993;6(1):39–54.

14. Wilson CA, Choromokos EA, Sheppard R. Acute posterior multifocal placoid pigment epitheliopathy and cerebral vasculitis. *Arch Ophthalmol.* 1988; 106:796–800.

15. Pagon RA. Retinitis pigmentosa. *Surv Ophthalmol.* 1988;33:137–186.

16. Lambert SR, Taylor D, Kriss A. The infant with nystagmus, normal appearing fundi, but an abnormal ERG. *Surv Ophthalmol.* 1989;34:173–186.

17. Weinstein JM, Kelman SE, Bresnick GH, Kornguth SE. Paraneoplastic retinopathy associated with antiretinal bipolar cell antibodies in cutaneous malignant melanoma. *Ophthalmology.* 1994;101:1236–1243.

18. Jacobson DM. Paraneoplastic disorders of neuro-ophthalmologic interest. *Curr Opin Ophthalmol.* 1996;7:30–38.

19. Buchanan TAS, Gardiner TA, Archer DB. An ultrastructural study of retinal photoreceptor degeneration associated with bronchial carcinoma. *Am J Ophthalmol.* 1984;97:277–287.

20. Klein R, Klein B, Linton KLP. Prevalence of age-related maculopathy: the Beaver Dam Eye Study. *Ophthalmology.* 1992;99:933–943.

21. Seddon JM, Willett WC, Speizer FE, Hankinson SE. A prospective study of cigarette smoking and age-related macular degeneration in women. *JAMA.* 1996;276:1141–1146.

22. Christen WG, Glynn RJ, Manson JE, Ajani UA, Buring JE. A prospective study of cigarette smoking and risk of age-related macular degeneration in men. *JAMA.* 1996;276:1147–1151.

23. Bressler NM, Bressler SB, Fine SL. Age-related macular degeneration. *Surv Ophthalmol.* 1988;31:375.

24. Zimmer-Galler IE, Bressler NM, Bressler SB. Treatment of choroidal neovascularization: updated information from recent Macular Photocoagulation Study Group reports. *Int Ophthalmol Cl.* 1995; 35(4):37–58.

25. Sherr DL, Finger PT. Radiation therapy for age-related macular degeneration. *Sem Ophthalmol.* 1997; 12(1):26–33.

26. Guyer DR, Adamis AP. Antiangiogenic drug therapy for macular degeneration. *Sem Ophthalmol.* 1997;12(1):10–13.

27. Delpriore LV, Kaplan HJ, Berger AS. Retinal pigment epithelial transplantation in the management of subfoveal choroidal neovascularization. *Sem Ophthalmol.* 1997;12(1):45–55.

28. Avila MP, Weiter JJ, Jalkh AE. Natural history of choroidal neovascularization in degenerative myopia. *Ophthalmology.* 1984;91:1573–1581.

29. Clarkson JG, Altman RD. Angioid streaks. *Surv Ophthalmol.* 1982;26:235–246.

30. Sahel JA, Brini A, Albert DM. Pathology of the retina and vitreous. In: Albert DM, Jakobiec FA, eds. *Principles and Practice of Ophthalmology.* Vol 4. Philadelphia: Saunders; 1994:2239–2280.

31. Condon GP, Brownstein S, Wang NS. Congenital hereditary (juvenile X-linked) retinoschisis: histopathologic and ultrastructural findings in three eyes. *Arch Ophthalmol.* 1986;104:576.

32. Foos RY, Wheeler NC. Vitreoretinal juncture: synchysis senilis and posterior vitreous detachment. *Ophthalmology.* 1982;89:1502–1512.

33. Tasman WS. Posterior vitreous detachment and peripheral retinal breaks. *Trans Am Acad Ophthalmol Otolaryngol.* 1968;72:217–224.

34. Tani P, Robertson DM, Langworthy A. Prognosis for central vision and anatomic reattachment in rhegmatogenous retinal detachment with macula detached. *Am J Ophthalmol.* 1981;92:611–620.

35. Smiddy WE, Maguire AM, Green WR. Idiopathic epiretinal membranes: ultrastructural characteristics and clinicopathologic correlation. *Ophthalmology.* 1989;96:811–821.

36. Pesin SR, Olk RJ, Grand MG. Vitrectomy for premacular fibroplasia; prognostic factors, long-term follow-up, and time course of visual improvement. *Ophthalmology.* 1991;98:1109–1114.

37. Smiddy WE, Green WR, Michels RG, Delacruz Z. Ultrastructural studies of vitreomacular traction syndrome. *Am J Ophthalmol.* 1989;107:177–185.

38. McDonald HR, Johnson RN, Schatz H. Surgical results in the vitreomacular traction syndrome. *Ophthalmology.* 1994;101:1397–1403.

39. Gass JDM. Reappraisal of biomicroscopic classification of stages of development of a macular hole. *Am J Ophthalmol.* 1995;119:752–759.

40. Gaudric A, Haouchine B, Massin P, Paques M, Blain P, Erginay A. Macular hole formation: new data provided by optical coherence tomography. *Arch Ophthalmol.* 1999;117:744–751.

41. Kim JW, Freeman WR, Azen SP. Prospective randomized trial of vitrectomy or observation for stage 2 macular holes. *Am J Ophthalmol.* 1996;121:605–614.

42. Ryan EH, Gilbert HD. Results of surgical treatment of recent-onset full-thickness idiopathic macular holes. *Arch Ophthalmol.* 1994;112:1545–1553.

43. Wendel RT, Patel AC, Kelly NE, Salzano TC, Wells JW, Novack GD. Vitreous surgery for macular holes. *Ophthalmology.* 1993;100:1671–1676.

44. Heckenlively JR, Martin D, Levy J. Chloroquine retinopathy. *Am J Ophthalmol.* 1980;89:150–151.

45. Johnson MW, Vine AK. Hydroxychloroquine therapy in massive doses without retinal toxicity. *Am J Ophthalmol.* 1987;104:139–144.

46. Miller FS 3d, Bunt-Milam AH, Kalina RE. Clinical-

ultrastructural study of thioridazine retinopathy. *Ophthalmology.* 1982;89:1478–1488.

47. Mehta AM, Engstrom RE Jr, Kreiger AE. Deferox-amine-associated retinopathy after subcutaneous injection. *Am J Ophthalmol.* 1994;118:260–262.

48. Pavlidis NA, Petris C, Briassoulis E, et al. Clear evidence that long-term low-dose tamoxifen treatment can induce ocular toxicity: a prospective study of 63 patients. *Cancer.* 1992;69:2961–2964.

49. Weleber RG, Shults WT. Digoxin retinal toxicity; clinical and electrophysiologic evaluation of a cone dysfunction syndrome. *Arch Ophthalmol.* 1981;99: 1568–1572.

50. Robertson DM, Hollenhorst RW, Callahan JA. Ocular manifestations of digitalis toxicity. *Arch Ophthalmol.* 1966;76:640–645.

51. Schneider T, Dahlheim P, Zrenner E. Experimental investigations of the ocular toxicity of cardiac glycosides in animals. *Fortschr Ophthalmol.* 1989;86: 751–755.

52. Piltz JR, Wertenbaker C, Lance SE, Slamovits T, Leeper HF. Digoxin toxicity: recognizing the varied visual presentations. *J Clin Neuro-ophthalmol.* 1993; 13:275–280.

53. Purvin VA. Visual disturbance secondary to clomiphene citrate. *Arch Ophthalmol.* 1995;113:482–484.

54. Shields JA, Shields SC. *Intraocular Tumors: A Text and Atlas.* Philadelphia: Saunders; 1992.

55. Whitcup SM, DeMet MD, Rubin BI, et al. Intraocular lymphoma: clinical and histopathologic diagnosis. *Ophthalmology.* 1993;100:1399–1406.

56. Qualman SJ, Mendelsohn G, Mann RB, Green WR. Intraocular lymphomas: natural history based on a clinicopathologic study of eight cases and review of the literature. *Cancer.* 1983;52:878–886.

57. Allen RA, Straastma BR. Ocular involvement in leukemia-allied disorders. *Arch Ophthalmol.* 1961;66: 490–508.

58. Kincaid MC, Green WR. Ocular and orbital involvement in leukemia. *Surv Ophthalmol.* 1983;27: 211–232.

59. Mukai S, Gragoudas ES. Diagnosis of choroidal melanoma. In: Albert DM, Jakobiec FA, eds. *Principles and Practice of Ophthalmology.* Vol 5. Philadelphia: Saunders; 1994:3209–3216.

60. Collaborative Ocular Melanoma Study. Accuracy of diagnosis of choroidal melanomas in the Collaborative Ocular Melanoma Study; COMS report no. 1. *Arch Ophthalmol.* 1990;108:1268–1273.

61. Ferry AP, Font RL. Carcinoma metastatic to the eye and orbit: I. A clinicopathologic study of 227 cases. *Arch Ophthalmol.* 1974;92:276–286.

62. Stephens RF, Shields JA. Diagnosis and management of cancer metastatic to the uvea: a study of 70 cases. *Ophthalmology.* 1979;86:1336–1344.

63. Freedman MI, Folk JC. Metastatic tumors to the eye and orbit: patient survival and clinical characteristics. *Arch Ophthalmol.* 1987;105:1215–1223.

64. Carr RE, Siegel IM. *Electrodiagnostic Testing of the Visual System.* Philadelphia: FA Davis; 1990.

65. Fishman GA, Sokol S. *Electrophysiologic Testing in Disorders of the Retina, Optic Nerve, and Visual Pathway.* San Francisco: American Academy of Ophthalmology; 1990.

Chapter 12

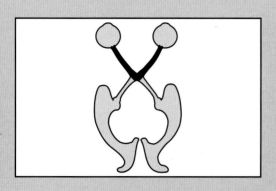

OPTIC NERVE AND CHIASM I: INFLAMMATORY, ISCHEMIC, AND INCREASED INTRACRANIAL PRESSURE DISORDERS

The optic nerves and chiasm are the prow of the diencephalon, white matter tracts made up of axons of retinal ganglion cells coated with oligodendroglial myelin. Damage to each component causes distinctive clinical features.

GENERAL CLINICAL MANIFESTATIONS

Optic Nerve Disorders

Impaired transmission within the optic nerves is typically reported as blurred, foggy, or dim vision. Less commonly, patients will describe positive phenomena, such as brief flashes of light. Examination discloses the following signs.

REDUCED VISUAL ACUITY

If the axon bundles carrying information from the foveal ganglion cells are affected, the ability to discriminate high-contrast stimuli (visual acuity) fails (Chapter 6).

ELEVATED FIXATION THRESHOLD

When visual acuity is reduced, an elevated static stimulus threshold is often found at the point of fixation on visual field testing (Chapter 7).

REDUCED COLOR VISION

Because the foveal ganglion cell axons carry most of the cone-mediated color information, a lesion of these axons will often impair color vision, reflected in poor performance on standard color vision tests and in the perception that colors appear "washed out," or desaturated (Chapter 6). Standard screening color vision tests are sensitive only to severe color dysfunction, but detailed tests are more accurate.

REDUCED CONTRAST SENSITIVITY

Lesions of the foveal ganglion cell axons interfere with contrast sensitivity, the ability to resolve low-contrast images. This capability is tested with black-and-white gratings or letters (Chapter 6).

REDUCED BRIGHTNESS SENSE

Vision appears dim, as if the lights have been turned down (Chapter 6). Placing a neutral density filter in front of a healthy eye mimics this sensation.

VISUAL FIELD LOSS

If the foveal ganglion cell axons are spared, and other axon bundles are damaged, visual field defects will appear despite normal visual acuity (Chapter 7). Visual field defects will have an arcuate, altitudinal, or radial shape, depending on which nerve fiber bundles have been principally lesioned (Chapters 1, 7).

AFFERENT PUPIL DEFECT

Because the optic nerve axons also serve as the afferent pathway for the pupillary reflex arc, interocularly asymmetric optic nerve defects will produce an afferent pupil defect (Chapter 8).

ABNORMAL VISUAL EVOKED POTENTIAL

The VEP is an objective and sensitive indicator of dysfunction of the retinocortical pathway mediated by foveal cones, but it is insensitive to damage of the nonfoveal pathway (Chapter 9). The VEP signal can also be degraded by inattention and deliberate noncompliance.

ABNORMAL OPTIC DISK

The four important structural alterations of the optic disk associated with optic neuropathy are pallor, elevation, excavation, and hypoplasia (Table 12-1):

Pallor

Pallor (Plates 41–44) describes a graying or whitening of the optic disk rim reflecting a death of axons. It arises from any process affecting the retinal ganglion cells or their axons on their way to the lateral geniculate body (LGB). It arises from lesions of the retrogeniculate pathway *only if they develop* in utero *or within the neonatal period.*[1]

Table 12–1. **The Abnormal Optic Disk**

Sign	Appearance	Pathogenesis	Causes
Pallor	Neuroretinal rim loses pink-orange color and turns gray-white	Death of retinal ganglion cell axons	Any optic neuropathy
Elevation	Acquired: blurred disk margins and peripapillary nerve fiber layer, surface hemorrhages/cotton-wool spots Congenital: elevated disk, loss of physiologic cup, epipapillary membrane, drusen	Acquired: axoplasmic stasis Congenital: overcrowding in small scleral opening, vascular anomalies, drusen, anomalies of fetal fissure closure	Acquired: increased ICP, infarction, inflammation, infiltration, oxidative phosphorylation failure Congenital: small eyes, failure of involution of hyaloid remnants, high myopia
Excavation	Erosion of neuroretinal rim so that cup diameter exceeds 1/2 disk diameter	Acquired: death of retinal ganglion cell axons Congenital: abnormal fetal fissure closure, high myopia	Acquired: any optic neuropathy but mainly glaucoma Congenital: embryonic anomalies
Hypoplasia	Small disk diameter; double-ring sign	Congenital lack of development of retinal ganglion cell axons	Uncertain

The optic disk color change from orange to gray-white probably results from a decrease in the caliber of its capillaries and a reorganization of its glial tissue as the axon bundles disappear.[2] This process requires a minimum of four weeks from the time of axon damage, and longer if the lesion is remote from the disk. Subtle uniocular pallor is best appreciated by comparison with the fellow eye. A media opacity, especially a nuclear cataract, may lend a golden glow to a white (atrophic) disk.

Elevation

Elevation (Plates 45–56) may be a reflection of axonal swelling (acquired disk elevation) or a congenital structural anomaly (congenital disk elevation). Axonal swelling results from stagnation of axoplasm as it flows toward the LGB (Fig. 12-1; Box 12-1).[3] Arrest of axoplasmic flow occurs most prominently as the axon bundles squeeze through the holes in the scleral lamina cribrosa. Any insult—regardless of its cause—compromises movement at this checkpoint.[4]

The degree of optic disk elevation associ-

Box 12–1

AXOPLASMIC STASIS, OPTIC DISK SWELLING, AND OPTIC NEUROPATHY

- Axoplasmic flow is a normal phenomenon in which metabolic products are carried along the axon both toward (retrograde) and away from (orthograde) the soma (cell body).

- If orthograde axoplasmic flow in retinal ganglion cell axons is impeded (axoplasmic stasis), the optic disk will swell. Neurotransmission may still occur at this stage. When axoplasmic flow stops altogether, neurotransmission fails.

- In papilledema, elevated intraocular pressure, and hypotony, experimental evidence shows that a block of orthograde flow occurs at the scleral lamina.[157] Such a block may also explain neurotransmission failure in ischemic optic neuropathy, optic neuritis, Leber's hereditary optic neuropathy, drusen optic neuropathy, or focal compression by mass lesions.

ated with axoplasmic stasis depends on the *nature and location of the insult.* For example, elevation is florid following a precipitous rise or a sustained, marked increase in intracranial pressure, large infarction at the nerve head (giant cell arteritis), neoplastic infiltration, or severe optic disk inflammation (Fig. 12-1). These conditions have in common a relatively focal injury at the lamina cribrosa to retinal ganglion cell axons. Disk elevation is less prominent in association with Leber's hereditary, toxic, and nutritional optic neuropathies, where the injury is to the ganglion cells (neuronopathy) rather than to the axons (axonopathy) (Chapter 15).

Disk elevation is pronounced when the intraocular portion of the optic nerve is involved by a focal lesion, because the axoplasm is held up at the lamina cribrosa. Elevation also occurs but is less pronounced when the intraorbital portion is involved within its sheath (meningioma, hemorrhage), at the orbital apex (Graves' disease, tumors), or within the optic canal, spaces that confine the optic nerve. Disk elevation does not occur when the optic nerve is compressed intracranially, where it has room to shift position.

The first hint of acquired optic disk elevation appears in the retina at the upper and lower disk borders, where swollen axons interfere with normal transparency. Severe axonal swelling obliterates the physiologic cup and compresses disk capillaries to cause peripapillary cotton-wool spots and hemorrhages. Although axonal enlargement is responsible for most of the disk swelling, there is also a component of vasogenic edema, evident as leakage of dye within the disk substance on fluorescein angiography.

Blurred optic disk margins and disk elevation are also features of congenital disk elevation. In this case, the axoplasm is flowing adequately to keep neurotransmission alive, the axons are not markedly swollen, and there is no vascular leakage. The elevation results mostly from tight packing within a small scleral opening (Plate 54). The bulging disk has a normal diameter, but at the sacrifice of its physiologic cup. In some cases, there is an excess of blood vessels and a buildup of calcified extra-axonal dead mitochondria called drusen, visible as chunks of yellow-white material on the disk sur-

face (see "Dysplastic Disorders," Chapter 13) (Plate 55). A congenital vitreous membrane may fail to regress normally and cover the disk surface (epipapillary membrane). Anomalies of fetal fissure closure and high myopia can tilt the optic disk so much that the nasal disk margin seen through the ophthalmoscope appears blurred (Plate 56).

Congenital and acquired optic disk elevation may be difficult to distinguish ophthalmoscopically, but congenital disk elevation should show none of the three cardinal signs of severe axoplasmic slowdown: thickening of the peripapillary nerve fiber layer, peripapillary retinal surface hemorrhages, and cotton-wool spots.

Excavation

Pathologic enlargement of the optic disk cup is referred to as excavation. The normal disk has a physiologic cup whose diameter should not exceed half the diameter of the disk. Any acquired process that kills axons may cause erosion of the disk rim tissue.[5] However, *glaucoma is the only acquired optic neuropathy that consistently causes marked excavation, or excavation that is out of proportion to the degree of visual loss* (Plate 57). A useful distinction between glaucomatous and nonglaucomatous cupping is that the preserved disk rim is typically of normal color in patients with glaucoma, whereas it is pale in those with other acquired optic neuropathies (Plate 58).[6] Improper fetal fissure closure and high myopia may cause striking optic nerve excavation that can be confused with glaucoma (Plate 59) (see Dysplastic Disorders, Chapter 13).[7]

Hypoplasia

Hypoplasia is a congenital lack of optic nerve tissue that produces a small disk diameter (Plate 60).[8] This sign can be hard to recognize because disk size normally varies greatly. Pathologically small nerve heads are invariably pale, but the correlation between structural abnormality and visual dysfunction is poor.

ABNORMAL IMAGING

Magnetic resonance imaging (MRI), the definitive means of visualizing the optic nerve

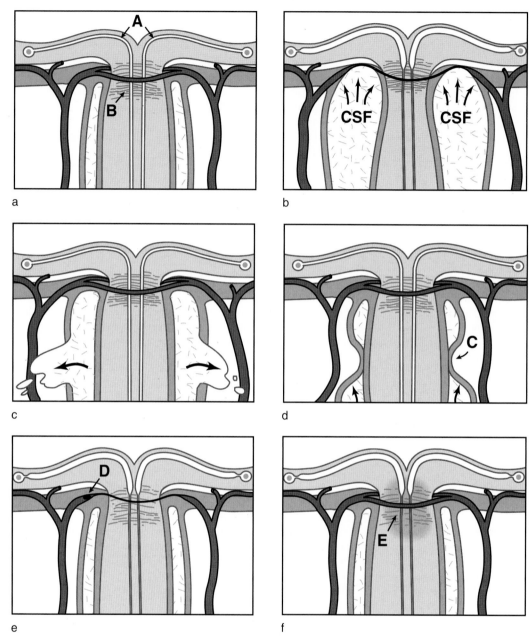

Figure 12–1. Axoplasmic stasis. (*a*) Normal. Retinal ganglion cell axons (A) are not distended because axoplasm flows normally past the scleral lamina cribrosa (B) toward the lateral geniculate body. (*b*) Increased intracranial pressure. CSF under pressure in the subarachnoid space compresses the fragile ciliary arterioles that supply the optic nerve head. Chronic ischemia retards axoplasmic flow at the scleral lamina and causes distention of prelaminar retinal ganglion cell axons. The optic disc swells (papilledema). (*c*) Optic nerve sheath fenestration: acute phase. Cutting a hole in the sheath allows CSF to escape (arrows) and relieve pressure on the ciliary blood supply. Normal axoplasmic flow is restored, and papilledema resolves. (*d*) Optic nerve sheath fenestration: chronic phase. The surgical window in the sheath has scarred down (C), but it acts as a buffer against direct pressure on the ciliary blood supply. Axoplasmic flow continues normally in spite of persistently elevated ICP (arrows). (*e*) Ischemic optic neuropathy. Occlusion of ciliary arterioles (D) causes ischemia to the optic nerve; axoplasmic flow dams up at the sclera lamina and the optic disk swells. (*f*) Optic neuritis. Inflammation of the optic nerve (E) impairs axoplasmic flow at the vulnerable "checkpoint"—the scleral lamina. The optic disk swells. (*continued*)

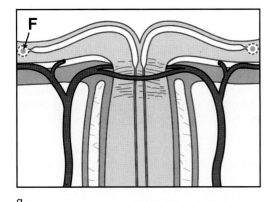

g

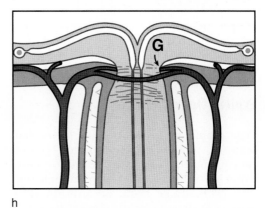

h

Figure 12–1. (*continued*) Axoplasmic stasis. (*g*) Leber's hereditary optic neuropathy. Oxidative phosphorylation fails within retinal ganglion cells (F), slowing axoplasmic flow at the scleral lamina. (*h*) Drusen optic neuropathy. A congenitally narrow scleral canal (G) makes passage of axoplasm across the scleral lamina even more difficult. Chronic slow flow eventually leads to axonal death and the accumulation of drusen.

behind the eye, is particularly helpful in revealing major dysplasias and compressive lesions. In addition, it can disclose signal abnormalities associated with inflammatory, neoplastic, or ischemic disorders owing to altered proton mobility, increased vascularity, or a breach in the blood–brain barrier. Generally MRI is normal in patients with toxic, nutritional, metabolic, or hereditary optic neuropathies.

Chiasmal Disorders

Chiasmal disorders cause disturbances of vision much like those of optic nerve disorders. In fact, most patients with chiasmal disorders present with uniocular visual loss. Examination typically shows an ipsilateral depression of visual acuity and an afferent pupil defect.[9] The optic nerve may appear normal (if the process is acute or mild) or pale (if the process is chronic), but never swollen. Inasmuch as most patients have no other neurologic manifestations and little or no explicit endocrine symptoms, *localization to the chiasm depends on finding the characteristic temporal hemianopic visual field loss.*

At the optic chiasm, axons originating from the nasal and temporal hemifields of each eye separate so that those conveying right hemifield signals enter the left optic tract and those conveying left hemifield signals enter the right optic tract (Fig. 1-8). The visual field loss of chiasmal lesions is based on the segregation of nasal and temporal axons and the fact that the nasal crossing fibers are selectively vulnerable to pathology of any type (Chapters 1, 7).

This vulnerability gives rise to a temporal hemianopic defect, the hallmark of chiasmal disorders. Defined as a temporal visual field defect whose border is aligned to the vertical meridian, it may exist in the visual field of one eye or both. However, it must not be coupled with a nasal hemianopic defect in the other eye, for then the localization would be to the retrochiasmal pathway (optic tract, lateral geniculate body, optic radiations, visual cortex) (Chapters 1, 7).

Lesions of the chiasm typically generate a bitemporal hemianopia. By contrast, those situated at the junction of one optic nerve and the chiasm generate hybrids of a nerve fiber bundle defect and a temporal hemianopic defect (Chapters 1, 7).

INFLAMMATORY DISORDERS

Optic neuritis is the term given to inflammation of the optic nerve.[10] In its typical form, it reflects primary destruction of the myelin sheath (demyelination) in an idiopathic autoimmune process affecting central nervous system white matter. Atypical forms of optic neuritis also involve demyelination, but the process is secondary to infection, a connective tissue disorder, posterior uveitis, or sarcoidosis.

Typical Optic Neuritis

Typical optic neuritis is defined by its characteristic presenting features and clinical course, and by a lack of evidence for an inflammatory disease other than multiple sclerosis (MS) (Table 12-2). Because the diagnosis is so dependent on clinical course, it cannot be made with certainty at onset if there are no other manifestations of MS.

PRESENTING CLINICAL FEATURES

The Optic Neuritis Treatment Trial (ONTT), enrolling 457 patients with acute optic neuritis between 1988 and 1992, has confirmed previous anecdotal information about the clinical profile of this condition.[11–16] Patients are usually aged between 15 and 45 years, and 75% are female. They usually complain of acute monocular vision loss and periocular pain (92%) exacerbated by eye movement. (Binocular optic neuritis is a more common presentation in children.) Visual scintillations (flashes) are relatively rare.[17] With probing, patients may complain of misjudging the position of moving objects, a fascinating visuospatial symptom based on a difference in the speed of conduction in the two optic nerves (the Pulfrich phenomenon; Fig. 4-3).[18]

In affected eyes, visual acuity ranges from 20/20 or better (11%) to no light perception (3%), with 55% having between 20/25 and 20/200. An afferent pupil defect is always present unless the fellow eye is, or has been, equivalently damaged. Optic disk edema, found in only one-third of affected eyes, is rarely dramatic. *Any abnormalities of the retina, choroid, or vitreous should cast doubt on the diagnosis of typical optic neuritis* (see "Atypical Optic Neuritis," below). Visual field defects are nonfocal in 50% of cases, focal with nerve fiber bundle configuration in 40%, and focal with hemianopic features in 10% (Chapter 7).[19,20] Among those with hemianopic defects, 50% have chiasmal features and 50% have retrochiasmal features (Chapter 7).

VISUAL EVOKED POTENTIALS

Visual evoked potentials provide objective—but nonspecific—support for optic nerve dysfunction (Chapter 9). In over 90% of optic neuritis cases, VEP signals from the affected eye will show prolonged latency.[21] Although VEPs are commonly ordered by neurologists in the evaluation of optic neuritis, they add no useful information if the classic clinical features—particularly the afferent pupil defect—are present.

NATURAL HISTORY

The natural history of this typical form of optic neuritis is favorable. Without treatment, vision stops worsening within one week, begins to recover in 85% within two weeks, and eventually reaches 20/20 or better in 70%, 20/40 or better in 93%.[14] Nearly all patients achieve maximum recovery within 30 days; a few stragglers continue to improve for up to one year. In the ONTT population, the only predictor of a poor visual outcome was a poor baseline visual acuity. Still, among those with finger counting or worse acuity at outset, 80% recovered to 20/40 or better.

Recurrent attacks of optic neuritis occurred in 28% of untreated patients over five years in the ONTT, with equal frequency in affected and fellow eyes. Fortunately, new bouts of optic neuritis also had a good outcome, so that visual function was not substantially lowered. Of patients who developed two or more recurrences of optic neuritis in the affected eye, 80% retained visual acuity of 20/30 or better.[15] Although recurrent optic neuritis was more frequent among patients who developed nonvisual neurologic manifestations of MS, 9% of the cohort had recurrent optic neuritis *without either clinical or imaging evidence of MS.*[15] Visual function declined slightly in some MS patients who did not have documented acute exacerbations of optic neuritis, affirming that a chronic progressive form of optic neuritis does exist in MS. (It is more common in later stages of the disease.) Still, after five years, only 1% of the entire cohort had a visual acuity worse than 20/40 in both eyes.[15]

Nearly one-third of patients who develop their first attack of typical optic neuritis have

Table 12–2. **Typical Optic Neuritis**

Risk Group	Manifestations	Imaging	Treatment	Clinical Course

Age 15–45
Female > Male
	Acute/subacute
	  monocular vision loss
	Pain on eye movement
	Visual field loss
	Afferent pupil defect
	Optic disk often normal
	History or evidence of
	  multiple sclerosis in 1/3
		1/2 are normal
		1/2 have signal
		  abnormalities
		  typical of
		  multiple sclerosis
			Intravenous methylprednisolone
			  (1 gm/day × 3 days)
			followed by prednisone
			  (1 mg/kg × 11 days)
				Untreated: vision stops getting worse
				  within 7 days, starts improving in
				  85% within 14 days; most recovery
				  attained within 30 days, but some
				  recovery up to 1 year; 70% recover 20/20
				Treated: no difference from untreated
				  except recovery is faster within first
				  2 weeks

had prior neurologic symptoms suggestive of MS.[22] Among those who have not, nearly one-third will develop other signs of MS within five years.[16] Beyond five years, the incidence of MS continues at a rate of 2% per year to reach 50%–60% by 40 years.[23] The degree of visual, motor, and cognitive impairment is low within the first five years.[16] During that time, only 4% of ONTT patients developed moderate disability and only 1% required assistance in ambulation or were wheelchair-bound. Earlier studies had suggested that MS ushered in by optic neuritis has a more benign prognosis than that initiated by brainstem or spinal cord findings.[24,25] Detailed information about long-term neurologic status after optic neuritis will be forthcoming as the ONTT patients are tracked further.

MAGNETIC RESONANCE IMAGING FINDINGS

Between 40% and 60% of patients with a first attack of optic neuritis have abnormalities on MRI that are consistent with multifocal demyelination.[26] Most of these abnormalities are located in the periventricular cerebral white matter. The prevalence of MRI enhancement of the affected optic nerve is high—84% among 37 eyes in one study.[27] The ONTT showed that the MRI "lesion load" (number and size of signal abnormalities) discovered at the time of acute optic neuritis is the single best predictor of the likelihood of future neurologic events typical of MS. After five years, only 16% of patients with normal MRIs had developed clinically definite MS, as compared to 51% of those with three or more signal abnormalities. Two earlier and smaller series had found a similarly powerful predictive value for MRI.[28,29]

TREATMENT

Prior to the ONTT, optic neuritis was usually treated with a two-week course of oral prednisone, despite the lack of any scientific evidence for its efficacy. In randomizing treatment with prednisone (1 mg/kg for 14 days), intravenous methylprednisolone (1 g for 3 days, followed by prednisone 1 mg/kg for 11 days), and placebo, the ONTT made a startling discovery: prednisone treatment

provided no benefit and actually doubled the recurrence rate of optic neuritis.[11] Intravenous methylprednisolone accelerated visual recovery within the first two weeks, but thereafter provided no benefit over placebo in terms of visual outcome. The hazards of treatment were minimal.[30]

If methylprednisolone treatment had no long-term effect on visual outcome, it did have an unexpected and dramatic impact on the short-term development of neurologic events that fulfilled the diagnosis of "clinically definite MS" (CDMS). Within the first two years of acute optic neuritis, CDMS developed in only 8% of patients treated with intravenous methylprednisolone, as compared to 17% of patients treated with placebo. Among patients with two or more MRI signal abnormalities, the chances of developing CDMS dropped from 36% with placebo to 16% with methylprednisolone. This protective effect was short-lived. By three years after optic neuritis, intravenous and placebo-treated patients had an equal cumulative incidence of CDMS. The temporary benefit of intravenous methylprednisolone is unexplained.

The ONTT findings have relegated prednisone treatment of acute optic neuritis to therapeutic oblivion. Most physicians have substituted intravenous methylprednisolone because even a temporary respite from advancing MS is considered a benefit.[31] Whether repeated intravenous treatment would prolong the hiatus is unknown. Periodic retreatment has not become a practice standard. (Randomized trials employing six-monthly pulsed methylprednisolone and interferon therapy are under way.) Some physicians restrict corticosteroid treatment to patients who have two or more MRI signal abnormalities; others offer treatment to all patients; some treat no one. About 40% of physicians do not order MRI as part of the management of acute optic neuritis.[31] Based on the available evidence, any of these options can be justified (Fig. 12-2).

A final alternative is to initiate chronic treatment with an immunomodulatory agent such as inteferon beta or glatiramer acetate. At the time of this writing, a large prospective randomized trial of patients with first attack optic neuritis (or incomplete transverse myelitis or brain stem deficits) found that intravenous methylprednisolone

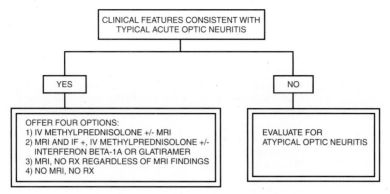

Figure 12–2. Management of optic neuritis.

1 gm/day for three days, followed by weekly intramuscular injections of interferon beta-1a 30 micrograms significantly reduced the 3-year development of a second clinical event that defined multiple sclerosis and the accumulation of MRI signal abnormalities.[31a] However, there are still no reports that any medical treatment alters the degree of disability in this illness. In considering their use at this early stage in the illness, clinicians must balance the beneficial effects of these agents against their high cost and side effects, the fact that many patients with monosymptomatic optic neuritis have a benign clinical course, and the possibility that the development of antibodies might nullify their immunomodulatory effects.

Based on this evidence, there are four reasonable options to managing first attack optic neuritis (Fig. 12-2): (*1*) IV methylprednisolone with or without MRI scan; (*2*) MRI scan and, if there are 2 or more 3 mm typical signal abnormalities, treat acutely with IV methylprednisolone and consider initiating chronic treatment with interferon beta or glatiramer acetate; (*3*) MRI for diagnostic and prognostic purposes, but defer treatment; (*4*) no MRI, defer treatment.

Atypical Optic Neuritis

A small but important subset of patients have optic neuritis related to a definable process other than MS, a condition here labeled as "atypical." Since typical and atypical optic neuritis often have identical presenting ophthalmic features, *the diagnosis of atypical optic neuritis depends on two features:*

- Baseline clinical or imaging evidence of a disease other than MS that could cause optic nerve inflammation.
- A clinical course that differs from that of typical optic neuritis.

Atypical optic neuritis may be associated with bacterial or fungal infections, presumed viral infections or vaccination, connective tissue diseases, or sarcoidosis, or it may be secondary to choroiditis or retinitis (Table 12-3).

INFECTIOUS OPTIC NEURITIS

In most cases of infectious optic neuritis, the patient is immune-compromised or has evidence of a systemic infection. Another clue is the frequent coexistence of uveitis, retinitis, or meningoencephalitis.

In infectious optic neuritis, damage may occur by direct invasion of organisms or thrombosis of the blood supply. The responsible pathogens are usually bacteria (hemophilus in children; streptococcus, staphylococcus, spirochetes,[32,33] and mycobacteria in adults), protozoa (toxoplasma),[34] fungi (cryptococcocus, aspergillus, mucormycosis),[35] or herpesviruses (cytomegalovirus, herpes simplex, herpes zoster).[35,36] Many of these specific optic neuritides occur in patients who are immunocompromised by HIV disease, organ transplantation, chronic corticosteroid therapy, alcoholism, severe burns, trauma, major surgery, or the neonatal state. They respond briskly to specific pharmacotherapy if it is given promptly.

Syphilitic optic neuritis occurs during any stage of the disease.[32,37,38] Visual loss may be rapid. In some cases, visual acuity is relatively

Table 12–3. **Atypical Optic Neuritis**

Condition	Causes	Comments
Infection	Strep/staph Hemophilus Syphilis/Lyme Tuberculosis Toxoplasmosis Cryptococcocus Aspergillosis Mucormycosis Herpesviruses Bartonella	Often coexisting retinitis, uveitis, or meningoencephalitis Must treat promptly
Viral illness, vaccination	Organisms not usually known	Optic neuritis often bilateral Recovery usually good
Connective tissue disease	Autoimmunity	Often improves dramatically following corticosteroid therapy
Sarcoidosis	Cranial base meningeal inflammation Chiasm, hypothalamus often involved	Slowly progressive Usually responds to corticosteroids but needs chronic treatment
Choroiditis, retinitis	Conditions associated with choroiditis or retinitis (Chapter 11)	Treatment aimed at underlying inflammation

preserved and pathologic examination discloses *perineuritis,* that is, the epicenter of inflammation is at the margins of the nerve, sparing the central macular bundle.[39] The rare optic neuritis of Lyme disease is associated with its secondary stage.[33,40] Optic neuritis in the context of toxoplasmosis and the herpesviruses often includes retinitis and uveitis.[34] In patients with tuberculosis, optic neuritis is part of a basal meningitis that often also affects the optic chiasm, a presentation mimicking sarcoidosis (see "Optic Neuritis in Sarcoidosis," below).

An ophthalmoscopically distinct form of optic neuritis called *Leber's stellate neuroretinitis* follows a flulike illness and has been linked to *Bartonella (Rochalimaea) henselae,* the organism responsible for cat-scratch disease.[41–44] Marked disk and peripapillary retinal edema give way within a week to a star-shaped collection of hard yellow exudates radiating from the fovea (Plate 49).[45,46] Many cases also display vitreous cells and focal areas of chorioretinitis near the optic disk.[47] Fluorescein angiography discloses profuse leakage from peripapillary retinal capillaries. Visual prognosis is generally good, and no patient with this pattern of optic neuritis has yet been reported to develop MS.[48]

Although optic neuritis has been blamed on an adjacent bacterial sinusitis, a cause-and-effect relationship is unlikely unless imaging shows a mucocoele, bone destruction, or a subperiosteal mass. On the other hand, *fungal sinusitis can compromise the optic nerve without showing any imaging abnormality* (Box 12-2).

POSTVIRAL OR POSTVACCINIAL OPTIC NEURITIS

Optic neuritis may appear within days to weeks of a systemic "influenzalike" illness or vaccination.[37,49–51] In these "para-infectious" cases, which are common in children, optic neuritis is often binocular, whereas in typical cases it is usually monocular. Good visual recovery is typical but not invariable.[50] Whether the pathogenesis is infectious or autoimmune is unsettled. For example, as yet unidentified pathogens may trigger the optic neuritis associated with acute disseminated encephalomyelitis and Guillain-Barre syndrome. Accepted treatment of this type of optic neuritis is high-dose corticosteroids, but no reliable study has demonstrated their value.

evident, but they may be subtle.[56] In this condition, optic neuritis is typically a component of a basilar meningitis that may involve the optic chiasm (producing hemianopic field loss), hypothalamus, and other cranial nerves (especially seventh and eighth; less often third, fourth, and sixth).[57] The differential diagnosis includes tuberculosis, histiocytosis, lymphoma, carcinoma, and idiopathic pachymeningitis.

Visual recovery can be impressive following corticosteroid therapy, especially if the visual loss has been recent. Regression is common, however, unless some level of therapy is maintained for months, possibly years. Noncorticosteroid immunosuppressive therapy is effective in some cases, but no pharmacologic agent can match corticosteroids. Radiation therapy has not worked.[54] In some cases, chronic basilar inflammation leads to hydrocephalus that requires shunting.

OPTIC NEURITIS IN CONNECTIVE TISSUE DISEASE

Optic neuritis is a rare but well documented feature of Crohn's disease, ulcerative colitis, Reiter's syndrome, Sjögren's syndrome, Behçet's disease, Wegener's granulomatosis, relapsing polychondritis, and lupus erythematosus.[49,52] Other parts of the eye, the orbit, and the sinuses are often inflamed. The optic nerve may be damaged by infarction rather than inflammation,[52] but because high-dose immunosuppressive treatment may bring about improvement, it should be tried.

Optic neuritis has also been reported in patients who have systemic and serologic signs of an autoimmune rheumatologic disorder that do not meet the full criteria for a named syndrome.[53] Their optic nerve function is alleged to improve only with very high corticosteroid or other immunosuppressive medication. Tapering of the dosage often leads to rapid recrudescence of the optic neuropathy, so the treatment must be long-term.

OPTIC NEURITIS IN SARCOIDOSIS

Optic neuritis is a rare manifestation of sarcoidosis.[54,55] The time course of visual loss is typically indolent. The optic disk may or may not be swollen. Pulmonary and extrapulmonary signs of sarcoidosis are usually

OPTIC NEURITIS SECONDARY TO CHOROIDITIS OR RETINITIS

Optic neuritis is an underrecognized component of an inflammation seated within the retina or choroid (Chapter 11).[49] In these cases, the optic disk is generally swollen. Accompanying findings are choroidal infiltrates, vitreous cells, anterior chamber inflammation, or retinal occlusive phenomena. Some patients have no obvious evidence of a systemic disorder, but a thorough evaluation is necessary.

An enigmatic condition that may fit into this category consists of acute unilateral optic disk swelling with marked engorgement of the retinal veins and perivenous hemorrhage (Plate 53). The patient, usually under age 45, complains of acute uniocular visual loss often accompanied by flickering. Visual acuity and field loss may be substantial, and there is often an afferent pupil defect. Systemic evaluation is typically unrevealing. Histopathologic study of one case disclosed lymphocytic infiltration of the intraoptic retinal veins,[58] leading to the designation *papillophlebitis.* Controversy prevails as to whether venous or optic nerve inflammation is primary. There is no treatment, but the fundus signs eventually disappear, and vision usually recovers substantially.

Five noninflammatory conditions imitate optic neuritis (Table 12-4). They are isch-

Table 12–4. Differential Diagnosis of Optic Neuritis

Entity	One Eye or Both?	Time Course	Pattern of Visual Field Loss	Ophthalmoscopy	Ancillary Findings
Optic neuritis	Usually one	Acute/subacute	Nerve fiber bundle or diffuse	Normal	MRI white matter changes of MS in 50%
Ischemic optic neuropathy	One	Acute	Nerve fiber bundle	Disk often swollen	Elevated ESR in giant cell arteritis form
Infiltrative optic neuropathy	One or both	Subacute	Nerve fiber bundle or diffuse or hemianopic	Normal, but disk sometimes swollen	Evidence of primary or metastatic (including meningeal) cancer
Compressive optic neuropathy	One or both	Chronic (but rarely acute)	Usually hemianopic; may be nerve fiber bundle	Disk pale, normal or rarely swollen	MRI evidence of intracranial or intraorbital mass
Leber's hereditary optic neuropathy	One followed by the other after weeks to months	Acute/subacute	Usually central/cecocentral	Peripapillary nerve fiber layer thickening and telangiectasia	Blood test reveals DNA mutation
Toxic optic neuropathy	Both	Acute/subacute/chronic	Usually central/cecocentral	Normal, but rarely mild swelling	Toxin in urine (sometimes)

emic optic neuropathy, infiltration by cancer, compression by masses, Leber's hereditary optic neuropathy, and toxic disorders. Distinguishing between these six entities depends principally on the time course of the visual loss, whether the affection is monocular or binocular, the pattern of the visual field loss, and the ophthalmoscopic findings. Ancillary tests, including brain imaging, may be necessary to make a definitive diagnosis.

ISCHEMIC DISORDERS

Ischemic optic neuropathy is the term applied to infarction of the optic nerve. A survey of ophthalmologists disclosed that this condition comprised 35% of acute optic neuropathies at all ages, and 66% among patients aged 50 years or older.[59] Ischemic optic neuropathy has several clinical variants (Table 12-5).

Nonarteritic Anterior Ischemic Optic Neuropathy

This variant, known as NAION, accounts for over 90% of all acute ischemic optic neuropathy cases. Infarction of the optic disk is believed to result from reduced perfusion of the postlaminar optic nerve, supplied by an anastomotic circle derived from medial and lateral branches of the posterior ciliary arterioles (Fig. 1-16).[60,61] These ciliary branch vessels are so small, and pathologic material so sparse, that it is still unclear whether NAION results from frank occlusion or watershed ischemia. Autopsies of elderly patients without NAION have shown intimal narrowing of posterior ciliary feeders,[62] and histopathologic material from three cases of NAION, marred by atypical clinical features, have shown segmental infarction immediately behind the lamina cribrosa[63,64] and occlusion of three ciliary feeder vessels.[65]

This variant is called *nonarteritic* to emphasize that its pathogenesis is noninflammatory, as distinct from the less common but more virulent arteritic form (see "Arteritic Ischemic Optic Neuropathy," below). It is called *anterior* to highlight the fact that the optic disk is always swollen, as distinct from the variant in which the infarct occurs far enough behind the optic nerve head that no edema is ever observed (see "Posterior Ischemic Optic Neuropathy," below).

PRESENTING FEATURES

The afflicted patient, aged 40 years or more (peak age 55–70 years), complains of acute, usually (>90%) painless,[66] sustained uniocular visual loss. The loss of vision is often first noticed upon awakening in the morning. It is almost never preceded by transient blackouts or hallucinations.[67-70] Visual loss may worsen for a few days, and uncommonly for a few weeks.[71,72] There are no other relevant visual, neurological, or constitutional symptoms.

Visual acuity ranges from normal to no light perception, but more than 50% of patients have better than 20/60 acuity. A nerve fiber bundle defect (most commonly inferonasal arcuate or altitudinal) or nonlocalizing defect (Chapter 7) is found on perimetry. Unless there has been equivalent optic nerve damage to the fellow eye in the past, an ipsilateral afferent pupil defect is present, albeit subtle if the damage is minimal.

The optic disk in the affected eye is diffusely or segmentally swollen. If the swelling is segmental, the edematous sector corresponds to the region of visual field loss. Flame hemorrhages and cotton-wool spots are often visible on the surface of the disk or at its margin (Plate 50). If the cotton wool spots are not contiguous with the disk margin, suspect combined optic disk and retinal infarction from markedly elevated blood pressure (see "Hypertensive Optic Neuropathy," below). Although the optic disk edema is often described as "pallid," (gray-white), red-orange (hyperemic) edema is nearly as common.[68]

The optic disk in the fellow eye typically has a below average cup-to-disk ratio.[73] In some cases, it discloses mild edema but normal visual function.[74] Because this finding has been associated with imminent development of NAION in the fellow eye,[68] it is called *preeruptive*. Perhaps chronic axoplasmic stasis (caused by chronic low-grade ischemia and a tight optic disk space) precedes actual infarction in these cases.

NATURAL HISTORY

Visual recovery is minimal, in sharp contrast to the course of typical optic neuritis. More than two-thirds of patients show little or no improvement; in the remaining third, recovery is modest.[75] The affected eye suffers virtually no recurrent attacks, but the fellow eye may suffer a similar event with an incidence of 19%[76] to 25%[77] within 5 years. The interval to involvement of the second eye varies from months to decades, with 25% of events occurring within 2.5 years.[77] Very rarely, both eyes become involved simultaneously or within days, a finding that should lead to the presumption of a preceding hypotensive event (including overtreatment with antihypertensive medications), a hypercoagulable state, or arteritis.

The future risk of myocardial infarction and stroke in patients with NAION is negligibly greater than expected for age.[78,79] Two small studies comparing the prevalence of multifocal deep cerebral white matter signal abnormalities in NAION and in age-matched controls without hypertension came to opposite conclusions. In one study, there was no difference,[80] whereas in the other, the number of such lesions was significantly greater in NAION than in an age-matched population.[81]

RISK FACTORS

Who is vulnerable to this condition? Conventional arteriosclerotic risk factors, including diabetes and essential hypertension, are present more often in afflicted patients than in age-matched controls, particularly among those aged 65 years or less.[78,79,82,83] In one study, smoking was significantly more prevalent among NAION patients than among age-matched controls.[84] Atheromatous disease of the cervical carotid arteries, cardiac sources of emboli, and retinal emboli are not prominent among patients with NAION.[85–87]

The fact that many patients report visual loss upon first awakening from nighttime sleep has suggested that NAION arises from low noctural perfusion. One uncontrolled study did find exaggerated noctural dips in systemic blood pressure in NAION patients,[88] and another study found that NAION patients had a relatively slow rise in daytime blood pressure compared to controls.[89] Intriguingly, a clinical syndrome almost exactly like that of NAION occurs after intraoperative hypotension (see "Hypotensive Ischemic Optic Neuropathy," below).[90–93] In the author's experience, NAION often follows within a week of an increase in blood pressure–lowering medications.

PATHOGENESIS

Any pathogenetic theory of NAION must take into account the following facts: (*1*) most attacks occur suddenly and painlessly, and the deficit, while briefly progressive and modestly reversible, is basically fixed; (*2*) most attacks occur upon awakening; (*3*) infarction is a one-time event in each eye; (*4*) the fellow eye, which often has a cupless disk, is highly vulnerable to attack after months to years; (*5*) arteriosclerotic risk factors are prominent, but future risk of MI and stroke is negligibly increased; (*6*) a nearly identical process follows acute hypotension or overtreated hypertension.

The hypothesis that best reconciles these data considers typical NAION a watershed microinfarction in an area that is vulnerable to brief diurnal falls in blood pressure because of tight tissue packing, exposure to intraocular pressure, and a flimsy blood supply with poor autoregulation. After all, the arterial feeders of the optic nerve unfairly compete with the dominant choroidal circulation, which drains most of the ciliary supply through a fast, low-pressure system designed to meet the high metabolic needs of the RPE (Chapter 1). Why do patients with NAION so rarely develop strokes elsewhere in the central nervous system? Perhaps because the stroke that causes optic neuropathy requires only a tiny area of ischemia, yet it affects an eloquent and topographically organized axon system that lacks the redundancy common to other brain regions.

TREATMENT

There is no effective treatment for NAION. A brief flurry of excitement over the efficacy of optic nerve sheath fenestration, based on uncontrolled information,[94–97] has been stilled by a large controlled study.[75] Not only

Table 12–5. Variants of Ischemic Optic Neuropathy

Variant	Setting	Findings	Management	Outcome
Non-arteritic anterior	Hypertension, diabetes, other arteriosclerotic risk factors	Variable degree of monocular vision loss with swollen disk	Correct discretionary arteriosclerotic risk factors, guard against overtreated hypertension	Stable or mild recovery; fellow eye sometimes involved later
Hypotensive	Hypotension, blood loss, dialysis surgery	Variable degree of visual loss, often binocular Disks normal or swollen	Probably no treatment works but try fluid loading to raise BP	Stable or mild recovery
Hypertensive	Diastolic pressures above 120 mm Hg	Peripapillary cotton-wool spots, retinal macroinfarcts	Lower BP slowly	Stable Visual decline if BP lowered too quickly
Arteritic	Polymyalgia rheumatica complex; patient usually aged over 65	Marked monocular visual loss with swollen disk, choroidal ischemia	Immediate high-dose corticosteroids	Stable if treated Fellow eye affected in 30%–50% within days to weeks if not treated
Posterior	Craniofacial irradiation, surgery; arteritis	Monocular visual loss with normal disk Sometimes chiasmal field loss	Imaging, LP, systemic evaluation to rule out treatable causes	Depends on cause
Acute cervical carotid artery occlusion	Atheroma, dissection	Concurrent signs of ipsilateral hemispheric ischemia	Imaging of neck and head Possible carotid surgery	Stable
Postcataract extraction	Cataract surgery preceding within hours to weeks	Visual loss immediately postop or weeks later; swollen disk	Delay cataract surgery on fellow eye as long as possible	50% incidence of similar event with cataract surgery on fellow eye
Migrainous	History of migraine	Monocular visual loss with swollen disk	Consider calcium channel blocker prophylaxis	Future stroke rate not known to be increased
Diabetic papillopathy	Diabetes mellitus	Subacute visual loss with chronic, often bilateral optic disk swelling with prominent surface telangiectasia	None	Gradual resolution of disk signs Visual loss usually mild and recovery better than in NAION
Chronic low perfusion states	Carotid stenosis Elevated ICP Carotid-cavernous fistula Glaucoma?	Depends on underlying condition	Depends on underlying condition	Depends on underlying condition

is sheath decompression useless, it actually harms patients by worsening their visual outcome.[75]

A retrospective study found that aspirin users got no protection from the severity of visual loss in NAION.[98] There is no study showing that aspirin reduces the incidence of fellow eye involvement. But aspirin is clearly preventive in TIA or stroke, so that it has become customary to prescribe it prophylactically after NAION has struck one eye. Arteriosclerotic risk factor reduction is, however, the governing principle of management, *with special attention directed at avoiding overtreatment of hypertension.* The preventive value of lowering intraocular pressure in the unaffected eye has not been explored.

Hypotensive Ischemic Optic Neuropathy

An acute optic neuropathy with many of the clinical features of the "spontaneous" form of NAION has been well documented following intraoperative hypotension, severe blood loss, or renal dialysis, which all share a sudden profound drop in blood pressure.[90–93,99,100] Postsurgical NAION cases are often marked by preexisting arteriosclerosis, anemia (hemoglobin <6 g/dL), ample intraoperative bleeding, prone position, pump oxygenation, long operative time (>6 hours), lower cardiac output requiring inordinate use of inotropic agents, or marked weight gain secondary to large fluid infusions required to maintain intraoperative blood pressure.[91,100] Notably, however, some postsurgical cases lack any recorded evidence of hypotension or extraordinary blood loss.

PRESENTING FEATURES

The ophthalmic characteristics of the hypotensive (shock-induced, blood loss) form of NAION differ from those of the spontaneous variety in three ways: (*1*) both eyes are often involved concurrently; (*2*) visual loss is usually more profound; and (*3*) optic disk edema is absent, mild, or delayed by several days after the hypotensive event (see "Posterior Ischemic Optic Neuropathy," below). When visual loss is profound and binocular, and the eye grounds appear normal, a mis-

diagnosis of cortical blindness may be entertained unless a lack of pupillary reaction to light is noted. Visual recovery is usually modest, but it may be impressive within days to weeks of the event.

PATHOGENESIS

The pathogenesis of this form of NAION is believed to be watershed infarction of the midorbital and anterior orbital optic nerve.[90] Intriguingly, pathologic examination of the rest of the brain and spinal cord shows no obvious ischemic areas.[90] This evidence suggests that *the extracranial optic nerve is exceedingly vulnerable to hypotension* for reasons that remain to be explained. The operative setting most commonly associated with this complication is coronary bypass surgery,[100] but it also follows coronary catheterization, hemodialysis, pneumonectomy, cholecystectomy, and spine surgery. In spine procedures, the face-down position may worsen perfusion by raising intraocular and retinal venous pressure.[91,101] In coronary bypass procedures, longer bypass times and higher use of inotropic agents may be contributory.[100]

Is the incidence or merely the awareness of this complication increasing? Perhaps both, although as improvements in surgical and anesthetic techniques have permitted procedures of longer duration and greater daring, they must be facilitated by deliberate intraoperative hypotension. Moreover, low hematocrits have often been tolerated in order to avoid the infectious complications of blood transfusions.

TREATMENT

No effective treatment has emerged, although one report describes substantial recovery of vision with prompt fluid loading, presumably to increase blood pressure and optic nerve perfusion.[93]

Hypertensive Optic Neuropathy

Severe (malignant) hypertension can cause optic disc edema,[102] but in most cases the visual loss is caused by infarction of the retina or choroid. The optic disk edema of malignant hypertension probably results from a breakthrough in autoregulation. This causes disk vessels to leak (vasogenic edema), but vision is usually preserved. Confronted with binocular disk swelling and preserved vision, the examiner may mistakenly diagnose papilledema.

Malignant hypertension can cause optic disk infarction in rhesus monkeys[103,104] and rarely in humans,[105] especially children.[106] In these cases, there is ischemic swelling of the endothelium and pericytes, vascular occlusion, and infarction of axons. The disk edema in such cases is not "vasogenic" but "cytotoxic"—reflecting ischemic arrest of axoplasmic flow with a massive distention of axons.[103,104]

Ophthalmoscopy should suggest malignant hypertension as the cause of optic disk infarction if it is accompanied by segmental ischemic retinal swelling or choroidal infarcts (focal elevations of the RPE) (Chapter 10). This type of ischemic optic neuropathy is characterized by many cotton-wool spots that are separated from the optic disk by one or more disk diameters.

This two-stage sequence of vasogenic edema resulting from autoregulatory breakthrough, followed by occlusive infarction of axons, recalls a process that occurs in the parieto-occipital branches of the posterior cerebral artery in patients with hypertensive encephalopathy (see "Hypertensive Encephalopathy," Chapter 15). It should alert clinicians to the importance of lowering blood pressure before an occlusive stage is reached and permanent visual loss occurs. On the other hand, *exuberant lowering of blood pressure in the presence of optic disk edema is dangerous:* it can lead to a disastrous loss of vision, presumably because imperfect autoregulation results in a precipitous drop in perfusion.[107,108] This cruel paradox—that either very high or very low blood pressure can cause ischemic optic neuropathy—is common to ischemic stroke anywhere in the nervous system. It reflects a common pathogenesis: poor perfusion.

Arteritic Ischemic Optic Neuropathy

Although the optic nerve is affected by a variety of inflammatory vasculopathies, including those associated with connective tissue diseases and fungi, the most important one to consider is giant cell (temporal) arteritis. The diamondback of optic neuropathies, it strikes quickly and unexpectedly with deadly effects.[109–111]

RISK GROUP

Patients over age 50 (female/male = 3/1) are at risk, but the prevalence rises rapidly over age 70.[112] All races are vulnerable, but most information comes from northern latitudes where Caucasians are overrepresented. In the face of unsound data on the relative prevalence of arteritic and nonarteritic ischemic optic neuropathy, estimates are that even among the elderly, the nonarteritic form is at least ten times as common.[59] Yet the arteritic form must always be excluded because the threat of involvement of the fellow eye is as high as 33% in untreated cases.[113]

PRESENTING FEATURES

The acute ophthalmic manifestations of arteritic ischemic optic neuropathy overlap those of NAION. In general, however, visual acuity loss is greater, and the optic disk has more pallid swelling. There are isolated case reports of bona fide giant cell arteritis without disk swelling, but they are precious.[109] Retinal arterial infarcts may uncommonly occur without optic nerve infarcts.[109]

Although not usually ophthalmoscopically visible, segmental hypoperfusion of the choroid is found on fluorescein angiography;[114] this may explain visual loss before optic disk edema appears (Fig. 12-3).[115] Color Doppler imaging is useful in showing the blatantly poor perfusion associated with giant cell arteritis and the relatively well-preserved flow of NAION.[116,117] In cases of arteritis, there may be coexisting cilioretinal artery and anterior ocular segment ischemia (hypotony, anterior chamber cell and flare) (Chapter 10).[109] Months later, chorioretinal atrophy, pathologic optic disk cupping, iris rubeosis, and cataract may occur. These devastating effects are based on proximal or multiple branch ciliary occlusions,[118] as opposed to the distal watershed ischemia of NAION.

Although most patients have symptoms of polymyalgia rheumatica (malaise, proximal joint and muscle ache, fatigue, fever, ano-

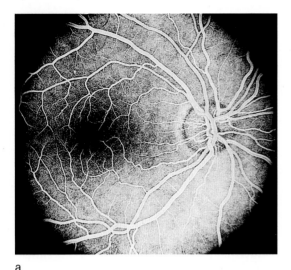
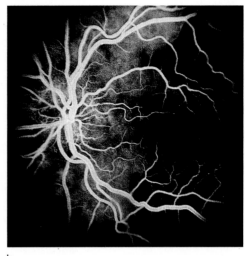

a   b

Figure 12–3. Ischemic optic neuropathy in giant cell arteritis: choroidal nonperfusion. In this retinal fluorescein angiogram, the unaffected right eye (*a*) displays a normal diffuse white background fluorescence at 33 seconds after injection, reflecting normal choroidal flow. The left eye (*b*) displays large areas of choroidal nonperfusion temporally (dark areas), owing to arteritic occlusion of the ophthalmic artery.

rexia) or cranial inflammation (headache, jaw claudication, scalp tenderness), an estimated 8%,[119] 21%,[120] or 38%[121] have no such constitutional manifestations. Patients who have arteritic ischemic optic neuropathy as an isolated manifestation (occult giant cell arteritis)[122,123] pose a stiff diagnostic challenge.

Acute-phase reactants, including sedimentation rate and C-reactive protein, are elevated in more than 80% of cases.[68,124] C-reactive protein elevation may be more specific for the disease than sedimentation rate elevation.[125]

A properly performed temporal artery biopsy has a sensitivity of at least 95%[126,127] and near-perfect specificity. The pathology specimen need not include giant cells, but it should show fragmentation of the internal limiting membrane with lymphocytic infiltration in the acute stage and fibrosis in the chronic stage.[128] These abnormalities are spotty, however, leaving intervals of undisturbed vessel wall in more than 25% of cases.[129] Thus the high sensitivity of biopsy depends on harvesting a segment of at least 2 cm and sectioning it into 1 mm segments with nine sections per segment.[130] Although corticosteroid treatment eliminates flagrant inflammation within weeks, macrophages persist for months.[131,132] To avoid equivoca-

tion, biopsy should be performed within days of beginning corticosteroid treatment.

DIFFERENTIAL DIAGNOSIS

In the elderly patient presenting with acute visual loss and a swollen optic disk, the challenge is to distinguish between the common nonarteritic and the rare but catastrophic arteritic form of ischemic optic neuropathy (Table 12-6). Advanced age, constitutional symptoms, severe visual loss, binocular involvement, presence of other signs of ocular ischemia, elevated acute-phase reactants, and lack of arteriosclerotic risk factors favor a diagnosis of arteritis. Ancillary tests such as fluorescein angiography and color Doppler orbital imaging may be helpful in demonstrating the reduced perfusion through large ciliary and choroidal branches typical of the arteritic form (Fig 12-3).

NATURAL HISTORY AND MANAGEMENT

The untreated clinical course of this disease is dismal. There is no recovery of vision in the affected eye, and in one-third of instances the fellow eye will succumb to optic disk infarction within four weeks of diagno-

Table 12–6. **Arteritic versus Nonarteritic Ischemic Optic Neuropathy**

Clinical Feature	Arteritic	Nonarteritic
Age	>65	45–70
Polymyalgia rheumatica (PMR) complex	Present in 50% or more	Absent
Erythrocyte sedimentation rate, C-reactive protein	Elevated in > 80%	Normal
Arteriosclerotic risk factors	Age appropriate	Elevated
Binocular involvement	Up to 50% with interval often less than one week	Up to 20% but interval rarely less than 6 months
Degree of visual loss	Severe	Variable, but milder than arteritic
Ophthalmoscopic findings	Disk edema pronounced and often pallid; may see retinal cotton-wool spots	Pallid disk edema less pronounced than in arteritic No retinal cotton-wool spots Unaffected eye has cupless disk
Choroidal perfusion on fluorescein angiography	Reduced	Normal
Arterial flow on orbital color Doppler imaging	Reduced	Normal
Temporal artery biopsy	Positive in 95% Very few false positives	Negative
Effect of corticosteroid treatment	Prompt recovery of PMR symptoms Normalization of acute phase reactants	None

sis.[133] Fellow eye infarctions are very rarely reported after that interval. Anecdotal data, but no formal prospective trial, support high-dose corticosteroid therapy (1–4 g/day intravenous methylprednisolone or 1.5–2 mg/kg prednisone). This therapy rarely improves vision in the affected eye but reduces the chances that the optic nerve in the fellow eye will become infarcted.[133,134] Regrettably, many fellow eyes that appear clinically uninvolved at outset will become infarcted inspite of high-dose regimens.[135] Even so, prompt institution of high-dose intravenous treatment is increasingly advocated once one optic nerve has become infarcted.[136]

A temporal artery biopsy should be performed within a few days of instituting corticosteroid therapy. Even in cases where the clinical diagnosis appears firm, a positive biopsy is a security worth having because of the hazards of chronic corticosteroid ther-

apy. Corticosteroid dose may be tapered gradually (by 10% of daily dose/week), with the acute-phase reactants and constitutional symptoms used as guidelines. To reduce corticosteroid side-effects, aim to have the patient converted to an every-other-day prednisone regimen within three months of diagnosis, as the chance of optic nerve infarction becomes acceptably low by this time. A regimen equivalent to prednisone 10 mg/day is continued for 12 months. In the instances where corticosteroid therapy fails to control the disease or is poorly tolerated, methotrexate is the next-best choice.[137]

Because polymyalgia rheumatica (PMR) and giant cell arteritis probably represent variants of the same condition, consideration should be given to performing a biopsy on all patients with PMR symptoms. If the biopsy shows features of arteritis, they should be treated aggressively.[138]

Posterior Ischemic
Optic Neuropathy

In this variant, known as PION, optic nerve infarction is remote from the disk and axoplasmic pileup at the nervehead is too minimal to be visible ophthalmoscopically. Apart from the absence of optic disk edema, the ophthalmic manifestations are like those of NAION.

The recognized causes of PION are hypotension (see "Hypotensive Ischemic Optic Neuropathy," above), surgical trauma to the optic nerve, radiation,[139] giant cell,[140] fungal, and nonspecific arteritis, migraine,[141] and arteriosclerosis.[142,143] Given the rarity of PION, however, *visual loss unassociated with optic disk edema should always be evaluated with thorough neurodiagnostic studies, particularly in older or immune-compromised individuals, unless it can be comfortably attributed to typical optic neuritis.*

RADIATION OPTIC NEUROPATHY AND CHIASMOPATHY

Ischemic damage to the optic nerves and chiasm from high-voltage external-beam therapeutic radiation is a well-documented phenomenon among patients treated for a variety of malignancies of the paranasal sinuses, nasopharynx, orbit, and anterior and middle cranial fossa,[144] even with highly focused modern techniques.[145] Visual loss is cataclysmic and untreatable. Fortunately, it happens rarely if proper dosimetry precautions are upheld.

The first episode occurs from 1 to 14 years after radiation, but mean latencies are 1.5 to 2 years. Thereafter, visual loss often has a stepwise downward course, as if successive infarcts were occurring. Visual field defects reflect involvement of either the optic nerve or chiasm. If the radiation has been centered near the eye, the fundus may disclose optic disk swelling or retinal infarcts. Following radiation centered more posteriorly, there are no fundus abnormalities until optic disk pallor appears months later. An MRI usually discloses enhancement of the lesioned region,[146,147] and sometimes the tissue is swollen enough to falsely suggest tumor. The pathology is that of infarction secondary to obliterative arteriopathy.

This complication occurs in fewer than 2% of cases at total doses of less than 6000 cGy[144,148] unless patients have substantial preexisting compression of the anterior visual pathways.[139] Other sensitizing factors are chemotherapy, diabetes, arteriosclerosis, and older age.[144] At total doses of 6000 cGy or greater, the incidence of visual pathway damage rises precipitously, and daily dose fraction size becomes critical. In one authoritative study, the 15 year actuarial risk of optic neuropathy was only 11% for fraction sizes of < 190 cGy but 47% for fraction sizes of ≥190 cGy.[144]

There is no effective treatment for radiation injury to the anterior visual pathway. Despite initial enthusiasm about hyperbaric oxygen and corticosteroids, neither has proved helpful.[149] A regimen of heparin followed by warfarin anticoagulation produced a modest improvement in nonvisual neurologic signs in a small cohort,[150] but there is no published experience with visual loss. In the absence of effective treatment, investigators stress reduced portal sizes in order to protect the visual apparatus. Three-dimensional conformal radiation protocols offer such a potential.

Cervical Carotid Artery Occlusion

Although NAION typically occurs in the absence of large vessel atheromatous disease, there are the very rare exceptions of patients who present with concurrent optic nerve stroke and ipsilateral hemispheric TIA or stroke (opticocerebral syndrome).[151–153] In such cases, angiography documents total cervical carotid occlusion or dissection and reversal of flow in the ophthalmic artery. Interestingly, the retinal circulation is spared.

Post–Cataract Extraction
Optic Neuropathy

A syndrome equivalent to NAION follows uncomplicated cataract surgery, either immediately[154] or weeks to months afterwards.[155] Anesthesia may have been administered retrobulbarly or endotracheally. Among those cases that are detected in the immediate postoperative period, patients of-

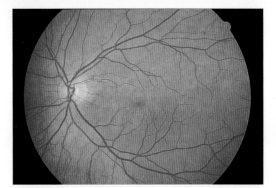

Plate 1. Normal fundus oculi.

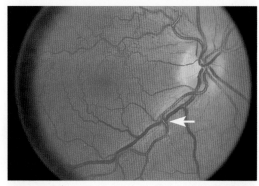

Plate 2. Arteriolar sclerosis. Chronic hypertension leads to a stiffening of the arteriolar walls, visible as a yellowing of the light reflection and a deviation of the veins as they cross arteries (arteriovenous nicking) (arrow).

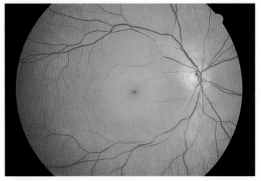

Plate 3. Acute central retinal artery occlusion. Note ischemic whitening except in the foveola, where the retina has only photoreceptors. The red reflection of the choroid shines through as a "cherry-red spot."

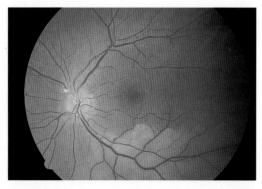

Plate 4. Acute large branch retinal artery occlusion. Note focal ischemic whitening in the distal field of the vessel occluded by an embolus.

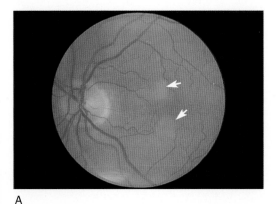

A

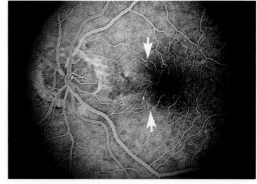

B

Plate 5. Acute small branch retinal arteriolar occlusions. Note tiny areas of ischemic whitening (arrows) (a); fluorescein angiogram pinpoints occluded segments (arrows) (b).

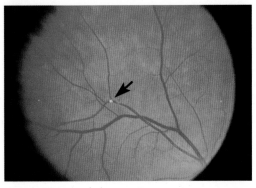

Plate 6. Hollenhorst plaque. The yellow plug (arrow) wedged at a distal arteriolar bifurcation did not cause infarction.

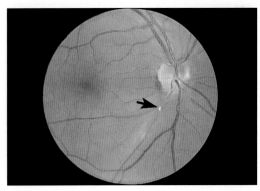

Plate 7. Calcific plaque (arrow). Whiter and larger than a Hollenhorst plaque, it usually originates from the aortic valve.

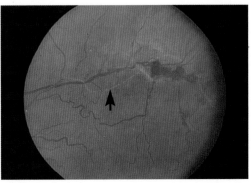

Plate 8. Longstanding branch retinal arteriolar occlusion. Note the sheathed distal arteriole (arrow); it often looks like a pipecleaner.

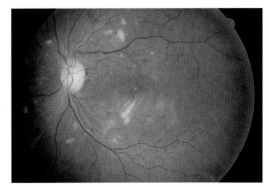

Plate 9. Precapillary arteriolar occlusion: cotton-wool spots. The fluffy yellow-white areas are nerve fiber layer microinfarcts.

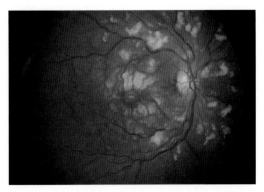

Plate 10. Precapillary arteriolar occlusion: Purtscher's-like retinopathy. A plethora of cotton-wool spots, as seen in malignant hypertension, chest or pelvic injury, pancreatitis, active lupus erythematosus, and hypercoagulable states.

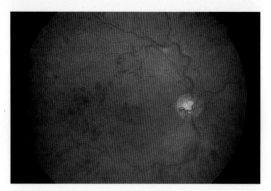

Plate 11. Venous stasis ("low-flow") retinopathy. Note distended retinal veins with perivenous hemorrhages.

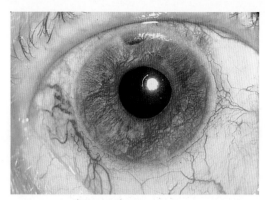

Plate 12. Ocular ischemic syndrome. Note conjunctival hyperemia and iris neovascularization, signs of chronic anterior ocular hypoperfusion.

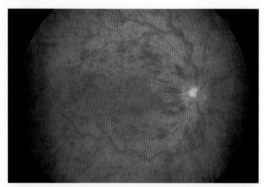

Plate 13. Central retinal vein occlusion. The retinal surface is covered with hemorrhages but there are no cotton-wool spots, an indication of relatively mild ischemia.

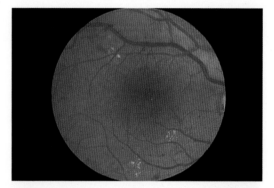

Plate 14. Inner blood–retinal barrier incompetence: hard exudates.

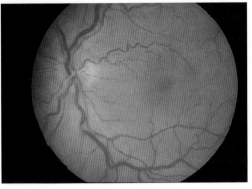

A

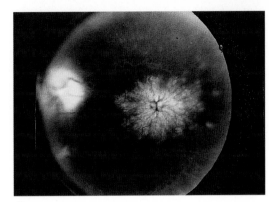

B

Plate 15. Inner blood–retinal barrier incompetence: cystoid macular edema. Clear, serous fluid escapes from retinal capillaries and collects in the inner plexiform layer of the macula in a petalloid distribution (a), seen best on fluorescein angiography (b).

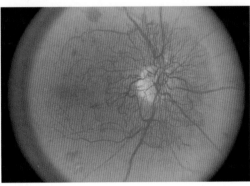

A

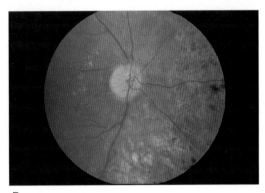

B

Plate 16. Retinal neovascularization. A tangle of immature vessels has sprouted on the retinal surface in response to chronic retinal ischemia (a); panretinal photocoagulation has caused the new vessels to regress completely (b).

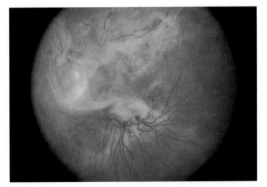

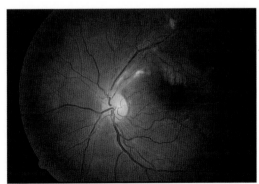

Plate 17. Proliferative retinopathy. A fibrovascular stalk has grown from the retinal surface onto the vitreous, detaching the retina.

Plate 18. Vasculitis. Segmental white cuffs around the vessels signify inflammation of retinal vessels.

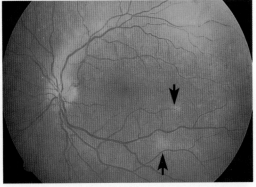

A

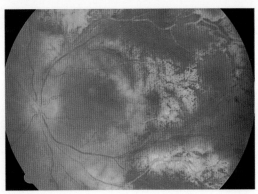

B

Plate 19. Cytomegalovirus retinitis. Initial signs of retinitis and retinal vasculitis (arrows) (a) evolve within 10 days to hemorrhagic necrosis (b).

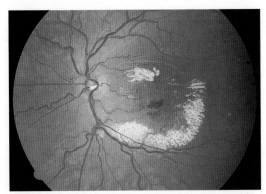

Plate 20. Vascular malformation: Coats' disease. Hard exudates around the fovea caused by exudation from incompetent, telangiectatic vessels.

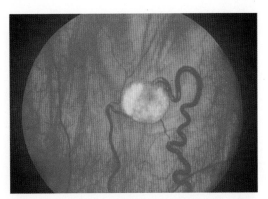

Plate 21. Vascular malformation: von Hippel-Lindau disease. Retinal angioma (yellow mound) with feeding arteriole and draining vein.

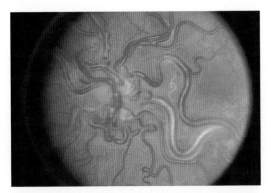

Plate 22. Wyburn-Masson syndrome. Enlarged, tortuous retinal arteries and veins emanating from the optic disk are part of an arteriovenous malformation.

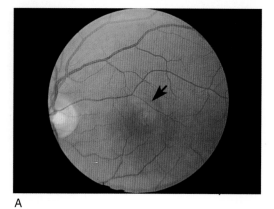

A

Plate 23. Choroidal neovascularization and submacular hemorrhage. The gray spot under the macula (arrow) is a sign of bleeding (a); fluorescein angiography highlights the submacular neovascular net (arrow) (b). See Fig. 10-1c.

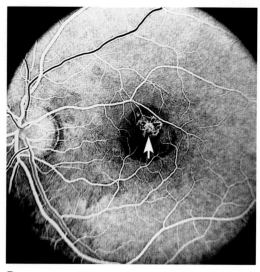

B

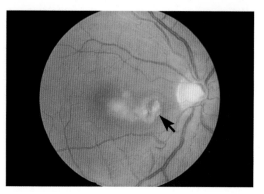

Plate 24. Toxoplasmosis, active. Fluffy, yellow patch of retinitis signifies reactivation of an adjacent congenital infection that had been quiescent (arrow).

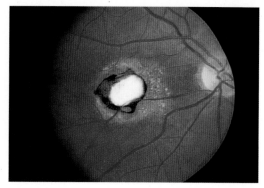

Plate 25. Toxoplasmosis, healed. White sclera is visible where infection has destroyed retina and choroid. Discrete margin indicates the lesion is inactive.

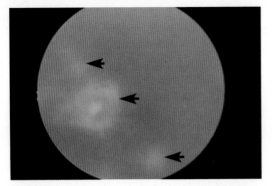

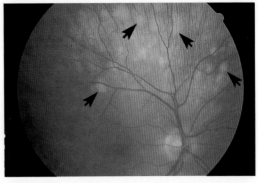

Plate 26. Candida vitritis. Multiple yellow-white round lesions (arrows) obscured by hazy vitreous.

Plate 27. Full thickness choroidopathy: sarcoidosis. Multiple faint round granulomatous nodules (arrows) are seen deep to the retina.

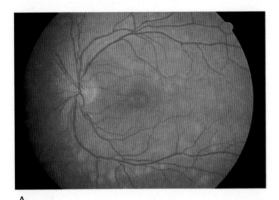

A

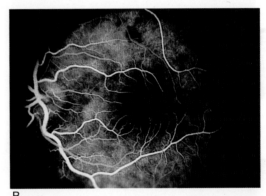

B

Plate 28. Superficial choroidopathy: multiple evanescent white dot syndrome (MEWDS). Faint cream-colored dots beneath the retina are patches of superficial choroidal and RPE inflammation (a); in the early phase of fluorescein angiography, they block fluorescence (b); in the late phase, they stain with fluorescein dye (c).

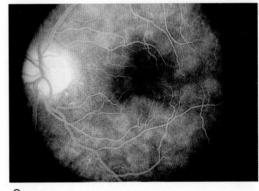

C

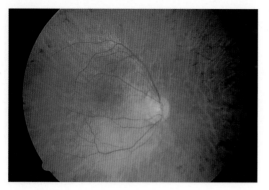

Plate 29. Retinitis pigmentosa. Retinal arteriolar attenuation, disk pallor, RPE atrophy, and spicular black pigmentation in the midperiphery.

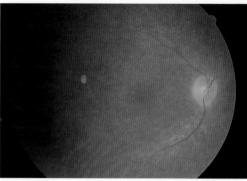

Plate 30. Cancer-associated retinopathy (CAR). Features are similar to retinitis pigmentosa, except that there are no black pigment spicules.

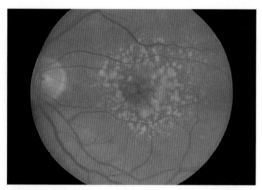

Plate 31. Retinal drusen. The yellow spots clustered around the fovea represent deposits in Bruch's membrane beneath the RPE. They signify focal dysfunction of the RPE in that region.

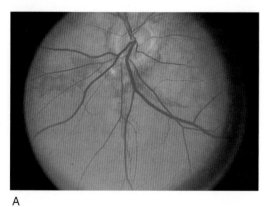

A

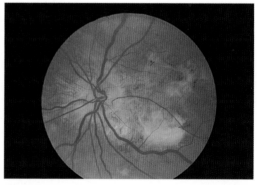

B

Plate 32. Angioid streaks. Jagged red lines radiating from optic disk represent tears in Bruch's membrane (a); choroidal neovascularization and subretinal bleeding have led to macular scarring (b).

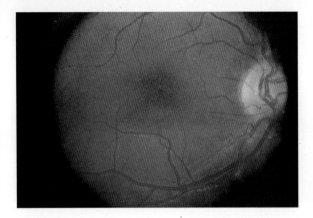

Plate 33. Juvenile retinoschisis. Fine lines radiate out of the fovea, a subtle finding that is easily overlooked.

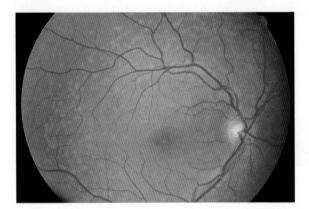

Plate 34. Stargardt's disease. Faint yellow flecks are visible throughout the posterior retina. These flecks may be absent in some cases.

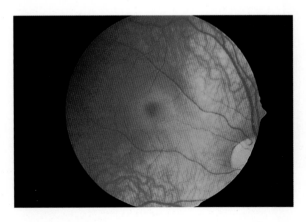

Plate 35. Cherry-red spot in Tay-Sachs disease. Accumulation of ganglioside in the dense ganglion cell layer of the perifoveal region produces a cherry-red spot. See Table 11-7 for differential diagnosis.

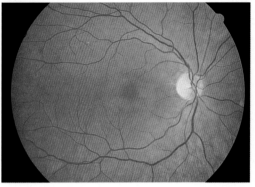

A

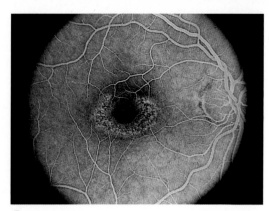

B

Plate 36. Bull's-eye maculopathy. The perifoveal RPE is relatively atrophic (a), producing a bull's eye that is better visualized with fluorescein angiography (b). See Table 11-7 for differential diagnosis.

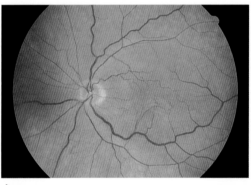

A

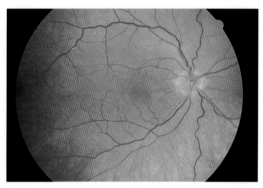

B

Plate 37. Cellophane (surface-wrinkling, epiretinal membrane, macular pucker, premacular fibroplasia) maculopathy. Retinal surface in the left eye in macular region is distorted by a fibroglial membrane, causing metamorphopsia (a). Compare with normal right eye (b).

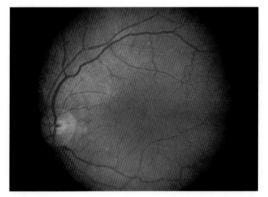

Plate 38. Macular hole. The superficial retinal tissue in the fovea has been torn away with the detaching vitreous.

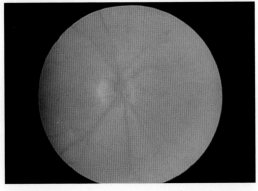

A

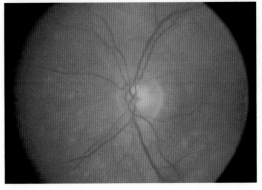

B

Plate 39. Primary CNS lymphoma: ocular manifestations. A. Hazy vitreous. B. Scattered round yellow deposits under the RPE.

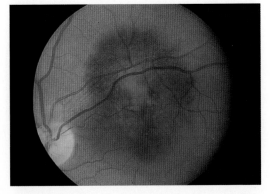

Plate 40. Choroidal melanoma. Note the dark brown mound under the retina. Some choroidal melanomas are nonpigmented and appear as white mounds.

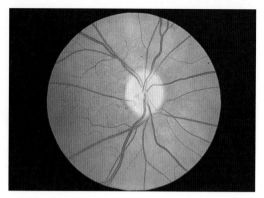

Plate 41. Optic disk pallor: diffuse. This is a nonspecific sign of optic neuropathy.

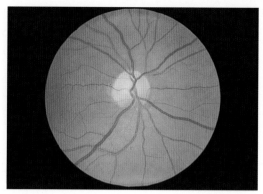

Plate 42. Optic disk pallor: altitudinal. Note pallor is restricted to the upper half of the disk. Altitudinal pallor is typical of ischemic optic neuropathy.

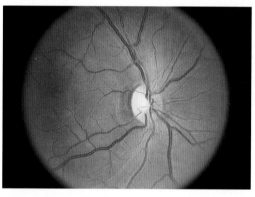

Plate 43. Optic disk pallor: temporal. Note pallor is restricted to the temporal wedge segment. This is typical of hereditary-toxic-metabolic-nutritional injury, but common on other conditions as well.

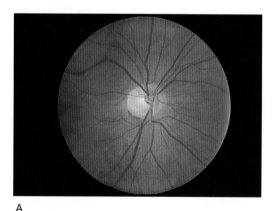

A

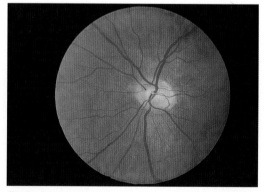

B

Plate 44. Optic disk pallor: bow tie (butterfly, band). The pallor in the left optic disk (b) involves its nasal and temporal midsection, sparing its superior and inferior sections. The pallor in the right optic disk (a) is restricted to the temporal section. This combination is specific for optic tract or lateral geniculate body injury. The patient had a right optic tract lesion.

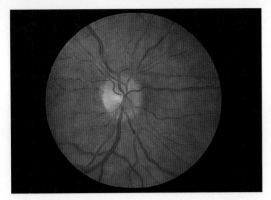

Plate 45. Papilledema: mild. Superior and inferior disk margins are blurred.

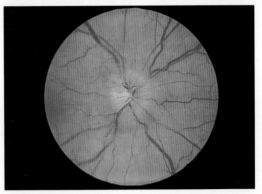

Plate 46. Papilledema: moderate. Superior, inferior, and nasal disk margins are elevated and blurred.

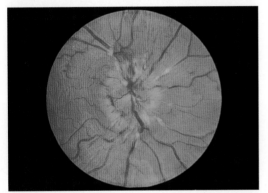

Plate 47. Papilledema: marked. All margins are elevated and blurred, and there are hemorrhages and cotton-wool spots.

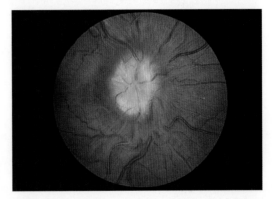

Plate 48. Papilledema: atrophic. Disk is elevated but pale, reflecting death of axons.

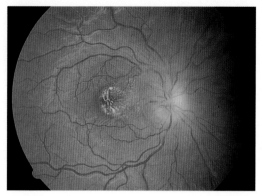

Plate 49. Leber's stellate neuroretinitis. Hard yellow exudates radiate from the fovea; the optic disk is swollen.

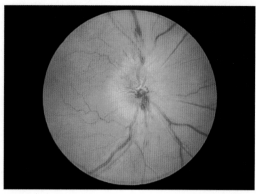

Plate 50. Acute ischemic optic neuropathy. The optic disk is swollen and there is a surface hemorrhage.

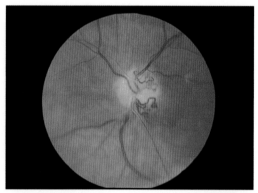

Plate 51. Optociliary shunt vessels: The optic disk is pale and slightly swollen; tortuous veins on its surface are shunting blood into peripapillary choroidal veins because exit routes through the optic disk are blocked. These findings often indicate an optic nerve sheath meningioma.

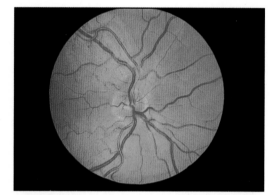

Plate 52. Acute Leber's hereditary optic neuropathy. The optic disk is hyperemic and the peripapillary nerve fiber layer is thickened, a sign of axoplasmic stasis.

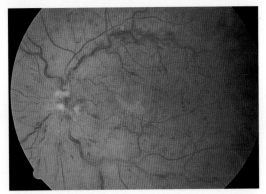

Plate 53. Papillophlebitis. The optic disk is swollen; retinal veins are distended and leaking blood.

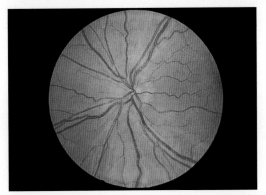

Plate 54. Congenital dysplasia. Disk margins are blurred and retinal vessels occupy a relatively large proportion of space.

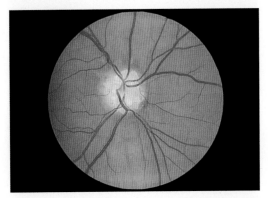

Plate 55. Optic disk drusen. Yellow concretions are partially buried within the optic disk. They represent calcified debris extruded from dysfunctional axons.

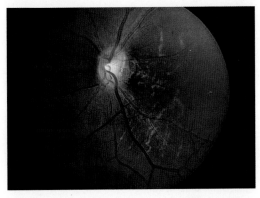

Plate 56. Tilted optic disk. The nerve head architecture is distorted, such that the nasal portion is relatively prominent and the temporal portion is shortened. Such a congenital deformity may be associated with normal function.

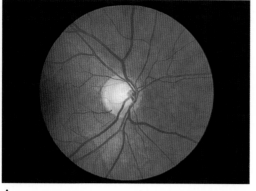

A

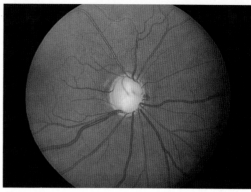

B

Plate 57. Glaucomatous excavation. A. Mild excavation: the disk rim is thinned. B. Marked excavation: the disk rim is nearly obliterated.

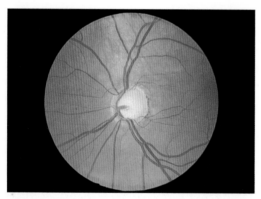

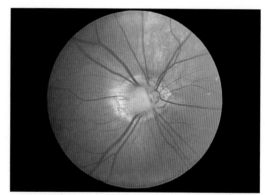

Plate 58. Nonglaucomatous excavation (by compression from pituitary tumor). The cup is enlarged and the rim is relatively pale. Rim pallor differentiates nonglaucomatous from glaucomatous optic disk excavation.

Plate 59. Optic disk coloboma. The cup is congenitally enlarged by a defect in closure of the fetal fissure.

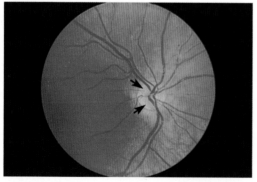

Plate 60. Optic disk hypoplasia. The disk is deceptively small and axon-poor. Its temporal margin (arrows) is enclosed by a pale crescent created by congenital absence of choroid in that region.

ten have arteriosclerotic risk factors, particularly hypertension.[154]

Post–cataract extraction optic disk infarction has been unconvincingly attributed to the well-recognized increase in intraocular pressure in the days following surgery, with the recommendation that patients be placed on acetazolamide for several days before and after surgery.[154] This regimen did not prevent fellow eye involvement in one reported case.[156] A more reasonable explanation is that the sudden intraoperative drop in intraocular pressure upsets a tenuous perfusion balance within the optic nerve in vulnerable subjects. Indeed, experimental ocular hypotony has produced optic disk edema and axoplasmic stasis at the lamina cribrosa.[157] As there is a 50% likelihood of the same catastrophe occurring in the fellow eye,[155] and no way to prevent it, surgeons should be wary of operating on the uninvolved eye.

Migrainous Optic Neuropathy

Ophthalmic manifestations identical to those of NAION have been reported rarely in the setting of migraine.[158–161] Fewer than a dozen cases have been reported, primarily involving women under age 50 with long histories of migraine that often lack a typical visual aura. The visual loss occurs suddenly during a severe headache; the mechanism is presumed to be vasospasm. Prophylactic treatment with calcium channel blockers is advised, based on anecdotal evidence that they reduce the frequency of monocular transient visual loss.[162]

Diabetic Papillopathy

Diabetic patients are at risk not only for typical NAION, but for an optic neuropathy that looks like a muted, protracted, and more reversible form of NAION.[163–167] Diabetic papillopathy has no relationship to poor blood sugar control or degree of retinopathy, and it is not a forerunner of proliferative retinopathy. It differs from NAION by:

- Affecting patients of all ages, regardless of the age of onset of diabetes or insulin dependence.
- Often occurring simultaneously in both eyes. This feature, together with relatively preserved vision, will raise the question of papilledema (see "Increased Intracranial Pressure," below).
- Causing visual loss that is milder and more reversible.
- Causing more protracted optic disk edema (average of six months).
- Causing very dilated optic disk vessels. They superficially resemble diabetic new blood vessels but differ in having a more orderly radial pattern, not rising above the disk surface, and not leaking fluorescein.

These clinical features are less suggestive of a watershed infarct typical of NAION than of a chronic ischemic or dysmetabolic process similar to that which affects the lumbosacral plexus in diabetic patients (diabetic amyotrophy).[168]

Chronic Low-Perfusion States

With the possible exception of diabetic papillopathy, each variant of ischemic optic neuropathy reviewed thus far results from an acute deprivation of blood flow. Impaired optic nerve function has also been documented in chronic low-flow states, including the "ocular ischemic syndrome" associated with high-grade stenosis of the carotid circulation[169] and high-flow carotid-cavernous sinus fistulas.[170] Since the retina is also chronically ischemic in these conditions, the contribution of optic nerve dysfunction is hard to assess, although afferent pupil defects have disappeared following the repair of fistulas.

The optic disk edema caused by increased intracranial pressure (see "Papilledema," below) could be another example of chronic hypoperfusion of the optic nerve.[3] Pressure transmitted through the dural cuff of the optic nerve may collapse the ciliary vessels supplying the laminar axons, leading to chronic axoplasmic stasis (Fig 12-1). If ischemia becomes severe, axoplasmic flow stops altogether and axons die. Whether tumorous compression also affects the optic nerves and chiasm via chronic ischemia or via direct mechanical interference with axoplasmic flow is unsettled. Chronic ischemia also has been posited as a mechanism for primary open-angle glaucoma (see "Glaucoma," Chapter 13).[171,172]

INCREASED INTRACRANIAL PRESSURE

Papilledema

Papilledema is the term reserved for optic disk edema consequent to increased intracranial pressure (ICP). The faster ICP rises, and the higher it gets, the sooner papilledema will appear, and the more florid it will be. Papilledema may be observed within three hours if ICP climbs precipitously as the result of intracranial bleeding, but it takes weeks to resolve after ICP normalizes.[173] There are four stages (Table 12-7):

- **Mild papilledema:** swelling of the superior and/or inferior disk margins, turbidity of the peripapillary nerve fiber layer, and absent central retinal venous pulsations (Plate 45). (Spontaneous venous pulsa-

tions, observed as the central retinal vein dives into the physiologic cup, are present in 80% of individuals whose ICP is 200 mm Hg or below. Therefore, their absence is not necessarily a sign of raised ICP. Their presence is, however, a sign that ICP is normal during the time of observation.) Visual acuity is normal; static perimetry may show mild nasal visual field loss.

- **Moderate papilledema:** obvious disk elevation throughout the rim with some preservation of the cup; no hemorrhages or cotton-wool spots (Plate 46). Visual acuity is normal; static perimetry often shows mild field loss.

- **Marked papilledema:** disk elevation, narrowing of the physiologic cup, dilation of disk surface vessels and the central retinal vein, and cotton-wool spots and hemorrhages on or near the disk surface (Plate 47). The cotton-wool spots indicate that axoplasmic flow has stopped completely in some axons. It is an omen that irreversible death will occur unless ICP is normalized,

Table 12–7. **The Four Stages of Papilledema**

Stage	Ophthalmoscopic Findings	Significance
Mild (Plate 45)	Superior and inferior disk swelling Turbidity of peripapillary nerve fiber layer Absent central retinal venous pulsations	Mild axoplasmic stasis Visual acuity normal Visual fields normal or mild inferonasal loss Probably tolerable for long periods
Moderate (Plate 46)	Circumferential disk elevation Partial preservation of the physiologic cup Absent central retinal venous pulsations	Moderate axoplasmic stasis Visual acuity usually normal Visual fields often show some loss
Marked (Plate 47)	Marked disc elevation Absence of the physiologic cup Absent central retinal venous pulsations Dilation of disk surface vessels and the central retinal vein Cotton-wool spots and hemorrhages on or near disk surface	Severe axoplasmic stasis with some axonal death Visual acuity may or may not be normal Visual fields always show loss Threat of further axonal death if not reversed soon
Atrophic (Plate 48)	Mild-moderate disk elevation Gray-white color of disk substance	Considerable axonal death with stasis in surviving axons Visual acuity may be abnormal Visual fields show marked constriction Rapid reduction in ICP may cause further visual loss Efficacy of any treatment in doubt at this stage

but there is no good information on how much ICP elevation a human optic nerve can withstand. Disk hemorrhages reflect the bursting of veins under increased pressure in the nerve head or immediately behind it. Visual acuity is usually normal but static perimetry always shows nasal loss.

- **Atrophic papilledema:** the disk is elevated but its color has changed from a plethoric pink-orange to an anemic gray-white (Plate 48). This change reflects the harmful effects of persistently high ICP—dead axons as well as swollen axons. Visual acuity may or may not be normal; static perimetry shows very constricted fields. If ICP remains high, visual field loss will gradually spread inward to close out all vision. In some cases, sudden deterioration occurs as the disk is infarcted and new segmental optic disk edema appears.[174]

Once atrophic papilledema has developed, relieving intracranial pressure may not stop the progression of visual loss. In fact, relieving pressure may even cause vision to worsen quickly. Sudden deterioration of vision is especially likely following craniotomy or ventriculostomy (postdecompression optic neuropathy).[175] The speculated mechanism of this postdecompression blindness is that a sudden drop in intracranial pressure shifts blood flow away from an already compromised optic nerve head. Vigorous pharmacologic measures aimed at gradually lowering intracranial pressure (corticosteroids, acetazolamide, mannitol) should be employed prior to shunting.

The relationship between papilledema and elevated ICP contains the following important nuances.

Elevated Intracranial Pressure May Exist Without Papilledema

The latency between ICP elevation and papilledema depends mostly on the rate of rise of ICP. With very slow increases, the development of papilledema will lag far behind.

Papilledema will not occur at all if the elevated ICP cannot be transmitted to the junction of the optic nerve and globe. A block may occur as an anatomic variant at the optic canal, accounting for the observation of unilateral or binocularly asymmetric papilledema. It may also occur as a result of orbital scarring following trauma, inflam-

mation, or surgery (including optic nerve sheath fenestration, see below). In one series of 59 patients with elevated ICP caused by dural sinus thrombosis and documented by LP, 8 (13%) did not have papilledema.[175a]

Prior death of optic nerve axons from another process (or from longstanding papilledema) will preclude the development of disk edema because nonfunctioning axons cannot expand. The most famous example of this phenomenon is the rare Foster-Kennedy syndrome, in which a unilateral subfrontal mass compresses the ipsilateral optic nerve to cause optic atrophy and raises intracranial pressure to cause papilledema in the contralateral eye.

Papilledema May Exist Without Elevated Intracranial Pressure

After normalization of ICP, it takes several weeks for papilledema to "unwind." In cases where papilledema has been longstanding, the disk surface may have a permanently glazed appearance from glial overgrowth.

DIFFERENTIAL DIAGNOSIS

Through the ophthalmoscope, the disk swelling of papilledema cannot be confidently distinguished from local optic disk disorders best remembered as beginning with the letter "i": inflammation, infarction, infiltration, and indentation (compression) (Table 12-8). The disk swelling of papilledema and the other "i" processes look alike because they share a common mechanistic pathway: arrest of axoplasmic flow at the scleral lamina (Box 12-1). Experimental models of raised ICP show that the pressure is transmitted through the dural envelope of the optic nerve, where it is believed to compress the tenuous ciliary blood supply of the optic nerve axons.[3] The resulting ischemia impedes axoplasmic flow at the lamina cribrosa, as has been found in the acute ischemic optic neuropathies. The disk swelling derives not so much from extracellular fluid as from distended axons whose organelles are dammed up anterior to the scleral lamina. The most vulnerable axons are those traveling at the outer margin of the optic nerve and originating in the retinal periphery.[176] This vulnerability of peripheral axons explains why disk margin blurring is

Table 12–8. **Causes of Acquired Optic Disk Edema**

Entity	Distinguishing Features
Papilledema	Visual acuity usually normal; binocular disk edema; headache or neurologic abnormalities may be present; evidence of increased ICP
Optic neuritis	Uniocular > binocular acute vision loss; sometimes pain on eye movement
Ischemic optic neuropathy	Usually uniocular, acute, painless vision loss, age over 50, arteriosclerotic risk factors or polymyalgia rheumatica syndrome; sometimes history of severe hypotension
Neoplastic infiltration	Uniocular or binocular progressive vision loss; disk(s) usually swollen; history of cancer usually present
Compression by orbital mass	Slowly progressive (may rarely be acute) uniocular or binocular vision loss, +/− proptosis, +/− optociliary shunt vessels on disk
Leber's hereditary optic neuropathy	Subacute uniocular or consecutively binocular (separated by weeks to months) painless vision loss; peripapillary nerve fiber layer edema, usually in males aged 15–35
Methanol intoxication	Acute binocular vision loss; peripapillary nerve fiber layer edema similar to Leber's; history of methanol ingestion; often encephalopathic
Retinal venous hypertension	Acute uniocular vision loss; dilated retinal veins and perivenous retinal hemorrhages; look for orbital or cavernous fistula, polycythemia, macroglobulinemia, superior vena cava syndrome

the initial ophthalmoscopic finding in papilledema and why the earliest visual field defects involve the peripheral field (inferonasally, for uncertain reasons). The postural blackouts (transient obscurations) of vision, so common in papilledema, may be caused by momentary drops in perfusion in a ciliary circulation already compressed by high pressure within the optic nerve sheath.

The finding of papilledema, even in the absence of neurologic symptoms, always implies present or prior elevation of intracranial pressure, which demands an urgent evaluation (Fig. 12-4). In most cases, other neurologic manifestations are present. The notable exception is the pseudotumor cerebri syndrome.

Pseudotumor Cerebri Syndrome

This syndrome is defined as: (*1*) increased ICP (opening pressure recumbent > 200 mm water if nonobese, >250 mm water if obese) with normal spinal fluid formula; (*2*) no imaging evidence of ventriculomegaly, mass effect, or cerebral edema; and (*3*) no pertinent neurologic manifestations apart from those attributable to the increased ICP.[177]

SYMPTOMS AND SIGNS

Symptoms of the pseudotumor cerebri syndrome include headache (>90%), neck and shoulder pain (30%–40%), tinnitus (60%), transient obscurations of vision (75%), and diplopia (35%).[185,186] Examination will disclose papilledema (nearly 100%), mild peripheral visual field loss (>90%), and sometimes esotropia owing to sixth nerve palsy or excessive convergence (10%–20%).[185] When the cause of this syndrome is dural sinus thrombosis, the symptoms are more acute and pronounced than when the cause is meningeal scarring or idiopathic.[180]

CAUSES

There are three known causes for the pseudotumor cerebri syndrome (Table 12-9):
1. **Increased cerebral venous pressure.** This results primarily from total or partial occlusion of dural venous sinuses[177–180] and convexity arteriovenous (AV) fistulas.[181] Less commonly, these manifestations result from increased pressure in the jugular veins, vena cava, and right heart. Magnetic resonance angiography (MRA) or MRI of the head is sufficient to diagnose the intracranial venous blockage and AV

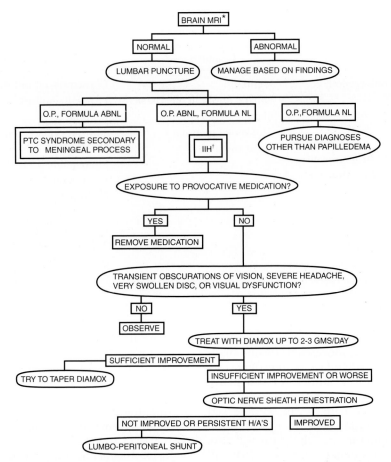

Figure 12–4. Management of papilledema. *Include neck if patient does not fit clinical profile of idiopathic intracranial hypertension. †IIH = Idiopathic intracranial hypertension (pseudotumor cerebri); O.P. = opening pressure; Formula = spinal fluid formula.

fistulas. However, unless imaging is extended to the neck and chest, obstruction there will be missed.

Dural (sagittal, transverse) sinus thrombosis is the most important variant to recognize because treatment is urgently required. It has been associated with active inflammations (meningitis, otitis media, Behcet's disease, connective tissue disorders), head trauma, hypercoagulable states (thrombocytosis, puerperium, dehydration, cancer, protein S and C deficiency), torcular mass lesions (meningioma, metastases, bone tumors), and intracranial surgery.[178,180] Diagnosis is established with MRI (absence of flow void) or MRA. Even partial obstruction of the

sagittal or transverse sinus may induce high enough ICP to produce florid papilledema and threatened vision. If dural sinuses appear normal by MRI or MRA, scanning should extend down through the neck and chest to rule out venous blockage there.

The pseudotumor cerebri syndrome caused by dural sinus thrombosis erupts suddenly with severe headache and vomiting; it may progress to seizures, encephalopathy, and hemiparesis if the thrombus backs up into the cortical veins or if ICP is profoundly elevated (>500 mm water). Because it is impossible to predict the course of acute dural sinus thrombosis, current recommendations

Table 12–9. **Causes of the Pseudotumor Cerebri Syndrome**

Increased Cerebral Venous Pressure	Damaged Arachnoid Granulations	Chemically Induced* Conditions
Dural sinus compression, thrombosis	Meningitis	Corticosteroid withdrawal
Jugular vein compression, radical neck dissection	Subarachnoid hemorrhage	Hypervitaminosis A
AV fistulas	Meningiomatosis	Uremia
Increased right heart pressure	Thickened meninges	Thyroid replacement in children
Superior vena cava syndrome	Head trauma	Tetracycline
		Minocycline
		Isotretinoin
		Cyclosporine
		Chlordecone
		Oral contraceptives
		Nalidixic acid
		Amiodarone

*The medications and conditions listed here may exacerbate a predisposition toward intracranial hypertension. In some cases, evidence for a cause-and-effect relationship is weak.[179]

are to undertake immediate heparin anticoagulation. Endovascular thrombolysis is an option in the face of neurologic decline.[178,178a] Prothrombotic or obstructive causes should be corrected, if possible. Otherwise, the patient can be observed either without intervention or with serial lumbar punctures, as the sinus will usually reopen spontaneously and ICP will normalize without damaging the optic nerves.[178,180] Acetazolamide, a carbonic anhydrase inhibitor that reduces CSF production, can be prescribed if the patient is anticoagulated, but otherwise should be used with caution because its dehydrating effects may promote thrombosis.

Dural AV fistulas and malformations that drain into the sagittal or transverse sinuses can increase cerebral venous pressure enough to cause the pseudotumor cerebri syndrome.[181] These vascular anomalies may elude detection even with MRA, and they therefore require conventional angiography.[181] The importance of diagnosing a fistula is that management is different: lumbar puncture and CSF diverting procedures must not be performed because of the high risk of tonsillar herniation and death.[181] The appropriate treatment is endovascular occlusion. If vision is impaired by high-grade papilledema, optic nerve sheath

fenestration should be performed (see below).

2. **Damaged arachnoid granulations.** Impaired CSF outflow across the arachnoid granulations may occur secondary to meningitis, subarachnoid hemorrhage, meningiomatosis, meningeal thickening, or head trauma.[177]

Meningeal disorders cause obstruction to CSF flow at the arachnoid granulations primarily along the cerebral convexity. Because the increased pressure affects the intraventricular and extraventricular CSF spaces equally, there is typically no enlargement of the ventricles. Although the spinal fluid may reveal a pathologic increase in cell count and protein, it is often normal.

A major diagnostic trap in this setting results from the fact that meningitis may cause both optic neuritis and the pseudotumor cerebri syndrome.[177] That is, inflammation can produce direct damage to the optic nerves and cause the disks to swell (papillitis). It can also inhibit filtration through the arachnoid granulations and raise ICP. The swollen disks may be misinterpreted as papilledema, especially when lumbar puncture reveals an elevated opening pressure. A correct diagnosis is reached by noting that visual acuity loss has occurred in the acute phase of disk swelling, which would be very unusual in patients with papilledema (Table 12-8). Surgical procedures, such as optic nerve sheath fenestration or CSF diverting procedures, are usually not indicated.

3. **Chemically induced conditions.** In this variant, the mechanism is unknown.[182–184] Several medical conditions and medications have been implicated (Table 12-9).[179,185] Withdrawal of the medication and elimination of the underlying condition often leads to complete recovery.

A majority of cases of pseudotumor cerebri syndrome have no known cause (idiopathic intracranial hypertension, IIH). Most adult patients are women. More than 90% are of childbearing age, are clinically obese, or have had a recent weight gain of 20 pounds or more.[185] Among the 7% of cases that occur in children, there is no sex bias and no excessive weight.[187,188]

Reliable natural history data do not exist in IIH because most patients are treated. Retrospective analyses are biased by the accrual of patients from centers that attract the most refractory or symptomatic cases.[189,190] They indicate a 12%–20% prevalence of disabling visual loss. Risk factors for visual loss have not been clearly established. Amalgated data suggest a recurrence rate of 40%.[191] Solid longitudinal information on the duration of clinical symptoms and visual outcomes does not exist.

Various medical and surgical treatments have been used, but there are no controlled trials to support their efficacy. Weight loss as an isolated intervention has been described as effective,[179] but sustaining it is difficult for these patients. Serial lumbar punctures have been largely abandoned because they hurt, cause post–lumbar puncture headaches, and have only a temporary pressure-lowering effect. Corticosteroids probably work, but chronic use causes many intolerable side-effects and withdrawal may itself induce ICP elevation. Acetazolamide, in doses of 2 g/day, is the pharmacologic agent of choice. It is considered safe during pregnancy but should be withheld during the first 20 weeks of gestation.[192] Furosemide is a weak alternative to acetazolamide.[179]

Among surgical treatment options, optic nerve sheath fenestration (ONSF)[193–203] and lumboperitoneal shunting (LPS)[204–206] are effective, but not always and not forever. According to large-series reports, ONSF will acutely improve visual function in 50%–90% of operated eyes, arrest visual loss in about 40%, and cause worsening in about 5%–10%. The success rate is higher in eyes with more acute papilledema,[197] but even patients with atrophic papilledema appear to benefit. Long-term visual results suggest that many patients continue to lose vision after ONSF.[196] It is not clear whether repeat ONSF is effective. It appears to increase risks more than benefits.[207]

What is ONSF and how does it work? It consists of cutting a 1 cm square window in the dura and arachnoid that envelops the optic nerve near its junction with the eye. Perhaps the window allows continuous venting of CSF. This might explain the improvement seen in the other eye after unilateral surgery. A more plausible hypothesis is that retrobulbar dural scarring creates a shield that protects the ciliary supply to the optic nerve from the effects of high CSF pressure (Fig 12-1).[3]

Optic nerve sheath fenestration carries a 40% complication rate,[207] but only 10% of complications create persistent visual deterioration. Eyes undergoing repeat ONSF appear to be at much higher risk of vision-threatening complications.[207]

An alternative surgical procedure to ONSF is lumboperitoneal shunting, in which the CSF is diverted from the lumbar subarachnoid space to the peritoneal cavity by means of a subcutaneous catheter. The ability of LPS to improve vision or forestall further visual loss appears to be between 60% and 80%,[204,205,208] a success rate equal to that of ONSF. The principal problem is shunt malfunction, usually owing to blockage, which may be expected in 50% of patients. Among those who develop blockage, an average of more than two revisions may be necessary to restore patency.[204] Less common complications include intracranial hypotension, meningitis, CSF leak, radiculopathy, abdominal pain, and bowel perforation.[204,205] Patients who are not effectively treated with LPS may achieve visual benefit from ONSF.

The following principles should be used in the management of IIH (Box 12-3):
- Exclude other causes of increased ICP.
- Eliminate medications that could exacerbate IIH.
- Document abnormalities with visual field examination and fundus photography.

Box 12–3

MANAGING IDIOPATHIC INTRACRANIAL HYPERTENSION

- Exclude other causes of increased intracranial pressure.

- Monitor clinical course with **visual field examinations** and **optic disk photographs.**

- Institute **weight loss program** and withhold pharmacologic therapy when disease is mild and patient is likely to be compliant.

- Treat moderately severe disease (severe headache, transient obscurations of vision, substantial disk swelling, or visual field loss) with **acetazolamide** up to 2–3 g/day (or furosemide if patient is sulfa-allergic or intolerant to acetazolamide) except if patient is within first 20 weeks of pregnancy (use repeated spinal taps if disease is severe).

- Perform **optic nerve sheath fenestration** (ONSF) before papilledema enters the atrophic phase if a trial of medical therapy fails to improve vision or halt progression.

- Perform **CSF diverting procedure** (usually lumboperitoneal shunt) if optic nerve sheath fenestration fails.

- Advise weight loss as only intervention if there are no transient obscurations of vision or persistent visual dysfunction, and if papilledema is mild.

- Prescribe oral acetazolamide if patient has transient obscurations of vision, persistent visual dysfunction, or moderate-marked papilledema.

- Perform ONSF for visual loss if medical therapy fails; LPS is a reasonable alternative.

- Perform LPS if ONSF fails. Prominent headache is not a compelling indication for a primary LPS. Headache can often be successfully managed with analgesic or tricyclic medications.

SUMMARY

The optic nerves and chiasm are forward extensions of the diencephalon that share many pathologic processes.

Lesions of the optic nerves produce subnormal vision and unformed hallucinations. Examination may disclose reduced visual acuity, nerve fiber bundle visual field defects, an afferent pupil defect (if the two nerves are damaged asymmetrically), and structural alterations of the optic disk—pallor, elevation, excavation, or hypoplasia.

Lesions of the optic chiasm produce bitemporal or junctional field loss, often combined with subnormal visual acuity. Visual deficits may be combined with endocrinologic manifestations.

Typical optic neuritis is a primary demyelinating process, often a component of multiple sclerosis, but this may be its initial manifestation. Unless there are clinical or imaging features of MS at outset, the diagnosis is presumptive. Although high-dose methylprednisolone can retard the development of MS, it does not affect the long-term course of the illness.

Atypical optic neuritis may be caused by infectious organisms and must be treated vigorously to preserve vision. Atypical optic neuritis may be indistinguishable from typical (primary demyelinating) optic neuritis at outset.

Ischemic optic neuropathy is the term given to infarction of the optic nerve. The nonarteritic anterior form is most common. Its pathogenesis may be reduced perfusion in pathologically narrowed vessels during a brief period of subclinical systemic hypotension. There is no treatment. Later involvement of the fellow eye is the major concern. Presently there are no accepted preventive measures, although arteriosclerotic risk factor management, aspirin, and avoidance of overtreatment of hypertension are recommended.

Arteritic ischemic optic neuropathy occurs primarily in giant cell arteritis. It causes abrupt, severe, and irreversible optic nerve infarction. Fellow eye involvement may occur within days, and high-dose corticosteroid treatment is effective in preventing that catastrophe. The diagnosis is suggested by eliciting symptoms of polymyalgia rheumatica and cephalic claudication, and by finding a high sedimentation rate or C-reactive protein in an elderly patient. However, none of these features need be present, so it is prudent to make a presumptive diagnosis in any patient aged over 70 years who has sustained optic nerve infarction. If performed correctly, temporal artery biopsy has a high sensitivity and specificity.

Increased intracranial pressure probably damages the optic nerves by compressing their delicate ciliary arterial supply. As chronic ischemia impairs axoplasmic flow, the axons swell and the disk appears elevated (papilledema). If the ICP persists at a high enough level, axoplasmic flow shuts down altogether, and the optic nerve axons die.

A common cause of persistent papilledema is the pseudotumor cerebri syndrome, which may result from dural sinus obstruction or thrombosis, meningeal processes that impair arachnoid granulations, certain medications and dysmetabolic states, and an idiopathic condition primarily affecting overweight young women (idiopathic intracranial hypertension). Treatment employs acetazolamide (a cerebrospinal fluid suppressant) and two surgical measures—optic nerve sheath fenestration and CSF diversion—if medical therapy fails.

REFERENCES

1. Miller NR, Newman SA. Transsynaptic degeneration. *Arch Ophthalmol.* 1981;99:1654.
2. Quigley HA, Anderson DR. The histologic basis of optic disk in experimental optic atrophy. *Am J Ophthalmol.* 1977;83:709–717.
3. Sanders MD. The Bowman Lecture. Papilloedema: "the pendulum of progress". *Eye.* 1997; 11:267–294.
4. Tso MO, Hayreh SS. Optic disc edema in raised intracranial pressure: IV. Axoplasmic transport in experimental papilledema. *Arch Ophthalmol.* 1977; 95:1458–1462.
5. Trobe JD, Glaser JD, Cassady JC. Optic atrophy: differential diagnosis by fundus observation alone. *Arch Ophthalmol.* 1980;98:1040–1045.
6. Trobe JD, Glaser JS, Cassady J, Herschler J, Anderson DR. Nonglaucomatous excavation of the optic disc. *Arch Ophthalmol.* 1980;98:1046–1050.
7. Brodsky MC. Congenital optic disk anomalies. *Surv Ophthalmol.* 1994;39:89–112.
8. Golnik KC. Congenital optic nerve anomalies. *Curr Opin Ophthalmol.* 1998;9(6):18–26.
9. Trobe JD, Tao AH, Shuster JJ. Perichiasmal tumors: diagnostic and prognostic features. *Neurosurgery.* 1984;15:391–399.
10. Purvin V. Optic neuritis. *Curr Opin Ophthalmol.* 1998;9(6):3–9.
11. Beck RW, Cleary PA, Anderson MM, Optic Neuritis Study Group. A randomized, controlled trial of corticosteroids in the treatment of acute optic neuritis. *N Engl J Med.* 1992;326:581–588.
12. Beck RW, Cleary PA, Trobe JD, Optic Neuritis Study Group. The effect of corticosteroids for acute optic neuritis on the subsequent development of multiple sclerosis. *N Engl J Med.* 1993; 329:1764–1769.
13. Beck RW, Cleary PA, Optic Neuritis Study Group. Optic neuritis treatment trial: one-year follow-up results. *Arch Ophthalmol.* 1993;111:773–775.
14. Beck RW, Trobe JD, Optic Neuritis Study Group. What we have learned from the Optic Neuritis Treatment Trial. *Ophthalmology.* 1995;102:1504–1508.
15. Optic Neuritis Study Group. Visual function 5 years after optic neuritis: experience of the Optic Neuritis Treatment Trial. *Arch Ophthalmol.* 1997; 115:1545–1552
16. Optic Neuritis Study Group. The 5-year risk of MS after optic neuritis: experience of the Optic Neuritis Treatment Trial. *Neurology.* 1997; 49:1404–1413.
17. Davis FA, Bergen D, Schauf C, McDonald I, Deutsch W. Movement phosphenes in optic neuritis: a new clinical sign. *Neurology.* 1976;26:1100–1104.
18. Sokol S. The Pulfrich stereo-illusion as an index of optic nerve dysfunction. *Surv Ophthalmol.* 1976;20:432–434.
19. Keltner JL, Johnson CA, Spurr JO, Beck RW. Baseline visual field profile of optic neuritis: the experience of the Optic Neuritis Treatment Trial. *Arch Ophthalmol.* 1993;111:231–234.
20. Keltner JL, Johnson CA, Spurr JO, Beck RW. Visual field profile of optic neuritis: one-year follow-up in the Optic Neuritis Treatment Trial. *Arch Ophthalmol.* 1994;112:946–953.
21. Chiappa KH. *Evoked Potentials in Clinical Medicine.* New York: Raven Press; 1983.
22. Beck RW. The clinical profile of optic neuritis: experience of the Optic Neuritis Treatment Trial. *Arch Ophthalmol.* 1991;109:1673–1678.
23. Rodriguez M, Siva A, Cross SA, O'Brien PC, Kurland LT. Optic neuritis: a population-based study in Olmsted County, Minnesota. *Neurology.* 1995;45: 244–250.
24. Weinshenker BG, Rice GPA, Noseworthy JH, Carriere W, Baskerville J, Ebers GC. The natural history of multiple sclerosis: a geographically based study. *Brain.* 1991;114:1045–1056.
25. Runmarker B, Andersen O. Prognostic factors in a multiple sclerosis incidence cohort with twenty-five years of follow-up. *Brain.* 1993;116:117–134.
26. Beck RW, Arrington J, Murtagh FR, Cleary PA, Kaufman DI. Brain magnetic resonance imaging in acute optic neuritis: experience of the Optic Neuritis Treatment Trial. *Arch Neurol.* 1993;50:841–846.
27. Miller DH, Newton MR, Van der Poel EPGH, et al. Magnetic resonance imaging of the optic nerve in optic neuritis. *Neurology.* 1988;38:175–179.
28. Miller DH, Ormerod IEC, McDonald WI, et al. The early risk of multiple sclerosis after optic neuritis. *J Neurol Neurosurg Psychiatry.* 1988;51:1569–1571.
29. Frederiksen JL, Larsson HBW, Henriksen O, Olesen J. Magnetic resonance imaging of the brain in patients with acute monosymptomatic optic neuritis. *Acta Neurol Scand.* 1989;80:512–517.

30. Chrousos GA, Kattah JC, Beck RW, Cleary PA. Side effects of glucocorticoid treatment: experience of the Optic Neuritis Treatment Trial. *JAMA.* 1993; 269:2110–2112.

31. Trobe JD, Sieving PC, Fendrick AM, Guire KE. The impact of the Optic Neuritis Treatment Trial on the practices of ophthalmologists and neurologists. *Ophthalmology.* 1999;106:2047–2053.

31a. Jacobs LD, Beck RW, Simon JH et al and the CHAMPS Study Group. Intramuscular interferon beta-1a therapy initiated during a first demyelinating event in multiple sclerosis. *N Engl J Med.* 2000;343:898–904.

32. Weinstein JM, Lexow SS, Ho P, Spickards A. Acute syphilitic optic neuritis. *Arch Ophthalmol.* 1981;99: 1392–1394.

33. Lesser RS, Kornmehl EW, Pachner AR, et al. Neuro-ophthalmologic manifestations of Lyme disease. *Ophthalmology.* 1990;97:699–706.

34. Fish RH, Hoskins JC, Kline LB. Toxoplasmosis neuroretinitis. *Ophthalmology.* 1993;100:1177–1182.

35. Winward KE, Hamed LM, Glaser JS. The spectrum of optic nerve disease in human immunodeficiency virus infection. *Am J Ophthalmol.* 1989;107: 373–380.

36. Lee MS, Cooney EL, Stoessel KM, Gariano RF. *Varicella zoster* virus retrobulbar optic neuritis preceding retinitis in patients with acquired immune deficiency syndrome. *Ophthalmology* 1998;105:467–471.

37. Hepler RS. Miscellaneous optic neuropathies. In: Albert DM, Jakobiec FA, eds. *Principles and Practice of Ophthalmology.* Vol 4. Philadelphia: Saunders; 1994:2604–2615.

38. Frohman L, Wolansky L. Magnetic resonance imaging of syphilitic optic neuritis/perineuritis. *J Neuro-ophthalmol.* 1997;17:57–59.

39. Toshniwal P. Optic perineuritis with secondary syphilis. *J Clin Neuro-ophthalmol.* 1987;7:6–10.

40. Jacobson DM, Marx JJ, Dlesk A. Frequency and clinical significance of Lyme seropositivity in patients with isolated optic neuritis. *Neurology.* 1991; 41:706–711.

41. Newsom RW, Martin TJ, Wasilauskas B. Cat-scratch disease diagnosed serologically using an enzyme immunoassay in a patient with neuroretinitis. *Arch Ophthalmol.* 1996;114:493–494.

42. Brazis P, Lee AG. Optic disc edema with a macular star. *Mayo Clin Proc.* 1996;71:1162–1166.

43. Golnik KC, Marotto ME, Fanous MM, et al. Ophthalmic manifestations of *Rochalimaea* species. *Am J Ophthalmol.* 1994;118:145–151.

44. Ghauri RR, Lee AG. Optic disk edema with a macular star. *Surv Ophthalmol.* 1998;43:270–274.

45. Dreyer RF, Hopen G, Gass JDM, Smith JL. Leber's idiopathic stellate neuroretinitis. *Arch Ophthalmol.* 1984:102:1140–1145.

46. Maitland CG, Miller NR. Neuroretinitis. *Arch Ophthalmol.* 1984;102:1146–1149.

47. Ormerod LD, Skolnick KA, Menosky MM, Pavan PR, Pon DM. Retinal and choroidal manifestations of cat-scratch disease. *Ophthalmology.* 1998;105: 1024–1031.

48. Parmley VC, Schiffman JS, Maitland CG, Miller NR, Dreyer RF, Hoyt WF. Does neuroretinitis rule out multiple sclerosis? *Arch Neurol.* 1987;44:1045–1048.

49. Miller NR. *Walsh and Hoyt's Clinical Neuro-ophthalmology.* Baltimore: Williams & Wilkins 4th ed. Vol 1. 1982:240–243.

50. Selbst RG, Selhorst JB, Harbison JW. Parainfectious optic neuritis: report and review following *Varicella. Arch Neurol.* 1983;40:347–351.

51. Ray CL, Dreizin IJ. Bilateral optic neuropathy associated with influenza vaccination. *J Neuro-ophthalmol.* 1996;16:182–184.

52. Jabs DA, Miller NR, Newman SA, Johnson MA, Stevens MB. Optic neuropathy in systemic lupus erythematosus. *Arch Ophthalmol.* 1986;104:564–568.

53. Kupersmith MJ, Burde RM, Warren FA, Kingele TG, Frohman LP, Mitnick H. Autoimmune optic neuropathy: evaluation and treatment. *J Neurol Neurosurg Psychiatry.* 1980;51:1381–1386.

54. Gelwan MJ, Kellen RI, Burde RM, Kupersmith MJ. Sarcoidosis of the anterior visual pathway: successes and failures. *J Neurol Neurosurg Psychiatry.* 1988;51:1473–1480.

55. Beardsley TL, Brown SVL, Sydnor CF. Grimson BS, Klintworth GK. Eleven cases of sarcoidosis of the optic nerve. *Am J Ophthalmol.* 1984;97:62–66.

56. Jordan DR, Anderson RL, Nerad JA, Patrinely JR, Scrafford DB. Optic nerve involvement as the initial manifestation of sarcoidosis. *Can J Ophthalmol.* 1988;23:232–237.

57. Stern BJ, Krumholz A, Johns C, Scott P, Nissim J. Sarcoidosis and its neurological manifestations. *Arch Neurol.* 1985;42:909–917.

58. Appen RE, DeVenecia G, Ferwerda J. Optic disk vasculitis. *Am J Ophthalmol.* 1980;90:352–359.

59. Johnson LN, Arnold AC. Incidence of nonarteritic and arteritic anterior ischemic optic neuropathy: population-based study in the state of Missouri and Los Angeles County, California. *J Neuro-ophthalmol.* 1994;14:38–44.

60. Olver JM, Spalton DJ, McCartney AC. Quantitative morphology of human retrolaminar optic nerve vasculature. *Invest Ophthalmol Vis Sci.* 1994;35: 5858–5866.

61. Onda E, Cioffi GA, Bacon DR, Van Buskirk EM. Microvasculature of the human optic nerve. *Am J Ophthalmol.* 1995;120:92–102.

62. Ellenberger C, Netsky MD. Infarction of the optic nerve. *J Neurol Neurosurg Psychiatry.* 1968;31:606–611.

63. Cogan DG. *Neurology of the Visual System.* Springfield, Ill: Charles C Thomas; 1966:263.

64. Knox DL, Duke JR. Slowly progressive ischemic optic neuropathy. *Trans Am Acad Ophthalmol Otolaryngol.* 1971;75:1065–1068.

65. Lieberman MF, Shahi A, Green WR. Embolic ischemic optic neuropathy. *Am J Ophthalmol.* 1978; 86:206–210.

66. Swartz NG, Beck RW, Savino PJ, et al. Pain in anterior ischemic optic neuropathy. *J Neuro-ophthalmol.* 1995;15:9–10.

67. Boghen DR, Glaser JS. Ischaemic optic neuropathy: the clinical profile and history. *Brain.* 1975; 98:689–708.

68. Hayreh SS. Anterior ischaemic optic neuropathy: differentiation of arteritic from non-arteritic type and its management. *Eye.* 1990;4:25–41.

69. Hayreh SS. *Anterior Ischemic Optic Neuropathy.* New York: Springer-Verlag; 1975.

70. Miller GR, Smith JL. Ischemic optic neuropathy. *Am J Ophthalmol.* 1966;62:103–115.

71. Kline LB. Progression of visual defects in ischemic optic neuropathy. *Am J Ophthalmol.* 1988;106: 199–203.

72. Rizzo JF III, Lessell S. Optic neuritis and ischemic optic neuropathy: overlapping clinical profiles. *Arch Ophthalmol.* 1991;109:1668–1672.

73. Beck RW, Servais GE, Hayreh SS. Anterior ischemic optic neuropathy: IX. Cup-to-disc ratio and its role in pathogenesis. *Ophthalmology.* 1987; 94:1503–1508.

74. Hayreh SS. Anterior ischemic optic neuropathy: V. Optic disc edema, an early sign. *Arch Ophthalmol.* 1981;99:1030–1040.

75. The Ischemic Optic Neuropathy Decompression Trial Research Group. Optic nerve decompression surgery for nonarteritic anterior ischemic optic neuropathy (NAION) is not effective and may be harmful. *JAMA.* 1995;273:625–632.

76. Beck RW, Hayreh SS, Podhajsky PA, Tan E-S, Moke PS. Aspirin therapy in non-arteritic anterior ischemic optic neuropathy. *Am J Ophthalmol.* 1997; 123:212–217.

77. Beri M, Klugman MR, Kohler JA, Hayreh SS. Anterior ischemic optic neuropathy. VII. Incidence of bilaterality and various influencing factors. *Ophthalmology.* 1987;94:1020–1028.

78. Guyer DR, Miller NR, Auer CL, Fine SL. The risk of cerebrovascular and cardiovascular disease in patients with anterior ischemic optic neuropathy. *Arch Ophthalmol.* 1985;103:1136–1142.

79. Repka MX, Savino PJ, Schatz NJ, Sergott RC. Clinical profile and long-term implications of anterior ischemic optic neuropathy. *Am J Ophthalmol.* 1983; 96:478–483.

80. Jay WM, Williamson MR. Incidence of subcortical lesions not increased in nonarteritic ischemic optic neuropathy on magnetic resonance imaging. *Am J Ophthalmol.* 1987;104:398–400.

81. Arnold AC, Hepler RS, Hamilton DR, Lufkin RB. Magnetic resonance imaging of the brain in nonarteritic ischemic optic neuropathy on magnetic resonance imaging. *J Neuro-ophthalmol.* 1995; 15:158–160.

82. Hayreh SS, Joos KM, Podhajsky PA, Long CR. Systemic diseases associated with nonarteritic anterior ischemic optic neuropathy. *Am J Ophthalmol.* 1994;118:766–780.

83. Jacobson DM, Vierkant RA, Belongia EA. Nonarteritic anterior ischemic optic neuropathy: a case-control study of potential risk factors. *Arch Ophthalmol.* 1997;115:1403–1407.

84. Chung SM, Gay CA, McCrary JA 3rd. Non-arteritic anterior ischemic optic neuropathy: the impact of tobacco use. *Ophthalmology.* 1994;101:779–782.

85. Fry CL, Carter JE, Kanter MC, Tegeler CH, Tuley MR. Anterior ischemic optic neuropathy is not associated with carotid artery atherosclerosis. *Stroke.* 1993;24:539–542.

86. Tomsak RL. Ischemic optic neuropathy associated with retinal embolism. *Am J Ophthalmol.* 1985;99: 590–592.

87. Portnoy SL, Beer PM, Packer AJ, Van Dyke HJ. Embolic anterior ischemic optic neuropathy. *J Clin Neuro-ophthalmol.* 1989;9:21–25.

88. Hayreh SS, Zimmerman MB, Podhajsky P, Alward WLM. Nocturnal arterial hypotension and its role in optic nerve head and ocular ischemic disorders. *Am J Ophthalmol.* 1994;117:603–624.

89. Landau K, Winterkorn JMS, Mailloux LU, Vetter W, Napolitano B. 24-Hour blood pressure monitoring in patients with anterior ischemic optic neuropathy. *Arch Ophthalmol.* 1996;114:570–575.

90. Johnson MW, Kincaid MC, Trobe JD. Bilateral retrobulbar optic nerve infarction after blood loss and hypotension: a clinicopathologic case study. *Ophthalmology.* 1987;94:1577–1584.

91. Katz DM, Trobe JD, Cornblath WT, Kline LB. Ischemic optic neuropathy after lumbar spine surgery. *Arch Ophthalmol.* 1994;112:925–931.

92. Rizzo JF III, Lessell S. Posterior ischemic optic neuropathy during general surgery. *Am J Ophthalmol.* 1987;103:808–811.

93. Connolly SE, Gordon KB, Horton JC. Salvage of vision after hypotension-induced ischemic optic neuropathy. *Am J Ophthalmol.* 1994;117:235–242.

94. Sergott RC, Cohen MS, Bosley TM, Savino PJ. Optic nerve decompression may improve the progressive form of nonarteritic ischemic optic neuropathy. *Arch Ophthalmol.* 1989;107:1743–1754.

95. Kelman SE, Elman MJ. Optic nerve sheath decompression for non-arteritic ischemic optic neuropathy improves multiple visual function parameters. *Arch Ophthalmol.* 1991;109:667–671.

96. Spoor TC, Wilkinson MJ, Ramocki JM. Optic nerve sheath decompression for the treatment of progressive nonarteritic ischemic optic neuropathy. *Am J Ophthalmol.* 1991;111:724–728.

97. Spoor TC, McHenry JG, Lau-Sickon L. Progressive and static nonarteritic ischemic optic neuropathy treated by optic nerve sheath compression. *Ophthalmology.* 1993;100:306–311.

98. Botelho PJ, Johnson LN, Arnold AC. The effect of aspirin on the visual outcome of nonarteritic anterior ischemic optic neuropathy. *Am J Ophthalmol.* 1996;121:450–451.

99. Williams EL, Hart WM Jr, Tempelhoff R. Post-operative ischemic optic neuropathy. *Anesth Analg.* 1995;80:1018–1029.

100. Shapira OM, Kimmel WA, Lindsey PS, Shahian DM. Anterior ischemic optic neuropathy after open heart operations. *Ann Thorac Surg.* 1996; 61:660–666.

101. Myers MA, Hamilton SR, Bogosian AJ. Visual loss as a complication of spine surgery. *Spine.* 1997; 22:1325–1329.

102. Keith NM, Wagener HP, Baker NW. Some different types of essential hypertension: their course and prognosis. *Am J Med Sci.* 1939;197:332–343.

103. Hayreh SS, Servais GE, Virdi PS. Fundus lesions in malignant hypertension: VI. Hypertensive choroidopathy. *Ophthalmology.* 1986;93:1383–1400.

104. Kishi S, Tso MOM, Hayreh SS. Fundus lesions in malignant hypertension II. A pathologic study of experimental hypertensive optic neuropathy. *Arch Ophthalmol.* 1985;103:1198–1206.

105. Beck RW, Gamel JW, Willcourt RJ, Berman G. Acute ischemic optic neuropathy in severe preeclampsia. *Am J Ophthalmol.* 1980;90:342–346.

106. Taylor D, Ramsay J, Day S, Dillon M. Infarction of the optic nerve in children with accelerated hypertension. *Br J Ophthalmol.* 1981;65:153–160.

107. Cove DH, Seddon M, Fletcher RF, Dukes DC.

Blindness after treatment for malignant hypertension. *Br Med J.* 1979;2:245–246.

108. Pryor JS, Davies PD, Hamilton DV. Blindness and malignant hypertension. *Lancet.* 1979;2:803.

109. Ghanchi FD, Dutton GN. Current concepts in giant cell (temporal) arteritis. *Surv Ophthalmol.* 1997;42:99–123.

110. Lee AG, Brazis PW. *Clinical Pathways in Neuro-ophthalmology: An Evidence-based Approach.* New York: Thieme; 1998.

111. McFadzean RM. Ischemic optic neuropathy and giant cell arteritis. *Curr Opin Ophthalmol.* 1998;9:10–17.

112. Hunder GG, Michet CJ. Giant cell arteritis and polymyalgia rheumatica. *Clin Rheum Dis.* 1985;11: 471–483.

113. Goodman BW. Temporal arteritis. *Am J Med.* 1979; 67:111–119.

114. Quillen DA, Cantore WA, Schwartz SR, Brod RD, Sassani JW. Choroidal nonperfusion in giant cell arteritis. *Am J Ophthalmol.* 1993;116:171–175.

115. Slavin ML, Barondes MJ. Visual loss caused by choroidal ischemia preceding anterior ischemic optic neuropathy in giant cell arteritis. *Am J Ophthalmol.* 1994;117:81–86.

116. Ghanchi FD, Williamson TH, Lim CS. Colour Doppler imaging in giant cell arteritis: serial examination and comparison with nonarteritic anterior ischemic optic neuropathy. *Eye.* 1996;10: 459–464.

117. Ho AC, Sergott RC, Regillo CD, et al. Color Doppler hemodynamics of giant cell arteritis. *Arch Ophthalmol.* 1994;112:938–945.

118. Henkind P, Charles NC, Pearson J. Histopathology of ischemic optic neuropathy. *Am J Ophthalmol.* 1970;69:78–90.

119. Bengtsson BA, Malmvall BE. The epidemiology of giant cell arteritis including temporal arteritis and polymyalgia rheumatica: incidences of different clinical presentations and eye complications. *Arthritis Rheum.* 1981;24:899–904.

120. Hayreh SS, Podhajsky PA, Zimmerman B. Ocular manifestations of giant cell arteritis. *Am J Ophthalmol.* 1998;125:509–520.

121. Desmet GD, Knockaert DC, Bobbaers HJ. Temporal arteritis: the silent presentation and delay in diagnosis. *J Intern Med.* 1990;227:237–240.

122. Simmons RJ, Cogan DG. Occult temporal arteritis. *Arch Ophthalmol.* 1962;68:8–13.

123. Jonasson F, Cullen JF, Elton RA. Temporal arteritis: a 14 year epidemiological, clinical and prognostic study. *Scott Med J.* 1979;11:111–1119.

124. Jacobson DM, Slamovits TL. Erythrocyte sedimentation rate and its relationship to hematocrit in giant cell arteritis. *Arch Ophthalmol.* 1987;105: 965–967.

125. Hayreh SS, Podhajsky PA, Raman R, Zimmerman B. Giant cell arteritis: validity and reliability of various diagnostic criteria. *Am J Ophthalmol.* 1997;123: 285–296.

126. Hedges TR III, Gieger GL, Albert DM. The clinical value of negative temporal artery biopsy specimens. *Arch Ophthalmol.* 1983;101:1251–1254.

127. Hall S, Persellin S, Lie JT, O'Brien PC, Kurland LT, Hunder GG. The therapeutic impact of temporal artery biopsy. *Lancet.* 1983;2:1217–1220.

128. McDonnell PJ, Moore W, Miller NR, Hutchins GM, Green WR. Temporal arteritis: a clinicopathologic study. *Ophthalmology.* 1986;93:518–530.

129. Klein RG, Campbell RJ, Hunder GG, Carney JA. Skip lesions in temporal arteritis. *Mayo Clin Proc.* 1976;51:504–510.

130. Chambers WA, Bernardino VB. Specimen length in temporal artery biopsies. *J Clin Neuro-ophthalmol.* 1988;8:121–125.

131. Achkar AA, Lie JT, Hunder GG, O'Fallon WM, Gabriel SE. How does previous corticosteroid treatment affect the biopsy findings in giant cell (temporal) arteritis? *Ann Intern Med.* 1994;120:987–992.

132. Allison MC, Gallagher PJ. Temporal artery biopsy and corticosteroid treatment. *Ann Rheum Dis.* 1984;43:416–417.

133. Burde RM, Savino PJ, Trobe JD. *Clinical Decisions in Neuro-ophthalmology.* 2nd ed. St. Louis: Mosby; 1992:54.

134. Turnbull J. Temporal arteritis and polymyalgia rheumatica: nosographic and nosologic considerations. *Neurology.* 1996;46:901–906.

135. Cornblath WT, Eggenberger ER. Progressive visual loss from giant cell arteritis despite high-dose intravenous methylprednisolone. *Ophthalmology.* 1997;104:854–858.

136. Finlay R. Diagnosing and managing polymyalgia rheumatica and temporal arteritis : oral prednisolone 40 mg daily is not adequate for temporal arteritis once vision is affected. *Br Med J.* 1997;315:549.

137. Wilke WS, Hoffman GS. Treatment of corticosteroid-resistant giant cell arteritis. *Rheum Dis Clin North Am.* 1995;21:59–71.

138. Hunder GG. Giant cell arteritis in polymyalgia rheumatica. *Am J Med.* 1997;102:514–516.

139. Kline LB, Kim JY, Ceballos R. Radiation optic neuropathy. *Ophthalmology.* 1985;92:1118–1126.

140. Wagner HP, Hollenhorst RW. The ocular lesions of temporal arteritis. *Am J Ophthalmol.* 1958;45: 617–630.

141. Lee AG, Brazis PW, Miller NR. Posterior ischemic optic neuropathy associated with migraine. *Headache.* 1996;36:506–510.

142. Hayreh SS. Posterior ischemic optic neuropathy. *Ophthalmologica.* 1981;182:29–41.

143. Isayama Y, Takahashi T, Inoue M, Jimura T. Posterior ischemic optic neuropathy. III. Clinical diagnosis. *Ophthalmologica.* 1983;187:141–147.

144. Parsons JT, Bova FJ, Fitzgerald CR, Mendenhall WM, Million RR. Radiation optic neuropathy after megavoltage external-beam irradiation: analysis of time-dose factors. *Int J Rad Oncol Biol Phys.* 1994;30:755–763.

145. Girkin CA, Comey CH, Lunsford LD, Goodman ML, Kline LB. Radiation optic neuropathy after stereotactic radiosurgery. *Ophthalmology.* 1997;104: 1634–1643.

146. Zimmerman CF, Schatz NJ, Glaser JS. Magnetic resonance imaging of radiation optic neuropathy. *Am J Ophthalmol.* 1990;110:389–394.

147. Young WC, Thornton AF, Gebarski SS, Cornblath WT. Radiation-induced neuropathy: correlation of MR imaging and radiation dosimetry. *Radiology.* 1992;185:904–907.

148. Goldsmith BJ, Rosenthal SA, Wara WM, Larson DA. Optic neuropathy after irradiation of meningioma. *Radiology.* 1992;185:71–76.

149. Roden D, Bosley TM, Fowble B, et al. Delayed radiation injury to the optic nerves and chiasm: clinical syndrome and treatment with hyperbaric oxygen and corticosteroids. *Ophthalmology.* 1990;97:346–351.

150. Glantz MJ, Burger PC, Friedman AH, Radtke RA, Massey EW, Schold SC. Treatment of radiation-induced nervous system injury with heparin and warfarin. *Neurology.* 1994;44:2020–2027.

151. Bogousslavsky J, Regli F, Zografos L, Uske A. Opticocerebral syndrome: simultaneous hemodynamic infarction of optic nerve and brain. *Neurology.* 1987;37:263–268.

152. Waybright EA, Selhorst JB, Combs J. Anterior ischemic optic neuropathy with internal carotid artery occlusion. *Am J Ophthalmol.* 1982;93:42–47.

153. Biousse V, Schaisson M, Touboul PJ, D'Anglejan-Chatillon J, Bousser MG. Ischemic optic neuropathy associated with internal carotid artery dissection. *Arch Neurol.* 1998;55:715–719.

154. Hayreh SS. Anterior ischemic optic neuropathy: IV. Occurrence after cataract extraction. *Arch Ophthalmol.* 1980;98:1410–1416.

155. Carroll FD. Optic nerve complications of cataract extraction. *Trans Am Acad Ophthalmol Otolaryngol.* 1973;77:623–629.

156. Serrano LA, Behrens MM, Carroll FD. Postcataract extraction ischemic optic neuropathy. *Arch Ophthalmol.* 1982;100:1177–1178.

157. Minckler DS, Tso MOM, Zimmerman LE. A light microscopic autoradiographic study of axoplasmic transport in the optic nerve head during ocular hypotony, increased intraocular pressure, and papilledema. *Am J Ophthalmol.* 1976; 82: 741–757.

158. O'Hara M, OConnor PS. Migrainous optic neuropathy. *J Clin Neuro-ophthalmol.* 1984;4:85–90.

159. Katz B. Bilateral sequential migrainous ischemic optic neuropathy. *Am J Ophthalmol.* 1985;99:489.

160. McDonald WI, Sanders MD. Migraine complicated by ischaemic papillopathy. *Lancet.* 1971;1:521–523.

161. Katz B, Bamford C. Migrainous ischemic optic neuropathy. *Neurology.* 1985;35:112–114.

162. Winterkorn JM, Burde RM. Vasospasm—not migraine—in the anterior visual pathway. *Ophthalmol Clin North Am.* 1996;9(3):393–405.

163. Lubow M, Makley TA. Pseudopapilledema of juvenile diabetes mellitus. *Arch Ophthalmol.* 1971;85:417–422.

164. Barr CC, Glaser JS, Blankenship G. Acute disc swelling in juvenile diabetes: clinical profile and natural history of 12 cases. *Arch Ophthalmol.* 1980;98:2185–2192.

165. Pavan PR, Aiello LM, Wafai MZ, Briones JC, Sebestyen JG, Bradbury MJ. Optic disc edema in juvenile-onset diabetes. *Arch Ophthalmol.* 1980;98:2193–2195.

166. Hayreh SS, Zahoruk RM. Anterior ischemic optic neuropathy: VI. In juvenile diabetics. *Ophthalmologica.* 1981;82:13–28.

167. Regillo CD, Brown GC, Savino PJ, et al. Diabetic papillopathy: patient characteristics and fundus findings. *Arch Ophthalmol.* 1995;113:889–895.

168. Layzer RB. *Neuromuscular Manifestations of Systemic Disease.* Philadelphia: FA Davis; 1985:121–125.

169. Brown GC. The ocular ischemic syndrome. In: Ryan SJ, ed. *Retina.* 2nd ed. Philadelphia: Mosby; 1994:1515–1527.

170. Kupersmith MJ, Berenstein A, Flamm E, Ransohoff J. Neuro-ophthalmologic abnormalities and intravascular therapy of traumatic carotid cavernous fistulas. *Ophthalmology.* 1986;93:906–912.

171. Drance SM, ed. International Symposium on Neuroprotection and Vascular Risk Factors in Glaucoma. *Surv Ophthalmol.* 1999(suppl 1):43.

172. Shields MB. *Textbook of Glaucoma.* 4th ed. Baltimore: Williams & Wilkins; 1998:77–82.

173. Miller NR. *Walsh & Hoyt's Clinical Neuro-Ophthalmology.* 4th ed. Vol 1. Baltimore: Williams & Wilkins; 1982:185–186.

174. Green GJ, Lessell S, Lowenstein JI. Ischemic optic neuropathy in chronic papilledema. *Arch Ophthalmol.* 1980;98:502–504.

175. Beck RW, Greenberg HS. Post-decompression optic neuropathy. *J Neurosurg.* 1985;63:196–199.

175a. Biousse V, Ameri A, Bousser M-G. Isolated intracranial hypertension as the only sign of cerebral venous thrombosis. *Neurology.* 1999;53:1537–1542.

176. Gu XZ, Tsai JC, Wurderman A, Wall M, Foote T, Sadun AA. Pattern of axonal loss in longstanding papilloedema due to idiopathic intracranial hypertension. *Curr Eye Res.* 1995;14:173–180.

177. Johnston I, Hawke S, Halmagyi M, Teo C. The pseudotumor syndrome. *Arch Neurol.* 1991;48:740–747.

178. Ameri A, Bousser M. Cerebral venous thrombosis. *Neurol Clin.* 1992;10:87–111.

178a. Bousser M-G. Cerebral venous thrombosis. Nothing, heparin, or local thrombolysis? *Stroke.* 1999;30:481–483.

179. Wall M. Idiopathic intracranial hypertension. *Neurol Clin.* 1991;9:73–95.

180. Purvin VA, Trobe JD, Kosmorsky GD. Neuro-ophthalmic features of cerebral venous obstruction. *Arch Neurol.* 1995;52:880–885.

181. Cognard C, Casasco A, Toevi M, Houdart E, Chiras J, Merland JJ. Dural arteriovenous fistulas as a cause of intracranial hypertension due to impairment of cranial venous outflow. *J Neurol Neurosurg Psychiatry.* 1998;65:308–316.

182. Fishman RA. The pathophysiology of pseudotumor cerebri: an unsolved puzzle. *Arch Neurol.* 1984;41:257–258.

183. Johnston I, Patterson A. Benign intracranial hypertension. II. CSF pressure and circulation. *Brain.* 1974;97:301–312.

184. Brazis PW, Lee AG. Elevated intracranial pressure and pseudotumor cerebri. *Curr Opin Ophthalmol.* 1998;9:27–32.

185. Wall M, George D. Idiopathic intracranial hypertension: a prospective study of 50 patients. *Brain.* 1991;114:155–180.

186. Round R, Keane JR. The minor symptoms of increased intracranial pressure: 101 patients with benign intracranial hypertension. *Neurology.* 1988;38:1461–1464.

187. Lessell S. Pediatric pseudotumor cerebri (idiopathic intracranial hypertension). *Surv Ophthalmol.* 1992;37:155–156.

188. Scott IU, Siatkowski RM, Eneyni M, Brodsky MC, Lam BL. Idiopathic intracranial hypertension in children and adolescents. *Am J Ophthalmol.* 1997;124:253–255.

189. Corbett JJ, Savino PJ, Thompson HS, et al. Visual loss in pseudotumor cerebri: follow-up of 57 patients from five to 41 years and a profile of 14 patients with permanent severe visual loss. *Arch Neurol.* 1982;39:461–474.

190. Wall M. Sensory visual testing in idiopathic intracranial hypertension: measures sensitive to change. *Neurology.* 1990;40:1859–1864.

191. Rush JA. Pseudotumor cerebri: clinical profile and visual outcome in 63 patients. *Mayo Clin Proc.* 1980;55:541–546.

192. Digre KB, Varner MW, Corbett JJ. Pseudotumor cerebri and pregnancy. *Neurology.* 1984;34:721–729.

193. Acheson JF, Green WT, Sanders MD. Optic nerve sheath decompression for the treatment of visual failure in chronic raised intracranial pressure. *J Neurol Neurosurg Psychiatry.* 1994;57:1426–1429.

194. Kelman SE, Heaps R, Wolf A, Elman MJ. Optic nerve decompression surgery improves visual function in patients with pseudotumor cerebri. *Neurosurgery.* 1992;30:391–395.

195. Sergott RC, Savino PJ, Bosley TM. Modified optic nerve sheath decompression provides long-term visual improvement for pseudotumor cerebri. *Arch Ophthalmol.* 1988;106:1384–1390.

196. Spoor TC, McHenry JG. Long-term effectiveness of optic nerve sheath decompression for pseudotumor cerebri. *Arch Ophthalmol.* 1993;111:632–635.

197. Spoor TC, Ramocki JM, Madison MP, Wilkinson MJ. Treatment of pseudotumor cerebri by primary and secondary optic nerve sheath decompression. *Am J Ophthalmol.* 1991;112:177–185.

198. Knight RS, Fielder AR, Firth JL. Benign intracranial hypertension: visual loss and optic nerve sheath fenestration. *J Neurol Neurosurg Psychiatry.* 1986;49:243–250.

199. Corbett JJ, Nerad JA, Tse DT, Anderson RL. Results of optic nerve sheath fenestration for pseudotumor cerebri: the lateral orbitotomy approach. *Arch Ophthalmol.* 1988;106:1391–1397.

200. Brourman MD, Spoor TC, Ramocki JM. Optic nerve sheath decompression for pseudotumor cerebri. *Arch Ophthalmol.* 1988;106:1378–1383.

201. Tse DT, Nerad JA, Anderson RL, Corbett JJ. Optic nerve sheath fenestration in pseudotumor cerebri: a lateral orbitotomy approach. *Arch Ophthalmol.* 1988;106:1458–1462.

202. Keltner JL. Optic nerve sheath decompression: how does it work? Has its time come? *Arch Ophthalmol.* 1988;106:1365–1369.

203. Goh KY, Schatz NJ, Glaser JS. Optic nerve sheath fenestration for pseudotumor cerebri. *J Neuro-ophthalmol.* 1997;17:86–91.

204. Eggenberger ER, Miller NR, Vitale S. Lumboperitoneal shunt for the treatment of pseudotumor cerebri. *Neurology.* 1996;46:1524–1530.

205. Rosenberg ML, Corbett JJ, Smith C, et al. Cerebrospinal fluid diversion procedures in pseudotumor cerebri. *Neurology.* 1993;43:1071–1072.

206. Johnston I, Besser M, Morgan MK. Cerebrospinal fluid diversion in the treatment of benign intracranial hypertension. *J Neurosurg.* 1988;69:195–202.

207. Plotnik JL, Kosmorsky GS. Operative complications of optic nerve sheath decompression. *Ophthalmology.* 1993;100:683–690.

208. Burgett RA, Purvin VA, Kawasaki A. Lumboperitoneal shunting for pseudotumor cerebri. *Neurology.* 1997;49:734–739.

209. Slavin ML, Glaser JS. Acute severe irreversible visual loss with sphenoethmoiditis—"posterior" orbital cellulitis. *Arch Ophthalmol.* 1987;105:345–348.

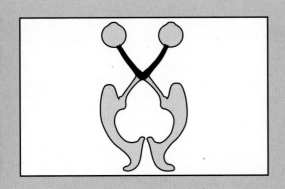

Chapter 13

OPTIC NERVE AND CHIASM II: DYSPLASTIC, NEOPLASTIC, ANEURYSMAL, HEREDITARY, TOXIC, NUTRITIONAL, TRAUMATIC, AND GLAUCOMATOUS DISORDERS

TRAUMATIC DISORDERS
    Precanalicular Optic Nerve Injury
    Intracanalicular Optic Nerve Injury
    Chiasmal Injury

GLAUCOMA
    Primary Open Angle Glaucoma
    Angle Closure Glaucoma
    Secondary Glaucoma
    Congenital Glaucoma

SUMMARY

This chapter considers disorders of the optic nerve and chiasm caused by congenital malformations (dysplasias), neoplasms, aneurysms, head trauma, glaucoma, as well as toxic, hereditary, and nutritional diseases.

DYSPLASTIC DISORDERS

There are four types of congenital optic disk malformations:[1,2] (*1*) small (hypoplastic), (*2*) cupped (colobomatous), (*3*) tilted (dysverted), and (*4*) elevated (pseudopapilledematous) (Table 13-1).

The Small (Hypoplastic) Disk

This sporadic anomaly is so axon-poor that its diameter is less than half of normal (Plate 60). But its diminutive size may be difficult to recognize because the disk margin is often hard to define, and even normal optic disks vary in diameter. The disk substance itself is pale and often surrounded by a light pink ring.[3] If the pink ring is mistakenly considered part of the disk, the hypoplasia may be overlooked. In most cases, vision is poor in the affected eye.

Optic disk hypoplasia may be monocular or binocular. In monocular cases, the abnormality typically declares itself with strabismus. Associated brain dysgeneses are rare. In binocular cases, the patient often presents with nystagmus, and *forebrain anomalies are common,* especially agenesis of the septum pellucidum (de Morsier's syndrome). Hypothalamic/pituitary dysfunction is present in about 15% of patients, highlighted by short stature (growth hormone deficiency) and life-threatening episodes of unexplained fever and hypotension (adrenocorticoid deficiency).[4-6]

An unusual variant of the hypoplastic disk occurs binocularly in children of diabetic

Table 13–1. **The Dysplastic Optic Disk**

Optic Disk Anomaly	Ophthalmoscopic Findings	Significance
Small (hypoplastic)	Small diameter Double-ring sign	Reduced number of axons Vision usually poor May be associated with mid-line cerebral dysgenesis and hypopituitarism, especially if binocular
Cupped (colobomatous)	Physiologic cup diameter <50% of disk diameter Focal deepening of cup	May be confused with glaucomatous cupping May be associated with forebrain or systemic anomalies
Tilted (dysverted)	Disk turned about 30 degrees clockwise Nasal margin excessively heaped Inferior retina atrophic	May produce pseudo bitemporal hemianopia Sometimes mistaken for acquired optic disk edema
Elevated (pseudopapilledematous)	Disk rises like dome with absent physiologic cup May have drusen, anomalous vessels	Often mistaken for acquired optic disk edema, especially papilledema Drusen variant associated with with progressive visual field loss

mothers.[7] Its ophthalmoscopic appearance is distinctive: the upper half of the disk is pale and shrunken, and the vessels emerge near the upper pole of the disk rather than from its center. Visual acuity is usually normal, but dense inferior altitudinal nerve fiber bundle visual field defects and profound atrophy of the superior nerve fiber layer are always present. Visual loss is not progressive.

The Cupped (Excavated) Disk

Colobomatous excavation of the optic disk is a *congenital* deepening and widening of the physiologic cup. This changes the optic disk appearance from that of a doughnut to that of a bean pot (Plate 59). The critical differential here is with an *acquired* widening of the cup, principally caused by primary open angle glaucoma (see below).

Colobomatous disk dysplasia is a manifestation of imperfect closure of the embryonic choroidal fissure, leaving behind a cleft of absent or malformed tissue.[6,8] The cleft usually involves the inferior part of the optic disk and may extend to the inferior choroid and iris. The degree of visual loss depends on the size of the cleft in the optic disk and choroidal tissue. This malformation may be uniocular or binocular, sporadic or familial. It is not associated with CNS malformations but may be part of a constellation of multiple skeletal and visceral anomalies.[6]

There are two relatively rare but clinically significant colobomatous variants: the morning glory disk and the optic pit. The morning glory disk consists of a funnel-shaped disk excavation ringed by dysplastic choroid and retina. Its critical association is with basal encephalocoele, a herniation of meninges and often optic chiasm and hypothalamus into the nasopharynx. This herniated mass which can cause obstructed breathing, may be mistaken for a nasal polyp and resected with disastrous consequences.[6] Midfacial anomalies, including hypertelorism and cleft palate may be tipoffs to its presence.[9]

The other coloboma variant, the optic pit, is a round or oval depression within the inferior part of the disk. *There are no associated brain anomalies.*[6,10] Often difficult to delineate against the background of the physiologic cup, the optic pit causes a dense arcuate field defect corresponding to the lost axons. Visual acuity is typically normal unless there is an associated serous detachment of the macula. The combination of focal excavation and field loss often leads to a misdiagnosis of glaucoma. The characteristic appearance of the pit, the normal intraocular pressure, as well as the steep margins and lack of progression of the field defect, are clues to the congenital nature of this condition. Notches in the neuroretinal rim that look like congenital pits may also be acquired in adults with normal-tension glaucoma following a flame hemorrhage on that part of the rim.[11]

The Tilted (Dysverted) Disk

The normal optic nerve has a nearly perpendicular entry to the back of the globe. Viewed through the ophthalmoscope, its nasal rim is slightly more elevated than its temporal rim. In patients with myopia of more than 5 diopters, the optic nerve enters the globe obliquely, so that its nasal rim appears abnormally thick, and its temporal disk rim is slightly pale, saucerized, and surrounded by a pale crescent of sclera (Plate 56). The thick nasal rim of this "myopic tilt" gives rise to the false impression of optic disk edema. The temporal disk abnormalities often suggest acquired optic disk pallor or excavation, inviting a false diagnosis of glaucoma or other optic neuropathies. Visual fields are usually normal except in extremely high myopia (>10 diopters), when retinal degeneration may cause various defects.

Another type of tilted disk, unassociated with myopia, is turned clockwise about 30 degrees so that retinal vessels no longer emerge at the 6 and 12 o'clock positions.[12] Associated atrophy of the inferior nasal retinal pigment epithelium and sclera may generate bitemporal visual field defects. The borders of these defects do not align themselves to the vertical fixational meridian and are therefore not true hemianopias. Nevertheless, casual interpretation of these visual field defects generates a false suspicion of a chiasmal-area lesion. In some cases, field defects are the result of local myopia, created by outpouching of the sclera (staphyloma). These defects will sometimes disappear if visual fields are performed with appropriate refractive correction.

The Elevated (Pseudopapilledematous) Disk

Congenitally elevated disks appear in four variants:[13]

- **Full but otherwise normal disk.** A normal complement of axons is crammed through a relatively small scleral opening. Such a small scleral opening is common in hyperopic eyes, but it may occur even without hyperopia. Rising well above the retinal surface, the disk tissue has no physiologic cup or spontaneous venous pulsations. It can be differentiated from acquired optic disk edema by the lack of peripapillary nerve fiber layer turbidity, surface hemorrhages, or cotton-wool spots. Mild hyperemia may be present. Some of these disks may be elevated by buried drusen (see below).
- **Full and anomalous disk.** On the surface of this elevated disk are an excessive number of large arteries and veins with anomalous branching patterns.
- **Epipapillary membrane.** The disk surface is covered with a white glial veil left over from incomplete atresia of a congenital vascular system that emerged from the disk, traversed the vitreous cavity, and perfused the developing lens. This veil can add considerable bulk to a normal disk.
- **Optic disk drusen.** These are yellow-white refractile chunks that poke above the disk surface, especially at its margins (Plate 55). Also called "hyaline bodies" or "colloid bodies" ("drusen" is German for crystalline bodies), they are composed of acid mucopolysaccharides, ribonucleic acid, iron, and calcium,[14] and they are believed to be mitochondrial debris ejected from dysfunctional axons.[15] Sometimes inherited dominantly, usually involving both eyes, they become more apparent with age.[16,17] Generally they remain buried until the second or third decade. Visual acuity is typically normal,[18] but progressive nerve fiber bundle field loss often oc-

curs.[19] Although one speculation has been that the drusen compress optic nerve axons, a more likely explanation is that axoplasmic flow is slowly strangulated by a tight scleral opening (or some other unknown process), and that the drusen are a secondary phenomenon (Fig. 12-1).[20] Curiously, drusen do not occur in any compressive optic neuropathies.

When ophthalmoscopic diagnosis of drusen is in doubt, ultrasound or CT scanning can readily identify calcium within the optic nerve. Unfortunately, there is no treatment for the associated optic neuropathy.

NEOPLASTIC DISORDERS

Mass lesions of the optic nerves and chiasm typically produce a slowly progressive decline in vision. However, an acute drop in vision may also occur if the mass expands suddenly (hemorrhage, ischemic necrosis, abscess, mucocoele, cyst) or the tissue has reached its compensatory limit. Improvement in vision and pain following treatment with corticosteroids offers false comfort, since tumors only shrink temporarily.

The mechanisms by which compressive and infiltrative lesions impair vision are not well understood. As they indent and distort neural tissue, mass lesions may cut off blood supply or mechanically block axoplasmic flow. Infiltrative lesions, which produce less tissue distortion, may cause damage by releasing toxins.

The degree of baseline visual loss and optic disk pallor are imperfect gauges of how much vision will recover after decompression. If recovery is to occur, it will be within days to weeks.

Anterior visual pathway tumors are largely intracranial in origin. Principal damage is to the optic chiasm; sometimes the contiguous intracranial optic nerves are damaged as well. Pilocytic astrocytoma, craniopharyngioma, and germinoma are the common tumors of childhood; pituitary adenoma, meningioma, craniopharyngioma, metastasis, and aneurysm are the common tumors of adulthood (Table 13-2).

Chiasmal-area lesions cause painless progressive monocular (or, less often, binocular) visual loss. Visual acuity loss, an afferent pupil defect, and optic disk pallor are the typical abnormalities. The finding of a hemianopic defect is necessary for clinical localization (Chapter 7). Unfortunately, the hemianopic nature of the defect may be hard to discern if field loss is subtle or extensive. Children with chiasmal mass lesions often ignore their visual problems, so that diagnosis is based on pituitary/hypothalamic dysfunction (failure to thrive, growth arrest, precocious puberty, polydipsia-polyuria), distortion of pain-sensitive basal cranial structures (headache), or hydrocephalus (headache, lethargy, diplopia).

Of the tumors that originate in the orbit, the major considerations in children are pilocytic astrocytoma, meningioma, and sarcoma (rhabdomyosarcoma). In adults, major considerations are optic nerve sheath meningiomas, other intraconal and extraconal masses, and enlarged extraocular muscles in Graves' disease. Orbital masses usually cause proptosis, or forward displacement of the eye. Exceptions are tumors tucked into the orbital apex or optic canal, or growing within the nerve sheath, where they harm vision without taking up much space. Indolent, scirrhous (sclerosing) masses, notably metastatic breast cancer, may actually cause globe retraction rather than proptosis.

Compressive lesions are readily detected with state-of-the-art MRI scanning, but abnormalities may not be distinctive enough to allow a diagnosis without biopsy. Infiltrative masses, including pilocytic astrocytomas and lymphoproliferative and hematopoietic malignancies, are somewhat more difficult to visualize with scanning because they may cause little or no distortion of brain tissue. They are visualized when they brighten signal on T2-weighted scans or enhance with contrast. Most elusive of all are leptomeningeal metastases, which may produce neither structural deformities nor signal alteration; they are detected only if they cause enough compromise of the blood–brain barrier to stain the meninges on enhanced images.

Pilocytic Astrocytoma

Low-grade (pilocytic, or "hairlike") astrocytomas affect the optic nerves and chiasm of children (optic glioma, visual pathway glioma).[21-25] About three-fourths of these tumors involve the chiasm as well as one or both nerves, and nearly half of those that involve the chiasm extend into the hypothalamus.[25] Diagnosis is usually made within the first decade of life.

PRESENTING FEATURES

Among pilocytic astrocytomas involving the optic nerve, important presenting findings are monocular visual loss, an afferent pupil defect, an inwardly or outwardly deviated eye (strabismus), a low-amplitude vertical pendular nystagmus, proptosis, and a pale or swollen optic disk. The child usually has no other physical abnormalities except those associated with neurofibromatosis (NF) Type 1, present in 10%–70% of patients (mean 30%).[25] Among patients with NF Type 1, between 2%[26] and 15%[27,28] have pilocytic astrocytomas, depending on the method of ascertainment. Only 50% of these lesions will ever become symptomatic. The presence of NF Type 1 has not been consistently associated with any difference in tumor histology or natural history of the illness.[21,29] When the glioma involves the chiasm, visual failure is joined by symptoms related to hypothalamic dysfunction (failure to thrive, precocious puberty, somnolence) or hydrocephalus (headache, lethargy, nausea, and vomiting).

IMAGING

Imaging of the orbital component discloses fusiform or bulbous enlargement of the nerve (Fig. 13-1). High-definition imaging reveals that this enlargement involves the optic nerve rather than its sheath, as would occur in cases of meningioma or schwannoma. However, this parenchymal enlargement is not specific for glioma; it may occur in patients with optic neuritis or nongliomatous neoplastic infiltrative disorders. Chiasmal enlargement, caused by tumor infiltration, is common (Fig. 13-2), as is extension along the optic tracts. If an imaging diagnosis is not secure, biopsy is advised, particularly if a portion of the mass appears to extend outside the optic chiasm (exophytic component).

Table 13–2. **Neoplasms Affecting the Optic Nerves and Chiasm**

Tumor	Risk Group	Clinical Features	Imaging Features	Management	Outcome
Pilocytic astrocytoma	First decade M = F Neurofibromatosis type I in 30%	Visual loss, proptosis, strabismus, nystagmus, failure to thrive, hypopituitarism, hydrocephalus	Fusiform or diffuse enlargement of nerves or chiasm; isointense on T1, variably hyperintense on T2, mild enhancement	Optic nerve only: observe, excise only if cosmetic blemish Chiasm: biopsy and observe, chemo, or x-ray; shunt for hydrocephalus	Confined to optic nerve: stable Involves chiasm: stable or slow growth, 10%–50% 15-year mortality
Craniopharyngioma	First decade; fifth to seventh decade M = F	Child: headache, growth arrest, visual loss, polydipsia Adult: visual loss, amenorrhea, impotence	Suprasellar mass with variable signal intensity, enhancing rim; calcification on CT	Biopsy or subtotal removal + x-ray Recurrences: reexcision or cyst aspiration, instillation of P 32	Recurrences common, often cystic with sudden visual loss Visual morbidity and mortality may be high with frequent recurrences
Germinoma	Under age 30 M = F	Visual loss, polydipsia, hypopituitarism	Suprasellar infiltrating mass; isointense to brain on T1W, slightly hyper on T2W, enhancing strongly; coexisting pineal mass; CSF dissemination common	X-ray and/or chemo	Good recovery but recurrences common; poor response suggests more malignant germ cell type
Optic nerve sheath meningioma	Any age F > M	Slowly progressive monocular visual loss Pale disk sometimes with edema and optociliary shunt vessels	Diffuse enlargement of optic nerve sheath (tram-track sign) Small intracranial component	Observe or x-ray	Untreated: complete monocular loss of vision Intracranial component does not grow X-ray may arrest progression of visual loss in some cases

Pituitary adenoma	Adults F > M	Progressive visual loss with chiasmal field defect. Endocrine symptoms uncommon except impotence, amenorrhea, galactorrhea	Discrete dumbbell (figure of 8) lesion on coronal view of mixed intensity signal, enhances strongly but inhomogeneously; sometimes signal of fresh intratumor hemorrhage	Trial of dopamine agonist for prolactinoma. Surgical (usually transphenoidal) excision. X-ray for residual tumor, recurrences, nonsurgical candidates	Dopamine agonist often improves vision. Surgery improves vision in 75%, stabilizes it in 25%, worsens it in 5%. Recurrences uncommon
Metastasis	Rare event; consider lymphoma, leukemia, histiocytosis more than solid tumors	Orbit: visual loss, often with swollen disk. Intracranial: visual loss, hypopituitarism	Solid: isointense on T1W, hyperintense on T2W, enhances moderately. Meningeal: not visible except as enhancement coating brain	Multiple lumbar punctures for cytology. Corticosteroids, x-ray, intrathecal or systemic chemo	Depends on tumor; usually a terminal sign in adults
Sphenoid meningioma	Any age F > M	Monocular (rarely binocular) visual loss	Isointense on T1W, variable signal on T2W; enhances strongly. CT: calcification and adjacent bone thickening	Surgical excision, x-ray. X-ray if tumor left behind or for recurrences	Post-op vision better in 50%, same in 30%, worse in 20%. X-ray can halt worsening in 50%

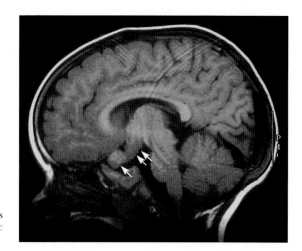

Figure 13–1. Pilocytic astrocytoma of optic nerves and chiasm. Sagittal T1 MRI shows thickened optic nerves (single arrow) and chiasm (double arrows).

NATURAL HISTORY

Pilocytic astrocytomas remain the same size or grow slowly.[29–31] Their indolence and benign histology have given rise to the contention that they are hamartomas rather than true neoplasms. But the astrocytes of these tumors have nucleolar features similar to those of neoplastic astrocytes,[32] and some cases show unequivocal growth. When they expand, it is by one of three mechanisms: cell division, induction of arachnoid hyperplasia, and production of mucin. Chiasmal gliomas can suddenly expand from hemorrhage.

Among patients whose tumor is confined to the orbit, vision may decline, but intracranial growth is rare, and nonvisual morbidity is low.[21] Those that involve the chiasm (and hypothalamus) have no greater visual morbidity than those confined to the optic nerve, but they pose a more serious threat to survival because even minor growth impairs vital functions. They have a 15 year 10%–50% mortality rate, with death caused largely by hypothalamic dysfunction.[25]

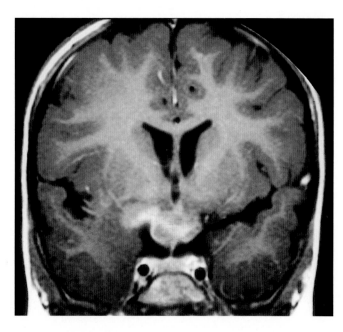

Figure 13–2. Pilocytic astrocytoma of optic chiasm and tracts. Coronal T1-enhanced MRI shows thickened chiasm and right optic tract.

MANAGEMENT

There is no solid evidence that any therapy alters the course of anterior visual pathway childhood gliomas.[21] Complete surgical excision of orbit-confined masses eliminates a chance of intracranial extension, but that likelihood is very low even without surgery. Complete surgical excision of chiasmal/hypothalamic masses is never a consideration. Surgery is limited to biopsy, debulking of exophytic components, and shunting for hydrocephalus. Anecdotal rather than prospective controlled trial data support both external x-irradiation (4500–5500 cGy in 150–180 cGy fractions) and chemotherapy (carboplatinum and vincristine) as ways to preserve vision, restrain growth, and improve survival.[21]

In the case of suspected glioma confined to the orbit by imaging, a presumptive diagnosis can be made without biopsy if imaging signs are distinctive and the patient has NF Type 1. No treatment is necessary unless the proptosis becomes a cosmetic blemish or there is imaging evidence of intracranial spread. Under these circumstances, the orbital and intracanalicular nerve may be excised if vision is poor or irradiated if vision is useful.

Definitive diagnosis of pilocytic astrocytomas of the chiasm/hypothalamus depends on obtaining a positive biopsy. Shunting is recommended for hydrocephalus, and chemotherapy is advised for children under age 8, particularly if there is visual deterioration or tumor growth. After age 8, the brain's limbic and endocrine systems are less vulnerable to radiation, which may then be more safely instituted.[21]

Malignant Glioma of Adulthood

In marked contrast to the relatively benign childhood pilocytic astrocytoma is the malignant glioma of adulthood (age range 22–79).[33] This rare tumor often presents with a rapid loss of vision and periocular pain, falsely suggesting optic neuritis. Imaging may show a mass or diffuse signal change in the optic nerve, chiasm, or other parts of the diencephalon.[34,35] There is no treatment, and unimpeded by any form of therapy, it spreads quickly through the brain in a pattern reminiscent of gliomatosis cerebri. Death comes within months.

Craniopharyngioma

This tumor arises from a congenital nest of squamous epithelial cells in the roof of the mouth (Rathke's pouch) trapped inside or above the sella turcica. The nest grows by cell division to form knots of tissue and cysts. The tumor eventually pushes down on the pituitary gland and up against the chiasm, hypothalamus, and anterior third ventricle.

CLINICAL FEATURES

In terms of age and mode of presentation, craniopharyngioma has a peculiar bimodal clustering. Some 50% of cases declare themselves before age 15 with headache, papilledema, visual loss, growth arrest, or polydipsia/polyuria. The remaining 50% are discovered in midadulthood with visual loss, optic disk pallor, impotence (males), or amenorrhea/galactorrhea (females).[36–38]

IMAGING

Craniopharyngioma can sometimes be recognized by its inhomogeneous MRI signal and the presence of cysts and calcium (Fig. 13-3).[39] In some cases, however, diffuse T2-weighted hyperintensity can look just like glioma or germinoma.[40] Sudden enlargement of a cyst usually accounts for a precipitous decline in vision.

MANAGEMENT

Craniopharyngiomas are difficult to manage because they cannot be completely excised without causing devastating effects on vision. Current recommendations are to undertake partial surgical removal with decompression of cysts and then treat with external beam radiation (about 5500–6000 cGy in children, 6000–6500 cGy in adults).[41] Radiation should be withheld in patients aged 8 years or under because of toxicity. Even with combined surgical and radiation therapy, tumor recurrence reaches about 20%.[42] Reoperation often causes blindness.[43] A less danger-

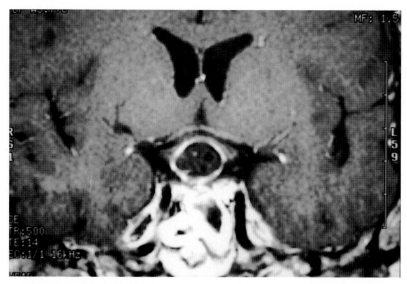

Figure 13–3. Craniopharyngioma. Coronal T1-enhanced MRI shows cystic mass elevating optic chiasm.

ous and more effective approach to recurrent cystic expansion is cyst aspiration or stereotactic instillation of bleomycin, phosphorus-32, or yttrium-90 to make the cyst walls stick together.[43,44]

GERMINOMA

This germ cell tumor (also called *dysgerminoma* and *ectopic pinealoma*) is most often found in the pineal gland, but it may also arise above the pituitary gland, in front of the infundibulum (Fig. 13-4). It presents in childhood with a triad of chiasmal field loss, diabetes insipidus, and hypopituitarism.[45,46]

This lesion is often so small that it is hard to see on unenhanced MRI, but it brightens prominently and homogeneously with contrast. Sometimes it appears to be intrinsic to the optic chiasm and may be mistaken for glioma.[47] Although it shrinks spectacularly following radiation,[48] recurrences are common, particularly in tumors with highly malignant features (embryonal or yolk sac components).[49] Chemotherapy may enhance control.

Meningioma

Two types of meningiomas compress the anterior visual pathways. Medial sphenoid menin-

gioma affects the intracranial optic nerve or chiasm (Fig. 13-5). Optic nerve sheath meningioma affects the intraorbital optic nerve (Fig. 13-6). A bone-hugging ("en plaque") medial sphenoid meningioma can grow into the optic canal and orbit and be confused with an optic nerve sheath meningioma.[29,50]

MEDIAL SPHENOID MENINGIOMA

This tumor is a slow-growing, benign excrescence of the dura of the anterior middle fossa that causes visual loss by compression and proptosis by inducing orbital bone growth (Fig. 13-5).[51] It may arise from the anterior clinoid process, medial sphenoid ridge, tuberculum sellae, diaphragma sellae, or planum sphenoidale, where it is very close to the intracranial optic nerve and chiasm. When it germinates in the dura of the anterior clinoid process or tuberculum, the tumor may exert very detrimental effects on vision for its small size because it wedges the optic nerve against tight fibrous and bony confines. Large tumors often extend into the ipsilateral cavernous sinus or superior orbital fissure to cause third, fourth, or sixth nerve palsies and Horner's syndrome. Women in early and midadulthood are most at risk. This sex bias may reflect the fact that many meningiomas have progesterone receptors, accounting for growth spurts in pregnancy.[52]

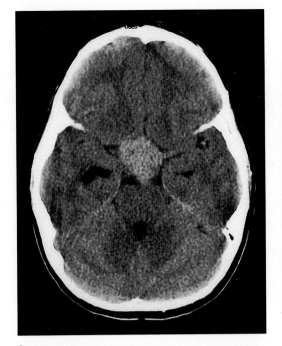

a

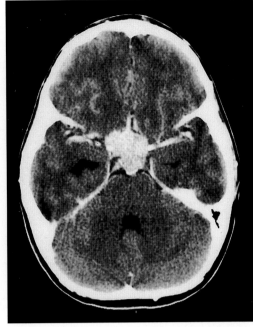

b

c

Figure 13–4. Germinoma of the chiasmal region. CT shows suprasellar mass (*a*) that enhances uniformly with contrast (*b*) and disappears after a course of chemotherapy (*c*).

Large meningiomas are readily visualized with MRI and CT scanning, but small tumors that do not alter bone may appear only after contrast injection.

The natural course of these meningiomas is to grow slowly and to inexorably depress vision. Meningiomas discovered late in life tend to be less aggressive than those found earlier. In the presence of surgically accessible lesions and visual loss, *intervention should not be deferred because visual decline can be abrupt.*

Surgical excision is the procedure of choice in young, otherwise healthy patients,

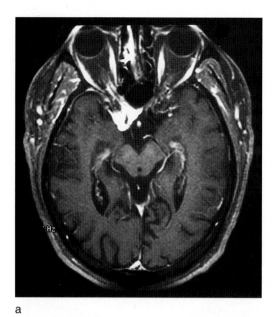
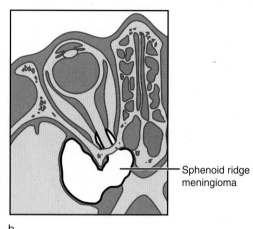

Sphenoid ridge
meningioma

Figure 13–5. Sphenoid ridge meningioma. Axial T1-enhanced MRI (*a*) shows mass based on sphenoid ridge with extension into the optic canal. These features are highlighted in the schematic illustration (*b*).

particularly if visual decline has been documented. Based on reported series, about 50% of patients will show visual improvement,[53] 30% will show no change,[51] and 20% will lose vision as a result of surgery.[29] The duration of visual loss and the degree of optic pallor adversely affect the visual result; the size and location of the tumor less reliably predict outcome. Meningiomas were formerly believed to be radioresistant. However, uncontrolled data disclose that while little recovery of vision occurs following treatment (standard dose = 5000 cGy), visual loss and tumor growth are halted in 50% of cases.[54]

OPTIC NERVE SHEATH MENINGIOMA

This tumor arises from the inner surface of the dural sheath of the intraorbital optic nerve (Fig. 13-6).[25,55] In most cases, it can be distinguished radiologically from the medial sphenoid wing meningioma, which may grow into the orbit through the optic canal but has a more prominent intracranial component and more bone-inducing effects.[56] Middle-aged women are most vulnerable, but this tumor also occurs in adult men and in children of either sex.

Patients complain of monocular visual loss

advancing so slowly that they are unable to date its onset. Occasionally they experience monocular scintillations or blackouts of vision, especially with extreme eye movements, reflecting compression of a kinked optic nerve. Examination discloses optic disk pallor or a swollen disk, sometimes accompanied by dilated veins at the disk margin. These dilated veins are retinochoroidal (optociliary) shunt vessels that have expanded in order to bypass an obstructed central retinal vein (Plate 51).

Orbital imaging discloses diffuse (tubular) or fusiform (focal) thickening of the intraorbital optic nerve. Contrast reveals cufflike enhancement ("tram-track sign"), indicating that the thickening derives from the sheath rather than the nerve. This finding should exclude intrinsic optic nerve inflammation or neoplastic infiltration, but not inflammatory or neoplastic meningeal processes (see "Pilocytic Astrocytoma," above).[56] A lump of enhancement is often present on the medial intracranial side of the optic canal. *Without fine-section MRI that includes a special protocol to suppress signal from orbital fat, optic nerve sheath meningiomas will often go unnoticed or be mistaken for other lesions.*

Without treatment, the sheath meningioma will completely destroy vision in the

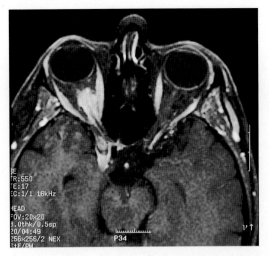

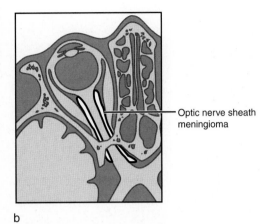

Optic nerve sheath meningioma

a   b

Figure 13–6. Optic nerve sheath meningioma. Axial T1-enhanced MRI (*a*) shows thickened meninges around the intraorbital optic nerve ("tram-track sign") with extension through the optic canal into the intracranial space, features highlighted on the schematic illustration (*b*).

affected eye by exerting a napkin-ring effect on the optic nerve. Remarkably, the lesion does not appear to enlarge very much as it kills the optic nerve, and the intracranial component has never been documented to grow toward the chiasm or across to the other optic nerve. Perhaps the intracranial component is a reactive rather than a neoplastic dural proliferation.

When clinical and radiologic examinations show features distinctive for optic nerve sheath meningioma, biopsy is not necessary. Even the most meticulous attempt at surgical extirpation will infarct the nerve because, unlike sphenoid meningiomas, optic nerve sheath meningiomas are enmeshed within the nerve's blood supply. *Surgery should be performed only if there is firm evidence of an enlarging intracranial component.* Anecdotal experience supports the efficacy of radiation therapy in arresting progression of visual loss, but data are limited.[57,58]

Pituitary Adenoma

Pituitary adenomas are generally benign neoplasms that arise from the anterior portion of the gland (adenohypophysis) (Fig. 13-7). By altering hormone production, these tumors cause endocrine dysfunction. To cause visual loss, they must grow up at

least 10 mm above the sella turcica and indent the optic chiasm, nerves, or tracts. If the overlying diaphragma sellae restrains upward growth, the tumors may expand sideways into the cavernous sinus to cause ophthalmoplegia. Less commonly, they erode through the floor of the sphenoid sinus to cause cerebrospinal fluid rhinorrhea and meningitis.

PRESENTING FEATURES

As a rule, corticosteroid and growth hormone–secreting tumors come to attention because of their endocrine manifestations before they attain enough height to compress the optic apparatus. Those that present with vision loss are usually nonsecreting or prolactin-secreting. (The principal effects of excess prolactin—amenorrhea/galactorrhea in women and impotence in men—are often initially attributed to other causes.)

Most patients complain of visual loss in one eye and will show unilateral or asymmetric visual loss, a temporal hemianopia, an afferent pupil defect, and pallor of the optic disk. A notable variant to this presentation is sudden visual loss with headache, the result of bleeding within the tumor (pituitary apoplexy; Fig. 13-8). Patients with an apoplectic presentation may require urgent corticosteroid replacement.

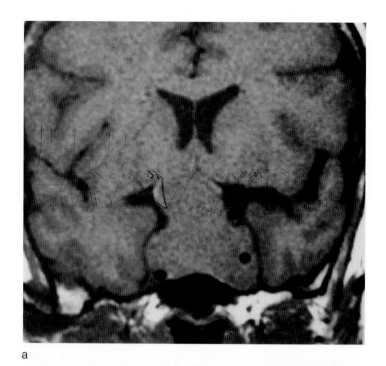

a

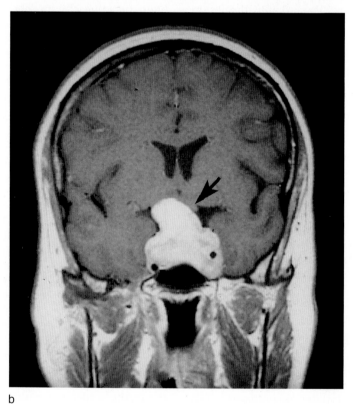

b

Figure 13–7. Pituitary adenoma. Coronal T1 MRI (*a*) shows a dumbbell-shaped mass involving the intrasellar, suprasellar, and cavernous sinus regions, which enhances uniformly (*b*). The mass caused bitemporal visual field loss as it elevated and stretched the optic chiasm (arrow).

250

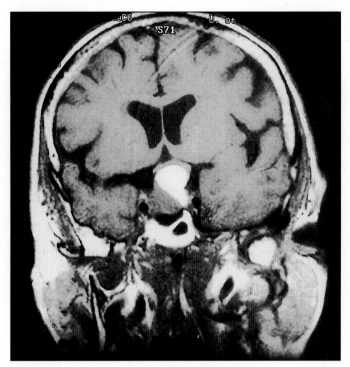

Figure 13–8. Pituitary apoplexy. Unenhanced coronal T1 MRI shows high signal in a sellar mass, indicating recent bleeding into a pituitary tumor.

IMAGING

Usually MRI will identify the pituitary tumor as distinct from other causes. A dumbbell-shaped ("figure-of-eight") mass arises within the sella, pinches through the diaphragma sellae, and elevates the optic chiasm, which is draped over its upper portion like a beret (Fig. 13-7). The tumor 's signal may be homogeneous or mixed, and it will enhance moderately. In apoplectic presentations, there is often a segment with signal characteristics of acute hemorrhage (Fig. 13-8). These features may sometimes fail to exclude craniopharyngioma, glioma, meningioma, germinoma, and even aneurysm.

MANAGEMENT

Surgical removal is the usual treatment for pituitary tumors causing vision loss. However, patients with markedly elevated prolactin levels should first be given a trial of dopamine agonists (such as bromocriptine 2.5–10 mg/day), which may bring about dramatic shrinkage of the tumor and restoration of vision.[59] A lifelong treatment, it is generally well tolerated.

Most pituitary tumors can be removed trans-sphenoidally; exceptions are those of very fibrous consistency and those with large suprasellar and parasellar extension. Patients can anticipate a 75% chance of regaining some vision after surgery and only a 5% risk of losing sight.[29] These odds become much less favorable if visual loss is profound and longstanding, as evidenced by intense pallor of the optic disk, and if the surgeon must approach the tumor transcranially. Recovery of sight after surgery is nearly instantaneous. In fact, lack of improvement or worsening compels urgent rescanning to see if something is causing compression of the chiasm. Most patients require multiple hormone replacement after surgery. If tumor is left behind, x-irradiation is often recommended because it reduces the rate of tumor recurrence from 30% to about 10%.[60] Primary x-irradiation is a viable alternative in treating nonsecreting adenomas for those patients who refuse surgery.[61]

Metastatic and Hematopoietic Neoplasms

Solid metastases and hematopoietic malignancies affect the anterior visual pathway as they do any aspect of the nervous system, by direct invasion or by raising intracranial pressure, causing abnormalities in coagulation, immunity, and general metabolism.[62]

MECHANISMS AND SOURCES

Invasion may occur by implantation within the parenchyma of the optic nerves or chiasm, or by external compression after landing in adjacent bone, dura, subarachnoid space, orbital soft tissues, cavernous sinus, or pituitary. Once the parenchyma is affected, the potential mechanisms of damage are impaired arterial perfusion or venous drainage, mechanical blockage of axoplasmic flow, or interference with tissue metabolism in some as yet unspecified way.

The lung, breast, and skin (melanoma) are the most common sources of solid tumor metastases, but virtually any tissue of origin has been implicated. These tumors reach the orbit, cranium, central nervous system, and meninges via the bloodstream.[62] Most appear to alight in the lungs first, so that pulmonary nodules are usually visible. However, some metastases slip past the lung through pulmonary shunts, a patent heart foramen, or paravertebral venous plexes.

How hematopoietic malignancies reach the head is less well understood, but pulmonary involvement is not a precondition (Table 13-3). Among the leukemias, optic nerve or chiasmal involvement occurs most often in relapses of acute lymphoblastic

Table 13–3. **Ophthalmic Manifestations of Hematopoetic Malignancies**

Entity	Optic Nerves and Chiasm	Retina	Uvea
Acute leukemia	Leptomeningeal infiltration or papilledema	Retinal hemorrhages, Roth spots, dilated veins	Iritis with hypopyon, subclinical choroidal infiltrates
Chronic leukemia	None	Peripheral capillary dropout, neovascularization	None
Hodgkin's lymphoma	Leptomeningeal infiltration	None	None
Non-Hodgkin's lymphoma: systemic type	Leptomeningeal infiltration	None	None
Non-Hodgkin's lymphoma: primary CNS type	Leptomeningeal infiltration	Sub-RPE yellow plaques	Anterior and posterior uveitis with vitritis
Non-Hodgkin's lymphoma: Burkitt's type	None	None	None
Plasma cell gammopathies	Adjacent bone, soft tissue masses, and direct infiltration	Venous stasis retinopathy	Ciliary body cysts
Histiocytosis	Adjacent bone, soft tissue masses, and direct infiltration	None	None

leukemia in children.[63] Leukemic aggregates (chloromas) may be found in the orbit. Among the lymphomas, the systemic non-Hodgkin's diffuse large cell type accounts for most direct invasion of the optic nerves and chiasm.[64]

An entirely different species of large cell lymphoma confined to the CNS (primary CNS lymphoma) may manifest in the eye as a predominantly posterior uveitis with vitritis, together with yellow, plaquelike deposits under the retinal pigment epithelium (Chapter 11).[65,66] *Optic nerve infiltration may sometimes occur without uveitis.*[67] Ocular findings may precede clinical or radiographic CNS involvement by months to years. In such cases, diagnosis must be made by vitreous biopsy.

Plasma cell neoplasms[29] and histiocytoses[68] are rare malignancies that involve the visual pathway in the orbit or middle cranial fossa. The suprasellar form of histiocytosis, which also causes diabetes insipidus, produces such nonspecific imaging abnormalities that the diagnosis will not be made until lytic calvarial defects are discovered or biopsy reveals the answer.

Metastatic and hematopoietic neoplasms of the optic nerves and chiasm share the following clinical features.

PRESENTING FEATURES

Visual loss is usually acute, progressive, and severe. The optic disk may appear normal, or swollen with an exuberant fluffiness pocked by hemorrhage. In most cases, the underlying neoplasm has already been diagnosed, but visual loss may be the most prominent or only manifestation. If the optic disk appears normal, and there are no systemic manifestations, the patient may initially be assumed to have optic neuritis. If the disk is swollen, a misdiagnosis of papillitis or ischemic optic neuropathy may occur. Only when vision continues to worsen, or systemic symptoms appear, will a correct diagnosis emerge.

IMAGING

Findings by MRI are dependent on the site of tumor. Parenchymal masses usually thicken the visual pathways, brighten T2 signal, and enhance with contrast. Dural-based masses are best seen with enhanced MRI, and bony metastases are best defined with CT. Metastases confined to the leptomeninges are most difficult to visualize. Evidence of meningeal, ependymal, cranial nerve/spinal root enhancement, or enlarged ventricles was found by MRI in only 55% of clinically suspected cases and in only 76% of those with positive CSF cytology.[69]

LUMBAR PUNCTURE

When no extra-axial or parenchymal masses are found with imaging, the examiner must presume that the visual pathway has been stealthily infiltrated from meningeal sources. A diagnosis can sometimes be made by lumbar puncture, but it may take several tries. The first lumbar puncture captures neoplastic cells in about 50% of cases; adding two additional taps raises the sensitivity to a maximum of 90%.[62] In one series, however, cytology was positive after multiple taps in only 64% of cases that demonstrated meningeal enhancement on MRI.[69] Flow cytometry enhances the diagnosis by detecting abnormal nuclear morphology in various metastatic tumors and monoclonality in lymphomatous meningitis. The sensitivity of biochemical CSF tumor markers is uncertain.

TREATMENT AND PROGNOSIS

Treatment with intensive corticosteroids, external x-irradiation, and intrathecal chemotherapy improves vision promptly and prolongs life. However, for metastases of solid malignancies, death usually ensues within a year. The prognosis is somewhat better for the hematopoietic malignancies, especially in children.

ANEURYSMAL DISORDERS

Saccular (berry) aneurysms occur as outpouchings at points where arteries suddenly change direction or bifurcate.[70] Weakened by a lack of an internal elastic lamina and media, these vascular turning points become ectatic from a constant pounding of blood. Although believed to be congenital anomalies, berry aneurysms are rare in childhood. They appear with peak frequency in middle age, and more readily in the presence of arteriosclerosis and hypertension. Harm comes from rupture or compression of adjacent tissue.

Anterior visual pathway deficits result mostly from compression by aneurysms of the infraclinoid (carotid–ophthalmic artery junction) carotid artery, and of the supraclinoid carotid artery, that portion of the carotid artery distal to the anterior clinoid process and prior to its division into anterior and middle cerebral arteries (Figs. 13-9, 10; Table 13-4).[71] Both types of aneurysm are predominantly found in women between ages 40 and 70 (peak age = 55 years).[71] Together, they make up about 10% of all intracranial aneurysms.

Ophthalmic Artery Aneurysm

This aneurysm balloons upward from the carotid artery at the point where it gives off its first intracranial branch, the ophthalmic artery (Fig. 13-9). Lying inferomedial to the anterior clinoid process, this aneurysm hoists and stretches the optic nerve, which is tethered at its entry to the optic canal. Visual loss may be sudden or insidiously progressive; it is usually painless. Ophthalmic manifestations are those of a nonspecific optic neuropathy. Although MRI will detect some of these lesions, conventional angiography is necessary to find all of them.

Supraclinoid Carotid Artery Aneurysm

This aneurysm arises at the junction of the carotid and superior hypophyseal arteries, a few centimeters distal to the carotid–ophthalmic junction and medial to the infundibulum (Fig. 13-10). Often growing to giant proportions (>25 mm diameter), it may compress one or both optic nerves, the optic chiasm, and the optic tracts. Visual loss can be sudden or slowly progressive; hemianopic defects are common. The complicated flow pattern in these gigantic, partially clotted aneurysms gives rise to a mixed MRI signal. Because this aneurym often lies directly above the sella turcica, it may be mistaken for a solid tumor. Rim calcification is a distinctive radiographic sign.

The preferred management for both types

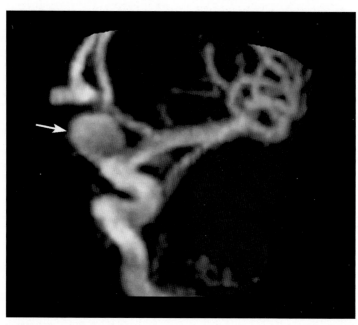

Figure 13–9. Ophthalmic artery aneurysm. Magnetic resonance angiogram (MRA) shows aneurysm (arrow) at junction of the carotid and ophthalmic arteries. It caused compression and dysfunction of the optic nerve.

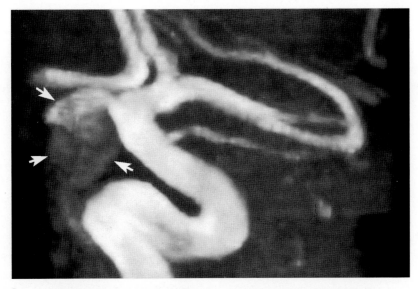

a

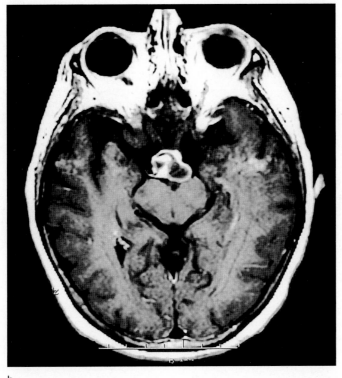

b

Figure 13–10. Supraclinoid aneurysm. (*a*) MRA shows partially clotted (arrows) large aneurysm originating from the supracavernous internal carotid artery. (*b*) T1-enhanced MRI shows enhancing walls of aneurysm which compress both optic nerves and cerebral peduncles.

Table 13–4. **Aneurysms Affecting the Optic Nerves and Chiasm**

Aneurym Type	Risk Group	Clinical Features	Imaging Features	Management	Outcome
Ophthalmic artery	Adults	Progressive or stepwise monocular visual loss with nerve fiber bundle defects, pale disk	Aneurysm sometimes missed on MRI; need MRA or angio	Attempt clipping but exposure difficult	Vision usually worsens after surgery May rupture or further compromise vision if left untreated
Supraclinoid carotid artery	Adults (especially women 40–70)	Progressive or stepwise monocular visual loss with chiasmal field defect	Often partially clotted, giant mass often mistaken for solid tumor; mixed signal on on MRI because of flow patterns; may be calcified	Clipping if neck not wide; otherwise endovascular occlusion, neck occlusion, or trapping	Vision may worsen after surgery May rupture or further compromise vision if left untreated

of aneurysms is direct clipping. For ophthalmic artery aneurysms, the challenge is exposure; for supraclinoid aneurysms, it is the broad aneurysmal neck. Alternative approaches include endovascular balloon or coil occlusion, progressive cervical carotid clamping, and trapping.[71] Although recovery of vision often occurs, some vision loss is common.[71]

HEREDITARY DISORDERS

The hereditary optic neuropathies may be divided into two groups—those in which the optic neuropathy is an isolated manifestation (Table 13-5) and those in which it is part of a more widespread neurologic or systemic disorder (Table 13-6). Among the disorders isolated to the eyes, there are two that follow a mendelian inheritance pattern and one that follows a mitochondrial inheritance pattern. These entities are distinguished from each other by genetic and clinical characteristics.[72]

Dominant Optic Atrophy

This dominantly inherited disorder (also known as the Kjer type) accounts for most cases of inherited optic neuropathy. Visual

acuity declines within the first decade of life—but so minimally and insidiously that diagnosis is often postponed until much later. Visual acuity loss is typically symmetric (within 2–3 Snellen lines), ranging between 20/25 and 20/400 (median 20/80).[73–75] When reliable visual fields can be performed, they disclose central or cecocentral scotomas. There is a tritan axis of color blindness, and optic disks show a characteristic wedge-shaped temporal pallor with its apex at the disk center (Plate 43). In some pedigrees, the degree of optic disk excavation is severe enough to suggest glaucoma.[76] Because of the symmetrical visual loss, there is no afferent pupil defect. Nystagmus may be present in patients with early or severe disease.

There is so much intrafamilial variation in the degree of acuity loss that mildly affected family members may not even suspect that they have the disease—until their optic disks are discovered to be pale and sensitive tests of visual function (contrast sensitivity, foveal thresholds, color vision, visual evoked potentials) show abnormalities. Pathology discloses a loss of retinal ganglion cells and their axons within the papillomacular bundle.[77] The genetic defect has been traced to the chromosome 3q region.[78] There is no treatment.

When the familial nature of this disorder

Table 13–5. **Hereditary Optic Neuropathies without Systemic Disorders**

Entity	General Features	Clinical Findings	Pathogenesis
Dominant optic atrophy (Kjer type)	First two decades M = F Autosomal dominant Accounts for most inherited optic neuropathies Large intrafamilial variance in severity	Symmetrical acuity loss 20/25–20/400, very slowly progressive Central or cecocentral scotomas Tritan color loss Wedge-shaped bitemporal disk pallor	? Abnormal gene on long arm of chromosome 3
Recessive optic atrophy	Very rare Discovered at birth or within first years owing to nystagmus Must be separated from conditions associated with systemic abnormalities	Nonprogressive, severe binocular visual loss Nystagmus Diffusely pale disks, attenuated retinal vessels Normal ERG	Unknown
Leber's hereditary optic neuropathy*	Age 15–40 (range 6–80, peak 23) M: F is 4:1 Maternal transmission but 50% cases have no known family history at time of genetic diagnosis	Acute/subacute monocular visual loss to 20/200 or worse Circumpapillary nerve fiber layer thickening and telangiectasia often seen at onset Optic disk pallor months later Second eye follows same pattern weeks to months later Visual recovery depends on type of mutation Some cases do not follow this classic consecutive attack pattern	Missense mutation in mitochondrial DNA, mostly causing abnormalities in NADH subunits Mutations at three sites responsible for 80% of LHON: 11778: 50% of cases, no visual recovery, 80% of affected males but only 8–32% of affected females get LHON 3460: 15% of cases, 22% recover some vision 14484: 15% of cases, 40% recover some vision

*Rarely may violate the rule of having no systemic or other neurologic features; see text.

is not known, the bilateral cecocentral visual field defects—which often resemble bitemporal hemianopic defects—may mislead an examiner into believing that this slowly progressive disorder is caused by a mass lesion in the chiasmal region.[79]

Recessive Optic Atrophy

This extremely rare disorder presents at birth or within the first years of life with severe visual loss, pendular nystagmus, intensely pale but normally configured optic disks, and an

attenuation of retinal vessels.[80] Parents are often consanguineous. The attenuated retinal vessels may falsely suggest a congenital photoreceptor dystrophy (Leber's congenital amaurosis) but electroretinography is normal (Chapter 11).

Leber's Hereditary Optic Neuropathy

Unlike dominant and recessive optic atrophies, which are caused by defects in nuclear DNA, Leber's hereditary optic neuropathy

(LHON) is a disorder of mitochondrial DNA which is transmitted through females to their children, mostly sons. The mitochondrial source explains why the disorder is maternally transmitted, since mitochondria are passed to offspring exclusively through the ovum. The preferential involvement of males is unexplained.

PATHOGENESIS

There are four mitochondrial genome mutation sites at DNA positions 11778, 3460, 14484, and 14459 (the latter causing dystonia in addition to optic neuropathy).[81] The relative prevalance of the different mutations varies from country to country, but the 11778 mutation accounts for over 50% of cases. The 14484 and 3460 sites are less common, and 14459 is rarest. Male preponderance varies from 8:1 with the 14484 mutation to 4:1 with the 11778 and 3460 mutations.[82]

Mutated mitochondrial DNA is unable to code for proper enzymes to mediate energy production (adenosine triphosphate) within the oxidative phosphorylation pathway of the mitochondria. Each mutation affects different aspects of the energy chain, although most abnormalities involve the first step (complex I). Energy failure dooms the retinal ganglion cells, but why these cells are selectively harmed remains a mystery, since the mutation affects mitochondria in cells everywhere in the body.

DIAGNOSTIC FEATURES

A diagnosis of LHON is confirmed biochemically by assessing the patient's whole blood for one of the recognized mutations. If no mutations are found, the patient probably does not have LHON. On the other hand, the presence of a mutation does not ensure that the patient will develop clinical signs of LHON. This discrepancy may be explained, at least in part, by the phenomenon of "heteroplasmy," in which patients carry a mixture of mutant and normal (wild-type) mitochondrial DNA.[83] If there is a sufficient amount of normal DNA, the patient will remain clinically free of disease. Heteroplasmy has been discovered in up to 14% of cases, primarily at the 11778 site. Perhaps a greater proportion of normal DNA protects the cells against energy failure. The mutant signature in the individual's blood gives no indication of the proportion of mutant DNA in the retinal ganglion cells. Genetically affected individuals may be more likely to develop clinical disease if they carry mutations at other mitochondrial DNA sites (secondary mutations).

The clinical phases of LHON are presymptomatic and symptomatic.[84] In the presymptomatic phase, which may be present for many years, ophthalmoscopy discloses a turbid thickening of the peripapillary retina, together with dilation of fine retinal surface vessels. This telangiectasia does not leak with fluorescein injection, indicating that the blood–retinal barrier is intact. Visual function is normal. These findings are present in many genetically positive LHON patients who never enter the symptomatic phase of the disorder.[85]

The symptomatic phase usually begins between ages 15 and 40 (but ranges from age 6 to 80 years) with painless acute or subacute monocular visual acuity loss. An afferent pupil defect is usually present.[86] Visual fields show a central or cecocentral scotoma. Peripapillary telangiectasia and nerve fiber layer thickening (Plate 52) are greater than in the presymptomatic phase. (In some cases, the fundus abnormalities are extremely subtle or even absent.[87] Visual loss progresses over days to weeks to reach 20/200 or worse. Months after symptoms begin, the optic nerve turns diffusely pale and the peripapillary opacities give way to an atrophic nerve fiber layer. Within weeks to months after the attack in the first eye, the second eye begins to lose vision and passes through a similar sequence. Visual improvement, which may be delayed for years, occurs in only 5% of patients with the 11778 mutation, in 22% with the 3460 mutation, and in 37% with the 14484 mutation.[88,89]

Frequently LHON is unsuspected, at least initially. If fundus abnormalities are obvious, young patients may be misdiagnosed as having papillitis, older patients as having NAION (Chapter 12). If fundus abnormalities are subtle or absent, young individuals will receive a diagnosis of retrobulbar optic neuritis, and older individuals will be investigated for compressive or infiltrative diseases. Using MRI to evaluate LHON may further mislead by disclosing optic nerve enlargement[90] or findings typical of MS (see below). In the presymptomatic phase, binocular peripapillary telangiectasia and nerve fiber layer thickening may be misinterpreted as mild papilledema.

Once LHON was genetically typed, its clinical spectrum was recognized as much wider than originally supposed. Some patients with bilateral visual loss and optic disk pallor, initially assumed to have a toxic-nutritional cause of optic neuropathy, have tested positive for a LHON mutation.[91] Another important feature of LHON has become clear: it may not be limited to the eyes. Some patients have features of multiple sclerosis, ataxia, peripheral neuropathy, and cardiac conduction abnormalities.[81,92] This spectrum of signs is reminiscent of other mitochondrial disorders.

TREATMENT

As with other mitochondrial disorders, there is no effective treatment. Because the disorder damages the oxidative phosphorylation pathway, patients have been treated with antioxidants (vitamins C and E, coenzyme Q) and are urged to avoid tobacco use and food with cyanide.

Leber's hereditary optic neuropathy is one condition among many in which visual loss occurs as the result of mitochondrial mutation (Box 13-1).

Optic Neuropathy in Hereditary Multisystem Disorders

Slowly progressive bilateral optic neuropathy with features akin to those of dominant optic atrophy is a component of many multisystem disorders (Table 13-6). In some of these disorders, mitochondrial missense mutations resembling those of LHON have been discovered.[72] Visual acuity may be relatively preserved (or even normal), but sensitive visual function tests disclose abnormalities and disks are often pale.

TOXIC AND NUTRITIONAL DISORDERS

Optic neuropathies associated with toxins and dietary deficiencies share a common clinical picture: *symmetrical optic neuropathy that targets the maculopapillar bundle,* causing visual acuity loss, central and cecocentral scotomas, and dyschromatopsia. The only hope of reversing visual dysfunction is early diagnosis, allowing prompt elimination of the toxin or correction of the dietary deficiency.

Many medications and substances are re-

MITOCHONDRIAL DNA MUTATION AND VISION LOSS

Vision loss is common in several mitochondrial DNA mutation syndromes. The retinal ganglion cells/axons and photoreceptors are the principal targets.[176]

Mitochondrial Disorder	Target Tissue
Kearns-Sayre syndrome	Photoreceptors
Leigh's disease	Retinal ganglion cells
	Photoreceptors
Leber's hereditary optic neuropathy	Retinal ganglion cells
Myoclonic epilepsy with ragged red fibers (MERRF)	Retinal ganglion cells
Mitochondrial encephalomyopathy with lactic acidosis and strokelike episodes (MELAS)	Vision-related cortex

Table 13–6. **Hereditary Optic Neuropathies with Systemic Disorders**

Entity	Associated Clinical Findings	Genetics
Behr's syndrome	Nystagmus Spasticity, ataxia, mental retardation, pes cavus	Autosomal recessive inheritance
Wolfram's syndrome (DIDMOAD)*	Diabetes insipidus, diabetes mellitus, deafness	Autosomal recessive inheritance
Hereditary sensorimotor neuropathies	Extremity numbness, weakness, atrophy, depressed reflexes	All Mendelian types
Hereditary ataxias	Ataxia	All Mendelian types
LHON + dystonia	Dystonia	?Mitochondrial mutation at 14459
LHON + myelopathy	Myelopathy	?Mitochondrial mutation at 7706, 15257

*DIDMOAD = diabetes insipidus, diabetes mellitus, optic atrophy, and deafness.

ported to be toxic to the optic nerves (Table 13-7), but cause-and-effect relationships have been definitively established in a very limited number (Table 13-8).[93] Among medications, the standouts are ethambutol and isoniazid. Among substances, the major offender is methanol. Alcohol and tobacco may be toxic to the optic nerves, but evidence is confounded by their interactions with each other and with malnutrition (see "Tobacco–Alcohol Amblyopia," below).

The principal dietary deficiencies implicated in optic neuropathy involve the B complex vitamins. Thiamine (B1) is a cofactor in the energy-yielding breakdown of glucose to acetyl coenzyme A. Cyanocobalamin (B12) and folate detoxify cyanide and formic acid, both of which interfere with oxidative phosphorylation. Some observers now consider B complex and folate deficiency (as well as tobacco, alcohol, and ethambutol ingestion) to be factors that precipitate optic neuropathy in individuals predisposed by having a mitochondrial mutation.[72,94,95] Indeed, the LHON mutation has been found among abusers of alcohol and tobacco who develop optic neuropathy.[91]

Table 13–7. **Toxins and Medications Associated with Optic Neuropathy**

Arsenicals	Hexachlorophene
Carbon disulfide	Isoniazid
Carbon tetrachloride	Lead
Chloramphenicol	Methanol
Chlorodinitrobenzene	Penicillamine
Cisplatin	Quinine
Cyclosporine	Streptomycin
Dinitrotoluene	Sulfonamides
Disulfiram	Thallium
Ethambutol	Tobacco
Ethyl alcohol	Toluene
Ethylene glycol	Trichloroethylene
Halogenated hydroxyquinolones	Vincristine

Methanol Optic Neuropathy

Methanol poisoning causes an apoplectic, profound, and largely irreversible binocular optic neuropathy in alcoholics seeking an ethyl alcohol substitute or in depressive individuals attempting suicide.[96,97] The methanol is metabolized to formic acid, causing a severe metabolic acidosis that leads to vomiting, reduced consciousness, delirium, and parkinsonism. Vision, when it can finally be assessed, is poor. Pupillary responses are usually symmetrically reduced, and ophthalmoscopy discloses either no abnormalities or mild optic disk edema, especially in the peri-

Table 13–8. **Established Toxic and Deficiency Optic Neuropathies**

Toxicity/Deficiency	Clinical Setting	Comments
Methanol	Ingested by alcoholics and during attempted suicide	Toxicity via formic acid poisoning of oxphos Also affects basal ganglia, parieto-occipital white matter Produces severe encephalopathy, parkinsonism Treatment with alcohol, metabolic support, dialysis
Ethambutol	Treatment of mycobacterial diseases	<5% of patients treated with <25 mg/kg/day get optic neuropathy except those with compromised renal function; findings often incompletely reversible
Isoniazid	Treatment of mycobacterial diseases	Toxicity less definite than for ethambutol; usually also causes peripheral neuropathy; pyridoxine may be protective
Tobacco	Heavy cigar > cigarette smoking	Optic neuropathy probably conditioned by genetic predisposition; may have Leber's-like mutation
Alcohol	Sustained heavy alcohol use	Uncertain whether alcohol is toxic or causes nutritional deficiency; effects may be conditioned by genetic predisposition, as with tobacco
Thiamine	Starvation	Will cause optic neuropathy even if diet otherwise fine
B12	Pernicious anemia, gastrectomy, fish tapeworm infestation	Optic neuropathy usually subclinical but may be a leading manifestation
Folate	Alcohol abuse and heavy tobacco use	Optic neuropathy is weakly documented

papillary region. The optic nerves eventually turn pale.

Magnetic resonance imaging signal abnormalities are concentrated in the basal ganglia and in the parietooccipital white matter (Fig. 15-18, Chapter 15).[98] Pathologic examination shows anoxic injury in these regions and in the retrobulbar optic nerve.[97,99] The pattern of brain involvement is so reminiscent of anoxic encephalopathy from asphyxiation and cardiopulmonary arrest[100] that the retrobulbar optic nerve is believed to be an oxygen watershed region.[99] Intriguingly, identical pathology is found in the optic nerve after acute hypotension (Chapter 13).[101] Treatment is aimed at correcting the acidosis, by providing intravenous ethyl alcohol, metabolic support, and dialysis. If the poisoning has been severe, blindness, parkinsonism, and memory loss may persist.

Ethambutol Optic Neuropathy

Ethambutol, an antituberculous agent, causes a slowly progressive binocular optic neuropathy.[102] In common with many toxins, it has a predilection for damaging the papillomacular fibers, causing cecocentral scotomas and poor color vision. It may also involve the optic chiasm to produce bitemporal hemianopia.[103,104] At currently recommended daily doses of 15–25 mg/kg/day, the incidence of clinical optic neuropathy is below 3%,[105] but patients with renal failure may be at unusual risk.[106]

Visual loss and dyschromatopsia develop insidiously after two to eight months of therapy, even at standard dose regimens.[107] Because no structural alterations are discernible in the globes at this stage, patients may be dismissed as having nonorganic visual loss. (No afferent pupil defect is present as the deficits are binocularly symmetric.) Contrast sensitivity is an early measure of visual dysfunction,[108] and visual evoked potentials are useful to document the organicity of the complaints.[109,110] If the medication is not discontinued, visual acuity continues to fall, and eventually temporal optic disk pallor appears. Once disks are pale and visual loss is profound, withdrawing the medication may not lead to substantial visual recovery.[107,111] In fact, vision may continue to worsen.

Isoniazid Optic Neuropathy

Evidence for optic nerve toxicity of isoniazid is less firm than it is for ethambutol because isoniazid is rarely administered without ethambutol. Nevertheless, isoniazid appears to have its own potential to damage the optic nerve,[105,112–115] in a pattern similar to that of ethambutol.[116] Peripheral neuropathy is a common but not necessary accompaniment. Pyridoxine may be protective against both effects.

Tobacco–Alcohol Optic Neuropathy

This traditional hybrid label applies to patients who develop slowly progressive binocular optic neuropathy in the setting of either heavy tobacco or heavy alcohol use, where other causes have been excluded. It is hard to establish separate toxicity of each, because most afflicted individuals seem to indulge in both.

Where tobacco use exists without heavy alcohol consumption, evidence for the independent toxicity of tobacco is weak. Many people smoke; few get optic neuropathy. Evidence that visual loss reverses with smoking cessation alone is unconvincing.[117] The proffered explanation for tobacco toxicity is accumulation of cyanide moieties, which impair oxidative phosphorylation and cause demyelination.[118] A genetically low level of vitamin B12, which binds cyanide ions, and poor dietary intake of amino acids (methionine, cysteine, and cystine) needed to detoxify cyanide may confer sensitivity to the toxic effects of tobacco.[119] This rationale has been used to justify treatment with hydroxycobalamin, a form of B12 that is especially effective in binding cyanide.

Is alcohol directly toxic to the optic nerves, or does alcoholism cause harm indirectly by engendering a variety of metabolic abnormalities, including poor diet and malabsorption? This debate continues to rage, although the direct neurotoxicity of alcohol has been established experimentally.[120] As with tobacco, however, many people abuse alcohol, yet few get optic neuropathy. Alcohol neurotoxicity seems to be conditioned by dietary or absorption deficiencies, particularly of B vitamins, and possibly by genetic predisposition.[121,122] In classic studies on prisoners of war conducted a half-century ago, optic neuropathy improved with dietary supplementation of thiamine or B complex vitamins even when heavy drinking and smoking continued.[123,124]

Vitamin B Deficiency Optic Neuropathy

Several lines of evidence now support the importance of B vitamin deficiency in the development of optic neuropathy, and in other neurologic deficits. In most cases, no single vitamin deficiency alone has been implicated. Dietary supplementation with riboflavin, nicotinic acid, and other B vitamins restored some vision in World War II prisoners who had been fed a poor diet.[125] Thiamine and multiple B vitamin treatment also resulted in visual improvement in Korean War prisoners.[123,124]

Among case reports of the restorative power of B vitamins on sight,[126,127] the 1991–1993 Cuban epidemic stands out. Poor nutrition triggered by a U.S. governmental food embargo set off an outbreak of optic neuropathy, myelopathy, sensorineural deafness, and peripheral neuropathy.[128] A case-control study eventually implicated two familiar toxins—tobacco (especially from cigars) and cassava, especially in individuals with poor diet.[129] Reduced risk was associated with consumption of foods high in antioxidants. Vitamin B complex and folate treatment improved sight. This modern case study epitomizes the complex interrelationships between dietary deficiencies and toxins. It suggests interference with oxidative phosphorylation as a common pathogenetic pathway[95] and justifies the use of antioxidants in prevention and treatment.

Strong experimental,[130] pathological,[131] electrophysiologic,[132] and clinical[133] observations have long supported the causative role of B12 deficiency in optic neuropathy. Although optic neuropathy is subclinical in most cases of B12 deficiency,[132] it may be a leading manifestation in pernicious anemia.[134,135] It is also reported after fish tapeworm infestation and gastrointestinal procedures that interdict B12 absorption.[136]

Folate Deficiency Optic Neuropathy

The independent toxicity of folate on the optic nerves or spinal cord has not been firmly established. However, there are isolated reports of folate-deficient alcohol and tobacco abusers whose optic neuropathy improves with folate therapy alone.[137]

Management of Suspected Toxic-Deficiency-Hereditary Optic Neuropathies

Toxic, deficiency, or hereditary optic neuropathy should be suspected in patients who present with slowly progressive binocular visual loss, dyschromatopsia, and maculopapillar bundle field loss (Fig. 13-11). An electroretinogram (ERG) is part of this evaluation because retinal receptor dystrophies can manifest optic disk pallor and central scotomas (Chapter 11). The ERG will be normal in optic neuropathies and abnormal in those with some occult retinal disorders.

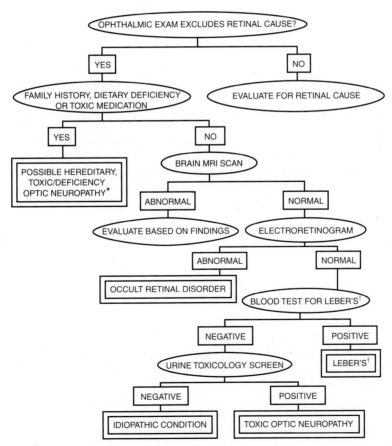

Figure 13–11. Evaluation of bilateral central scotomas. *Confirm with examination of family members, blood test, urine toxicology. †Leber's = Leber's hereditary optic neuropathy (LHON).

If no diagnosis appears, patients may be treated empirically for a period of months with thiamine, multivitamins, and possibly hydroxycobalamin. Alcohol and tobacco ingestion, if present, must be eliminated.

TRAUMATIC DISORDERS

The optic nerves and chiasm may be damaged by blunt injuries or penetrating trauma to the orbits and cranium.[138–140] An estimated 0.5%–5% of closed head injuries involve the optic nerve;[138] damage to the optic chiasm is much rarer (Table 13-9).

Precanalicular Optic Nerve Injury

The intraorbital (precanalicular) segment of the optic nerve is rarely injured in trauma because its laxity allows it to be displaced rather than contused. But a stab wound, a finger jabbed into the orbit,[141] or severe blunt injury to the eye may avulse the optic nerve from its attachment to the eye. If retinal and vitreous hemorrhage do not obscure the view, a gray hole ringed by hematoma will appear where the optic disk should be. Vision is usually lost completely at the time of injury and does not improve. There is no treatment.

If the intraorbital optic nerve is injured within a centimeter of the back of the globe, the central retinal artery is often occluded. If so, the ophthalmoscope will show ischemic retinal swelling with a cherry-red spot. Injury

more posterior within the orbit causes no ophthalmoscopic abnormality. The mechanism of damage is contusion, shearing, or compression by subperiosteal, intraconal, or intrasheath hematoma. Vision may continue to deteriorate after the time of injury. Extrasheath compression is suggested by proptosis and high intraocular pressure. Lateral canthotomy and cantholysis, which are surgical cuts in the tendons that attach the eyelid to the lateral orbital rim, are useful if globe pressure is above 40 mm Hg. On the other hand, the following surgical procedures, recommended on the basis of anecdote, cannot be justified in the absence of more rigorous data:

1. Orbitotomy to relieve mass effect from subperiosteal bleeding.
2. Optic nerve sheath fenestration to decompress an intrasheath hematoma.[142,143]
3. Removal of a foreign body impinging on the optic nerve near its entrance to the optic canal.[139,140]

Intracanalicular Optic Nerve Injury

Most optic nerve damage in patients with closed head injuries affects the intracanalicular segment of the nerve.[144,145] As opposed to precanalicular optic nerve injury, which results from a direct blow to the nerve, intracanalicular optic nerve injury results from indirect injury transmitted by deformation of surrounding bone. Visual loss is immediate and rarely progressive. If the eye has escaped injury, it appears normal. An afferent

Table 13–9. **Trauma to the Optic Nerves and Chiasm**

Site	Mechanism	Treatment
Intraorbital	Avulsion	None
Intraorbital	Extrasheath hemorrhage	Lateral canthotomy and cantholysis
Intraorbital	Intrasheath hemorrhage	None
Intraorbital	Impinging foreign body	None
Intracanalicular	Contusion transmitted via orbital bones	"Spinal cord" doses of IV corticosteroids*
		Surgical optic canal decompression*
Intracranial optic nerve and chiasm	Shearing from brain movement or basal fractures	None

*Customary treatment, but found to be ineffective in a large nonrandomized prospective trial.[158]

pupil defect is the clue to optic nerve damage (unless damage is binocular and symmetrical—a rare eventuality).

The pathology in the intracanalicular optic nerve is ischemic necrosis,[146,147] presumably owing to compression or shearing of nutrient vessels. In many cases of intracanalicular necrosis, similar changes are found in the intracranial segment of the optic nerve.[146]

Intracanalicular optic nerve injury is especially common after a blow to the brow or midface.[148] Profound optic nerve injury may occur with a seemingly trivial blow to the forehead.[149] Fractures of the sphenoid bone are demonstrated by CT in only about 50% of cases,[138] optic canal fractures are uncommon, and evidence of displaced canalicular bone fragments impaling the optic nerve are even rarer.[138] Compelling experimental interferometric evidence suggests that a deforming force on the brow is transmitted to the bone of the optic canal.[150] The relatively elastic bone of the optic canal compresses the optic nerve as the bone bends. The less elastic portions of the sphenoid bone may break, but they probably have nothing to do with optic nerve injury.[151]

The management of intracanalicular optic nerve injury is controversial. Based on retrospective studies,[138,139,152,153] high-dose corticosteroid therapy and surgical optic canal decompression[154] have become widely used approaches. Considering that vision improves spontaneously in up to 57% of cases,[155] however, the value of anecdote in judging efficacy of any intervention is questionable.

Apart from anecdote, the rationale of treating with high-dose corticosteroids is founded on their antioxidant properties and demonstrated efficacy in an acute spinal cord injury study.[156] In that study, a beneficial effect relative to placebo was found if intravenous methylprednisolone was administered within eight hours of injury in massive doses: a 30 mg/kg loading dose, followed by 5.4 mg/kg/hr continuous intravenous infusion each day for three days. This dose—tenfold greater than that recommended for acute optic neuritis and for organ transplant rejection—was selected because doses below this range do not have antioxidant protective properties. In a follow-up report,[157] investigators disclosed that *if this high-dose regimen was instituted after eight hours had elapsed from the time of injury, treatment actually worsened neurologic outcome.*

The lone prospective study addressing treatment of presumed intracanalicular traumatic optic neuropathy found no benefit of either corticosteroid therapy or surgical optic canal decompression.[158] This study was a *nonrandomized* trial enrolling 133 patients to observation, high-dose corticosteroid treatment (100–5400 mg/day) or optic canal decompression, according to patient and physician choice. Although the study is not definitive, it supports the contention that *these medical or surgical interventions can no longer be considered the standard of care in presumed intracanalicular traumatic optic neuropathy.*

Chiasmal Injury

Chiasmal injury accounts for about 12% of cases of visual loss following closed head injury,[144] which means that it is far less common than optic nerve injury. The head injury is always severe. Once consciousness is regained, the patient will manifest a dense bitemporal hemianopia, as if the median bar of the chiasm had been sliced anteroposteriorly. In fact, the mechanism of damage may be shearing of the vulnerable inferior perforators that supply the median bar[144,159,160] or mechanical splitting of the chiasm.[161] The setting for chiasmal injury is blunt injury to the midbrow or face with basilar skull fractures, coma, diabetes insipidus, or CSF rhinorrhea.[162,163] Although there is no treatment for the vision loss, attention must be paid to the diabetes insipidus and CSF rhinorrhea.

GLAUCOMA

Glaucoma consists of a series of conditions in which the optic nerve deteriorates with progressive enlargement and deepening of its physiologic cup (Plate 57; Table 13-10).[164] Other optic neuropathies—especially arteritic ischemic optic neuropathy[165]—can produce pathologic cupping of the disk that looks like glaucoma (Plate 58),[166,167] but

Table 13–10. **The Glaucomas**

Variant	Relative Prevalence	Pathogenesis	Treatment
Primary open angle	80% of cases; 1% of individuals aged over 40 in United States	Uncertain; First theory: abnormal trabecular meshwork impedes aqueous outflow, raising IOP; Second theory: optic nerve undergoes programmed death independent of IOP	Medications and surgery to lower IOP*
Angle closure	10% of cases	Iris blocks meshwork, raises IOP	Emergent reduction of IOP by medication, followed by laser or surgical iridectomy
Secondary	5%–10% of cases	Meshwork debris, inflammation, trauma, elevated episcleral venous pressure raise IOP	Elimination of precipitants, medical and surgical measures to lower IOP
Congenital	<1% of cases	Meshwork covered by obstructing veil of tissue, raising IOP	Surgical incision of meshwork veil (goniotomy)

*No rigorous, large-scale prospective trial is available to support efficacy of lowering IOP in retarding progression of primary open angle glaucoma.

none with such disproportionate cupping to vision loss as is seen in glaucoma (Box 13-2). The cupping of nonglaucomatous optic neuropathies can usually be differentiated from glaucoma by the presence of neuroretinal rim pallor and a lack of complete obliteration of the neuroretinal rim (Plate 58).[166,168]

Elevated intraocular pressure (IOP) is believed to be a major causative factor in glaucoma. Experimental elevation of IOP stops axoplasmic flow at the scleral lamina, either by compression or by interruption of blood supply.[169] In patients with angle closure, secondary, and congenital glaucomas (see be-

---

Box 13–2

WHY IS THE GLAUCOMATOUS DISK SO CUPPED?

- The most distinctive feature of glaucoma is the degree of enlargement and deepening of the physiologic cup. Why does this happen in glaucoma and so rarely in other acquired optic neuropathies?
- Loss of large-caliber axons is greater than in most other optic neuropathies. Many other optic neuropathies preferentially damage small-caliber axons vulnerable to compressive and metabolic insults.
- The lamina cribrosa bends backward. This results either because of a defect in collagen or because of persistently elevated IOP, more likely the former since it also occurs even when elevated IOP cannot be documented.
- Glia do not proliferate to fill gaps. The glial proliferation that replaces dead axons in inflammatory or ischemic optic neuropathies is not seen in glaucoma.

low), elevated IOP is considered the full explanation for optic nerve damage. But in the preponderant form of glaucoma—primary open angle (see below)—IOP is not consistently elevated, so that alternative theories of pathogenesis have been advanced, such as abnormal susceptibility to "normal" intraocular pressure owing to defective collagen in the scleral lamina or a degenerative condition entirely unrelated to IOP.[170]

In all forms of glaucoma, the first axons to die are those that enter the optic disk at its superior and inferior poles. Why should these bundles, which contain relatively large axons, be so vulnerable? A favored theory is that a defective extracellular matrix of the lamina cribrosa in these regions of the optic disk provides less protection against the effects of elevated intraocular pressure.[171,172] Axons of the maculopapillar bundle are spared until the disease is advanced.

There are four forms of glaucoma: primary open angle, angle closure, secondary, and congenital.

Primary Open Angle Glaucoma

This form of glaucoma accounts for more than 80% of all cases, with a prevalence estimated at about 1% of individuals over age 40, increasing gradually with age. It is the most common of all optic neuropathies among the elderly. Family history, myopia, and black race are risk factors.

The earliest sign is vertical elongation of the optic disk physiologic cup, which normally forms a horizontally oriented oval.[173] Eventually, the neuroretinal rim is etched away, first at the superior and inferior portion, and later at the nasal and temporal portion (Plate 57). Once extensive cupping has occurred, the visual field begins to show patchy deficits in the arcuate bundles arching over fixation in the nasal visual field (Chapter 7). At this stage, the patient is usually oblivious to the vision loss, because it evolves slowly and spares acuity. Only when the field loss encroaches upon fixation does it come into awareness.

In primary open glaucoma, structural changes in the trabecular meshwork impair aqueous outflow (Fig. 13-12a,b). Treatment is aimed first at lowering intraocular pressure by means of topically applied medica-

tions that reduce aqueous secretion or improve aqueous outflow. If that does not work, a surgical window is fashioned to bypass the trabecular meshwork (Fig. 13-12c). Whereas these maneuvers usually succeed in lowering intraocular pressure, the efficacy of lowered intraocular pressure in arresting glaucoma rests on a century of anecdote and faith. The single large-scale controlled study that examined the effect of lowering IOP in patients with normal-tension glaucoma found no relationship between IOP lowering and progression of visual field loss.[174,175]

Angle Closure Glaucoma

This form of glaucoma occurs when the iris covers the trabecular meshwork and impedes aqueous outflow (Fig. 13-12d). Most cases occur spontaneously in adults whose eyes have small anterior chambers or who are developing lens swelling from cataract. Only rarely is angle closure precipitated by pupil-dilating medications. Intraocular pressure rises precipitously to levels above 40 mm Hg, enough to stanch blood flow to the optic nerve and to cause severe periocular and brow pain, photophobia, conjunctival injection, and foggy vision from corneal edema. The conjunctival redness may lead to a misdiagnosis of conjunctivitis. Treatment must be emergent and is devoted to lowering the pressure, first by reducing aqueous production and constricting the pupil, and later by fashioning a hole (usually by laser) in the peripheral iris (iridectomy) to reestablish normal aqueous outflow (Fig. 13-12e). The degree of persisting optic neuropathy depends on the level and duration of intraocular pressure prior to treatment.

Secondary Glaucoma

In this form of glaucoma, intraocular pressure rises because the trabecular meshwork is clogged with cellular debris, scarred shut by inflammation or neovascularization, damaged by contusion, or subjected to hydrostatic forces from high episcleral venous pressure. If the precipitants cannot be quelled enough to open the meshwork, surgical procedures to bypass the meshwork ("filtering surgery") must be performed as

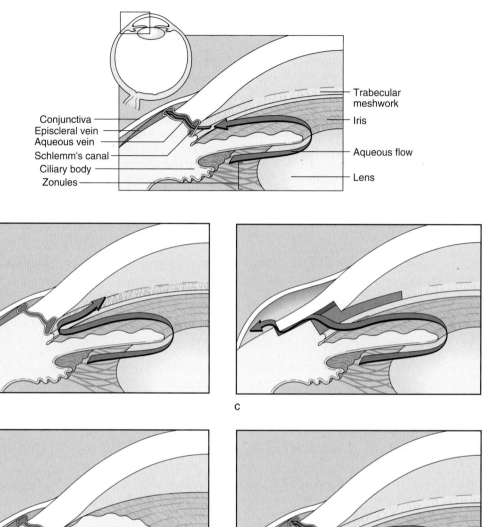

Conjunctiva
Episcleral vein
Aqueous vein
Schlemm's canal
Ciliary body
Zonules

Trabecular meshwork
Iris
Aqueous flow
Lens

a

b

c

d

e

Figure 13–12. Aqueous dynamics in glaucoma. (*a*) Normal. Aqueous fluid secreted by the ciliary body courses through the posterior chamber, around the pupil into the anterior chamber, and exits the eye via the trabecular meshwork, Schlemm's canal, aqueous veins, and episcleral veins. (*b*) Primary open angle glaucoma. Dysfunction of the trabecular meshwork impedes the outflow of aqueous, raising intraocular pressure. (*c*) Filtering surgery. A surgically created hole in the sclera bypasses the dysfunctional trabecular meshwork and restores normal aqueous outflow and intraocular pressure. (*d*) Angle closure glaucoma. The iris root blocks the entrance to the trabecular meshwork, raising intraocular pressure. (*e*) Iridectomy. A laser burn has created a hole in the peripheral iris, which relieves the blockage of the trabecular meshwork by creating new aqueous flow patterns. If the meshwork has not been damaged, intraocular pressure will normalize. (Reprinted with permission from Trobe JD, *The Physician's Guide to Eye Care,* American Academy of Ophthalmology, San Francisco, 1993.)

in primary open angle glaucoma. The ability to restore normal intraocular pressure depends on the nature of the underlying condition.

Congenital Glaucoma

In this rare form of glaucoma, the infant's trabecular meshwork is covered internally by an obstructing veil that impedes aqueous flow. Because the neonatal sclera is distensible, high intraocular pressure enlarges the globe and, by disabling the corneal endothelial pump that maintains cornea deturgescence, causes corneal clouding. Secondary signs are conjunctival injection, tearing, photophobia, and blepharospasm.

In most cases, congenital glaucoma is a sporadic and isolated anomaly, but other ocular or systemic dysgeneses may be present. Treatment consists of incision of the trabecular meshwork to pierce the malformed tissue (goniotomy). Several surgeries may be necessary to normalize intraocular pressure. The degree of optic nerve damage depends, as in secondary and angle closure glaucomas, on how long the eye has been under high intraocular pressure.

SUMMARY

The optic nerve head may be congenitally malformed in four ways: it may be small (hypoplastic), cupped (colobomatous), tilted (dysverted), or elevated (pseudopapilledematous). Some anomalies are associated with depressed vision, but it rarely worsens. Recognizing these anomalies is important in associating them with other systemic disorders and avoiding confusion with acquired neuro-ophthalmic disorders.

Compressive and infiltrative lesions affecting the anterior visual pathway may originate in the orbit or anterior middle fossa. Pilocytic astrocytoma, craniopharyngioma, and germinoma are the common intracranial tumors of childhood, whereas pituitary adenoma, meningioma, craniopharyngioma, metastasis, and aneurysm are the common tumors of adulthood. Among orbital tumors, the major considerations in children are pilocytic astrocytoma, meningioma, and sarcoma (rhabdomyosarcoma); in adults, the major considerations are optic nerve sheath meningiomas, a variety of other intraconal and extraconal masses, and enlarged extraocular muscles in Graves' disease. Nearly all masses respond to treatment, which can be complex and depends on the nature of the process.

The hereditary optic neuropathies are divided into those in which the optic nerve damage is an isolated finding and those in which it is part of neurologic and systemic disorders. Among the disorders limited to the eyes, dominant and recessive optic atrophy follow a mendelian inheritance pattern, and Leber's hereditary optic neuropathy follows a mitochondrial inheritance pattern.

Dominant optic atrophy, the most common variant, presents within the first decade as slowly progressive, symmetrical visual acuity loss, central scotomas, and optic disk pallor. Recessive optic atrophy, the rarest, presents at birth or within the first years of life with severe visual loss, pendular nystagmus, intensely pale but normally configured optic disks, and attenuation of retinal vessels. Leber's hereditary optic neuropathy principally affects males aged between 15 and 40 with acute or subacute monocular vision loss, followed months later by similar involvement of the other eye. A swollen peripapillary nerve fiber layer is often found during the phase of visual loss. Four different mitochondrial DNA mutations are responsible. Visual loss is generally irreversible and there is no treatment for any hereditary optic neuropathy.

Toxins and vitamin deficiencies cause a progressive symmetrical optic neuropathy. Timely elimination of the precipitant may reverse the damage if it is not too profound. The principal toxins are methanol and ethambutol. Alcoholism may affect the optic nerves by toxicity or concurrent nutritional deficiency. The independent toxicity of tobacco remains unverified. Optic neuropathies also result from deficiencies of vitamin B1 (thiamine) and B12 (cyanocobalamin) and perhaps other vitamins. Predisposition to nutritional (vitamin) deficiency, alcohol, and tobacco-related optic neuropathy may be based on one or more mitochondrial DNA mutations as yet undiscovered.

Traumatic optic neuropathy is usually the result of concussive injury to the frontal bone that is transmitted like a shock wave to the optic canal, where the optic nerve is contused. Although surgical decompression of the optic canal and high-dose corticosteroids (in doses equivalent to those found effective in traumatic spinal cord injury) have been recommended as therapy, a prospective trial provided no support for their efficacy.

Primary open angle glaucoma, the most common of all optic neuropathies in adulthood, produces a very slowly progressive binocular deterioration of vision and distinctive excavation of the optic disk. Although elevated intraocular pressure is considered a major causative factor, pathogenesis remains obscure. Elevated intraocular pressure may cause chronic ischemia or indirectly impair axoplasmic flow by deforming the scleral lamina cribrosa, made vulnerable by a weak extracellular matrix. Sustained lowering of intraocular pressure sometimes retards or halts the progression of the optic neuropathy.

REFERENCES

1. Brodsky MC. Congenital optic disk anomalies. *Surv Ophthalmol.* 1994;39:89–112.
2. Golnik KC. Congenital optic nerve anomalies. *Curr Opin Ophthalmol.* 1998;9(6):18–26.
3. Walton DS, Robb RM. Optic nerve hypoplasia: a report of 20 cases. *Arch Ophthalmol.* 1970;84:572–578.
4. Brodsky MC. Septo-optic dysplasia: a reappraisal. *Semin Ophthalmol.* 1991;6:227–232.
5. Lambert SR, Hoyt CS, Narahara MH. Optic nerve hypoplasia. *Surv Ophthalmol.* 1987;32:1–9.
6. Brodsky MC. Congenital anomalies of the optic disk. In: Miller NR, Newman NJ, eds. *Walsh & Hoyt's Clinical Neuro-ophthalmology.* 5th ed. Vol 1. Baltimore: Williams & Wilkins; 1998:775–826.
7. Kim RY, Hoyt WF, Lessell S, Narahara MH. Superior segmental optic hypoplasia: a sign of maternal diabetes. *Arch Ophthalmol.* 1989;107:1312–1315.
8. Robb RM. Developmental abnormalities of the eye affecting vision in the pediatric years. In: Albert DM, Jakobiec FA, eds. *Principles and Practice of Ophthalmology.* Vol 4. Philadelphia: Saunders; 1994.
9. Eustis HS, Sanders MR, Zimmerman T. Morning glory syndrome in children: association with endocrine and central nervous system anomalies. *Arch Ophthalmol.* 1994;112:204–207.
10. Brown GC, Shields JA, Goldberg RE. Congenital pits of the optic nerve head: II. Clinical studies in humans. *Ophthalmology.* 1980;87:51–65.
11. Javitt JC, Spaeth GL, Katz LJ. Acquired pits of the optic nerve; increased prevalence in patients with low-tension glaucoma. *Ophthalmology.* 1990;97:1038–1043.
12. Apple DJ. New aspects of colobomas and optic nerve anomalies. *Int Ophthalmol Clin.* 1984;24(1):109–115.
13. Kline LB. Developmental and hereditary optic nerve disorders. In: Kline LB, ed. *Optic Nerve Disorders.* San Francisco: American Academy of Ophthalmology; 1996:139–161.
14. Friedman AH, Henkind P, Gartner S. Drusen of the optic disk: a histopathological study. *Trans Ophthalmol Soc UK* 1975;95:4–9.
15. Tso MOM. Pathology and pathogenesis of drusen of the optic nervehead. *Ophthalmology.* 1981;88:1066–1080.
16. Lorentzen SE. Drusen of the optic disk: a clinical and genetic study. *Acta Ophthalmol Suppl.* 1966;90:1–181.
17. Rosenberg MA, Savino PJ, Glaser JS. A clinical analysis of pseudopapilledema: I. Population, laterality, acuity, refractive error, ophthalmoscopic characteristics, and coincident disease. *Arch Ophthalmol.* 1979;97:65–70.
18. Knight CL, Hoyt WF. Monocular blindness from drusen of the optic disk. *Am J Ophthalmol.* 1972;73:890–892.
19. Lansche RK, Rucker CW. Progression of defects in visual fields produced by hyaline bodies in optic disks. *Arch Ophthalmol.* 1957;58:115–121.
20. Spencer WH. Drusen of the optic disk and aberrant axoplasmic transport. *Am J Ophthalmol.* 1978;85:1–12.
21. Listernick R, Louis DN, Packer RJ, Gutmann DH. Optic pathway gliomas in children with neurofibromatosis: 1. Consensus statement from the NF1 optic pathway glioma task force. *Ann Neurol.* 1997;41:143–149.
22. Wright JE, McNab AA, McDonald WI. Optic nerve glioma and the management of optic nerve tumors in the young. *Br J Ophthalmol.* 1989;73:967–974.
23. Alvord EC Jr, Lofton S. Gliomas of the optic nerve of chiasm: outcome by patients' age, tumor site, and treatment. *J Neurosurg.* 1988;68:85–98.
24. McDonnell P, Miller NR. Chiasmatic and hypothalamic extension of optic nerve glioma. *Arch Ophthalmol.* 1983;101:1412–1415.
25. Dutton JJ. Optic nerve gliomas and meningiomas. *Neurol Clin.* 1991;9:163–177.
26. Huson SM, Harper PS, Compston DAS. Von Recklinghausen neurofibromatosis: a clinical and population study in southeast Wales. *Brain.* 1988;111:1355–1381.
27. Lewis RA, Gerson LP, Axelson KA. Von Recklinghausen neurofibromatosis. II. Incidence of optic gliomata. *Ophthalmology.* 1984;91:929–935.
28. Listernick R, Charrow J, Greenwald MJ, Esterly NB. Optic gliomas in children with neurofibromatosis type I. *J Pediatr.* 1989;114:788–792.
29. Miller NR. *Walsh & Hoyt's Clinical Neuro-ophthalmology.* 4th ed. Vol 3. Baltimore: Williams & Wilkins; 1988:1243–1747.
30. Listernick R, Charrow J, Greenwald MJ, Mets M. Natural history of optic pathway tumors in children with neurofibromatosis type 1: a longitudinal study. *J Pediatr.* 1994;125:63–66.

31. Imes RK, Hoyt WF. Childhood chiasmal gliomas: update on the fate of patients in the 1969 San Francisco Study. *Br J Ophthalmol.* 1986;70:179–182.

32. Burnstine MA, Levin LA, Louis DN, et al. Nucleolar organizer regions in optic gliomas. *Brain.* 1993;116:1465–1476.

33. Spoor TC, Kennerdell JS, Martinez AJ, Zorub D. Malignant gliomas of the optic nerve pathways. *Am J Ophthalmol.* 1980;89:284–292.

34. Millar WS, Tartaglino LM, Sergott RC, Friedman DP, Flanders AE. MR of malignant optic glioma of adulthood. *AJNR Am J Neuroradiol.* 1995;16:1673–1676.

35. Felsberg GJ, Glass JP, Tien RD, McLendon R. Gliomatosis cerebri presenting with optic nerve involvement: MRI. *Neuroradiology.* 1996;38:774–777.

36. Bartlett JR. Craniopharyngiomas: an analysis of some aspects of symptomatology, radiology, and histology. *Brain.* 1971;94:725–732.

37. Baskin DS, Wilson CB. Surgical management of craniopharyngiomas: a review of 74 cases. *J Neurosurg.* 1986;65:22–27.

38. Petito CK, DeGirolami U, Earle KM. Craniopharyngiomas: a clinical and pathological review. *Cancer.* 1976;37:1944–1952.

39. Harwoodnash DC. Neuroimaging of childhood craniopharyngioma. *Pediatr Neurosurg.* 1994;21 (suppl 1):2–10.

40. Brummit ML, Kline LB, Wilson ER. Craniopharyngiomas: pitfalls in diagnosis. *J Clin Neuro-ophthalmol.* 1992;12:77–81.

41. Graham PH, Gattamaneni HR, Birch JM. Paediatric craniopharyngiomas: a regional review. *Br J Neurosurg.* 1992;6:187–193.

42. Regine WF, Mohiuddin M, Kramer S. Long-term results of pediatric and adult craniopharyngiomas treated with combined surgery and radiation. *Radiother Oncol.* 1993;27:13–21.

43. Wisoff JH. Surgical management of recurrent craniopharyngiomas. *Pediatr Neurosurg.* 1994;21 (suppl 1):108–113.

44. Vandenberge JH, Blaauw G, Breeman WA, Rahmy A, Wijngaarde R. Intracavitary brachytheraphy of cystic craniopharyngiomas. *J Neurosurg.* 1992;77:545–550.

45. Bowman CB, Farris BK. Primary chiasmal germinoma: a case report and review of the literature. *J Clin Neuro-Ophthalmol.* 1990;10:9–17.

46. Sugiyama K, Uozumi T, Kiya K, et al. Intracranial germ-cell tumor with synchronous lesions in the pineal and suprasellar regions: report of six cases and review of the literature. *Surg Neurol.* 1993;38:114–120.

47. Wilson JT, Wald SL, Aitken PA, Mastromateo J, Vieco PT. Primary diffuse chiasmatic germinomas: differentiation from optic chiasm gliomas. *Pediatr Neurosurg.* 1995;23:1–5.

48. Isayama Y, Takahashi T, Inoue M. Ocular findings of suprasellar germinoma: long-term follow-up after radiotherapy. *Neuro-ophthalmology.* 1980;1:53–.

49. Sawamura Y, Ikeda J, Shirato H, Tada M, Abe H. Germ cell tumours of the central nervous system: treatment considerations based on 111 cases and their long-term clinical outcomes. *Eur J Cancer.* 1998;34:104–111.

50. Trobe JD, Glaser JS, Post JD, Page LK. Bilateral optic canal meningiomas: a case report. *Neurosurgery.* 1978;3:68–74.

51. Andrews BT, Wilson CB. Suprasellar meningiomas: the effect of tumor location on postoperative visual outcome. *J Neurosurg.* 1988;69:523–528.

52. Black PM. Meningiomas. *Neurosurgery.* 1993;32:643–657.

53. Rosenberg LF, Miller NR. Visual results after microsurgical removal involving the anterior visual system. *Arch Ophthalmol.* 1984;102:1019–1023.

54. Kupersmith MJ, Warren FA, Newall J, Ransohoff J. Irradiation of meningiomas of the intracranial anterior visual pathways. *Ann Neurol.* 1987;21:131–137.

55. Sibony PA, Krauss HR, Kennerdell JS, Maroon JC, Slamovits TL. Optic nerve sheath meningiomas: clinical manifestations. *Ophthalmology.* 1984;91:1313–1326.

56. Mafee MF, Goodwin J, Dorodi S. Optic nerve sheath meningiomas: role of MR imaging. *Radiol Clin North Am.* 1999;37:37–58.

57. Kennerdell JS, Maroon JC, Malton M, Warren FA. The management of optic nerve sheath meningiomas. *Am J Ophthalmol.* 1988;106:450–457.

58. Smith JL, Vuksanovic MM, Yates BM, Bienfang DC. Radiation therapy for primary optic nerve sheath meningiomas. *J Clin Neuro-Ophthalmol.* 1981;1:85–99.

59. Grimson BS, Bowman ZI. Rapid decompression of anterior intracranial visual pathways with bromocriptine. *Arch Ophthalmol.* 1983;101:604–606.

60. Ciric I, Mikhael M, Stafford T, Lawson L, Garces R. Transsphenoidal microsurgery of pituitary macroadenomas with long term follow-up results. *J Neurosurg.* 1983;59:395–401.

61. Benbow SJ, Foy P, Jones B, Shaw D, MacFarlane IA. Pituitary tumors presenting in the elderly: management and outcome. *Clin Endocrinol.* 1997;46:657–660.

62. Posner JB. *Neurologic Complications of Cancer.* Philadelphia: FA Davis; 1995.

63. Kincaid MC, Green WR. Ocular and orbital involvement in leukemia. *Surv Ophthalmol.* 1983;27:211–232.

64. Kay MC. Optic neuropathy secondary to lymphoma. *J Clin Neuro-ophthalmol.* 1986;6:31–34.

65. Freeman IN, Schachat AP, Knox DL, Michels RG, Green WR. Clinical features, laboratory investigations, and survival in ocular reticulum cell sarcoma. *Ophthalmology.* 1987;94:1631–1639.

66. Ridley ME, McDonald R, Sternberg P, Blumenkranz MS, Zarbin MA, Schachat AP. Retinal manifestations of ocular lymphoma (reticulum cell sarcoma). *Ophthalmology.* 1992;99:1153–1161.

67. Kline LB, Garcia JH, Harsh GR III. Lymphomatous optic neuropathy. *Arch Ophthalmol.* 1984;102:1655–1657.

68. Moore AT, Pritchard J, Taylor DS. Histiocytosis X: an ophthalmological overview. *Br J Ophthalmol.* 1985;69:7–14.

69. Freilich RJ, Krol G, Deangelis LM. Neuroimaging and cerebrospinal fluid cytology in the diagnosis of leptomeningeal metastasis. *Ann Neurol.* 1995;38:51–57.

70. Rhoton AL Jr. Anatomy of saccular aneurysms. *Surg Neurol.* 1980;14:59–66.

71. Day AL. Aneurysms of the ophthalmic segment: a clinical and anatomical analysis. *J Neurosurg.* 1990; 72:677–691.

72. Johns DR, Newman NJ. Hereditary optic neuropathies. *Sem Ophthalmol.* 1995;10:203–213.

73. Mantyjarvi MI, Nerdrum K, Tuppurainen K. Color vision in dominant optic atrophy. *J Clin Neuro-Ophthalmol.* 1992;12:89–93.

74. Kline LB, Glaser JS. Dominant optic atrophy; the clinical profile. *Arch Ophthalmol.* 1979;97:1680–1686.

75. Kjer P. Infantile optic atrophy with dominant mode of inheritance: a clinical and genetic study of 19 Danish families. *Acta Ophthalmol Suppl.* 1959;54.

76. Sandvig K. Pseudoglaucoma of autosomal dominant inheritance: a report on three families. *Acta Ophthalmol.* 1961;39:33–43.

77. Johnston PB, Gaster RN, Smith VC, Tripathi RC. A clinicopathologic study of autosomal dominant optic atrophy. *Am J Ophthalmol.* 1979;88:868–875.

78. Eiberg H, Kjer B, Kjer P, Rosenberg T. Dominant optic atrophy (OPA1) mapped to chromosome 3q region: I. Linkage analysis. *Hum Mol Genet.* 1994;3: 977–980.

79. Manchester PT, Calhoun FP. Dominant hereditary optic atrophy with bitemporal field defects. *Arch Ophthalmol.* 1958;60:479–484.

80. Waardenburg PJ. Different types of hereditary optic atrophy. *Acta Genet.* 1957;7:287–290.

81. Newman NJ. Leber's hereditary optic neuropathy: new genetic considerations. *Arch Neurol.* 1993;50: 540–548.

82. Harding AE, Sweeney MG, Govan GG. Pedigree analysis in Leber hereditary optic neuropathy families with a pathogenic mtDNA mutation. *Am J Hum Genet.* 1995;57:77–86.

83. Smith KH, Johns DR, Heher KL, Miller NR. Heteroplasmy in Leber's hereditary optic neuropathy. *Arch Ophthalmol.* 1993;111:1486–1490.

84. Newman NJ, Wallace DC. Mitochondria and Leber's hereditary optic neuropathy. *Am J Ophthalmol.* 1990;109:726–730.

85. Nikoskelainen E, Hoyt WF, Nummelin K. Ophthalmoscopic findings in Leber's hereditary optic neuropathy: II. The fundus findings in the affected family members. *Arch Ophthalmol.* 1983;101: 1059–1068.

86. Wakamura M, Yokoe J. Evidence for preserved direct pupillary light response in Leber's hereditary optic neuropathy. *Br J Ophthalmol.* 1995;79:442–446.

87. Smith Jl, Hoyt WF, Susac JO. Ocular fundus in acute Leber optic neuropathy. *Arch Ophthalmol.* 1973;90:349–354.

88. Johns DR, Heher KL, Miller NR, Smith KH. Leber's hereditary optic neuropathy: clinical manifestations of the 14484 mutation. *Arch Ophthalmol.* 1993;111:495–498.

89. Stone EM, Newman NJ, Miller NR, Johns DR, Lott MT, Wallace DC. Visual recovery in patients with Leber's hereditary optic neuropathy and the 11778 mutation. *J Clin Neuro-Ophthalmol.* 1992;12: 10–14.

90. Kermode AG, Moseley IF, Kendall BE, Miller DH, MacManus DG, MacDonald WI. Magnetic reso-

91. nance imaging in Leber's optic neuropathy. *J Neurol Neurosurg Psychiatry.* 1989;52:671–674.

91. Cullom ME, Heher KL, Miller NR, Savino PJ, Johns DR. Leber's hereditary optic neuropathy masquerading as tobacco–alcohol amblyopia. *Arch Ophthalmol.* 1993;111:1482–1485.

92. Johns DR. Mitochondrial DNA and disease. *N Engl J Med.* 1995;333:638–644.

93. Lessell S. Toxic and deficiency optic neuropathies. In: Albert DM, Jakobiec FA, eds. *Principles and Practice of Ophthalmology.* Vol 4. Philadelphia: Saunders; 1994:2599–2604.

94. Sadun AA, Rubin RM. Annual (almost) review in neuro-ophthalmology: the anterior visual pathways: II (Part One). *J Neuro-Ophthalmol.* 1996;16: 137–151.

95. Rizzo JF. Adenosine triphosphate deficiency: a genre of optic neuropathy. *Neurology.* 1995;45:11–16.

96. Stelmach MZ, Oday J. Partly reversible visual failure with methanol toxicity. *Aust N Z J Ophthalmol.* 1992;20:57–64.

97. Naeser P. Optic nerve involvement in a case of methanol poisoning. *Br J Ophthalmol.* 1988;72:778–781.

98. McLean DR, Jacobs H, Mielke BW. Methanol poisoning: a clinical and pathological study. *Ann Neurol.* 1980;8:161–167.

99. Sharpe JA, Hostovsky M, Bilbao JM, Rewcastle NB. Methanol optic neuropathy: a histopathologic study. *Neurology.* 1982;32:1093–1100.

100. Mascalchi M, Dalpozzo GC, Pinto F. MRI demonstration of the cerebellar damage in diffuse hypoxic-ischemic encephalopathy: case report. *Ital J Neurol Sci.* 1992;13:517–519.

101. Johnson MW, Kincaid MC, Trobe JD. Bilateral retrobulbar optic nerve infarction after blood loss and hypotension: a clinicopathologic case study. *Ophthalmology.* 1987;94:1577–1584.

102. Carr RE, Henkind P. Ocular manifestations of ethambutol: toxic amblyopia after administration of an experimental antituberculous drug. *Arch Ophthalmol.* 1962;67:566–571.

103. Lessell S. Histopathology of experimental ethambutol intoxication. *Invest Ophthalmol.* 1976;15:765.

104. Asayama T. Two cases of bitemporal hemianopsia due to ethambutol. *Jpn J Clin Ophthalmol.* 1969; 23:1209–1212.

105. Leibold JE. Drugs having a toxic effect on the optic nerve. *Int Ophthalmol Clin.* 1971;11:137–157.

106. Devita EG, Miao M, Sadun AA. Optic neuropathy in ethambutol-treated renal tuberculosis. *J Clin Neuro-Ophthalmol.* 1987;7:77–86.

107. Kumar A, Sandramouli S, Verma L, Tewari HK, Khosla PK. Ocular ethambutol toxicity: is it reversible? *J Clin Neuroophthalmol.* 1993;13:15–17.

108. Salmon JF, Carmichael TR, Welsh NH. Use of contrast sensitivity measurement in the detection of subclinical ethambutol toxic optic neuropathy. *Br J Ophthalmol.* 1987;71:192–196.

109. Kakisu Y, Adachi E, Mizota A. Pattern electroretinogram and visual evoked cortical potential in ethambutol optic neuropathy. *Doc Ophthalmol.* 1987;67:327–334.

110. Petrera JE, Fledelius HC, Trojaborg W. Serial pattern evoked potential recording in a case of toxic

optic neuropathy due to ethambutol. *Electroencephalogr Clin Neurophysiol.* 1988;71:146–149.

111. Woung LC, Jou JR, Liaw SL. Visual function in recovered ethambutol optic neuropathy. *J Ocul Pharmacol Ther.* 1995;11:411–419.

112. Martin SG, Weidle PJ, Rismondo V, Bever S, Wheeler DA. A case of isoniazid (INH) induced optic neuropathy in an asymptomatic HIV-infected woman and review of the literature. *Int Conf AIDS.* 1996;11:88.

113. Boulanouar A, Abdallah E, Elbakkali M, Benchrifa F, Berrahohamani A. Severe toxic optic neuropathies caused by isoniazid: apropos of 3 cases. *J Fr Ophthalmol.* 1995;18:183–187.

114. Kass K, Mandel W, Cohen H, Dressler SH. Isoniazid as a cause of optic neuritis and atrophy. *JAMA.* 1957;164:1740–1743.

115. Karmon G, Savir H, Zevin D, Levi J. Bilateral optic neuropathy due to combined ethambutol and isoniazid treatment. *Ann Ophthalmol.* 1979;11:1013–1017.

116. Kiyosawa M, Ishikawa S. A case of isoniazid-induced optic neuropathy. *Neuro-Ophthalmology.* 1981;2:67–70.

117. Rizzo JF, Lessell S. Tobacco amblyopia. *Am J Ophthalmol.* 1993;116:84–87.

118. Wilson J. Cyanide in human disease: a review of clinical and laboratory evidence. *Fundam Appl Toxicol.* 1983;3:397–399.

119. Woon C, Tang RA, Pardo G. Nutrition and optic nerve disease. *Sem Ophthalmol.* 1995;10:195–202.

120. Lancaster FE. Alcohol, nitric oxide, and neurotoxicity: is there a connection? A review. *Alcohol Clin Exp Res.* 1992;16:539–541.

121. Filley CM, Kelly JP. Alcohol- and drug-related neurotoxicity. *Curr Opin Neurol Neurosurg.* 1993;6:443–447.

122. Manzo L, Locatelli C, Candura SM, Costa LG. Nutrition and alcohol neurotoxicity. *Neurotoxicology.* 1994;15:555–565.

123. Carroll FD. Nutritional amblyopia. *Arch Ophthalmol.* 1966;76:406–411.

124. King JH, Passmore JW. Nutritional amblyopia: a study of American prisoners of war in Korea. *Am J Ophthalmol.* 1955;39:173–186.

125. Ridley H. Ocular manifestations of malnutrition in released prisoners of war from Thailand. *Br J Ophthalmol.* 1945;29:861–865.

126. Dang CV. Tobacco-alcohol amblyopia: a proposed biochemical basis for pathogenesis. *Med Hypoth.* 1981;7:1317–1328.

127. Lessell S. Nutritional disorders: ophthalmological aspects. *Bull Soc Belge Ophthalmol.* 1983;208:469–472.

128. Sadun AA, Martone JF, Muci-Mendoza R, et al. Epidemic optic neuropathy in Cuba: Eye findings. *Arch Ophthalmol.* 1994;112:691–699.

129. The Cuba Neuropathy Field Investigation Team. Epidemic optic neuropathy in Cuba: clinical characterization and risk factors. *N Engl J Med.* 1995;333:1176–1182.

130. Chester EM, Agamanopolis DP, Harris JW. Optic atrophy in experimental vitamin B12 deficiency in monkeys. *Acta Neurol Scand.* 1980;61:9–26.

131. Adams RD, Kubik CS. Subacute combined degeneration of the brain in pernicious anemia. *N Engl J Med.* 1944;131:1–10.

132. Troncoso J, Mancall EL, Schatz NJ. Visual evoked responses in pernicious anemia. *Arch Neurol.* 1979;36:168–169.

133. Hamilton HE, Ellis PP, Sheets RF. Visual impairment due to optic neuropathy in pernicious anemia: report of a case and review of the literature. *Blood.* 1959;14:378–385.

134. Lerman S, Feldman AL. Centrocecal scotomata as the presenting sign in pernicious anemia. *Arch Ophthalmol.* 1961;65:381–385.

135. Cohen H. Optic atrophy as the presenting sign in pernicious anemia. *Lancet.* 1936;2:1202.

136. Haag JR, Smith JL, Susac JO, Byrne SF. Optic atrophy following jejunoileal bypass surgery. *J Clin Neuro-Ophthalmol.* 1985;5:9–15.

137. Golnik KC, Schaible ER. Folate-responsive optic neuropathy. *J Neuroopthalmol.* 1994;14:163–169.

138. Steinsapir KD, Goldberg RA. Traumatic optic neuropathy. *Surv Ophthalmol.* 1994;38:487–518.

139. Bilyk JR, Joseph MP. Traumatic optic neuropathy. *Semin Ophthalmol.* 1994;9:200–211.

140. McCann JD, Seiff S. Traumatic neuropathies of the optic nerve, optic chiasm, and ocular motor nerves. *Curr Opin Ophthalmol.* 1994;5:3–10.

141. Sanborn GE, Gonder JR, Goldberg RE, Benson WE, Kessler S. Evulsion of the optic nerve: a clinicopathological study. *Can J Ophthalmol.* 1984;19:10–16.

142. Anderson RL, Panje WR, Gross CE. Optic nerve blindness following blunt forehead trauma. *Ophthalmology.* 1982;89:445–455.

143. Guy J, Sherwood M, Day AL. Surgical treatment of progressive visual loss in traumatic optic neuropathy: report of two cases. *J Neurosurg.* 1989;70:799–801.

144. Hughes B. Indirect injury of the optic nerves and chiasma. *Bull Johns Hopkins Hosp.* 1962;111:98–126.

145. Turner JWA. Indirect injury to the optic nerves. *Brain.* 1943;66:140–151.

146. Crompton MR. Visual lesions in closed head injury. *Brain.* 1970;93:785–792.

147. Pringle JH. Atrophy of the optic nerve following diffused violence to the skull. *Br Med J.* 1922;2:1156–1157.

148. Volpe NJ, Lessell S, Kline LB. Traumatic optic neuropathy: diagnosis and management. *Int Ophthalmol Clin.* 1991;31(4):142–156.

149. Sullivan G, Helveston EM. Optic atrophy after seemingly trivial trauma. *Arch Ophthalmol.* 1969;81:159–161.

150. Gross CE, DeKock JR, Panje WR, Hershkowitz N, Newman J. Evidence for orbital deformation that may contribute to monocular blindness following minor frontal head trauma. *J Neurosurg.* 1981;55:963–966.

151. Spetzler RF, Spetzler H. Holographic interferometry applied to the study of the human skull. *J Neurosurg.* 1980;52:825–828.

152. Cook MW, Levin LA, Joseph MP, Pinczower EF. Traumatic optic neuropathy: a meta-analysis. *Arch Otolaryngol Head Neck Surg.* 1996;122:389–392.

153. Chou PI, Sadun AA, Chen YC, Sy WY, Lin SZ, Lee CC. Clinical experiences in the management of traumatic optic neuropathy. *Neuro-ophthalmology.* 1996;18:325–336.

154. Joseph MP, Lessell S, Rizzo J, Momose KJ. Ex-

tracranial optic nerve decompression for traumatic optic neuropathy. *Arch Ophthalmol.* 1990; 108:1091–1093.

155. Berestka JS, Rizzo JF. Controversy in the management of traumatic optic neuropathy. *Int Ophthalmol Clin.* 1994;34:87–96.

156. Bracken MB, Shepard MJ, Collins WF, et al. A randomized controlled trial of methylprednisolone or naloxone in the treatment of acute spinal-cord injury: results of the second National Acute Spinal Cord Injury Study. *N Engl J Med.* 1990;322:1405–1411.

157. Bracken MB, Holford TR. Effects of timing of methylprednisolone or naloxone on recovery of segmental and long-tract neurological function in NASCIS 2. *J Neurosurg.* 1993;79:500–517.

158. Levin LA, Beck RW, Joseph MP, Seiff S, Kraker R. The treatment of traumatic optic neuropathy: the International Optic Nerve Trauma Study. *Ophthalmology.* 1999;106:1268–1277.

159. Laursen AB. Traumatic bitemporal hemianopsia: survey of the literature and report of a case. *Acta Ophthalmol.* 1971;49:134–142.

160. Traquair HM, Dott NM, Russell WR. Traumatic lesions of the optic chiasma. *Brain.* 1935;58:398–411.

161. Domingo Z, DeVilliers JC. Post-traumatic chiasmatic disruption. *Br J Neurosurg.* 1993;7:141–148.

162. Tang RA, Kramer LA, Schiffman J, Woon C, Hayman LA, Pardo G. Chiasmal trauma: clinical and imaging considerations. *Surv Ophthalmol.* 1994;38: 381–383.

163. Heinz GW, Nunery WR, Grossman CB. Traumatic chiasmal syndrome associated with midline basilar skull fractures. *Am J Ophthalmol.* 1994;117: 90–96.

164. Alward WLM. Medical management of glaucoma. *N Engl J Med.* 1998;339:1298–1307.

165. Sebag J, Thomas JV, Epstein DL, Grant WM. Op-

tic disk cupping in arteritic anterior ischemic optic neuropathy resembles glaucomatous cupping. *Ophthalmology.* 1986;93:357.

166. Trobe JD, Glaser JS, Cassady J, Herschler J, Anderson DR. Nonglaucomatous excavation of the optic disk. *Arch Ophthalmol.* 1980;98:1046–1050.

167. Trobe JD, Glaser JD, Cassady JC. Optic atrophy: differential diagnosis by fundus observation alone. *Arch Ophthalmol.* 1980;98:1040–1045.

168. Greenfield DS. Glaucomatous versus nonglaucomatous optic disk cupping: clinical differentiation. *Semin Ophthalmol.* 1999;14(2):95–108.

169. Anderson DR. Introductory comments on blood flow autoregulation in the optic nerve head and vascular risk factors in glaucoma. *Surv Ophthalmol.* 1999;43(suppl):85–89.

170. Shields MB. *Textbook of Glaucoma.* 4th ed. Baltimore: Williams & Wilkins; 1998:77–82.

171. Quigley HA, Addicks EM. Regional differences in the structure of the lamina cribrosa and their reaction to glaucomatous nerve damage. *Arch Ophthalmol.* 1981;99:137–143.

172. Hernandez MR, Andrzejewska WM, Neufeld AH. Changes in the extracellular matrix of the human optic nerve head in primary open angle glaucoma. *Am J Ophthalmol.* 1990;109:180–186.

173. Kirsch RE, Anderson DR. Clinical recognition of glaucomatous cupping. *Am J Ophthalmol.* 1973;75: 442–454.

174. Collaborative, Normal-Tension Glaucoma Study Group. The effectiveness of intraocular pressure reduction in the treatment of normal-tension glaucoma. *Am J Ophthalmol.* 1998;126:498–505.

175. Leske MC, Hyman L, Hussein M, Heijl A, Bengtsson BO. Letter. *Am J Ophthalmol.* 1999;127:625.

176. Shoffner JM, Wallace DC. Oxidative phosphorylation diseases. In: Scriver CR, Beaudet AL, Sly SW, eds. *The Metabolic and Molecular Bases of Inherited Disease.* 7th ed. New York: McGraw-Hill; 1995:1535.

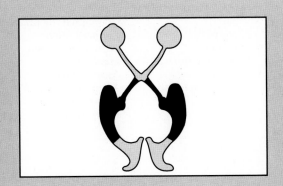

Chapter 14

OPTIC TRACT, LATERAL GENICULATE BODY, AND ANTERIOR OPTIC RADIATIONS

The optic tract, lateral geniculate body, and anterior optic radiations make up the rostral portion of the retrochiasmal visual pathway (Figs. 1-8, 1-22). A familiarity with the clinical features of lesions in this region is useful because imaging may not always disclose an obvious abnormality.

OPTIC TRACT

The optic tract, the first segment of the retrochiasmal visual pathway, arches upward around the cerebral peduncles to connect the optic chiasm to the lateral geniculate body (Fig. 1-8). Its proximity to the sella turcica makes it subject to compression by mass lesions that affect the optic chiasm. Alternatively, the optic tract may be infarcted by occlusion of branches of the anterior choroidal artery (AChA) or compressed by anterior temporal lobe masses.

Clinical Manifestations

The clinical diagnosis of an optic tract lesion depends on combining visual field, pupillary, and ophthalmoscopic findings (Table 14-1).

Table 14–1. **Optic Tract Lesions: Neuro-Ophthalmic Features**

Visual Field Defects	Pupils	Optic Disks	Causes
Complete hemianopia or Incongruous hemianopia	Normal or Afferent defect ipsilateral to field defect or Afferent defect contralateral to field defect*	Normal or Contralateral bow-tie pallor and ipsilateral temporal pallor†	Craniopharyngioma Pituitary tumor Carotid aneurysm Meningioma Astrocytoma Anterior choroidal artery occlusion Head trauma Hematoma

*Suggests optic nerve damage ipsilateral to the tract damage.
†Provided at least six weeks has elapsed from time of initial injury.

VISUAL FIELDS

The homonymous hemianopias of optic tract lesions may be complete or incomplete (Chapters 1, 7). In cases of incomplete hemianopia, field defects in the two eyes are typically *incongruous*, that is, unequal in size and shape. Incongruity is explained by the fact that axons from corresponding retinal points in the two eyes have not yet become contiguous (as they eventually will be in the posterior portion of the retrochiasmal pathway, where defects are *congruous*). Partial optic tract damage will therefore differentially affect fibers originating in the two eyes and produce very asymmetric field loss. In fact, when visual field defects are mild, the examiner is likely to overlook the defect in the less involved eye and mislocalize the lesion to the prechiasmal pathway.[1]

PUPILS

Because the optic tract is part of the afferent pupillary reflex arc (Fig. 8-1), lesions affecting one optic tract may cause a relative afferent pupil defect (RAPD). Two possible types of RAPDs are found in patients with unilateral optic tract lesions (Box 14-1; Fig. 14-1):

1. *A relative afferent pupil defect may be ipsilateral to the homonymous hemianopia.* This occurs if a tract lesion spares the optic nerve, and if the hemianopia is complete or nearly complete (Fig. 14-1a).[2-5] The RAPD results from the fact that the lesioned optic tract contains more axons

coming from the contralateral than from the ipsilateral eye. If the hemianopia is extensive, there will be enough difference between the pupillomotor inputs from the two eyes to generate a RAPD. The RAPD is always of low intensity (0.3–0.6 log units neutral density filter) and therefore easy to miss.[2]

2. *A relative afferent pupil defect may be contralateral to the homonymous hemianopia.*

Box 14–1

RELATIVE AFFERENT PUPIL DEFECTS AND OPTIC TRACT LESIONS

- A relative afferent pupil defect (RAPD) together with a homonymous hemianopia suggests an optic tract lesion.
- An RAPD in the eye *ipsilateral* to the field defect suggests a lesion limited to the optic tract (Fig. 14-1a). The RAPD is always of low intensity.
- An RAPD in the eye *contralateral* to the field defect suggests a lesion (usually a mass) that involves both the optic tract and the ipsilateral optic nerve (Figs. 14-1b, 14-2a). The RAPD is often of high intensity.
- These axioms hold only if the examiner can exclude an entirely separate lesion in the optic nerve or retina as a cause for the RAPD.

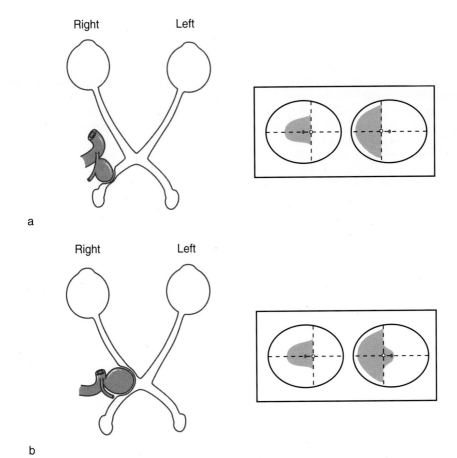

Figure 14–1. The two optic tract syndromes. (*a*) Pure optic tract syndrome. An aneurysm compresses the right optic tract, causing an incongruous left homonymous hemianopia and a low-intensity left afferent pupil defect. (*b*) Optic tract–optic nerve syndrome. An anteriorly positioned aneurysm compresses the optic tract and the optic nerve, causing a right centrocecal scotoma, a left homonymous hemianopia, and a high-intensity right afferent pupil defect.

This occurs when a lesion damages both the optic tract *and the ipsilateral optic nerve,* as happens commonly with mass lesions (craniopharyngiomas, meningiomas, and aneurysms) of the perisellar region (Fig. 14-1*b*).[6] The explanation for the contralateral RAPD is that a prechiasmal lesion causes a more profound asymmetry in signal input to the two Edinger-Westphal nuclei than does a postchiasmal lesion.

OPTIC DISKS

Damage to the optic tract will cause retrograde degeneration of its axons ("dying back") and produce optic disk pallor with a distinctive configuration. In the eye contralateral to the lesion, the pallor has the shape of a bow tie (butterfly or band) (Plate 44).[7] This is because its degenerated axons originate in the radial bundle that enters the nasal side of the optic disk, and in the maculopapillar bundle that enters the temporal side of the disk. As a result, both the nasal and temporal midsections of the optic disk will become pale, while its superior and inferior poles remain of normal pink color. In the eye ipsilateral to the optic tract lesion, optic disk pallor is limited to the temporal side, because atrophy affects only those axons originating in the temporal hemiretina and entering the temporal portion of the optic disk.

A combination of ipsilateral temporal pallor and contralateral bow-tie pallor is specific for optic tract and lateral geniculate body (LGB) lesions, with one exception: congenital[8] or neonatal[9] damage to the retrogeniculate pathways may cause transsynaptic degeneration across the LGB and produce the very same combination of optic nerve abnormalities seen in optic tract/LGB lesions. Transsynaptic degeneration does not occur if the damage is acquired after the neonatal period.[10] Caution: when bow-tie pallor *affects both optic disks,* the pathology does not lie in the optic tract, but in the optic chiasm, where damage initially affects only the nasal crossing fibers (Chapters 1, 12, 13). Once the enlarging chiasmal lesion has impaired the noncrossing fibers as well, bow-tie pallor will give way to diffuse pallor of the optic disks.

There are two limitations to the optic disk signs of optic tract and LGB lesions. First, no ophthalmoscopic findings may be expected within the first six weeks after an acute injury such as trauma, surgery, or stroke.[4] Second, bow-tie pallor is hard to recognize without experienced observation of the optic fundus, and even then it may be difficult when the ocular media are not clear. For these reasons, the hunt for a RAPD is critical to localization.

Lesions

Optic tract lesions make up less than 10% of cases in large series of isolated homonymous hemianopias,[11–13] which are dominated by pathology in posterior optic radiations and visual cortex. The nature of optic tract lesions collected in these earlier series has reflected their accrual from ophthalmology clinics. That is, the lesions have largely been perisellar masses—neoplasms and aneurysms—which have extended anteriorly enough to compress the optic nerves and chiasm (Fig. 14-2a).[6]

The optic tract may be an isolated target of temporal lobe or diencephalic tumors, extra-axial hematomas, closed head trauma, and demyelination.[11,14] With the advent of high-definition MRI, infarction in the domain of the anterior choroidal artery has also been recognized as an important cause of optic tract damage (Figs. 1-17, 1-22).[4,15] Infarcts of the AChA appear in three settings:[16]

1. Spontaneous occlusion when the AChA becomes occluded by thrombosis within vessel walls affected by lipohyalinosis.[17–19] In spontaneous AChA occlusion, the prevalence of hypertension is high and the prevalence of cardiac and cervical carotid embolic sources is low. Such occlusion has also been documented in conjunction with hypotension and hypercoagulable states, supporting small vessel disease as the underlying pathology.[16,20,21]
2. Compression by adjacent brain swelling or shift from head trauma, tumors (Fig. 14-2a), or hematomas.[14]
3. Surgical manipulation during temporal lobectomy for intractable seizures[5,15,22] or clipping of supraclinoid artery aneurysms (Fig. 14-2b).

Because the AChA domain includes the lateral thalamus and posterior limb of the internal capsule, infarction may produce a triad of contralateral hemiparesis, hemisensory loss, and hemianopia. Dysarthria, ataxia, neglect (nondominant infarction), and aphasia (dominant infarction) occur less commonly.[16] Hemiparesis, especially severe in the upper extremity and face, is the most prominent deficit.[17,19] Hemianopia is the least common of the three basic deficits, its prevalence varying from 6% to 50%.[17,19] It can be an isolated finding in association with a limited infarct.[5,19,20]

Interestingly, when the AChA was deliberately ligated in 12 patients to treat parkinsonism,[23] persistent hemianopia occurred only once, and there were no other neurologic deficits. In performing temporal lobectomy, infarction is extraordinarily rare, despite the fact that the AChA is often traumatized during the operation.[5] One explanation for this apparent discrepancy is the ample collateral circulation of this region, provided by branches of the posterior cerebral and posterior communicating arteries.[24] It is likely that AChA infarcts occur only when collaterals are poor or there is ample small vessel disease.

Because surrounding tissue densities are so heterogeneous, small lacunar infarcts caused by AChA-region occlusion are hard to find on MRI. Recognizing the visual fea-

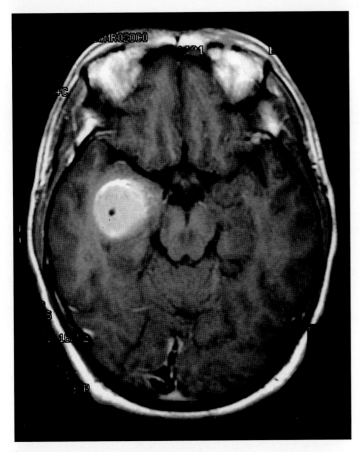

a

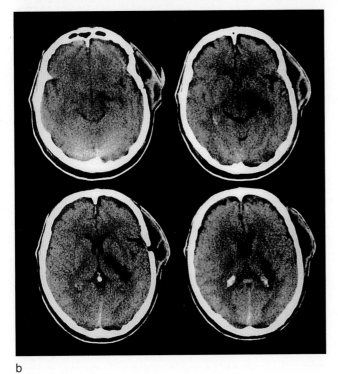

b

Figure 14–2. Optic tract lesions. (*a*) Temporal lobe astrocytoma compresses the right optic tract and, although not clearly shown here, the right optic nerve. (*b*) Anterior choroidal artery infarct following aneurysm repair. Axial CT scans at four levels.

279

tures of optic tract damage then becomes critical (Table 14-1).

LATERAL GENICULATE BODY

Lying on the lateral edge of the pulvinar in the posterior thalamus (Fig. 1-22), the lateral geniculate body contains the first synapses of the retinal ganglion axons (Fig. 1-20). Therefore, lesions here will eventually cause pallor of the optic disk and attenuation of the retinal nerve fiber layer, just as optic tract lesions do.

Within the LGB, the inferior visual field is represented medially, the superior field is represented laterally, and a horizontal wedge of visual field is represented in a V-shaped middle region (Chapter 1). The AChA, a branch of the carotid artery, supplies the medial and lateral sectors of the LGB. The posterior lateral choroidal artery (PLChA), a branch of the posterior cerebral artery, supplies the V-shaped central region (Fig. 1-21). Occlusion of each vessel gives rise to sector visual field defects that are the mirror images of one other (Figs. 1-21, 7-16).

Clinical Manifestations

Lesions of the lateral geniculate body share with optic tract lesions the tendency to produce homonymous hemianopias and contralateral bow-tie optic disk pallor (Plate 44). However, two clinical features are helpful in differentiating LGB from optic tract lesions (Table 14-2).

PUPILS

Unlike optic tract lesions, those restricted to the LGB *do not produce a RAPD* because the LGB lies posterior to the pupillary reflex arc. However, the brachium of the superior colliculus, which carries afferent input to the pretectum, branches off from the optic tract less than 2 mm anterior to the LGB, passing adjacent to the LGB on its way to the brainstem (Fig. 8-1). Thus only those lesions that are narrowly confined to the LGB will fail to produce an RAPD.

VISUAL FIELDS

Damage to the LBG may produce two incomplete, congruous, sectoral homonymous patterns of visual field loss that are not found in optic tract lesions.

- **Homonymous horizontal sectoranopia** describes wedge-shaped defects located near the horizontal meridian whose apices are pointed at fixation (Figs. 7-21*c*, 7-16*b*).[25–27] These defects are associated with occlusions (Fig. 14-3*a*), AVMs, and tumors believed to interrupt flow in the posterior lateral choroidal artery. This vessel supplies the middle portion of the LGB, which receives input from the horizontal sector of the visual field.
- **Homonymous horizontal sector-sparing hemianopia** is the mirror defect of homonymous horizontal sectoranopia. It involves the superior and inferior quadrants in the two homonymous fields (misleadingly described as "quadruple sectoranopia"),[28,29] sparing the central wedge or tongue-

Table 14–2. **Lateral Geniculate Body Lesions: Neuro-Ophthalmic Features**

Visual Field Defects	Pupils	Optic disks	Causes
Complete hemianopia	Normal*	Normal or	Anterior choroidal artery occlusion
Horizontal sectoranopia		Contralateral bow-tie pallor and	Posterior lateral choroidal artery occlusion
Horizontal sector-sparing hemianopia		ipsilateral temporal pallor†	Hypoxia Head trauma Cerebral hemispheric mass

*Unless lesion extends rostral enough to involve optic tract (see Table 14–1).
†If at least six weeks have elapsed from time of initial injury.

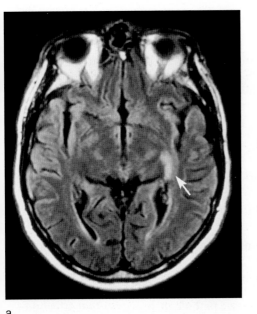

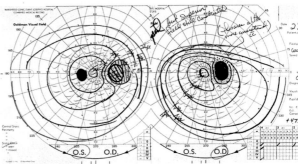

a

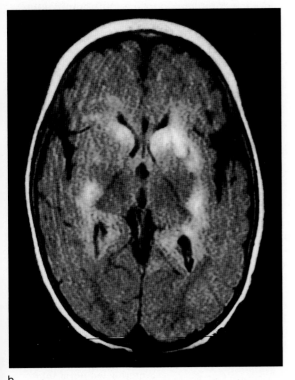

b

Figure 14–3. Lateral geniculate lesions. (*a*) Unilateral infarct. In a 66-year-old hypertensive man with sudden onset of a visual disturbance, MRI (FLAIR sequence) shows high signal in the region of the left LGB (*left*) and a corresponding right homonymous horizontal sectoranopia (*right*). (Courtesy of Daniel M. Jacobson, MD.) (*b*) Bilateral hypoxia. T2 MRI shows high signal in the basal ganglia and LGB bilaterally following cardiopulmonary arrest in a six-month-old boy who became completely blind after the event. Pupillary reactions to light were intact.

shaped region (Figs. 1-21*b* and Fig. 9-16*a*). It is caused by occlusion of the AChA, the vessel supplying the medial and lateral regions of the LGB.[20]

The evidence that links these two visual field patterns to selective occlusions of the AChA or PLChA is tenuous. Neither the AChA nor the PLChA is large enough to be consistently visualized on cerebral angiography,[20] so occlusion must be presumed.[25,26]

Pathologic specimens of the LGB have been obtained at necropsy from patients whose lesions had become so widely destructive that selective vascular occlusion could not be demonstrated.[30] If vascular occlusion cannot explain the sector defects, perhaps there is a nonvascular explanation for selective vulnerability of the two LGB regions, inasmuch as a case of LGB myelinolysis produced classic bilateral sector-sparing defects.[31] These sector field defects are not, however, specific to LGB damage, having been demonstrated in lesions in the anterior optic radiations (see below)[32–35] and the visual cortex.[36]

Lesions

Apart from infarction, LGB damage may be caused by hypoxia (Fig. 14-3b), invasion of adjacent glial tumors, head trauma, and compression by an arteriovenous malformation (AVM) or a cerebral hemisphere displaced by intra-axial or extra-axial mass effect.[14,37] Because the LGB is so small, it is often difficult to determine whether the primary damage caused by mass lesions is to the optic tract, the LGB, the root of the optic radiations, or all three regions.

ANTERIOR OPTIC RADIATIONS

As the root of the optic radiations exits posteriorly from the LGB, the expanding temporal horn of the lateral ventricle splays the inferior bundles anteriorly as Meyer's loop, which reaches within 4–8 mm of the anterior temporal tip (Chapter 1). As it courses posteriorly, Meyer's loop eventually merges with the rest of the radiations to form a vertically oriented pancake along the ventricular trigone (Fig. 1-22). Caudal to that point, the posterior optic radiations split into superior and inferior fascicles to enter the upper and lower banks of primary visual cortex (Fig. 1-24). The manifestations and causes of anterior radiation damage depend on whether a lesion lies in the root, Meyer's loop, or trigonal region (Table 14-3).

Root Lesions

Nourished primarily by the AChA (Fig. 1-22), the root of the optic radiations is subject to the same pathologic processes that affect the optic tract and LGB. Lesions (Fig. 14-4a) produce a complete contralateral homonymous hemianopia, often combined with hemiparesis and hemisensory loss.

Meyer's Loop Lesions

This anteriorly detoured segment of the anterior optic radiations is damaged predominantly by anterior temporal lobe tumors and during lobectomy for intractable epilepsy (Fig. 14-4b). Stroke is rare in this region.

The typical Meyer's loop "pie-in-the-sky" superior quadrant visual field defects are

Table 14–3. **Anterior Optic Radiation Lesions: Neuro-Ophthalmic Features**

Region	Visual Field Defects	Other Neurologic Manifestations	Causes
Root	Complete hemianopia	Hemiparesis Hemisensory loss	Anterior choroidal artery occlusion Cerebral tumor
Meyer's loop	Pie-in-the-sky hemianopia	Partial seizures	Anterior temporal lobectomy Anterior temporal tumor Head trauma
Trigone	Complete hemianopia or congruous hemianopia	Hemiparesis Hemisensory loss Neglect Aphasia	Middle cerebral artery stroke Cerebral tumor Head trauma Hematoma Leukoencephalopathy

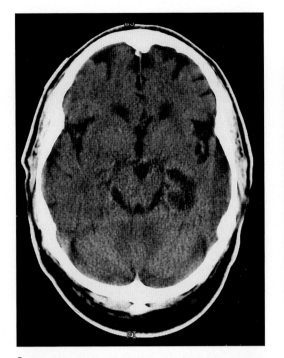

a

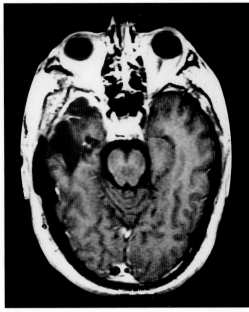

b

c

Figure 14–4. Optic radiation lesions. (*a*) Root lesion caused by a large anterior choroidal artery infarct. The patient had contralateral homonymous hemianopia, hemiparesis, and hemisensory loss. (*b*) Meyer's loop lesion. T1 axial MRI shows hypodense signal in the left anterior temporal region where the anterior temporal lobe had been extirpated for intractable seizures. Damage to Meyer's loop caused a left "pie-in-the-sky" homonymous hemianopia (Fig. 7-17). (*c*) Trigone lesion. CT shows parenchymal blood and edema in the right peritrigonal region following a depressed parietal skull fracture. The patient had a left homonymous hemianopia owing to damage to optic radiations.

homonymous and wedge-shaped, one border aligned to the vertical meridian, the other extending radially up from fixation. The radial border distinguishes these defects from the quadrantanopias characteristic of posterior radiation and visual cortex lesions

(see below). The defects are slightly incongruous, the larger defect belonging to the eye ipsilateral to the lesion.[38] A patient rarely notices these Meyer's loop defects spontaneously, probably because they cancel only a small portion of the upper field, which is irrelevant for walking or reading. Visual field loss is, therefore, not a presenting symptom of anterior temporal lobe masses unless the lesions lean medially to compress the optic tract.

A 4 cm surgical amputation of temporal lobe rarely affects Meyer's loop; a 5–7 cm amputation usually produces a pie-in-the-sky defect, while an 8 cm amputation will extend into the trigonal portion of the optic radiations and produce a complete homonymous hemianopia.[38,39]

Trigone

At the level of the ventricular trigone, where the optic radiations have become a more compact layer lining the lateral ventricular border, they are subject to damage by trauma (Fig. 14-4c),[34] tumors, nontraumatic intraparenchymal hemorrhage,[32] and occlusion of the temporal branches[40] and centrum semiovale penetrators[41] of the middle cerebral artery.

Visual field defects may be sectoranopias similar to those found in LGB lesions[32–35] but more commonly they will be complete homonymous hemianopias. In most cases, visual field defects are obscured by other neurologic deficits, including aphasia (left hemisphere) and spatial-attentional disorders (right hemisphere). Neglect is a common finding in patients with right hemisphere trigonal lesions, and it may be confused with hemianopia (Chapter 17).[40]

SUMMARY

The optic tract, LGB, and anterior optic radiations make up the rostral portion of the retrochiasmal visual pathway. As with all lesions affecting the retrochiasmal pathway, homonymous hemianopic field loss is a shared manifestation. Other clinical features, together with imaging, allow for more precise localization.

Optic tract lesions are often associated with relative afferent pupil defects, characteristic configurations of optic disk pallor, and complete or incomplete incongruous hemianopias. They are caused by perisellar and temporal lobe tumors, aneurysms, and,

less commonly, anterior choroidal artery occlusion.

Lesions confined to the LGB do not affect pupillary reactions, but they are associated with hemianopias and optic disk changes identical to those of optic tract lesions. Lateral geniculate body infarcts may produce sector field defects not seen in conjunction with optic tract lesions. Apart from infarction, other causes of the LGB damage are hypoxia, trauma, and tumor.

Anterior optic radiation damage occurs at three locations: the root, Meyer's loop, and the trigonal region. At the root, clinical manifestations and causes are similar to those of optic tract and LGB lesions. A triad of hemianopia, hemiparesis, and hemisensory loss is characteristic of optic radiation root lesions. Meyer's loop is injured by anterior temporal lobe masses, trauma, and surgical lobectomy for intractable epilepsy. The trigonal portion of the radiations is subject to damage by hemispheric masses and middle cerebral artery strokes. In patients with left hemisphere lesions, aphasia is common; in those with right hemisphere lesions, neglect is common and is often difficult to separate from hemianopia. Other nonvisual neurologic manifestations may also obscure the visual phenomena.

REFERENCES

1. Hedges TR. Retrochiasmal disorders. In: Albert DM, Jakobiec FA, eds. *Principles and Practice of Ophthalmology*. Vol 4. Philadelphia: Saunders; 1994: 2630.
2. Bell RA, Thompson HS. Relative afferent pupillary defect in optic tract hemianopias. *Am J Ophthalmol.* 1978;85:538–540.
3. O'Connor P, Mein C, Hughes J. The Marcus Gunn pupil in incomplete optic tract hemianopias. *J Clin Neuro-ophthalmol.* 1982;2:227–234.
4. Newman SA, Miller NR. Optic tract syndrome: neuro-ophthalmologic considerations. *Arch Ophthalmol.* 1983;101:187–193.
5. Anderson DR, Trobe JD, Hood TW, Gebarski SS. Optic tract injury after anterior temporal lobectomy. *Ophthalmology.* 1989;96:1065–1072.
6. Savino PJ, Paris M, Schatz NJ, Orr LS, Corbett JJ. Optic tract syndrome: a review of 21 patients. *Arch Ophthalmol.* 1978;96:656–663.
7. Unsold R, Hoyt WF. Band atrophy of the optic nerve: the histology of temporal hemianopsia. *Arch Ophthalmol.* 1980;98:1637–1638.
8. Hoyt WF, Rios-Montenegro EN, Behrens MM, Eckelhoff RJ. Homonymous hemioptic hypoplasia: fun-

doscopic features in standard and red-free illumination in three patients with congenital hemiplegia. *Br J Ophthalmol.* 1972;56:537–545.

9. Haddock JN, Berlin L. Transsynaptic degeneration of the visual system: report of a case. *Arch Neurol Psychiatr.* 1950;64:66–73.

10. Miller NR, Newman SA. Transsynaptic degeneration. *Arch Ophthalmol.* 1981;99:1654.

11. Fujino T, Kigazawa K, Yamada R. Homonymous hemianopia: a retrospective study of 140 cases. *Neuro-ophthalmology.* 1986;6:17–21.

12. Trobe JD, Lorber MI, Schlezinger NS. Isolated homonymous hemianopia. *Arch Ophthalmol.* 1973; 89:377–381.

13. Smith JL. Homonymous hemianopia: a review of 100 cases. *Am J Ophthalmol.* 1962;54:616–622.

14. Lindenberg R, Walsh FB, Sacks JG. *Neuropathology of Vision: An Atlas.* Philadelphia: Lea & Febiger; 1973:315–334.

15. Helgason C, Caplan LR, Goodwin J, Hedges T. Anterior choroidal artery territory infarction: report of cases and review. *Arch Neurol.* 1986;43:681–686.

16. Helgason CM. Anterior choroidal artery. In: Bogousslavsky J, Caplan L, eds. *Stroke Syndromes.* Cambridge, UK: Cambridge University Press; 1995:270–275.

17. Bruno A, Graff-Radford NR, Biller J, Adams HP. Anterior choroidal artery territory infarction: a small vessel disease. *Stroke.* 1989;20:616–619.

18. Hupperts RMM, Lodder J, Heutsvanraak EPM, Kessels F. Infarcts in the anterior choroidal artery territory: anatomical distribution, clinical syndromes, presumed pathogenesis, and early outcome. *Brain.* 1994;117:825–834.

19. Decroix JP, Graveleau P, Masson M, Cambier J. Infarction in the territory of the anterior choroidal artery. *Brain.* 1986;109:1071–1085.

20. Helgason CM. A new view of the anterior choroidal artery territory infarction. *J Neurol.* 1988;235:387–391.

21. Pertuiset B, Aron D, Dilenge D, Mazalton A. Les syndromes de l'artère choroidienne antérieure. Étude clinique et radiologique. *Rev Neurol.* 1962; 106:286–294.

22. Helgason CM, Bergen D, Bleck TP, Morrell F, Whisler W. Infarction after surgery for focal epilepsy: manipulation hemiplegia revisited. *Epilepsia.* 1987;28:340–345.

23. Morillo A, Cooper IS. Occlusion of the anterior choroidal artery. *Am J Ophthalmol.* 1955;40:796–801.

24. Rhoton AL Jr, Fujii K, Fradd B. Microsurgical anatomy of the anterior choroidal artery. *Surg Neurol.* 1979;12:171–187.

25. Frisen L, Holmegaard L, Rosencrantz M. Sectorial optic atrophy and homonymous horizontal sec-

toranopia: a lateral choroidal artery syndrome? *J Neurol Neurosurg Psychiatry.* 1978;4:374–380.

26. Shacklett DE, O'Connor PS, Dorwart RH, Linn D, Carter JE. Congruous and incongruous sectoral visual field defects with lesions of the lateral geniculate nucleus. *Am J Ophthalmol.* 1984;98:283–290.

27. Neau JP, Bogousslavsky J. The syndrome of the posterior choroidal artery territory infarction. *Ann Neurol.* 1996;39:779–788.

28. Frisen L. Quadruple sectoranopia and sectorial optic atrophy—a syndrome of the distal anterior choroidal artery. *J Neurol Neurosurg Psychiatry.* 1979;42:590–594.

29. Luco C, Hoppe A, Schweitzer M, Vicuna X, Fantin A. Visual field defects in vascular lesions of the lateral geniculate body. *J Neurol Neurosurg Psychiatry.* 1992;55:12–15.

30. Gunderson CH, Hoyt WF. Geniculate hemianopia: incongruous homonymous field defects in two patients with partial lesions of the lateral geniculate nucleus. *J Neurol Neurosurg Psychiatr.* 1971;34:1–6.

31. Donahue SP, Kardon RH, Thompson HS. Hourglass-shaped visual fields as a sign of bilateral lateral geniculate myelinolysis. *Am J Ophthalmol.* 1995; 119:378–380.

32. Carter JE, Oconnor P, Schacklett D, Rosenberg M. Lesions of the optic radiations mimicking lateral geniculate nucleus visual field defects. *J Neurol Neurosurg Psychiatry.* 1985;48:982–988.

33. Grochowski M, Vighetto A. Homonymous horizontal sectoranopia: report of four cases. *Br J Ophthalmol.* 1991;75:624–628.

34. Spalding JMK. Wounds of the visual pathway: I. The visual radiation. *J Neurol Neurosurg Psychiatry.* 1952; 15:99–109.

35. Smith RJS. Horizontal sector hemianopia of nontraumatic origin. *Br J Ophthalmol.* 1970;54:208–210.

36. Grossman M, Galetta SL, Nichols CW, Grossman RI. Horizontal homonymous sectoral field defect after ischemia infarction of the occipital cortex. *Am J Ophthalmol.* 1990;109:234–236.

37. Borruat FX, Maeder P. Sectoranopia after head trauma: evidence of lateral geniculate body lesion on MRI. *Neurology.* 1995;43:1430–1432.

38. Hughes TS, Abou-Khalil B, Lavin PJM, Fakhoury T, Blumenkopf B, Donahue SP. Visual field defects after temporal lobe resection: a prospective quantitative analysis. *Neurology.* 1999;53:167–172.

39. Miller NR. *Walsh & Hoyt's Clinical Neuro-ophthalmology.* 4th ed. Vol 1. Baltimore: Williams & Wilkins; 1982:134–136.

40. Caplan LR, Kelly M, Kase CS, et al. Infarcts of the inferior division of the right middle cerebral artery. *Neurology.* 1986;36:1015–1020.

41. Bogousslavsky J, Regli F. Centrum semiovale infarcts. *Neurology.* 1992;42:1992–1998.

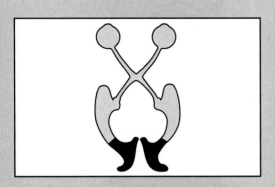

POSTERIOR OPTIC RADIATIONS AND PRIMARY VISUAL CORTEX

The posterior optic radiations and visual cortex form the caudal portion of the retrochiasmal visual pathway. Situated at the terminus of the posterior cerebral artery, this region is prone to transient ischemic attack and stroke. Because of this region's high metabolic rate and location within a vascular watershed area, it is selectively injured in association with hypotension, hypoxia, metabolic derangements, and systemic chemotherapy. The gray matter of this region is the origin of the visual hallucinations of migraine, some forms of epilepsy, mitochondrial encephalopathy, Alzheimer's disease, and Creutzfeldt-Jakob disease. The posterior hemispheric white matter is damaged in accelerated systemic hypertension, cerebral angiography, adrenoleukodystrophy, and progressive multifocal leukoencephalopathy.

The transition from anterior to posterior optic radiations occurs at the caudal ventricular trigone area. There, the radiations split into two forks. The superior fibers (subserving the inferior field) lie in the upper fork, and the inferior fibers (subserving the superior field) lie in the lower fork (Figs. 1-22, 1-24). The upper fork enters the upper bank of the calcarine fissure, and the lower fork enters the lower bank. The macular projections, representing the central 5 degrees of the hemifield, are allotted the caudal 50% of visual cortex. The projections from the rest of the visual field are crowded into the rostral 50% (Fig. 1-26).[1-3]

The blood supply of this portion of the visual pathway comes largely from the calcarine branches of the posterior cerebral artery (PCA), but the occipitoparietal and occipitotemporal branches may also contribute. The caudal part of the visual cortex receives a variable blood supply from occipital branches of the middle cerebral artery (MCA) (Figs. 1-17, 1-22).[4]

SHARED CLINICAL MANIFESTATIONS

Damage to the posterior optic radiations and primary visual cortex gives rise to visual field defects (Chapter 7), visual illusions, and visual hallucinations (Chapter 4). If a lesion extends into adjacent parietal vision-related cortex, visual spatial deficits will arise

(Chapter 16). If it extends to temporal vision-related cortex, visual recognition deficits will arise (Chapter 17). As with all lesions of the retrochiasmal pathway, visual acuity remains normal unless the macular projection fibers *in both hemispheres* are destroyed.

Hemianopic Visual Field Loss

Lesions of this region nearly always produce homonymous hemianopias. A *complete* homonymous hemianopia permits localization to the retrochiasmal pathway, but it does not permit localization to specific sites within it. On the other hand, the following *incomplete* hemianopic patterns are specific for lesions of the posterior radiations or visual cortex (Figs. 7-14 to 7-18).

CONGRUOUS HEMIANOPIA

These subtotal hemianopic field defects are identical in size and shape, reflecting the fact that axons from corresponding retinal points have come to lie next to one another in the terminal portion of the retinocortical pathway. (See Fig. 7-17b.)

PARACENTRAL DEFECTS

Hemianopic field loss is limited to the central 5–10 degrees. Even relatively large visual cortex lesions (Fig. 15-1a) can give rise to these tiny defects, because so much visual cortex area decodes the central few degrees of field (the magnification factor).[1-3] Often missed on standard perimetric protocols (Fig. 15-1b), these defects may be discovered only with special protocols that test intensively within the central ten degrees (Fig. 15-1c). Properly instructed, the patient can sometimes map these defects on a standard (Amsler) grid (Chapter 7) (Fig. 15-1d). (See Fig. 7-18c)

MACULAR SPARING

This pattern is the mirror image of homonymous paracentral defects. In these cases, the hemifield loss *spares* the central 5 degrees of field (Fig. 15-2b). This pattern results when

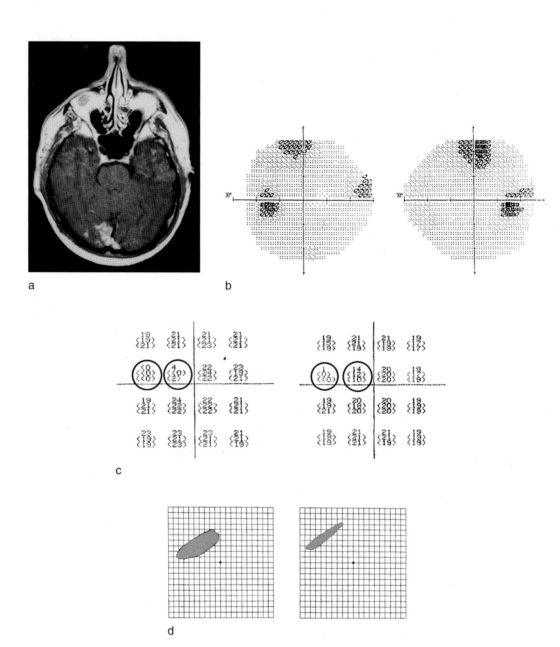

Figure 15–1. Homonymous paracentral scotomas caused by posterior visual cortex infarction. (*a*) Enhanced T1-weighted MRI shows a lesion (arrow) in the right posterior (caudal) visual cortex. (*b*) Standard (24-2) Humphrey automated perimetry fails to detect the field defects, which are small and close to fixation. (*c*) Special (macular) Humphrey automated perimetric protocol, which samples thresholds intensively within 5 degrees of fixation, finds two elevated threshold points (circled) to the left of fixation and above the horizontal meridian. (*d*) The patient maps his left homonymous defects on a standard (Amsler) grid. These tiny defects are very disabling because they are so close to fixation.

288

the lesion—usually a posterior cerebral artery infarct—leaves intact a large portion of the caudal 50% of the visual cortex (Fig. 15-2a).[5,6] Such sparing may reflect the extra protection of the caudal portion of the visual cortex by virtue of its dual supply from the PCA and MCA.[4] Notably, macular sparing does not occur when the lesion lies in the posterior radiations. (See Fig. 7-18d.)

QUADRANTANOPIC DEFECTS

These field defects have borders along both the vertical and horizontal meridians (Fig. 15-3). The square-edged pattern derives from the fact that the upper and lower segments of the posterior radiations and peristriate visual cortex can be selectively lesioned. (See Figs. 7-18a, 7-18b.)

CRESCENT-SPARING

In this defect pattern, the nasal hemifield of one eye is completely destroyed, together with the matching portion of the temporal hemifield of the other eye. However, in the eye with the temporal hemifield cut, the peripheral 30 degrees (the monocular or unpaired temporal crescent) is spared. This pattern reflects sparing of the anterior (rostral) 10% of visual cortex devoted to the unpaired temporal crescent of field. A rare occurrence, it is usually caused by infarction.[9,10] (See Fig. 7-18f.)

BILATERAL HEMIANOPIA

The posterior optic radiations or primary visual cortex may be involved bilaterally in association with hypoxia, hypotension, basilar artery thrombosis or emboli, bilateral posterior cerebral artery compression by brain herniation, sagittal sinus thrombosis, trauma, occipital tumor, demyelination, meningitis, or Alzheimer's disease.[11,12] Bilateral lesions create diagnosticially confusing defects of both homonymous fields. There are four variants:

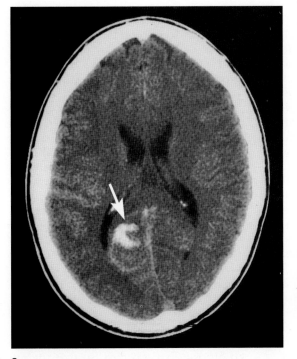

a

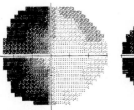

b

Figure 15–2. Macular-sparing from an anterior visual cortex lesion. (a) CT shows hemorrhage (arrow) in the right visual cortex that spares the posterior (caudal) 50%. (b) Visual fields disclose sparing of the central 5 degrees within the left homonymous hemianopia.

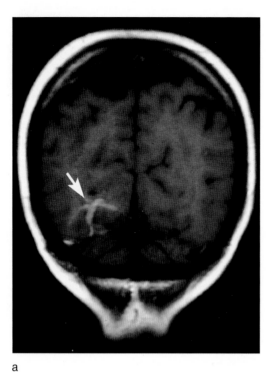

a

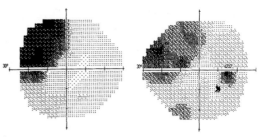

b

Figure 15–3. Superior homonymous quadrantanopia from an inferior trigonal lesion. (*a*) T1-weighted MRI shows hemorrhage (arrow) from an arteriovenous malformation in the right inferior trigonal area, damaging the posterior optic radiations leading into the inferior visual cortex. (*b*) The visual fields show a superior left homonymous quadrantanopia.

1. Altitudinal. When homonymous quadrantanopias occur on both sides of the visual field, the result is an altitudinal defect.[13] Bilateral parietooccipital PCA branch occlusions affect the dorsal regions to cause lower altitudinal defects, often together with spatial defects (Balint-Holmes syndrome, Chapter 16). Bilateral occipitotemporal PCA branch occlusions affect the ventral regions to cause upper altitudinal defects, often combined with recognition defects (Chapter 17). The altitudinal pattern may falsely suggest a binocular retinal or optic nerve disorder, particularly if the visual field loss is isolated and visual recognition or spatial deficits are not appreciated.

2. Central scotomatous. When paracentral defects in both hemifields are put together, they look like binocular central scotomas. They will cause loss of visual acuity in both eyes. Understandably, such findings misdirect attention toward a binocular macular or optic nerve disorder.

3. Keyhole. Extensive defects in both upper and lower quadrants may spare the fixation region in both hemifields (Fig. 15-4; see Fig. 7-18g). The resulting composite looks like a severely constricted visual field. The patient gropes about but has normal visual acuity and is mistakenly believed to be malingering or hysterical (Chapter 18). Carefully performed manual kinetic perimetry will disclose the feature that localizes the defect to the visual cortex: the degree of macular sparing on the two sides of the vertical meridian is not identical in size and shape.

4. Complete blindness. Complete destruction of the posterior radiations or visual cortex on both sides (usually by hypoxia, hypotension, or thrombosis)[14] renders the patient sightless. The eye grounds and pupillary reactions are normal, there are often no other neurologic deficits, and imaging may show no abnormalities within the first two days, so that the examiner may falsely conclude that the condition is psychogenic.

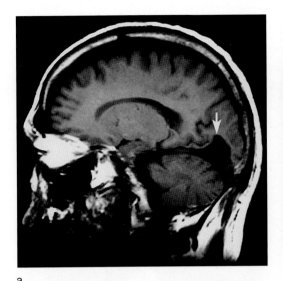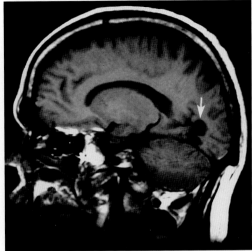

a

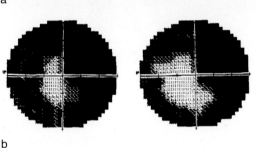

b

Figure 15–4. Bilateral homonymous hemianopias from bilateral visual cortex lesions. (*a*) T1-weighted sagittal MRIs show a large left visual cortex lesion (arrow) (*left*) and a smaller right visual cortex lesion (arrow) (*right*) from old infarcts. (*b*) The visual fields show bilateral homonymous hemianopias with large macular sparing on the left.

Nonhemianopic Visual Field Loss

There are two exceptions to the rule that retrochiasmal lesions always produce homonymous visual field loss. The first exception is the monocular crescent defect. The second exception is amblyopia.

MONOCULAR CRESCENT DEFECT

In this very rare pattern, the visual field is intact except for the most peripheral portion of the temporal field in the eye contralateral to the lesion. This crescent-shaped field defect is caused by a lesion restricted to the anterior 10% of visual cortex (Fig. 15-5).[7,8] Such defects will go undetected clinically with standard automated perimetry, which does not explore outside 30 degrees from fixation. (See Fig. 7-18*e*.)

AMBLYOPIA

Amblyopia is defined as subnormal visual acuity owing to early childhood visual deprivation (Chapter 1). Affecting about 5% of the population, it occurs in three settings: strabismus, anisometropia, and a media opacity occurring by age 6 years.[15,16] Each can impair the delivery of a clear image from the fovea of the affected eye to corresponding ocular dominance columns in the contralateral primary visual cortex. If the visual deprivation is not eliminated within the first half-decade of life, the cortical neurons fail to remain activated and visual acuity remains reduced in the amblyopic eye.

Visual fields fail to show a discrete scotoma in patients with amblyopia,[17] and there are no specific clinical or electrophysiologic markers. Amblyopia must therefore be regarded as a diagnosis of exclusion and considered only when one or more of the three

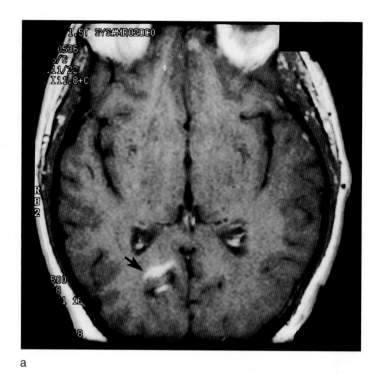

a

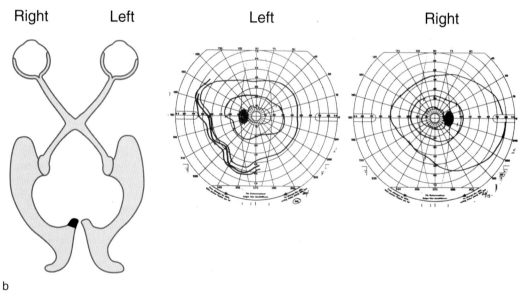

b

Figure 15–5. Monocular crescent loss from a very anterior visual cortex lesion. (*a*) T1-weighted MRI shows hemorrhage (arrow) in far right anterior visual cortex. (*b*) Visual fields show loss of the unpaired peripheral temporal field in the left eye.

predisposing conditions is (or has been) present. It is usually found only in one eye, although bilateral infantile media opacities or persistently uncorrected high hyperopia or astigmatism can cause bilateral amblyopia.

Illusions and Hallucinations

Binocular positive visual phenomena are a common signal of injury to the posterior radiations and visual cortex (Chapter 4). Transient cortical ischemia may cause stationary flickers that last only seconds. Focal seizures usually evoke similar symptoms that last for several minutes. Migraine causes a flickering that lasts 20 to 30 minutes and often spreads (marches) across the hemifield. Visual cortex infarcts cause flickering that may persist for weeks to months.

This chapter considers both transient and persistent visual disturbances associated with the posterior optic radiations and primary visual cortex. We turn first to the leading causes of *transient* visual disturbances (Table 15-1).

MIGRAINE

Definition

Migraine usually consists of episodic headaches preceded by neurologic disturbances (auras), which may include positive and negative visual phenomena, altered mood, paresthesias, motor weakness, or aphasia.[18]

In most individuals, migraine is a physiologic response conditioned by hereditary factors that are as yet unknown ("primary" or "idiopathic" migraine). It affects nearly 20% of women and 10% of men in the United States.[19] Some features of migraine also occur with unexpectedly high frequency in patients with lupus erythematosus, primary antiphospholipid antibody syndrome, mitochondrial encephalopathy, cerebral autosomal dominant arteriopathy with subcortical infarcts and leukoencephalopthy (CADASIL), and structural disorders of the occipital lobe. Migraine that occurs in association with these underlying conditions may be considered secondary.

Table 15–1. **Transient Binocular Visual Disturbances**

Clinical Feature	Migraine	Partial Seizure	Vertebrobasilar TIA	Closed Head Injury
Typical visual symptoms	Hemifield marching	Hemifield stationary	Hemifield or total	Binocular blindness
Duration of visual symptoms	20–30 minutes	Up to 5 minutes but variable	Seconds to minutes	Hours
Positive visual phenomena	Usual	Usual	Rare	Never
Provoking circumstance	None or stress	Usually none	None	Head trauma after a fall or heading a soccer ball
Headache	Usual; follows visual symptoms	Sometimes; no relation to visual symptoms	Rare	Usual; persistent
Other manifestations	Sonophobia, photophobia, dysphoria	Blinking, gaze deviation, nystagmus, altered consciousness	Dysequilibrium diplopia, dysarthria, dysphagia, drop attacks*	Amnesia, somnolence

*Also paresthesias, vertigo, nausea, amnesia, circumoral or extremity numbness, extremity weakness, tinnitus, and hearing loss. However, visual symptoms may be isolated in 10% of attacks (see text).

Pathogenesis

The pathogenesis of migraine remains uncertain. Current theories focus on discharge in a pathway that connects brainstem aminergic nuclei to the occipital lobe. This discharge leads to a spreading neuronal depression across the primary visual cortex that may be the physiologic counterpart to the migraine aura.[20–22] There is controversy as to whether the well-documented reduction in blood flow characteristic of migraine triggers the neuronal events or is merely a secondary phenomenon.[20] The headache phase is attributed to a release of nociceptive factors that activate trigeminal receptors.[23]

Clinical Features

About 20% of migraineurs have auras,[20] of which 75% are visual hallucinations of simple shapes.[24] About 50% of patients who have migrainous visual hallucinations report the following three-phase sequence:
1. Vague sense that vision is blurred in both eyes.
2. Twinkling dots, heat waves, kaleidoscopes, cut-glass distortions, or zigzag lines appearing to one side of the fixation.
3. Expansion of these flickering patterns toward the hemifield periphery within a period of 20–30 minutes (march, buildup), leaving a translucent scotomatous residue that temporarily obscures vision (Fig. 4-7).

This characteristic sequence is often violated. The hallucinations may not twinkle; they may merely shine. They may involve both hemifields rather than one hemifield, or be limited to one eye ("retinociliary migraine," see below). Quite often, the hallucinations are stationary. Or they may consist of scotomas without any positive phenomena.[25] Such purely negative visual auras, often described as "looking through water," were reported in 37% of adult migraineurs in one series[24] and in 100% of children in another.[26]

Although the typical visual disturbance of migraine usually ends after 20–30 minutes, patients may report shorter or longer periods. Headache centered on the cranial side opposite to the involved hemifield usually follows the visual aura, but many patients—particularly those aged over 40 years—describe a visual aura without headache (acephalgic migraine, migraine equivalent, migraine accompaniment, dissociated migraine).[27]

Differential Diagnosis

The visual aura of migraine accounts for most episodes of binocular unformed visual hallucinations in youth, and perhaps in late adulthood.[24] Confronted with this symptom, the physician must consider (1) whether the patient is suffering from migraine, TIA, seizure, or papilledema; and (2) if this really is migraine, is it primary (idiopathic) or secondary to an underlying illness?

MIGRAINE, TRANSIENT, ISCHEMIC ATTACK, SEIZURE, OR PAPILLEDEMA?

The differentiation of migraine from TIA, seizure, or papilledema depends on eliciting the zigzag shape of the scintillation, its march across the hemifield, and other accompanying neurologic manifestations (Table 15-1).

A twinkling zigzag pattern (scintillating scotoma) appears in about one-third of the visual auras of migraine.[24] The distinctive outline of the scintillation, resembling a medieval fortress, has led to its designation as *teichopsia*, from the Greek word *teichos*, meaning city wall. Because it appears spectral, or ghostlike, it has been called a *fortification spectrum*.[28] This vivid zigzag sensation has never been described in association with TIA,[29] posterior hemispheric surface electrode stimulation,[30] or electrographically documented spontaneous occipital seizures.[31,32]

If visual hallucinations lack this zigzag shape, TIAs and seizures remain diagnostic considerations unless the hallucinations are described as marching across the hemifield over a 20–30 minute period. Like the zigzag scintillation, this "buildup"[24] does not occur in TIA or in electrographically verified partial seizures.

Nonvisual features can also differentiate migraine from TIA and seizure.[20,24] The paresthesias of migraine typically follow the visual aura with a latency of 5–30 minutes. They progress from hand to mouth with a time course similar to that of the marching scintillation. Dysphasia may follow the paresthesias. By contrast, TIAs generally do not cause marching symptoms. The marching scintillations of seizures are much more rapid than those of migraine and lack the long latency typical of migraine.[24] Seizures are likely to be the cause of scintillations in the presence of gaze deviation, nystagmus, automatisms, and altered consciousness.[31–33]

Transient obscurations of vision associated with papilledema can be distinguished from migraine because they are ultra-brief and often provoked by the Valsalva maneuver or assumption of the upright posture (Chapters 3, 4, and 12). Also, they usually consist of loss of vision rather than scintillations. Ultimately, however, the only certain way to rule out papilledema as a cause of transient visual disturbance is by carefully examining the optic fundus.[29]

PRIMARY (IDIOPATHIC) OR SECONDARY MIGRAINE?

The visual features of primary and secondary migraine are indistinguishable. For example, the classic features of the visual aura of migraine have been reported by patients who have occipital lobe masses, particularly arteriovenous malformations.[34–37] Migraine-like marching scintillations were described by 21% of 70 patients with occipital lobe AVMs.[38] In two separate single-case reports, these phenomena disappeared after AVM excision.[34,36] Classic visual aura also occurs in association with lupus erythematosus[39] and cerebral autosomal dominant arteriopathy with subcortical infarcts and leukoencephalopathy (CADASIL).[40] The three most reliable clues that suggest migraine is primary rather than secondary are (1) attacks have been present since adolescence, (2) no persistent homonymous hemianopias after the attack, and (3) no clues of an underlying disease that predisposes to migraine.

Migrainous Infarction

A migraineur's greatest fear is that the "aura" will be permanent. Neurologic deficits that

persist beyond 48 hours after an attack of migraine imply that brain infarction (ischemic stroke) has occurred. Fortunately, these events are extremely rare.

Migraine does not appear to increase stroke risk in the population at large, probably because conventional risk factors overwhelm it.[41,42] However, when older patients without hypertension, diabetes, or smoking are excluded, migraine increases the risk of stroke three- to fivefold.[43] If *all three* factors are missing, the odds ratio for stroke in migraine jumps to 31:1.[43–45] Oral contraceptive medication, abrupt cessation of antimigrainous treatment, and excessive use of ergot derivatives probably contribute to stroke risk, but epidemiological studies are limited.[20]

Infarction following a migraine attack makes up a vanishingly small fraction of stroke, with an incidence of no more than 3 per 100,000 per year.[41,46–51] Infarction usually occurs in patients with a previous history of auras.[43,48,49] The frequency of prior migraine attacks, the intensity of the headache, and the type of aura are not predictive of the likelihood of stroke.

Most strokes in migraineurs lie within the posterior cerebral artery (PCA) domain and cause persistent homonymous hemianopias. Middle cerebral artery (MCA)-distribution strokes are next most common. Nonspecific features of brain infarction are seen on MRI. Cerebral angiography is often normal but may show vasospasm or complete proximal or distal occlusion.[42] Reduced perfusion is well documented in migraine with aura,[52] as is platelet hyperaggregability. These factors are believed to cause downstream stasis and clot formation.[53] The role of antiphospholipid antibodies in migrainous stroke is uncertain.[54]

Mitochondrial Encephalomyopathy

When seizures and migraine occur together in an adolescent or preadolescent, one consideration is a mitochondrial DNA-mutant condition known as mitochondrial encephalomyopathy, lactic acidosis, and stroke-like (MELAS) episodes.[55,56]

In this maternally inherited condition, migraine and seizure episodes occur in clusters. Migraine is accompanied by fierce headache but no visual aura; it often leaves behind a homonymous hemianopia or cortical blindness, owing to infarction of the occipital region. Visual loss may linger for days to weeks, or it may last forever. The refractory seizures are typically partial, involving visual loss, hemiparesis, or hemisensory loss.[57,58] Other clinical features of MELAS are muscle weakness and cramping, dementia, short stature, and hearing loss.[55] Family members of MELAS patients may have features resembling other mitochondrial cytopathies, including ptosis, ophthalmoplegia, and retinal pigmentary degeneration.[59]

Brain magnetic resonance imaging shows hyperintense signal on T2-weighted scans in the basal ganglia, cerebral and cerebellar cortex, and adjacent white matter (Fig. 15-6).[60] The prevalence of visual manifestations is explained by predominant involvement of occipital cortex. Parietal abnormalities probably explain the seizures. In mild cases, clinical and imaging abnormalities often resolve over time, but once the disease becomes more advanced, the defects become permanent. Their pathogenesis is uncertain. Pathologic study of cortical vessels discloses endothelial mitochondrial abnormalities but thrombosis has not been found.[61,62] The fact that imaging abnormalities lie primarily in gray matter and do not respect the distribution of arterial territories supports a primary intracellular oxidative phosphorylation failure rather than a vascular occlusive mechanism.[63,64]

The diagnosis of MELAS is made by finding a high blood lactate level (88% of cases), ragged red fibers on muscle biopsies (90%), and an A-to-G point mutation at the 3243 nucleotide position in the mitochondrial transfer ribonucleic acid that codes for leucine (80%). This mutation seems to impair complexes I and IV in the electron transport chain.

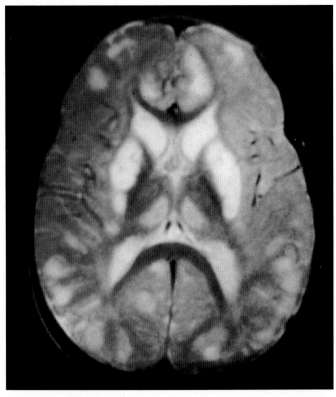

Figure 15–6. Mitochondrial encephalomyopathy. T2-weighted MRI shows high signal in the basal ganglia and parietal, occipital, and frontal lobes of a 12-year-old boy with mitochondrial encephalomyopathy, lactic acidosis, and strokelike episodes (MELAS).

Retinociliary Migraine

Although the typical migrainous visual aura is binocular and attributed to dysfunction in the primary visual cortex, many patients insist that the visual disturbance is seen by only one eye. Most of these individuals are actually experiencing a binocular hemifield disturbance, but they attribute it to the eye with the temporal field disturbance. Still, one must acknowledge that the visual disturbance is truly monocular if patients report that during the episode, they covered one eye at a time and noted that visual acuity was depressed in one eye only. (A binocular hemianopic disturbance would depress visual acuity equally in the two eyes.)

The relationship of such transient monocular disturbances to migraine is unsettled. Most episodes last less than five minutes, do not have positive phenomena or buildup, and are either painless or lack a constant temporal relationship to headache.[25,65,66] Ophthalmoscopic examination during an attack has sometimes disclosed arterial or venous spasm.[67,68] Infarction of the retina, optic nerve, and choroid rarely occur.[25]

Because such episodes often occur in young individuals with a history of other migraine manifestations, no conventional stroke risk factors, and a low likelihood of subsequent stroke, they have been labeled as migrainous.[42,69] However, identical visual symptoms can occur in association with systemic hypotension and preexisting tight carotid stenosis, carotid or cardiac source embolism, or a hypercoagulable state (Chapters 3, 4).[70] For this reason, "retinal migraine" (or, more properly "retinociliary migraine" since ischemia may affect both the retinal and ciliary circulations) should not be diagnosed unless *other causes have been excluded.*[71]

SEIZURES

A mere 5% of all partial seizures originate in the primary visual cortex.[33] A congenital lesion, trauma, neoplasm, inflammation, or infarction is usually responsible. In children, the visual cortex may appear structurally normal, yet partial seizures occur as part of an idiopathic condition called "benign epilepsy with occipital paroxysms."[72] The visual manifestations of primary visual cortex seizures are usually hallucinations,[73,74] although visual loss without hallucinations may also occur.[33]

Positive Visual Phenomena

Positive visual phenomena (hallucinations) typically appear before or during the epileptic discharges;[31] they usually consist of a single cluster of stationary colored or white lines, squares, stars, circles, disks, or dots.[31,32,75–78] Their duration is usually between one and five minutes.

Migrainelike zigzag scintillations are not reported after cortical stimulation[75,76] or in electrographically recorded occipital seizures.[31,32] On the other hand, typical zigzag fortification scotomas that march across the hemifield do occur in patients harboring occipital lobe AVMs[34,36,38] and stop after the AVM is surgically removed.[34,36] *Perhaps these lesions trigger migrainous rather than epileptic auras* (see "Migraine," above).

Negative Visual Phenomena

Visual loss without positive phenomena has been described in 15%[79] to 40%[33] of patients with primary visual cortex seizures. Coincident EEG recordings indicate that seizure-related visual loss occurs during or after the epileptic discharge.[31,73,78,80,81] Ranging from blurred vision to homonymous hemianopias to complete blindness, *visual loss may be the principal or only neurologic deficit.* It occurs in three settings:

- **Occipital lobe lesion.** A unilateral occipital lobe lesion gives rise to a partial seizure that spreads into the opposite visual cortex, and vision is lost throughout. Eye deviation, blinking, hemisensory loss or hemiparesis, aphasia, or confusion often accompany this "status epilepticus amauroticus." It may explain the temporary bilateral blindness in patients who suffer infarctions of one occipital lobe.[80]
- **Occipital absence.** Complete blindness occurs for several minutes during bioccipital spike and wave discharges in a type of prolonged "occipital absence."[72,74,82,83]

Nearly all cases involve individuals aged under 20 years.

- **Visual "Todd's paralysis."** Prolonged blindness may follow status epilepticus if the focus is an occipital lesion.[84] In rare instances, hemianopias or total blindness may be permanent if the status epilepticus has been protracted.[82] These phenomena are attributed to the relative vulnerability of the occipital cortex to hypoxia associated with status epilepticus. As a general rule, if visual recovery is delayed more than a few hours beyond return of consciousness following a generalized seizure, one should suspect either continuing occipital seizures or hypoxic injury to the visual cortex.

The diagnosis of seizures as a cause of transient visual hallucinations or visual loss is suggested by noting gaze deviation or frequent blinking, features present in more than 50% of patients.[33] These accompaniments are especially important in diagnosing benign childhood epilepsy with occipital paroxysms, which may falsely suggest migraine because it causes severe headaches with protracted vomiting.[85]

TRANSIENT ISCHEMIC ATTACKS

Definition

Transient ischemic attacks (TIAs) are defined as episodes of focal brain dysfunction attributable to reduced perfusion. They differ from strokes in that clinical manifestations last less than 24 hours and there is no imaging evidence of brain infarction.

Pathogenesis

Most TIAs affecting binocular vision are presumed to reflect ischemia within the vertebrobasilar circuit. More commonly than anterior circulation TIAs, posterior circulation TIAs often persist for many years without leading to stroke. The pathogenesis of posterior circulation TIAs is considered similar to that of anterior circulation TIAs, with a heavy emphasis on embolism. But posterior circulation TIAs are much more commonly precipitated by standing up suddenly, so that hemodynamic factors are probably very important.[86]

Visual Symptoms

Visual disturbances may consist of momentary blackouts or blurring of vision, as well as flickering, oscillating, or reduplicated images. These visual symptoms are prominent manifestations in about 50% of attacks accompanied by other vertebrobasilar ischemic phenomena (dysequilibrium, diplopia, dysarthria, dysphagia, drop attacks, paresthesias, vertigo, nausea, amnesia, circumoral or extremity numbness, extremity weakness, tinnitus, and hearing loss).[87,88] Transient visual disturbances have been reported as the *first or only symptoms* in 2%,[24] 7%,[87,89] and 16%[88] of vertebrobasilar TIAs.

Negative visual phenomena predominate over positive visual phenomena in cases of vertebrobasilar TIA. They may affect one or both hemifields, typically lasting only seconds. Because they are so brief, the patient hardly notices that something has interfered with vision.[29] Typical comments are that "my glasses fogged up," "my eyes suddenly went out of focus," "someone turned off the lights," or "part of my vision blanked out."

Positive phenomena occur in only 3%[90] to 10%[88] of vertebrobasilar TIA cases that involve vision. Hallucinations consist of tadpoles, soapflakes, snowflakes, sparklers, pinwheels, or glowing lights[29] or illusions of multiple or distorted objects. When these sensations persist beyond a few minutes, suspect a structural abnormality such as an infarct (see "Posterior Cerebral Artery Occlusion," below) or tumor that is causing partial seizures (see "Seizures," above).

CLOSED HEAD INJURY

Mild closed head injury may trigger profound but temporary binocular visual loss, accompanied by irritability and mild confusion.[91–93] Children will usually have fallen a short distance off a swing, wall, or bicycle. Soccer players have headed the ball vigorously.[94] Brain imaging is always normal, but EEG may show bihemispheric posterior slow waves. Vision spontaneously recovers fully within 24 hours. Affected individuals have had a higher than expected history of migraine or seizures.[92] A relative vulnerability of the youthful visual cortex may underlie this phenomenon.

We turn now to causes of *persistent* visual loss owing to lesions of the posterior radiations and visual cortex (Table 15-2).

POSTERIOR CEREBRAL ARTERY OCCLUSION

Mechanisms

Most PCA trunk occlusions are caused by atherosclerotic emboli originating in the vertebral or basilar arteries;[95] cardiac embolism is considered less common.[96] The midbrain and diencephalic PCA branches may be occluded by emboli that lodge in the PCA trunk at the takeoff of the perforating vessels, but small branch occlusions probably

Table 15–2. Important Causes of Persistent Dysfunction in Posterior Optic Radiations and Primary Visual Cortex

Ischemic/Hypoxic
Posterior cerebral artery occlusion
Middle cerebral artery occlusion
Hypoxia and hypotension*
Superior sagittal sinus thrombosis
Migrainous infarction
Mitochondrial encephalomyopathy†

Blood–Brain Barrier Breakthrough
Hypertensive encephalopathy
Cerebral angiography

Inflammatory/Infectious
Progressive multifocal leukoencephalopathy
Multiple sclerosis/acute disseminated
  encephalomyelitis
Hemophilus influenzae meningitis
Creutzfeldt-Jakob disease*
Toxoplasmosis
Subacute sclerosing panencephalitis

Leukodystrophic
Childhood X-linked adrenoleukodystrophy

Neoplastic
Parenchymal
Meningeal

Developmental
Malformation
Porencephaly
Delayed visual maturation*
Amblyopia*

*Toxic**
Intrathecal methotrexate
Vincristine
CCNU
Cyclosporine
FK506 (tacrolimus)
Interferon alpha
Methanol
Mercury
X-irradiation

*Dysmetabolic**
Hyperglycemia
Hypoglycemia
Correction of hyponatremia
Hepatic encephalopathy

Degenerative
Alzheimer's and unspecified dementias*

*Epileptic**
Status epilepticus
"Visual" Todd's paralysis

Traumatic
Closed head injury*
Penetrating injury
Electrical injury*
Electroshock*

*Few or no MRI abnormalities.
†Mechanism may be metabolic energy failure rather than ischemia.

Table 15–3. **Conditions Associated with Posterior Cerebral Artery Occlusion**

Vertebrobasilar atheroma, trauma, dissection	Tentorial herniation
Cardiac valve or wall abnormality	Hypertensive encephalopathy
Migraine	Cerebral angiography
Behçet's disease	Blood dyscrasias*
Lupus erythematosus	Acute intermittent porphyria
Fibromuscular dysplasia	

*Anemia, polcythemia, coagulation inhibitor deficiency, paraproteinemia, sickle cell disease.

also result from *in situ* thrombosis owing to hypotension, hypercoagulability, and local endothelial disease (Table 15-3).[97,98] The quadrigeminal (P3) segment of the PCA trunk (see below) is vulnerable to compression by a herniating temporal lobe.[99,100]

Anatomy

The PCA has three segments that provide deep branches to the paramedian midbrain and thalamus, the lateral midbrain and thalamus, and superficial branches to the inferomedial temporal lobes, posteromedial parietal lobes, and medial occipital lobes (Fig. 15-7).[4,101]

PRECOMMUNAL SEGMENT

This segment (P1, peduncular) extends from the top of the basilar artery to the junction of the PCA and posterior communicating artery. Lying ventral to the brainstem, it gives rise to the paramedian arterial supply of the midbrain and thalamus. The paramedian mesencephalic and thalamoperforating (thalamic subthalamic) branches supply the paramedian midbrain (medial cerebral peduncle, third cranial nerve nucleus and fascicles, red nucleus, superior cerebellar peduncle, tectum) and posteromedial thalamus (rostral interstitial nucleus of medial longitudinal fasciculus, and dorsomedial, parafascicular, and intralaminar thalamic nuclei). One P1 segment is often dominant (Percheron's artery) and supplies both sides of the posterior paramedian thalamus.

AMBIENT SEGMENT

This segment (P2) extends from the posterior communicating artery–PCA junction to the takeoff of the anterior temporal artery. Lying lateral to the brainstem in the ambient cistern, it gives rise to the arterial supply of the lateral midbrain and thalamus. The pedunculoperforating branch nourishes the cerebral peduncle, substantia nigra, lemnisci, and tectum; the thalamogeniculate branches nourish the posterolateral thalamus. The most distal branch, the medial and lateral posterior choroidal arteries, supply the pulvinar and the LGB, respectively.

QUADRIGEMINAL SEGMENT

This segment (P3) extends from the takeoff of the anterior temporal artery to the terminal hemispheric PCA branches. Lying dorsal to the midbrain, it gives rise to five major "superficial" branches that supply the inferior and medial temporal lobes, splenium, medial parieto-occipital junction, and medial and inferior occipital lobes. The anterior temporal artery nourishes the anteroinferior temporal lobe (hippocampal and parahippocampal gyri); the posterior temporal (occipitotemporal) artery nourishes the posteroinferior temporal and occipital lobes (lingual and fusiform gyri and inferior calcarine cortex); the splenial artery nourishes the splenium; the parieto-occipital artery nourishes the posteromedial parietal lobe (precuneus) and part of the medial occipital lobe (superior cuneus, superior calcarine cortex); the calcarine artery nourishes the medial occipital lobe (inferior cuneus,

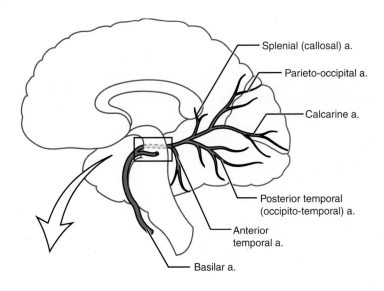

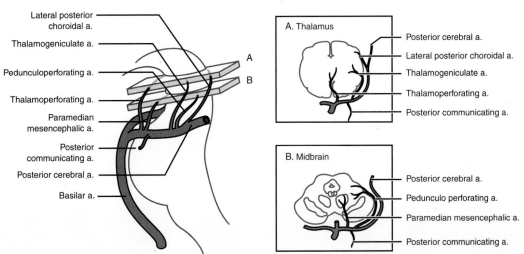

Figure 15–7. Posterior cerebral artery. *Top:* Cerebral branches. *Bottom:* Brainstem branches. At the pons–midbrain junction, the basilar artery bifurcates into two posterior cerebral arteries (PCAs). Before the takeoff of the posterior communicating artery, in the precommunal segment (P1), the PCA gives off the thalamoperforating and paramedian mesencephalic arteries. After the takeoff of the posterior communicating artery, in the postcommunal (P2) segment, the PCA gives off the more lateral supply: the thalamogeniculate, pedunculoperforating, and lateral posterior choroidal branches. After the takeoff of the anterior temporal artery, the cerebral PCA segment (P3) gives off the posterior temporal (occipitotemporal), splenial (callosal), parieto-occipital, and calcarine branches (top).

upper and lower calcarine cortex, superior lingual gyrus).

Occlusive Syndromes

The clinical features of PCA infarcts are best understood in terms of the branches that are occluded.[101a,102]

PROXIMAL POSTERIOR CEREBRAL ARTERY TRUNK OCCLUSION

By affecting the blood supply of the midbrain, thalamus, temporal and occipital lobes, occlusion of the proximal PCA produces a bewildering array of neurologic manifestations dubbed the "top of the basilar" syndrome (Fig. 15-8).[103] Because they often cause hemiplegia, these occlusions are frequently misdiagnosed clinically as MCA occlusions (see below).[104,105] The presence of hemifield loss without neglect or aphasia favors PCA territory infarction. However, *thalamic damage in association with PCA stroke may cause neglect and aphasia.* In such cases, the presence of vertical gaze abnormalities is the best clue that proximal PCA occlusion, rather than MCA occlusion, has occurred.

Components of the "top of the basilar" syndrome occur with occlusions of each of the deep branches of the PCA, as follows (Table 15-4).

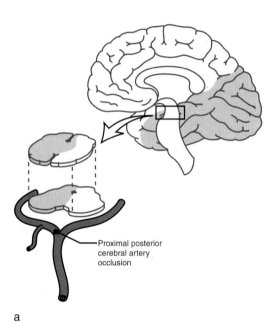

Proximal posterior cerebral artery occlusion

a

Figure 15–8. Proximal posterior cerebral artery ("top of the basilar") occlusion. (*a*) Schematic shows regions that would be infarcted in a right PCA trunk occlusion: the ipsilateral midbrain, posterior thalamus, and infero-omedial temporal and occipital lobes. In reality, infarction is usually patchy. (*b*) T2-weighted MRI of a patient with a "top of the basilar" occlusion, showing patchy high signal (white) abnormalities reflecting bilateral infarction of the thalamus and midbrain (*left*) and inferior temporo-occipital regions (*right*).

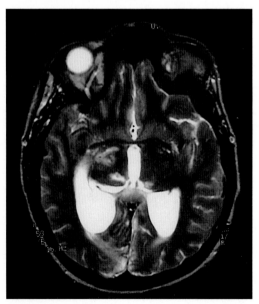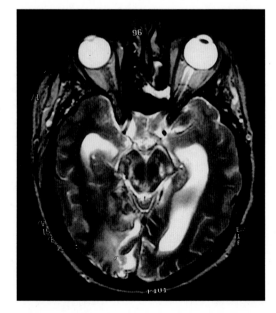

b

Table 15–4. **Posterior Cerebral Artery Infarcts: Deep Branch Territory***

Artery	Tissues Supplied	Principal Manifestations
Paramedian mesencephalic	Third cranial nerve Red nucleus Superior cerebellar peduncle Medial cerebral peduncle Midbrain tectum	Third cranial nerve palsy Contralateral hemiparesis Contralateral tremor and ataxia Visual hallucinations
Thalamoperforating (thalamic subthalamic)	Rostral interstitial nucleus of MLF Medial thalamus Sometimes anterior thalamus	Vertical gaze palsies[†] Hypersomnolence Amnesia Abulia
Pedunculoperforating	Lateral cerebral peduncle Substantia nigra Lemnisci	Contralateral hemiparesis
Thalamogeniculate	Posterolateral thalamus	Contralateral hemisensory loss (sometimes dysesthetic) Homonymous hemianopia (uncommon)
Posterior lateral choroidal	Lateral geniculate body	Homonymous horizontal sectoranopia

*Proximal PCA occlusion ("top of the basilar syndrome") gives rise to various combinations of the findings produced by individual branch occlusions.

[†]Less commonly, hyperconvergence, bilateral abduction deficits, skew deviation, internuclear ophthalmoplegia, lid retraction, retractory nystagmoid movements on attempted upgaze, seesaw nystagmus, fourth nerve palsy, monocular elevation paresis, and vertical one-and-one-half syndrome.[106]

Paramedian Mesencephalic and Thalamoperforating (Thalamic-Subthalamic) Artery Occlusion

Occlusions of these two vessels, which branch off the PCA prior to the posterior communicating artery takeoff ("precommunal" occlusions), may occur separately, but they often occur together (Fig. 15-9).

Occlusion of the paramedian mesencephalic arteries causes ipsilateral third cranial nerve palsy, contralateral hemiplegia (medial cerebral peduncle), contralateral tremor and/or ataxia (red nucleus/superior cerebellar peduncle).[106] There may be accompanying vivid visual hallucinations, often of animals or familiar humans, which the patient recognizes as being unreal (peduncular hallucinosis) (Chapter 4).[103]

Occlusion of the thalamoperforating artery frequently causes *bilateral* posteromedial thalamic infarction, because the blood supply to both sides often derives from a single vessel (the artery of Percheron). The classic triad of clinical signs is vertical gaze paralysis, hypersomnolence, and amnesia.[107] Other ophthalmic signs are hyperconvergence, bilateral abduction deficits, skew deviation, internuclear ophthalmoplegia, lid retraction, retractory nystagmoid movements on attempted upgaze, seesaw nystagmus, and fourth nerve palsy.[103,106] When infarction is unilateral, the patient may display a dissociated vertical gaze palsy such as a monocular elevation paresis or vertical one-and-one-half syndrome.[108] In some cases, these vessels also supply the anterior thalamus, so that occlusion will cause the patient to be apathetic or even abulic.[107]

In the initial stages of a stroke in this domain, the patient's clinical state may be dominated by depressed consciousness. If vertical gaze pareses (or other neuroophthalmic abnormalities) are not recognized, the examiner will undertake a fruitless search for a toxic-metabolic-infectious cause.

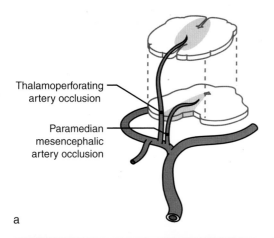

Thalamoperforating
artery occlusion

Paramedian
mesencephalic
artery occlusion

a

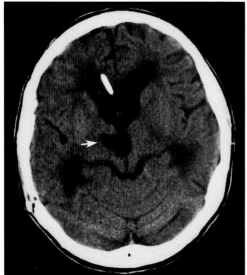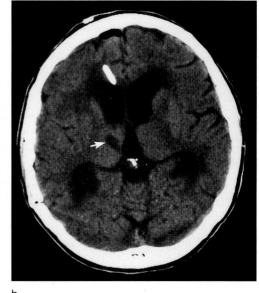

b

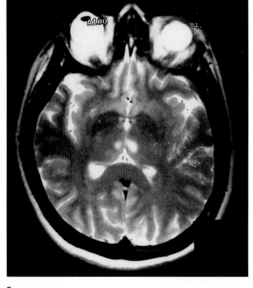

Figure 15–9. Paramedian mesencephalic and thalamoperforating (thalamic–subthalamic) artery occlusion. (*a*) Schematic shows infarction of the right paramedian midbrain and the posteromedial thalamus. Because the thalamic supply is often from one vessel, both sides are often infarcted. (*b*) Noncontrast CT shows low attenuation infarcted areas (arrows) in the right paramedian midbrain (*left*) and thalamus (*right*). (*c*) T2-weighted MRI of the patient shows high signal abnormalities (arrows) in both posterior paramedian thalamic regions, reflecting occlusion of a single thalamoperforating artery.

c

304

Pedunculoperforatoring and Thalamogeniculate (Thalamic-Subthalamic) Artery Occlusion

As with precommunal PCA occlusions, occlusions of these two early postcommunal branches often occur together (Fig. 15-10).

Occlusion of the pedunculoperforating artery causes infarction of the cerebral peduncle, sometimes producing a contralateral hemiplegia.[109] Occlusion of the thalamogeniculate artery causes infarction of the posterolateral thalamus, producing a pure contralateral hemisensory loss that may become dysesthetic (Dejerine-Roussy syndrome). A contralateral athetoid hemiparesis, ataxia, and hemisensory loss result when there is extension into the posterior limb of the internal capsule.[109]

Posterior Lateral Choroidal Artery Occlusion

Infarction in the domain of this branch is confined to the LGB (Fig. 15-11); it classically produces a horizontal sector homonymous hemianopia (Chapter 15). Sparing of a portion of the hemifield results from having a complementary arterial supply from the anterior choroidal artery (AChA), a branch of the carotid artery. There are also cases of complete homonymous hemianopia associated with proximal PCA branch occlusions in which, by imaging criteria, the LGB appears to be the only part of the retrochiasmal visual pathway that has been infarcted.[110,111]

SUPERFICIAL POSTERIOR CEREBRAL ARTERY INFARCTS

A different clinical syndrome develops as the result of occlusions of the superficial, or cerebral, branches of the PCA, as follows (Table 15-5).

Anterior Temporal Artery Occlusion

Isolated infarction in this branch is uncommon (Fig. 15-12); more typically, it occurs in combination with infarction in calcarine and occipitotemporal arteries.[86] Typical manifestations are visual recognition disorders, amnesia, and agitated delirium.[112]

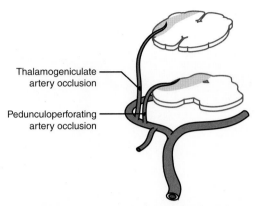

a

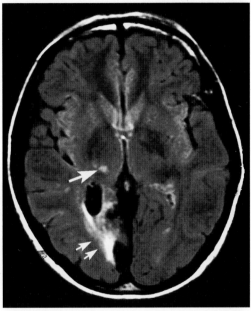

b

Figure 15–10. Pedunculoperforating and thalamogeniculate artery occlusion. (*a*) Schematic shows infarction of the lateral and dorsal midbrain and lateral thalamus. (*b*) T2-weighted MRI shows high signal (arrow) in the right lateral thalamus, reflecting occlusion of the thalamogeniculate branch, and infarction of the posteromedial occipital region (arrows), reflecting occlusion of the calcarine branch.

In the schematic:
Thalamogeniculate artery occlusion
Pedunculoperforating artery occlusion

Posterior Temporal (Occipitotemporal) Artery Occlusion

Bilateral blockage of this vessel (Fig. 15-13) gives rise to visual recognition and naming disturbances for objects (visual object agnosia and optic aphasia), a disturbance in

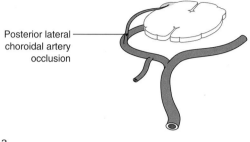

Posterior lateral choroidal artery occlusion

a

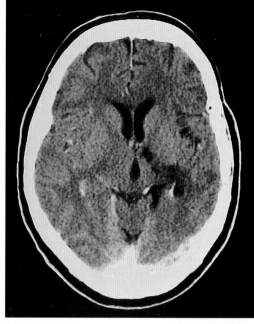

b

Figure 15–11. Posterior lateral choroidal artery occlusion. (*a*) Schematic shows isolated infarction of a portion of the lateral geniculate body (LGB). (*b*) CT shows a low attenuation infarction defect (arrow) in the region of the LGB.

Table 15–5. Posterior Cerebral Artery Infarcts: Superficial Branch Territory

Artery	Tissues Supplied	Manifestations
Anterior temporal	Anterior temporal lobe	Visual recognition deficits, amnesia, agitated delirium
Posterior temporal (occipitotemporal)	Posterior and inferior temporal lobe	Bilateral: visual recognition deficits, achromatopsia, amnesia, agitated delirium, superior altitudinal visual field loss
		Left: pure alexia, contralateral hemifield achromatopsia, verbal recent memory loss, right superior quadrantanopia
		Right: topographical agnosia, prosopagnosia, visual recent memory loss, left superior quadrantanopia
Splenial (callosal)	Splenium of corpus callosum	Pure alexia*
Parieto-occipital	Posteromedial parietal lobe, precuneus	Bilateral: optic ataxia, gaze deficits simultanagnosia, inferior altitudinal field loss
		Left: minimal effects
		Right: left hemispatial neglect
Calcarine	Posterior optic radiations, primary visual cortex	Visual field loss,† visual hallucinations and illusions, ipsilateral periocular pain

*Only if combined with ipsilateral calcarine or lateral geniculate infarction.
†Nearly always homonymous hemianopia, with many variants (see text).

306

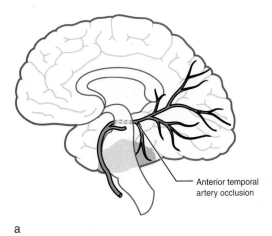

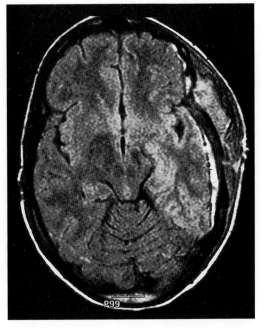

Figure 15–12. Anterior temporal artery occlusion. (*a*) Schematic shows infarction of the right anteroinferior temporal lobe. (*b*) FLAIR MRI shows high signal in the left anterior temporal lobe.

b

recognizing faces (prosopagnosia), inability to discriminate among different colored hues (cerebral achromatopsia), loss of recent memory, and sometimes an agitated delirium.[112]

Occlusion of the left posterior temporal artery causes an acquired inability to read (pure alexia) and contralateral hemiachromatopsia. Verbal recent memory loss is sometimes present, particularly if the ante-

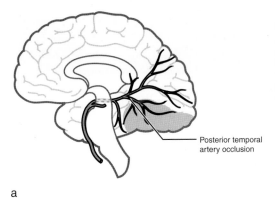

Figure 15–13. Posterior temporal (occipitotemporal) artery occlusion. (*a*) Schematic shows infarction of the lingual, fusiform, and inferior temporal gyri. (*b*) T2 MRI shows high signal in the inferior temporal and occipital lobes bilaterally.

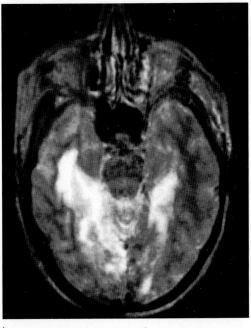

b

rior temporal artery is also occluded (see be-low).[113] Visual object agnosia and inability to name objects by sight (optic aphasia) may also occur.[113]

Occlusion of the right posterior temporal artery causes a visual recognition distur-bance for familiar places (topographical ag-nosia), visual recent memory loss, and some-times prosopagnosia (Chapter 17). In some patients, the posterior temporal branch nourishes a considerable part of the cal-carine cortex, so that its occlusion gives rise to contralateral superior quadrantanopia (unilateral infarct) or superior altitudinal hemianopia (bilateral infarct).[4]

Splenial (Callosal) Artery Occlusion

In combination with infarction in the do-main of the left calcarine artery, left splenial artery occlusion (Fig. 15-14) causes pure alexia (splenio-occipital alexia).[114] Infarc-tion in the domain of the splenial and cal-carine arteries is not the only way to produce pure alexia. Alternatives include (1) left splenial and thalamogeniculate or LPChA infarction (spleniogeniculate alexia)[110] and (2) left occipitotemporal artery[115] or occip-itoparietal artery[116] infarction, either of which affects the white matter subjacent to the left angular gyrus (subangular alexia). The splenio-occipital and spleniogeniculate types of pure alexia are always accompanied by right homonymous hemianopia. The sub-angular type may not exhibit this visual field defect.

Parietooccipital Artery Occlusion

Bilateral occlusion results in variants of the Balint-Holmes syndrome, consisting of im-paired volitional eye movements, visually guided misreaching in all directions (optic ataxia), and piecemeal perception (simul-tanagnosia) (Chapter 16). Occlusion of the right hemisphere branch leads to visuospa-tial disturbances involving left hemispace, in-cluding sensory neglect and misreaching; oc-clusion in the left hemisphere causes right hemispatial dysfunction but with far less pro-found clinical effects (Fig. 15-15). In some individuals, parieto-occipital branches sup-ply much of the superior calcarine cortex,[4]

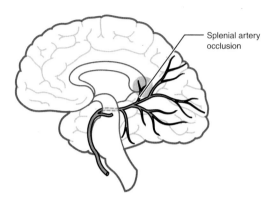

a

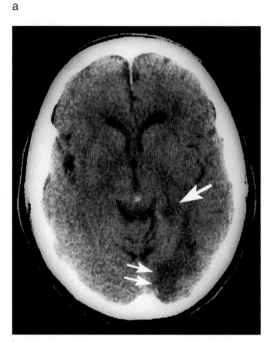

b

Figure 15–14. Splenial (callosal) artery occlusion. (a) Schematic shows infarction in the splenium and a portion of the parahippocampal gyrus. (b) CT shows low attenuation (arrow) in the left parasplenial region and in the domain of the calcarine branch (arrows).

so that occlusion causes a contralateral in-ferior quadrantanopia (unilateral infarct) or inferior altitudinal hemianopia (bilateral infarct).[13]

Calcarine Artery Occlusion

Among the cerebral branches, this one is the most often occluded (Fig. 15-16).[102] Clinical

(In image 2: Splenial artery occlusion)

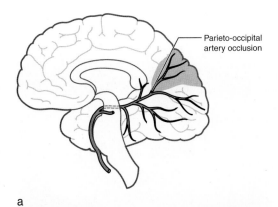

Parieto-occipital
artery occlusion

a

upper face occurs in association with any focal occipital process that also affects the meninges; for example, it is regularly reported after occipital lobar hemorrhages.[119]

MIDDLE CEREBRAL ARTERY OCCLUSION

The posterior radiations may also be infarcted by occlusion of the angular or temporo-occipital branches of the middle cere-

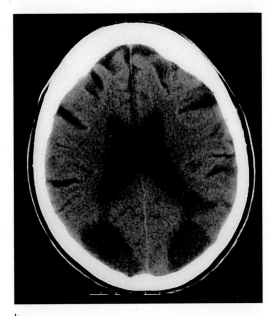

b

Figure 15–15. Parietooccipital artery occlusion. (*a*) Schematic shows infarction in the parieto-occipital region (precuneus). (*b*) CT shows low attenuation lesions (arrows) in the precuneus bilaterally.

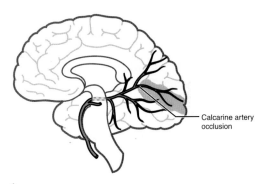

Calcarine artery
occlusion

a

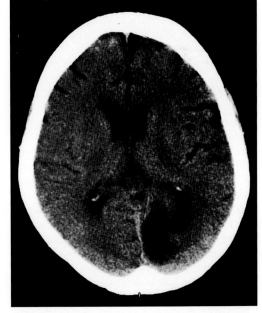

manifestations include homonymous hemianopia, visual hallucinations, and visual illusions. Patients are typically aware of their visual deficit, particularly once it has been pointed out to them (Chapter 3).[117] Referral of trigeminal pain generated by irritation of the occipital meninges[118] may lead to a common accompaniment to calcarine artery occlusion: *severe ipsilateral periocular or brow pain, which may be severe enough to distract both the patient and the physician from the underlying visual deficits.* Referral of occipital pain to the

b

Figure 15–16. Calcarine artery occlusion. (*a*) Schematic shows infarction of the calcarine banks (inferior cuneus, superior lingual gyrus). (*b*) CT shows low signal (arrow) in the left paramedian occipital lobe.

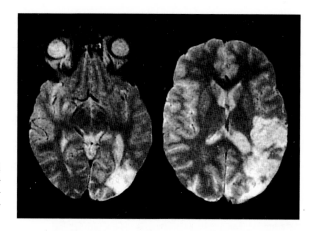

Figure 15–17. Homonymous hemianopia caused by a large middle cerebral artery (MCA) occlusion. Low axial (left) and high axial (right) T2-weighted MRIs show infarction in the left parieto-occipital region.

bral artery (MCA), which supply the posterior parietotemporal-occipital convexity (Fig. 15-17).[120] However, many MCA infarcts are densest at the cortical margin and do not reach deep enough into the hemispheric white matter to affect the radiations, which hug the ventricular surface. When full-thickness infarcts of the right hemisphere extend down to the radiations, they tend to cause hemispatial neglect, which is easily confused with hemianopia (Chapter 16). Deep MCA infarcts of the left hemisphere invariably cause aphasia, which complicates the assessment of visual pathway injury.[121]

HYPOTENSION AND HYPOXIA

A temporary fall in global arterial perfusion or oxygenation of the central nervous system may lead to infarction in tissue that is relatively active metabolically or poorly supplied.[122] In some cases, the oxygen deprivation occurs without a concomitant drop in perfusion (asphyxiation, mitochondrial disorders, Wernicke's encephalopathy, carbon monoxide and methanol poisoning). In other cases, there is a primary perfusion failure (cardiac arrest, exsanguination) or combined oxygenation–perfusion failure (cardiopulmonary arrest). The distribution of CNS tissue damage is similar in all three situations but will differ somewhat depending on whether the primary problem is oxygenation or perfusion failure, on whether high-grade carotid stenosis is present, and

on whether the event occurred in a preterm infant.

If oxygenation is the chief problem, with maintained perfusion, then the metabolically active tissues—the visual cortex, thalamus (including LGB), hippocampus, globus pallidus, and deep cerebellar nuclei—will suffer most (Fig. 15-18). In profound neonatal hypoxia, the LGB is frequently damaged, leading to blindness (Fig. 14-3b).[123] If perfusion is the chief problem, the damaged tissues will lie in the relatively vasodeprived regions—the vascular "watershed regions," which consist of the cerebral arterial border zones, the cerebral and cerebellar cortex, and the basal ganglia. In preterm infants, the watershed region lies in the periventricular white matter.

The posterior cerebral arterial border zone, lying between the domains of the MCA and PCA, is particularly vulnerable to hypotension. It consists of a white and gray matter strip that extends from the midparietal convexity backward toward the occipital pole, curving forward along the lateral temporal lobe.[124,125] Ischemia to this region produces the visuospatial and oculomotor deficits of Balint-Holmes syndrome (Fig. 15-19) (Chapter 16).[126]

Among patients who have high-grade carotid stenosis, infarction following systemic hypotension often primarily affects the anterior border zone, lying between the domains of the anterior cerebral artery (ACA) and MCA. It consists of a strip of gray and white matter extending parasagittally

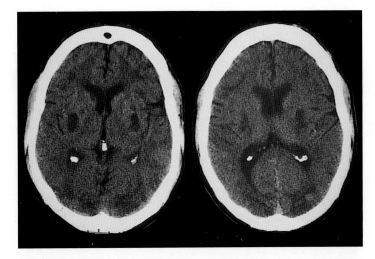

Figure 15–18. Methanol poisoning. This suicidal 40-year-old patient became cortically blind and parkinsonian after consuming methanol. Low axial (left) and high axial (right) CT sections show low signal foci in basal ganglia and medial occipital lobes, tissues with high metabolic demand. This injury pattern also occurs in mitochondrial encephalopathy (Fig. 15-6), and after global cerebral hypoperfusion (Fig. 15-20).

along the cerebral convexity in the frontal and anterior parietal lobes. Patients who sustain anterior border zone ischemia will manifest impaired volitional saccades, bibrachial weakness, and integrative somatosensory deficits.[124]

Hypotension also damages the cerebral cortex (third, fifth, and sixth laminae), particularly in the striate and peristriate regions, the hippocampus, and the basal ganglia, especially the globus pallidus. (The thalamus and brainstem nuclei are typically less often involved.[127]) These regions are vulnerable, not so much because they are remote from an arterial supply, but because their metabolic rates are relatively high.

If the brain is hypoperfused before term, the border zone shifts to the periventricular trigonal white matter, lying between ventricular and cortical arterial perforators. Damage appears as substance loss called "periventricular leukomalacia." The posterior optic radiations, which pass through this region, may become severely damaged (Fig. 15-20). *This is probably the mechanism of persistent blindness in many preterm infants.*[128]

When border zone damage is mild, CT typically shows no abnormalities, but MRI usually reveals T2-weighted hyperdensities.[129] If the insult is mild, MRI findings may be subtle or nonexistent. Blood flow deprivation may be evident only with xenon diffusion studies or single proton emission tomography (SPECT), and metabolic dysfunction may be apparent only with positron emission tomography (PET).[130] Clinical manifestations of border zone ischemia are more reversible than those associated with MCA or PCA occlusion.[14,124]

An alternative pattern of damage may follow hypotension in the presence of extremely high-grade arterial stenosis. Rather than being centered in arterial border zones, the *damage may lie in the domain of a*

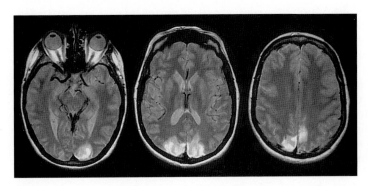

Figure 15–19. Bilateral posterior watershed zone infarctions. Low, mid, and high axial T2-weighted MRI sections reveal high signal areas in the parieto-occipital junctions, owing to severe hypotension after myocardial infarction. This pattern of infarction led to Balint Holmes syndrome (Chapter 16).

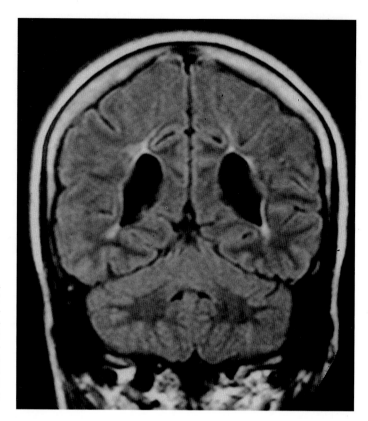

Figure 15–20. Periventricular leuko-malacia. T2-weighted coronal MRI shows *ex vacuo* ventricular enlarge-ment, corrugation of ventricular bor-ders, periventricular high signal, and atrophy of white matter. This 35-year-old patient, born prematurely, had lifelong binocular subnormal visual acuity and diffuse bilateral visual field loss from hypoxic damage to the optic radiations.

major cerebral artery. For example, in hy-potension superimposed on high-grade ver-tebrobasilar stenosis, an ischemic stroke may occur in the distribution of the PCA.[14,124,131] Hemianopias and complete blindness will be the prominent clinical findings. If the PCA–MCA border zone is also affected, ele-ments of the Balint-Holmes syndrome may be evident, and the patient may be unaware of visual loss (Anton's syndrome) (Chapter 5).[117] PCA-distribution ischemia may lead to the incorrect assumption that the mecha-nism was embolic occlusion.

Given this complicated interplay among vascular watershed zones, metabolically de-manding tissues, and preexisting arterial stenosis, one cannot confidently assign a pathogenesis to an occipital lobe stroke based purely on the location of MRI signal abnormalities. Consider how the following facts make it difficult to decide between hy-potension and thromboembolism as a cause of PCA stroke: (*1*) posterior border zone in-farctions are found on imaging in the ab-sence of documented systemic hypotension after coronary angiography, coronary bypass surgery, and heart valve surgery;[14] (*2*) PCA territorial infarctions are seen on scans when hypotension is the only likely cause; and (*3*) the posterior border zone overlaps the territory supplied by the parieto-occipital branch of the PCA.

SUPERIOR SAGITTAL SINUS THROMBOSIS

Superior sagittal sinus (SSS) thrombosis[132] and cortical vein thrombosis[133] are rare causes of visual cortex infarction (Fig. 15-21). The frontal and parietal lobes are much more commonly the targets.[134] Patients have hemiparesis and hemisensory loss, seizures, neglect, aphasia, and depressed conscious-ness. Visuospatial deficits may be prominent. Less commonly, there is damage to the vi-sual cortex, causing visual field loss and hal-lucinations. If damage is mild, the visual fields remain intact but the patient is dis-turbed by scintillations.[135] Because head-ache is often intense, this complex may falsely suggest migraine.

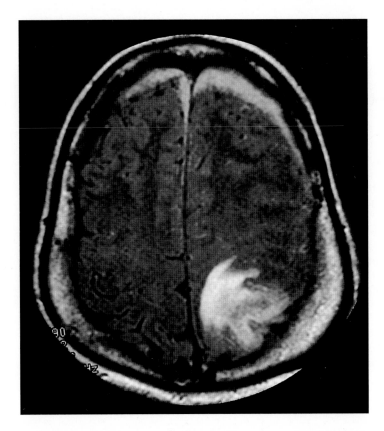

Figure 15–21. Posterior sagittal sinus thrombosis. T2-weighted MRI shows a large left posterior parieto-occipital hemorrhage (white), the result of venous hypertension due to sagittal sinus thrombosis.

The visual symptoms caused by SSS thrombosis are usually related to the "pseudotumor cerebri syndrome," that is, the effect of increased intracranial pressure on the optic nerves (Chapter 12).[136] Initial symptoms may include transient visual obscurations or scintillations, often precipitated or exacerbated by assuming an upright posture. If intracranial pressure remains high, visual loss quickly becomes persistent. Papilledema is a critical tipoff, but it may not have had time to develop if intracranial pressure rise is explosive. In that case, the examiner must avoid the presumption of migraine, particularly in the face of a normal brain CT scan. Diagnostic studies should include both an MRI and an MR venogram. In patients with cortical vein thrombosis but without SSS thrombosis, conventional cerebral angiography may be necessary for diagnosis.[133]

Superior sagittal sinus thrombosis occurs in the puerperium, in association with prothrombotic states such as dehydration, malignancy, trauma, burn, and sepsis; inflammatory conditions such as Behçet's and connective tissue diseases (especially lupus erythematosus); otitic/mastoid infections; and hereditary coagulation inhibitor deficiencies (protein S, protein C, antithrombin III).[134] Tumors in the torcular region may rarely cause SSS thrombosis, and oral contraceptive use has been implicated.[134] Still, 20%–35% of cases remain idiopathic.[134]

In the pre-MRI era, SSS thrombosis was often invoked as a cause of retrochiasmal visual loss during the postpartum period when hypercoagulability may occur.[137] Now that it has become possible to demonstrate patency of the cerebral venous sinuses noninvasively by MRI, it is clear that an alternative cause of these findings is hypertensive encephalopathy (see below).

OCCIPITAL LOBAR HEMORRHAGE

Spontaneous (nontraumatic) hemorrhages of the cerebral hemispheres usually affect the basal ganglia and thalamus in patients with preexisting hypertension. They may also occur more peripherally, and they are then designated as "lobar." The occipital lobe may be the site of a substantial proportion of lobar hemorrhages (42% in one series)[119] (Fig. 15-22). Hemorrhages in this location, as in other cerebral lobes, may result from an occult vascular malformation, metastatic tumor, warfarin anticoagulation, blood dyscrasias, amyloid angiopathy, aminergic substance abuse, or hypertensive angiopathy. Aneurysmal bleeding is not a consideration in this region. In many cases, no definite cause in determined. Lobar hemorrhages are often difficult to distinguish from hemorrhagic infarction. Two clues are that they spare the gray matter and do not conform to the supply region of large arteries. Visualization of an underlying mass lesion may be delayed for several weeks until the blood has resorbed.

The presenting features of occipital hemorrhages depend on the extent of hemorrhage. The principal manifestations are homonymous hemianopia and *severe head pain localized to the ipsilateral eye.*[119] This eye pain, which represents referral from trigeminal afferents in the occipital pole meninges, is also reported after occipital infarction. *Eye pain is not a feature of stroke in the other cerebral lobes.*

Controversy surrounds the advisability of evacuating lobar hemorrhages. Most sources recommend that they be left undisturbed, particularly in eloquent brain regions, unless their expansion is associated with deteriorating neurologic function or brain herniation.

LEUKOENCEPHALOPATHIES

Leukoencephalopathies are disorders that affect the cerebral white matter. The following conditions have a predilection for the white matter of the posterior cerebral hemispheres.

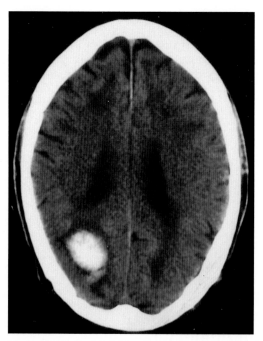 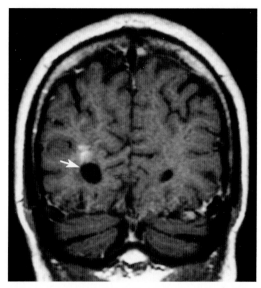

Figure 15–22. Occipital lobar hemorrhage. The radiodense high signal on this CT (*left*) signifies a right occipital lobar hemorrhage. It caused a congruous left homonymous hemianopia—the only neurologic deficit. The field defect shrank as the hemorrhage absorbed, leaving a small area of encephalomalacia (arrow) on coronal MRI three months later (*right*).

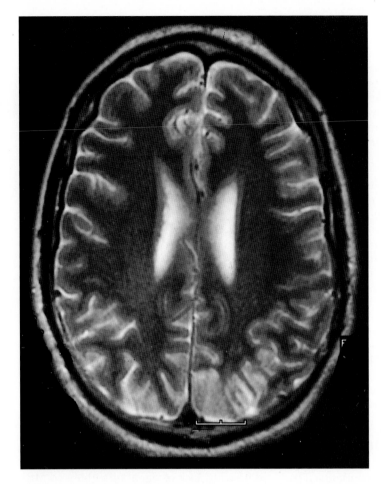

Figure 15–23. Hypertensive Encephalopathy. T2-weighted MRI shows bilateral high signal in the occipital white matter. This 24 year old with malignant hypertension from glomerulonephritis developed bilateral homonymous hemianopias. Following blood pressure normalization, the visual deficits and MRI signal abnormalities disappeared within one week. Such rapid clearing suggests that the high signal reflects vasogenic rather than cytotoxic edema.

Hypertensive Encephalopathy

A rapid rise in systolic blood pressure can bring about the syndrome of hypertensive encephalopathy, consisting of headache, alterations in consciousness, seizures, and binocular visual loss, illusions, and hallucinations.[138–140] *The absolute systolic level is less important than the rate of rise and the variance from the patient's usual systolic blood pressure.*

Visual alterations may be the first, the most prominent, or even the only manifestations. Although the eyes sometimes show vaso-occlusive retinopathy, optic neuropathy, or choroidopathy, they are often normal. The visual symptoms originate elsewhere: in the occipital and parieto-occipital white matter, which appears edematous on brain imaging (Fig. 15-23).[141]

Occurring at any age, hypertensive encephalopathy is particularly common in youth, in late pregnancy,[142,143] and in the postpartum period.[144] Although it may arise in a setting of chronic hypertension, it is more common in normotensive individuals whose blood pressure suddenly rises from acute renal disease, the use of monoamine oxidase inhibitors, or pregnancy.[140] The clinical and imaging features of hypertensive encephalopathy and eclampsia are identical.

In the early stages of hypertensive encephalopathy, the tissue is merely edematous (vasogenic edema), not infarcted (cytotoxic edema). If blood pressure is brought down promptly, clinical deficits will resolve totally within days and imaging abnormalities will disappear within weeks.[141,145] The pathogenesis of the blood–brain barrier breakdown is unsettled. An earlier hypothesis was that excessive vasospasm led to ischemic vascular injury and increased permeability.[140] Current belief is that the posterior hemispheric transudate results from a premature failure of cerebrovascular autoregulation. High blood pressure forces the vessels to dilate and leak.[146,147] This selective autoregulatory failure in the domain of the PCA has been attributed to its relatively poor sympathetic innervation.[148] If excessively high blood pressure is not relieved, the PCA branches become occluded and the brain infarcted. The pathogenesis of the vaso-occlusion remains unclear.

The combination of binocular visual loss, hallucinations, seizures, and posterior hemispheric white matter signal abnormalities may falsely suggest the diagnosis of PCA territory or posterior border zone infarction or of superior sagittal sinus thrombosis.[132,135,137] The relative sparing of gray matter on imaging and the rapid reversibility of clinical and imaging signs weigh against the diagnosis of arterial territory or border zone infarction. A normal lumbar puncture opening pressure and the presence of a flow void in the dural sinuses on MRI are evidence against a diagnosis of SSS thrombosis. Moreover, cortical visual dysfunction is extremely rare in patients with SSS thrombosis.

Toxic Leukoencephalopathy

A clinical and imaging complex identical to that of hypertensive encephalopathy has also been documented in patients taking cyclosporine.[145,149–152] The same findings occur in patients treated with two other immunosuppressive medications—tacrolimus[153] and alpha interferon.[145] Some of these patients have had elevated blood pressure. Acute intermittent porphyria,[154] cerebral angiography,[155,156] and cisplatinum chemotherapy[157] have provoked similar self-limited phenomena. Whether each of these agents exerts its effects through hypertension or through other mechanisms is unknown. For example, lipophilic agents could escape through the relatively weak blood–brain barrier of the PCA, become attached to myelin, and damage it. Alternatively, the target could be the endothelium of PCA vessels.

Whatever its pathogenesis, there appears to be a high susceptibility for leakage in the distal PCA domain that gives rise to a "reversible posterior leukoencephalopathy"

provoked by accelerated hypertension, cyclosporine, tacrolimus, alpha interferon, or angiographic dye.[145]

Progressive Multifocal Leukoencephalopathy

Progressive multifocal leukoencephalopathy is a white matter infection caused by a papovavirus known as JC. The virus infects oligodendroglial cells, the source of central nervous system myelin. Nearly all cases arise in individuals whose cell-mediated immunity is compromised by AIDS, lymphoproliferative disorders, and immunosuppressive therapy.[158] Approximately 1%[159] to 4%[160] of AIDS patients will develop presumptive PML.

Infection occurs by reactivation of dormant JC virus, as antibody titers to this virus are present in 90% of healthy adults.[160] Stored in the kidney, the JC virus is carried to the brain by infected B lymphocytes, enters oligodendroglia, and destroys their myelin-producing ability. The virus probably also enters astrocytes, turning them into bizarre shapes, but no JC particles have yet been identified within astrocytes. There is an impressive macrophage response, but oddly, the blood–brain barrier remains intact, as evidenced by lack of signal on enhanced MRI. Infection begins deep in the occipitoparietal white matter and spreads to the rest of the brain. On occasion, the lesions arise in the cerebellar, perithalamic, or basal ganglionic regions.

The five cardinal manifestations of PML are limb weakness, dementia, ataxia, dysarthria, and visual loss. The visual loss, which derives from damage to posterior optic radiations, is typically homonymous, often bilateral, but rarely symmetrical.[158,161] Found in about one-fourth of cases,[158] it may be the first or leading manifestation of PML.[161] The visual field defects may be combined with integrative visual deficits involving spatial (Chapter 16) and recognition dysfunction (Chapter 17).[162,163]

A diagnosis of PML is supported by MRI findings of nonenhancing, patchy T2 high signal centered in the deep posterior white matter, and sparing the white matter subjacent to the cortex (Fig. 17-3b). In early cases, the imaging abnormalities may be extremely subtle but should exclude other common causes of posterior white matter disease in immunocompromised patients, such as toxoplasmosis, primary CNS lymphoma, tuberculosis, syphilis, cryptococcomas, fungal abscesses, CMV encephalitis (all of which should enhance), herpes simplex encephalitis, which preferentially strikes temporal, insular, cingulate, and subfrontal cortex, and HIV encephalitis, which typically shows faint high signal in the frontal rather than occipitoparietal regions.

Definitive diagnosis depends on brain biopsy, which will reveal demyelination, eosinophilic intranuclear inclusions in oligodendrogliocytes that react with stains impregnated with antibody against papovavirus, and giant, irregular astrocytes. Unfortunately, there is no effective treatment for PML, which usually progresses to death within 18 months of diagnosis.

Childhood X-linked Adrenoleukodystrophy

The childhood X-linked form of adrenoleukodystrophy causes early and profound destruction of the white matter of the posterior hemispheres. Visual loss can be the presenting manifestation, although dementia and gait disturbance usually precede it.[164,165] The visual loss is slowly progressive and symmetric; the optic disks are pale. Early in the disease, MRI findings are striking and distinctive: diffuse high signal on T2-weighted scans in peritrigonal regions, splenium, and occipital lobes, eventually extending forward into the rest of the cerebrum.[166] The central portions of the lesions have low T1 signal, reflecting necrosis, and the advancing edges of the lesion enhance strongly (Fig. 15-24).

Childhood X-linked adrenoleukodystrophy is associated with the abnormal accu-

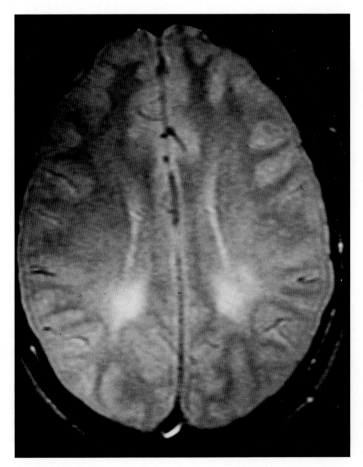

Figure 15–24. X-linked childhood adrenoleukodystrophy. T2-weighted MRI shows high signal in the retrotrigonal regions and frontal lobes. This 8-year-old boy had progressive binocular visual loss and personality change.

mulation of very long (22 to 26 carbon) chain fatty acids. They pile up because of impaired peroxisomal oxidative degradation, owing to deficiency of a membrane transport protein. The defective gene has been mapped to the long arm of the X chromosome (Xq28).[62] Once the disease has begun, there is no effective therapy. For presymptomatic family members, a mixture of glyceryl trioleate and trierucate ("Lorenzo's oil") may lessen the pace of progression.[167]

Acute Disseminated Encephalomyelitis and Multiple Sclerosis

Acute disseminated encephalomyelitis (ADEM) is a monophasic and MS a recurrent inflammatory demyelinating process of the central nervous system. In patients with either illness, MRI often shows lesions located in the posterior radiations, along the ventricular trigone border (Fig. 15-25). In-

deed, homonymous hemianopias have been reported in association with both conditions.[168–170] Considering how often posterior radiation imaging abnormalities are observed in these diseases, it is a mystery that homonymous field defects are reported so infrequently!

POLIOENCEPHALOPATHIES

Polioencephalopathies are disorders of the central gray matter. The conditions discussed in this section affect the visual cortex out of proportion to other cerebral gray matter.

Metabolic Encephalopathy

Cortical blindness has been anecdotally reported following hypoglycemia,[171] hepatic encephalopathy,[172] and dialysis.[173] The blindness generally occurs in a setting of global encephalopathy, but is its most promi-

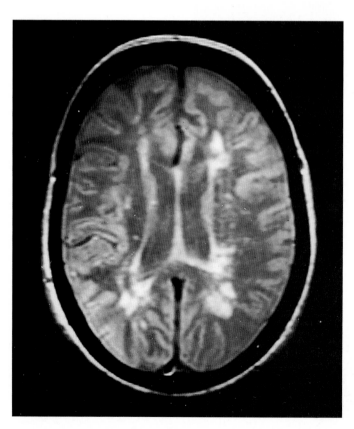

Figure 15–25. Multiple sclerosis. T2-weighted MRI shows periventricular high signal especially in the peritrigonal regions, affecting the posterior optic radiations bilaterally.

nent feature. Imaging that detects structural abnormalities may be expected to be normal. Generally, EEG shows diffuse background slowing and VEPs disclose reduced amplitude and increased latency. Blindness resolves once the metabolic abnormality is corrected. The temporary visual loss reflects the vulnerability of the visual cortex to metabolic derangements in view of its relatively high metabolic activity.

Hemophilus influenzae Meningitis

Cortical blindness is a frequent late complication of *Hemophilus influenzae* meningitis in children.[174] Its precise incidence unknown, cortical blindness appears relatively late in the course of the illness and often eventually disappears. The most likely mechanism is septic thrombophlebitis of dural sinuses with secondary infection or venous infarction of the visual cortex region.

Creutzfeldt-Jakob Disease

Creutzfeldt-Jakob Disease (CJD) is a dementing disorder of the elderly (age > 60 years) distinguished from more common forms of dementia (Alzheimer's disease, multi-infarct dementia) by relatively rapid progression over a period of weeks to months. In addition to cognitive decline, many patients have weakness, ataxia, and visual loss.

Now recognized as an infectious disease primarily involving the CNS gray matter, CJD is caused by an abnormal protein called a prion. How the prion enters brain tissue and causes cell death remains unclear. About 85% of cases are sporadic in origin, about 10% are familial, and 5% are iatrogenic—acquired through corneal transplantation, dural grafts, and growth hormone drawn from human pituitary glands.[175]

Magnetic resonance imaging may disclose subtle T2 high signal abnormalities in the cerebral cortex and basal ganglia but is *often normal*.[176] Diffusion-weighted MRI may highlight these abnormalities.[177] Spinal fluid examination often contains abnormal proteins found only in one other neurologic disease: herpes simplex encephalitis.[178,179] Initially

EEG discloses nonspecific background slowing, and eventually develops 1–2 triphasic sharp waves per second, which look electrocardiographic. Diagnosis is confirmed by brain biopsy, which reveals loss of neurons, vacuolation of the gray matter astrocytes and neuronal dendrites (spongioform encephalopathy), and a prominent reactive astrocytosis without evidence of inflammation.[180] Most brain specimens show amyloid precursor protein called "prion protein" by Western blot analysis.[175]

Many patients with CJD have visual spatial and recognition defects (Chapters 16, 17) in a setting of global cognitive decline. A minority of patients have depressed visual acuity, hemianopia, visual illusions, or visual hallucinations.[175,181,182] In a form of CJD known as the Heidenhain variant, cortical visual loss is the first or most prominent manifestation.[183–185] Spongioform cortical abnormalities are most pronounced in occipital regions. There is no treatment for any form of CJD.

Alzheimer's Disease and Nonspecific Dementias

The pathologically characterized chronic dementias are notable in sparing the primary visual cortex. Alzheimer's disease (AD) has a predilection for the parieto-occipital regions, causing prominent visuospatial deficits (Chapter 16), but visual acuity and fields are usually relatively intact if cognitive function permits adequate testing. However, pathologic study has shown that the primary visual cortex is not entirely spared in AD,[186] and as the disease advances, cortical blindness may set in. Among dementias of uncertain nosology, blindness may be a prominent feature, and the calcarine region is more heavily involved by pathologic abnormalities.[187]

DELAYED VISUAL MATURATION

Delayed visual maturation designates a phenomenon observed in infants who have extremely poor vision for the first 4 to 7 months of life and then catch up quickly to have normal vision by 12 months of age.[188]

Some have had perinatal distress with lingering neurologic abnormalities, but others have had normal birth histories and appear neurologically intact apart from poor vision. Given the presence of binocular vision loss, normal-appearing ocular structures, electroretinograms, and pupillary reactions, the deficits have been attributed to delayed development of some portion of the retrochiasmal visual pathway.[189] One theory is that the delay lies in synapse formation within the visual cortex, although no histologic material has been examined.[190] An alternative hypothesis is that the delayed development affects the retinocollicular pathway, believed to mediate rudimentary vision in the first months of life.[188]

SUMMARY

Damage to the posterior optic radiations and visual cortex typically produces homonymous hemianopias, visual illusions, and visual hallucinations. The homonymous hemianopias may display configurational features that are distinctive for this region: congruity, paracentral scotomas, macular sparing, quadrantic defects, crescent sparing, and bilateral defects.

The two exceptions to the rule that visual field loss from damage to this region is homonymous and hemianopic are (*1*) the monocular crescent defect, resulting from unilateral anterior calcarine cortex damage, and (*2*) amblyopia, a monocular visual acuity depression associated with cortical atrophy of ocular dominance columns owing to early childhood visual deprivation in the affected eye.

The posterior optic radiations and visual cortex are subject to temporary dysfunction by migraine, transient ischemic attack, seizure, and closed head injury. Distinguishing between them depends on the nature of the visual disturbance and the presence of accompanying neurologic manifestations.

Permanent optic radiation or visual cortex damage is most commonly the result of stroke from occlusion of branches of the posterior cerebral artery. The constellation of neurologic accompaniments to visual loss depends on the territory of the infarct. Less common causes of stroke in this region are occlusion of posterior branches of the middle cerebral artery, hypotension and hypoxia, venous sinus thrombosis, and lobar hemorrhage.

The posterior optic radiations are preferentially damaged by hypertensive encephalopathy, toxicity of certain systemically administered agents, progressive multifocal leukoencephalopathy, and childhood X-linked adrenoleukodystrophy. Acute disseminated encephalomyelitis and multiple sclerosis often create imaging abnormalities in this region but field loss is surprisingly uncommon.

The visual cortex is especially vulnerable to hypoxia, hypoglycemia, hepatic injury, mitochondrial encephalomyopathy, and some forms of meningitis. Some variants of Creutzfeldt-Jakob disease and chronic dementias may cause prominent visual disturbances.

REFERENCES

1. Horton JC, Hoyt WF. The representation of the visual field in human striate cortex: a revision of the classic Holmes map. *Arch Ophthalmol.* 1991;109: 816–824.
2. Wong AM, Sharpe JA. Representation of the visual field in the human occipital cortex: a magnetic resonance imaging and perimetric correlation. *Arch Ophthalmol.* 1999;117:208–217.
3. Kollias SS, Landau K, Khan N, et al. Functional evaluation using magnetic resonance imaging of the visual cortex in patients with retrochiasmal lesions. *J Neurosurg.* 1998;89:780–790.
4. Smith CG, Richardson WFG. The course and distribution of the arteries supplying the visual (striate) cortex. *Am J Ophthalmol.* 1966;61:1391–1396.
5. McFadzean R, Brosnahan D, Hadley D, Mutlukan E. Representation of the visual field in the occipital striate cortex. *Br J Ophthalmol.* 1994;78:185–190.
6. Gray LG, Galetta SL, Siegal T, Schatz NJ. The central visual field in homonymous hemianopia: evidence for unilateral foveal representation. *Arch Neurol.* 1997;54:312–317.
7. Landau K, Wichmann W, Valavanis A. The missing temporal crescent. *Am J Ophthalmol.* 1995;119: 345–349.
8. Chavis PS, Alhazmi A, Clunie D, Hoyt WF. Temporal crescent syndrome with magnetic resonance imaging. *J Neuro-ophthalmol.* 1997;17:151–155.
9. Benton S, Levy I, Swash M. Vision in the temporal crescent in occipital infarction. *Brain.* 1980; 103:83–97.
10. Meienberg O. Sparing of the temporal crescent in homonymous hemianopia and its significance for visual orientation. *Neuro-ophthalmology.* 1981;2: 129–134.

11. Nepple EW, Appen RE, Sackett JF. Bilateral homonymous hemianopia. *Am J Ophthalmol.* 1978; 86:536–543.

12. Miller NR, Newman NJ. Topical diagnosis of lesions in the visual sensory pathway. In: Miller NR, Newman NJ, eds. *Walsh & Hoyt's Clinical Neuro-ophthalmology.* 5th ed. Vol 1. Baltimore: Williams & Wilkins; 1998:237–386.

13. Newman RP, Kinkel WR, Jacobs L. Altitudinal hemianopia caused by occipital infarctions: clinical and computerized tomographic correlations. *Arch Neurol.* 1984;41:413–418.

14. Aldrich MS, Alessi AG, Beck RW, Gilman S. Cortical blindness: etiology, diagnosis and prognosis. *Ann Neurol.* 1987;21:149–158.

15. Brooks SE. Amblyopia. *Ophthalmol Clin North Am.* 1996;9(2):171–184.

16. Daw N. Critical periods and amblyopia. *Arch Ophthalmol.* 1998;116:502–505.

17. Donahue SP, Wall M, Kutzko KE, Kardon RH. Automated perimetry in amblyopia: a generalized depression. *Am J Ophthalmol.* 1999;127:312–321.

18. Lance JW. Current concepts of migraine pathogenesis. *Neurology.* 1993;43(suppl 3):S11–S15.

19. Stewart WF, Lipton RB, Celentano DD, Reed ML. Prevalence of migraine headache in the United States: relation to age, income, race, and other sociodemographic factors. *JAMA.* 1992;267:64–69.

20. Davidoff RA. *Migraine: Manifestations, Pathogenesis, and Management.* Philadelphia: FA Davis; 1995.

21. Welch KM. Pathogenesis of migraine. *Semin Neurol.* 1997;17:335–341.

22. Goadsby PJ. Current concepts of the pathophysiology of migraine. *Neurol Clin.* 1997;15:27–42.

23. Moskowitz MA. The neurobiology of vascular head pain. *Ann Neurol.* 1984;16:157–168.

24. Fisher CM. Late-life migraine accompaniments as a cause of unexplained transient ischemic attacks. 1980;7:9–17.

25. Hupp SL, Kline LB, Corbett JJ. Visual disturbances of migraine. *Surv Ophthalmol.* 1989;33:221–236.

26. Hachinski VC, Porchawka J, Steele JC. Visual symptoms in the migraine syndrome. *Neurology.* 1973; 23:570–579.

27. Alvarez WC. The migrainous scotoma as studied in 618 persons. *Am J Ophthalmol.* 1960;49:489–504.

28. Plant GT. The fortification spectra of migraine. *Br Med J.* 1986;293:1613–1617.

29. Hoyt WF. Transient bilateral blurring of vision: considerations of an episodic ischemic symptom of vertebro-basilar insufficiency. *Arch Ophthalmol.* 1963;70:746–751.

30. Penfield W, Jasper H. *Epilepsy and the Functional Anatomy of the Human Brain.* Boston: Little Brown; 1954.

31. Ludwig BI, Ajmone C. Clinical ictal patterns in epileptic patients with occipital electroencephalographic foci. *Neurology.* 1975;25:463–471.

32. Panayiotopoulos CP. Elementary visual hallucinations in migraine and epilepsy. *J Neurol Neurosurg Psychiatry.* 1994;57:1371–1374.

33. Williamson PD, Thadani VM, Darcey TM, Spencer DD, Spencer SS, Mattson RH. Occipital lobe epilepsy: clinical characteristics, seizure spread patterns, and results of surgery. *Ann Neurol.* 1992; 31:3–13.

34. Troost BT, Mark LE, Maroon JC. Resolution of classic migraine after removal of an occipital lobe AVM. *Ann Neurol.* 1979;5:199–201.

35. Riaz G, Hennessey JJ. Meningeal lesions mimicking migraine. *Neuro-ophthalmology.* 1991;11:41–48.

36. Kattah JC, Luessenhop AJ. Resolution of classic migraine after removal of an occipital lobe AVM. *Ann Neurol.* 1980;7:93.

37. Weiskrantz L, Warrington EK, Sanders MD, Marshall J. Visual capacity in the hemianopic field following a restricted occipital ablation. *Brain.* 1974; 97:709–728.

38. Kupersmith MJ, Vargas ME, Yashar A, et al. Occipital arteriovenous malformations: visual disturbances and presentation. *Neurology.* 1996;46:953–957.

39. Honda Y. Scintillating scotoma as the first symptom of systemic lupus erythematosus. *Am J Ophthalmol.* 1985;99:607–610.

40. Bousser MG, Tournier E. Summary of the proceedings of the first international workshop on CADASIL. *Stroke.* 1994;25:704–707.

41. Henrich JB, Sandercock PAG, Warlow CP, Jones LN. Stroke and migraine in the Oxfordshire Community Stroke Project. *J Neurol.* 1986;233:257–262.

42. Tatemichi TK, Mohr JP. Migraine and stroke. In: Barnett HJM, Mohr JP, Stein BM, Yatsu FM, eds. *Stroke. Pathophysiology, Diagnosis, and Management.* New York: Churchill Livingstone; 1992:761–785.

43. Henrich JB, Horwitz RI. A controlled study of ischemic stroke risk in migraine patients. *J Clin Epidemiol.* 1989;8:773–780.

44. Bousser MG. Migraine, female hormones, and stroke. *Cephalalgia.* 1999;19:75–79.

45. Becker WJ. Migraine and oral contraceptives. *Can J Neurol Sci.* 1997;24:16–21.

46. Connor RC. Complicated migraine: a study of permanent neurological and visual defects caused by migraine. *Lancet.* 1962;2:1072–1075.

47. Boisen E. Strokes in migraine: report on seven strokes associated with severe migraine attacks. *Danish Med Bull.* 1975;22:100–106.

48. Broderick JP, Swanson JW. Migraine-related strokes: clinical profile and prognosis in 20 patients. *Arch Neurol.* 1987;44:868–871.

49. Rothrock JF, Walicke P, Swenson MR, Lyden PD, Logan WR. Migrainous stroke. *Arch Neurol.* 1988; 45:63–67.

50. Bogousslavsky J, Regli F, Vanmelle G, Payot M, Uske A. Migraine stroke. *Neurology.* 1988;38:223–227.

51. Moen M, Levine SR, Newman DS, Dullbaird A, Brown GG, Welch KMA. Bilateral posterior cerebral artery strokes in a young migraine sufferer. *Stroke.* 1988;19:525–528.

52. Olesen J, Friberg L, Olsen TS, et al. Timing and topography of cerebral blood flow, aura, and headache during migraine attacks. *Ann Neurol.* 1990;28:791–798.

53. Welch KMA, Levine SR. Migraine-related stroke in the context of the International Headache Society classification of head pain. *Arch Neurol.* 1990; 47:458–462.

54. Levine SR, Joseph R, D'Andrea G, Welch KMA. Migraine and the lupus anticoagulant. *Cephalalgia.* 1987;7:93–99.

55. Goto Y, Horai S, Matsuoka T, et al. Mitochondrial myopathy, encephalopathy, lactic acidosis, and stroke-like episodes (MELAS): a correlative study of the clinical features and mitochondrial DNA mutation. *Neurology.* 1992;42:545–550.

56. Montagna P, Galassi R, Medori R, et al. MELAS syndrome: characteristic migrainous and epileptic features and maternal transmission. *Neurology.* 1988;38:751–754.

57. Shapira Y. Clinical aspects of mitochondrial encephalomyopathies. *Int Pediatr.* 1993;8:225–232.

58. Pavlakis SG, Phillips PC, DiMauro S, DeVivo DC, Rowland LF. Mitochondrial myopathy, encephalopathy, lactic acidosis, and stroke-like episodes: a distinctive clinical syndrome. *Ann Neurol.* 1984; 16:481–488.

59. Stroh EM, Winterkorn JMS, Jalkh AE, Lessell S. MELAS syndrome: a mitochondrially inherited disorder. *Int Ophthalmol Clin.* 1993;33:169–178.

60. Matthews PM, Tampieri D, Berkovic SF, et al. Magnetic resonance imaging shows specific abnormalities in the MELAS syndrome. *Neurology.* 1991; 41:1043–1046.

61. Sakuto R, Nonuka I. Vascular involvement in mitochondrial encephalomyopathy. *Ann Neurol.* 1989; 25:594–601.

62. Repka MX. Degenerative and metabolic diseases in infants and children. In: Miller NR, Newman NJ, eds. *Walsh & Hoyt's Clinical Neuro-Ophthalmology.* 5th ed. Vol 2. Baltimore: Williams & Wilkins; 1998:2811–2866.

63. Sue CM, Crimmins DS, Soo YS, et al. Neuroradiological features of six kindreds with MELAS tRNA (Leu) A2343G point mutation: implications of pathogenesis. *J Neurol Neurosurg Psychiat.* 1998;65: 233–240.

64. Kim IO, Kim WS, Hwang YS, Yeon KM, Han MC. Mitochondrial myopathy–encephalopathy lactic acidosis and stroke-like episodes (MELAS) syndrome: CT and MR findings in seven children. *AJR Am J Roentgenol.* 1996;166:641–645.

65. Carroll D. Retinal migraine. *Headache.* 1970;10:9–16.

66. Winterkorn JM, Burde RM. Vasospasm—not migraine—in the anterior visual pathway. *Ophthalmol Clin North Am.* 1996:393–405.

67. Burger SK, Saul RF, Selhorst JB, Thurston SE. Transient monocular blindness caused by vasospasm. *N Engl J Med.* 1991;325:870–873.

68. Winterkorn JMS, Kupersmith MJ, Wirtschafter JD, Forman S. Brief report: treatment of vasospastic amaurosis fugax with calcium-channel blockers. *N Engl J Med.* 1993;329:396–398.

69. Tippin J, Corbett JJ, Kerber RE, Schroeder E, Thompson HS. Amaurosis fugax and ocular infarction in adolescents and young adults. *Ann Neurol.* 1989;26:69–77.

70. Goodwin JA, Gorelick PB, Helgason CM. Symptoms of amaurosis fugax in atherosclerotic carotid artery disease. *Neurology.* 1987;37:829–833.

71. Headache Classification Committee, International Headache Society. Classification and diagnostic criteria for headache disorders, cranial neuralgias and facial pain. *Cephalalgia.* 1988;7(suppl 8):1–4.

72. Panayiotopoulos CP. Benign childhood epilepsy with occipital paroxysms: a 15-year prospective study. *Ann Neurol.* 1989;26:51–56.

73. Joseph JM, Louis S. Transient ictal cortical blindness during middle age: a case report and review of the literature. *J Neuro-ophthalmol.* 1995;15:39–42.

74. Jaffe SJ, Roach ES. Transient cortical blindness with occipital lobe epilepsy. *J Clin Neuro-ophthalmol.* 1988;8:221–224.

75. Penfield W, Perot P. The brain's record of auditory and visual experience. *Brain.* 1963;86:595–696.

76. Dobelle WH, Mladejovsky MG, Givin JP. Artificial vision for the blind: electrical stimulation of visual cortex offers hope for functional prosthesis. *Science.* 1974;183:440–444.

77. Brindley GS, Lewin WS. The sensations produced by electrical stimulation of the visual cortex. *J Physiol.* 1968;196:479–493.

78. Engel JL. *Seizures and Epilepsy.* Philadelphia: FA Davis; 1989:146.

79. Russell WR, Whitty WM. Studies in traumatic epilepsy: 3. Visual fits. *J Neurol Neurosurg Psychiatry.* 1955;18:79–96.

80. Barry E, Sussman NM, Bosley TM, Harner RN. Ictal blindness and status epilepticus amauroticus. *Epilepsia.* 1985;26:577–584.

81. Huott AD, Madison DS, Niedermeyer E. Occipital lobe epilepsy: a clinical and electroencephalographic study. *Neurology.* 1974;11:325–339.

82. Aldrich MS, Vanderzant CW, Alessi AG, Abou-Khalil B, Sackellares JC. Ictal cortical blindness with permanent visual loss. *Epilepsia.* 1989;30:116–120.

83. Zung A, Margalith D. Ictal cortical blindness: a case report and review of the literature. *Dev Med Child Neurol.* 1993;35:921–926.

84. Kosnik E, Paulson GW, Laguna JF. Post-ictal blindness. *Neurology.* 1976;26:248–250.

85. Panayiotopoulos CP. Difficulties in differentiating migraine and epilepsy based on clinical and EEG findings. In: Andermann F, Lugaresi E, eds. *Migraine and Epilepsy.* Boston: Butterworths; 1987:31–46.

86. Caplan LR. Vertebrobasilar occlusive disease. In: Barnett HJM, Mohr JP, Stein BM, Yatsu FM, eds. *Stroke.* Vol 1. Philadelphia: Churchill Livingstone; 1986:565.

87. Minor RH, Kearns TP, Millikan CH, Siekert RG, Sayre GP. Ocular manifestations of occlusive disease of the vertebro-basilar arterial system. *Arch Ophthalmol.* 1959;62:112–124.

88. Williams D, Wilson TG. The diagnosis of the major and minor syndromes of basilar insufficiency. *Brain.* 1962;85:741–774.

89. Dennis MS, Sandercock PAG, Bamford JM, Warlow CP. Lone bilateral blindness: a transient ischaemic attack. *Lancet.* 1989;1:185–189.

90. Fisher CM. The posterior cerebral artery syndrome. *Can J Neurol Sci.* 1986;13:232–239.

91. Griffith JF, Dodge PR. Transient blindness following head injury in children. *N Engl J Med.* 1968; 278:648–651.

92. Greenblatt SH. Posttraumatic transient cerebral blindness: association with migraine and seizure diatheses. *JAMA.* 1973;225:1073–1076.

93. Hochstetler K, Beals RD. Transient cortical blindness in a child. *Ann Emerg Med.* 1987;16:218–219.

94. Matthews WB. Footballer's migraine. *Br Med J.* 1972;2:326–327.

95. Castaigne P, Lhermitte F, Gautier JC, et al. Arterial occlusions in the vertebro-basilar system: a study of 44 patients with post-mortem data. *Brain.* 1973;96:133–154.

96. Pessin MS, Lathi ES, Cohen MB, Kwan ES, Hedges TR, Caplan LR. Clinical features and mechanism of occipital infarction. *Ann Neurol.* 1987;21:290–299.

97. Caplan LR, Tettenborn B. Vertebrobasilar occlusive disease: review of selected aspects: 2. Posterior circulation embolism. *Cerebrovasc Dis.* 1992;2:320–326.

98. Mehler MF. The rostral basilar artery syndrome: diagnosis, etiology, prognosis. *Neurology.* 1989;39:9–16.

99. Lindenberg R, Walsh FB, Sacks JG. *Neuropathology of Vision: An Atlas.* Philadelphia: Lea & Febiger; 1973:315–334.

100. Soza M, Tagle P, Kirkham T, Court J. Bilateral homonymous hemianopia with sparing of central vision after subdural hematoma. *Can J Neurol Sci.* 1987;14:153–155.

101. Margolis MT, Newton TH, Hoyt WF. Cortical branches of the posterior cerebral artery: anatomic–radiologic correlation. *Neuroradiology.* 1971;2:127–135.

101a. Mohr JP. Posterior cerebral artery. In Barnett HJM, Mohr JP, Stein BM, Yatsu FM eds. *Stroke. Pathophysiology, Diagnosis, and Management.* New York, 1986, Churchill-Livingston, pp. 451–474.

102. Kinkel WR, Newman RP, Jacobs L. Posterior cerebral artery branch occlusions: CT and anatomic considerations. In: Berguer R, Bauer RB, eds. *Vertebrobasilar Arterial Occlusive Disease: Medical and Surgical Management.* New York: Raven Press; 1984:117.

103. Caplan LR. "Top of the basilar" syndrome. *Neurology.* 1980;30:72–79.

104. Chambers BR, Brooder RJ, Donnan GA. Proximal posterior cerebral artery occlusion simulating middle cerebral artery occlusion. *Neurology.* 1991;41:385–390.

105. Hommel M, Besson G, Pollak P, Kahane P, Lebas JF, Perret J. Hemiplegia in posterior cerebral artery occlusion. *Neurology.* 1990;40:1496–1499.

106. Mehler MF. The neuro-ophthalmologic spectrum of the rostral basilar artery syndrome. *Arch Neurol.* 1988;45:966–971.

107. Barth A, Bogousslavsky J, Caplan LR, Thalamic infarcts and hemorrhages. In: Bogousslavksy J, Caplan L, eds. *Stroke Syndromes.* Cambridge, UK: Cambridge University Press; 1995:276–283.

108. Hommel M, Bogousslavsky J. The spectrum of vertical gaze palsy following unilateral brainstem stroke. *Neurology.* 1991;41:1229–1234.

109. Caplan LR, Dewitt LD, Pessin MS, Gorelick PB, Adelman LS. Lateral thalamic infarcts. *Arch Neurol.* 1988;45:959–964.

110. Stommel EW, Friedman RJ, Reeves AG. Alexia without agraphia associated with splenio-geniculate infarction. *Neurology.* 1991;41:587–588.

111. Caplan LR. Posterior cerebral artery. In: Bogousslavsky J, Caplan L, eds. *Stroke Syndromes.* Cambridge, UK: Cambridge University Press; 1995:290–299.

112. Devinsky O, Bear D, Volpe BT. Confusional states following posterior cerebral artery infarction. *Arch Neurol.* 1988;45:160–163.

113. DeRenzi E, Zambolin A, Crisi G. The pattern of neuropsychological impairment associated with left posterior cerebral artery infarcts. *Brain.* 1987;110:1099–1116.

114. Ajax ET, Schenkenberg T, Kosteljanetz M. Alexia without agraphia and the inferior splenium. *Neurology.* 1977;27:685–688.

115. Damasio AR, Damasio H. The anatomic basis of pure alexia. *Neurology.* 1983;33:1573–1583.

116. Iragui V, Kritchevsky M. Alexia without agraphia or hemianopia in parietal infarction. *J Neurol Neurosurg Psychiatry.* 1991;54:841.

117. Koehler PJ, Endtz LJ, Tevelde J, Hekster RE. Aware or non-aware: on the significance of awareness for the localization of the lesion responsible for homonymous hemianopia. *J Neurol Sci.* 1986;75:255–262.

118. Ross Russell RW. The posterior cerebral circulation. *J Royal Coll Phys.* 1973;7:331–336.

119. Ropper AH, Davis KR. Lobar cerebral hemorrhages: acute clinical syndromes in 26 cases. *Ann Neurol.* 1980;8:141–147.

120. Saver JL, Biller J. Superficial middle cerebral artery. In: Bogousslavsky J, Caplan L, eds. *Stroke Syndromes.* Cambridge, UK: Cambridge University Press; 1995:247–258.

121. Caplan LR, Kelly M, Kase CS, et al. Infarcts of the inferior division of the right middle cerebral artery. *Neurology.* 1986;36:1015–1020.

122. Myers RE. A unitary theory of causation of axonic and hypoxic brain pathology. In: Davis JN, Rowland LP, eds. *Advances in Neurology: Cerebral Hypoxia and Its Consequences.* New York: Raven Press; 1979.

123. Barkovich AJ. MR and CT evaluation of profound neonatal and infantile asphyxia. *AJNR Am J Neuroradiol.* 1992;13:79–83.

124. Howard R, Trend P, Ross Russell MD. Clinical features of ischemia in cerebral arterial border zones after periods of reduced cerebral blood flow. *Arch Neurol.* 1987;44:934–940.

125. Adams JH, Brierley JB, Connor RCR, Treip CS. The effects of systemic hypotension upon the human brain: clinical and neuropathological observations in 11 cases. *Brain.* 1966;89:235–268.

126. Monteiro J, Pena J, Genis D, Rubio F, Peres-Serra, Barraquer-Bordas L. Balint's syndrome: report of four cases with watershed parieto-occipital lesions from vertebrobasilar ischemia or systemic hypotension. *Acta Neurol Belg.* 1982;82:270–280.

127. Okazaki H. *Fundamentals of Neuropathology.* Tokyo: Igaku-Shoin; 1979:27–70.

128. Lambert SR, Hoyt CS, Jan JE, Barkovich J, Flodmark O. Visual recovery from hypoxic cortical blindness during childhood: computed tomographic and magnetic resonance imaging predictors. *Arch Ophthalmol.* 1987;105:1371–1377.

129. Osborne AG. *Diagnostic Neuroradiology.* St. Louis: Mosby; 1994:355–360.

130. Moster ML, Galetta SL, Schatz NJ. Physiologic functional imaging in "functional" visual loss. *Surv Ophthalmol.* 1996;40:395–399.

131. Gilman S. Cerebral disorders after open-heart operations. *N Engl J Med.* 1965;272:489–498.

132. Beal MF, Chapman PH. Cortical blindness and homonymous hemianopia in the postpartum period. *JAMA.* 1980;244:2085–2088.

133. Jacobs K, Moulin T, Bogousslavsky J, et al. The stroke syndrome of cortical vein thrombosis. *Neurology.* 1996;47:376–382.

134. Ameri A, Bousser M. Cerebral venous thrombosis. *Neurol Clin.* 1992;10(1):87–111.

135. Newman DS, Levine SR, Curtis VL, Welch KM. Migraine-like visual phenomena associated with cerebral venous thrombosis. *Headache.* 1989;29:82–85.

136. Purvin VA, Trobe JD, Kosmorsky GD. Neuro-ophthalmic features of cerebral venous obstruction. *Arch Neurol.* 1995;52:880–885.

137. Monteiro LR, Hoyt WF, Imes RK. Puerperal cerebral blindness: transient bilateral occipital involvement from presumed cerebral venous thrombosis. *Arch Neurol.* 1984;41:1300–1301.

138. Oppenheimer BS, Fishberg AM. Hypertensive encephalopathy. *Arch Intern Med.* 1928;41:264–278.

139. Jellinek EH, Painter M, Prineas J, RossRussell RW. Hypertensive encephalopathy with cortical disorders of vision. *Q J Med.* 1964;33:239–256.

140. Dinsdale HB. Hypertensive encephalopathy. In: Barnett HJM, Mohr JP, Stein BM, Yatsu FM, eds. *Stroke. Pathophysiology, Diagnosis, and Management.* Vol 2. New York: Churchill Livingstone; 1986:869–874.

141. Schwartz RB, Jones KM, Kalina P, et al. Hypertensive encephalopathy: findings on CT, MR imaging, and SPECT imaging in 14 cases. *AJR Am J Roentgenol.* 1992;159:379–383.

142. Digre KB, Varner MW, Osborn AG, Crawford S. Cranial magnetic resonance imaging in severe preeclampsia vs eclampsia. *Arch Neurol.* 1993;50:399–406.

143. Duncan R, Hadley D, Bone I, Symonds EM, Worthington BS, Rubin PC. Blindness in eclampsia: CT and MR imaging. *J Neurol Neurosurg Psychiatry.* 1989;52:899–902.

144. Raps EC, Galetta SL, Broderick M, Atlas SW. Delayed peripartum vasculopathy: cerebral eclampsia revisited. *Ann Neurol.* 1993;33:222–225.

145. Hinckey J, Chaves C, Appignani B, et al. A reversible posterior leukoencephalopathy syndrome. *N Engl J Med.* 1996;334:494–500.

146. Nag S, Robertson DM, Dinsdale HB. Cerebral cortical changes in acute experimental hypertension: an ultrastructural study. *Lab Invest.* 1977;36:150–161.

147. Beausang-Linder M, Bill A. Cerebral circulation in acute arterial hypertension: protective effects of sympathetic nervous activity. *Acta Physiol Scand.* 1981;111:193–199.

148. Edvinsson L, Owman C, Sjoberg N. Autonomic nerves, mast cells, and amine receptors in human brain vessel: a histochemical and pharmacological study. *Brain Res.* 1976;115:377–393.

149. DeGroen PC, Aksamit AJ, Rakela J, Forbes GS, Krom RAF. Central nervous system toxicity after liver transplantation: the role of cyclosporine and cholesterol. *N Engl J Med.* 1987;317:861–866.

150. Rubin AM, Kang H. Cerebral blindness and encephalopathy with cyclosporine A toxicity. *Neurology.* 1987;37:1072–1076.

151. Schwartz RB, Bravo SM, Klufas RA, et al. Cyclosporine neurotoxicity and its relationship to hypertensive encephalopathy: CT and MR findings in 16 cases. *AJR Am J Roentgenol.* 1995;165:627–631.

152. Bhatt BD, Meriano FV, Buchwald D. Cyclosporine-associated central nervous sytem toxicity. *N Engl J Med.* 1988;318:788.

153. Shutter LA, Green JP, Newman NJ, Hooks MA, Gordon RD. Cortical blindness and white matter lesions in a patient receiving FK506 after liver transplantation. *Neurology.* 1993;43:2417–2418.

154. Kupferschmidt H, Bont A, Schnorf H, et al. Transient cortical blindness and bioccipital brain lesions in two patients with acute intermittent porphyria. *Ann Intern Med.* 1995;123:598–600.

155. Lantos G. Cortical blindness due to osmotic disruption of the blood–brain barrier by angiographic contrast material: CT and MRI studies. *Neurology.* 1989;39:567–571.

156. Studdard WE, Davis DO, Young SW. Cortical blindness after cerebral angiography: case report. *J Neurosurg.* 1981;54:240–244.

157. Cohen RJ, Cuneo RA, Cruciger MP, Jackman AE. Transient left homonymous hemianopsia and encephalopathy following treatment of testicular carcinoma with cisplatinum, vinblastine, and bleomycin. *J Clin Oncol.* 1983;1:392–393.

158. Berger JR, Kaszovitz B, Post JD, Dickinson G. Progressive multifocal leukoencephalopathy associated with human immunodeficiency virus infection. *Ann Intern Med.* 1987;107:78–87.

159. Gillespie SM, Chang Y, Lemp G, et al. Progressive multifocal leukoencephalopathy in persons infected with human immunodeficiency virus, San Francisco, 1981–1989. *Ann Neurol.* 1991;30:597–604.

160. Chaisson RE, Griffin DE. Progressive multifocal leukoencephalopathy in AIDS. *JAMA.* 1990;264:79–82.

161. Slavin ML, Mallin JE, Jacob HS. Isolated homonymous hemianopsia in the acquired immunodeficiency syndrome. *Am J Ophthalmol.* 1989;108:198–200.

162. Butter CM, Trobe JD. Integrative agnosia following progressive multifocal leukoencephalopathy. *Cortex.* 1994;30:145–158.

163. Ormerod LD, Rhodes RH, Gross SA, Crane LR, Houchin KW. Ophthalmologic manifestations of acquired immune deficiency syndrome-associated progressive multifocal leukoencephalopathy. *Ophthalmology.* 1996;103:899–906.

164. Traboulsi EI, Maumenee IH. Ophthalmologic manifestations of childhood X-linked adrenoleukodystrophy. *Ophthalmology.* 1987;94:47–52.

165. Schaumburg HH, Powers JH, Raine CS, Suzuki K, Richardson EP Jr. Adrenoleukodystrophy: a clinical and pathological study of 17 cases. *Arch Neurol.* 1975;32:577–591.

166. Kendall BE. Disorders of lysosomes, peroxisomes, and mitochondria. *AJNR. Am J Neuroradiol.* 1992;13:621–653.

167. Moser HW, Kok F, Neumann S. Adrenoleukodystrophy update: genetics and effect of Lorenzo's oil therapy in asymptomatic patients. *Int Pediatr.* 1994;9:196–204.

168. Sedwick LA, Klingele TG, Burde RM, Fulling KH, Gado MH. Schilder's (1912) disease: total cerebral

blindness due to acute demyelination. *Arch Neurol.* 1986;43:85–87.

169. Hawkins K, Behrens MM. Homonymous hemianopia in multiple sclerosis. With report of bilateral case. *Br J Ophthalmol.* 1975;59:334–337.

170. Beck RW, Savino PJ, Schatz NJ, Smith CH, Sergott RC. Plaque causing homonymous hemianopsia in multiple sclerosis identified by computed tomography. *Am J Ophthalmol.* 1982;94:229–234.

171. Garty BZ, Dinari G, Nitzan M. Transient acute cortical blindness associated with hypoglycemia. *Pediatr Neurol.* 1987;3:169–170.

172. Miyata Y, Motomura S, Tsuji Y, Koga S. Hepatic encephalopathy and reversible cortical blindness. *Am J Gastroenterol.* 1988;83:780–782.

173. Moel DI, Kwun YA. Cortical blindness as a complication of hemodialysis. *J Pediatr.* 1978;93:890–891.

174. Ackroyd RS. Cortical blindness following bacterial meningitis: a case report with reassessment of prognosis and aetiology. *Dev Med Child Neurol.* 1984;26:227–230.

175. Brown P, Gibbs CJ, Rodgers-Johnson P, et al. Human spongiform encephalopathy: the National Institutes of Health series of 300 cases of experimentally transmitted disease. *Ann Neurol.* 1994; 35:513–529.

176. Finkenstaedt M, Szudra A, Zerr I, et al. MR imaging of Creutzfeldt-Jakob disease. *Radiology.* 1996; 199:793–798.

177. Demaerel P, Heiner L, Robberecht W, Sciot R, Wilms G. Diffusion-weighted MRI in sporadic Creutzfeldt-Jakob disease. *Neurology.* 1999;52:205–208.

178. Harrington MG, Merril CR, Asher DM, Gajdusek DC. Abnormal proteins in the cerebrospinal fluid of patients with Creutzfeldt-Jakob disease. *N Engl J Med.* 1986;315:279–283.

179. Blisard KS, Davis LE, Harrington MG, Lovell JK, Kornfeld M, Berger ML. Pre-mortem diagnosis of Creutzfeldt-Jakob disease by detection of abnormal cerebrospinal fluid proteins. *J Neurol Sci.* 1990;99:75–81.

180. Brown P, Cathala F, Castaigne P, Gajdusek DC. Creutzfeldt-Jakob disease: clinical analysis of a consecutive series of 230 neuropathologically verified cases. *Ann Neurol.* 1986;20:597–602.

181. Vargas ME, Kupersmith MJ, Savino PJ, Petito F, Frohman LP, Warren FA. Homonymous field defect as the first manifestation of Creutzfeldt-Jakob disease. *Am J Ophthalmol.* 1995;119:497–504.

182. Purvin V, Bonnino J, Goodman J. Palinopsia as a presenting manifestation of Creutzfeldt-Jakob disease. *J Clin Neuro-ophthalmol.* 1989;9:242–246.

183. Heidenhain A. Klinische und anatomische Untersuchungen über eine eigenartige organishce Erkrankung des Zentralnervensystems im Praesenium. *Z Gesamte Neurol Psychiatr.* 1928;118:49–114.

184. Meyer A, Leigh D, Bagg CT. A rare presenile dementia associated with cortical blindness (Heidenhain's syndrome). *J Neurol Neurosurg Psychiatry.* 1954;17:129–133.

185. Kropp S, Schulz-Schaeffer WJ, Finkenstaedt M, et al. The Heidenhain variant of Creutzfeldt-Jakob disease. *Arch Neurol.* 1999;56:55–61.

186. Hof PR, Bouras C, Constantinidis J, Morrison JH. Balint's syndrome in Alzheimer's disease: specific disruption of the occipito-parietal visual pathway. *Brain Res.* 1989;493:368–375.

187. Nadeau SE, Bebin J, Smith E. Nonspecific dementia, cortical blindness, and Congophilic angiopathy: a clinicopathological report. *J Neurol.* 1987;234:14–18.

188. Tresidder J, Fielder AR, Nicholson J. Delayed visual maturation: ophthalmic and neuro-developmental aspects. *Dev Med Child Neurol.* 1990;32: 872–881.

189. Lambert SR, Kriss A, Taylor D. Delayed visual maturation: a longitudinal clincial and electrophysiological assessment. *Ophthalmology.* 1989;96:524–528.

190. Hoyt CS, Jastrzebski G, Marg E. Delayed visual maturation in infancy. *Br J Ophthalmol.* 1983;67:127–130.

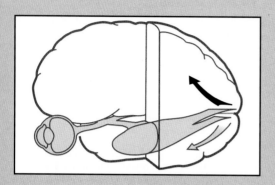

PARIETAL VISION-RELATED CORTEX

Lesions of the parietal vision-related cortex and its incoming pathways (Fig. 1-29) cause visual illusions (Chapter 4) and deficits related to the distribution of visual attention and the perception and manipulation of items in space (Table 16-1).

Patients with attentional deficits fail to notice parts of objects. As a result, the objects may not be recognized, even though feature analysis of their components may be correctly performed. The spatial relationships of objects, parts of objects, and moving objects often appear so disordered that they create a jumbled impression.

These deficits also create very abnormal behavior. Patients with *unilateral* occipito-parietal lesions may confine their attention and actions to ipsilesional hemispace. Those

with *bilateral* lesions may keep their eyes fixed on a target, walking cautiously with outstretched arms, yet colliding with obstacles slightly eccentric to fixation. Based on standard visual acuity and visual field tests, such patients would not be considered blind. Yet they behave as if they had searchlight vision, or "blinders" that interfere with peripheral vision.

HEMISPATIAL NEGLECT

Clinical Features

Patients with hemispatial neglect fail to "report, respond, or orient to novel or meaningful stimuli presented to the side opposite

Table 16–1. **Parieto-Occipital Vision Disorders**

Condition	Impairment	Localization	Mechanism
Hemispatial neglect	Ignoring stimuli in one hemispace Reduced movements in one hemispace Low arousal state	Unilateral parietal (mainly right)	Unilateral damage to parietal attentional center or its inputs
Bilateral visual inattention*	Not attending to more than one object at a time	Bilateral occipitoparietal	Bilateral damage to parietal attentional centers or their inputs
Acquired ocular motor apraxia*	Loss of pursuit and most saccades (spontaneous and reflexive saccades spared)	Bilateral parietal	Bilateral damage to parietal centers for generating eye movements
Optic ataxia*	Visually guided misreaching for objects	Parietal	Loss of retinotopic-craniotopic transformation or visuomotor disconnection
Impaired spatial relations*	Misjudging distance and size of objects	Occipitoparietal (mainly right)	Damage to parietal center governing space sense
Akinetopsia	Not detecting motion	Bilateral occipito-temporoparietal junction (MT, V5)	Damage to motion center

*Components of the Balint-Holmes syndrome.

a brain lesion when this failure cannot be attributed to either sensory or motor defects."[1](p 279)

In acute and extreme cases, patients do not acknowledge their own body parts or their neurologic deficits (anosognosia) on the contralesional side, and they keep their eyes deviated away from that side. In less extreme and resolving cases, they ignore sensory stimuli in the contralesional hemispace, leave out details that belong in that space when drawing or copying pictures, make fewer movements into that space, and misreach and navigate toward the lesioned side. In the mildest cases, the deficit may be merely a response bias in favor of the ipsilesional hemispace elicited by double simultaneous visual, auditory, or tactile stimulation (extinction), line or letter cancellation, or horizontal line bisection.

Hemispatial neglect may invade mental imagery. Asked to describe from memory the details of the Duomo (main cathedral) in Milan, two Milanese patients with right parietal lesions omitted all the features visible on the Duomo's left side when they were told to imagine they were facing it and omitted all the details on its right side when they were told to imagine the cathedral behind them.[2]

Five features of hemispatial neglect are crucial to diagnosis. Neglect is

- **Lateralized.** Attentional and intentional responses are reduced in one hemispace. Responses may be slightly reduced within the intact hemispace,[3] but the discrepancy between the affected and unaffected hemispaces is basic.
- **Body-centered rather than visual field–centered.** Hemispheric control of attention is governed by hemispaces (one-half of the body and extrapersonal space) rather than hemifields. The coordinates of hemispaces are based on the orientation of the head and body (craniotopic).

By contrast, the coordinates of hemifields are defined by the visual fixation point of the eyes (retinotopic). To execute accurate limb movements into extrapersonal space, the brain must convert retinotopic to craniotopic information. This occurs in the posterior parietal cortex, where neuronal firing adjusts for eye position.[4] When eyes are fixating a target straight ahead, craniotopic and field coordinates are aligned; when the eyes are gazing eccentrically, the coordinates are not aligned. This dissociation provides the rationale for a clinical test to distinguish visual field defects from hemispatial visual neglect (see below).

- **Multimodal.** Auditory, tactile, and visual perception are all damaged, although not necessarily to the same degree.
- **Manifested in sensory, motor, and motivational deficits.** The sensory deficit consists of ignoring stimuli in the contralesional hemispace; the motor deficit involves performing reduced movements and tasks in that hemispace; the motivational deficit is a reduced arousal to stimuli presented anywhere, but particularly in contralesional space.
- **Influenced by priming.** Neglect can be reduced by stimulating the inattentive hemispace[1,5–7]and increased by stimulating the intact hemispace.[8]

Hemispatial neglect occurs most commonly after acute stroke. Its intensity is related to the size of the infarct and the degree of preexisting brain atrophy.[9] Manifestations become less pronounced within the first few weeks after the stroke, after which there is little change.[9] Rehabilitative efforts based on stimulating the affected hemispace have had impressive short-term effects within the laboratory milieu but no sustained impact on activities of daily living.[5]

Pathophysiology

Hemispatial neglect usually derives from unilateral lesions of the posterior parietal region (Brodmann's areas 39 and 40) (Fig. 16-1), but lesions in the cingulate and dorsolateral frontal gyri, neostriatum, thalamus, and mesencephalic reticular formation can cause it as well.[1]

What do these lesions have in common? They all lie within the brain's arousal–attention circuit, which primes the posterior parietal cortex. Neurons in this region in monkeys fire in response to the presence of rewarding objects in contralateral hemispace.[10,11] Clinical, pathological, and experimental data favor the theory that neglect is a disorder of spatially directed attention caused by a lesion of the posterior parietal region or its activator circuits.[1,12]

Hemispatial neglect is more profound and enduring in patients with right-sided than left-sided cerebral lesions.[13] This phenomenon is explained by positing that the right cerebral hemisphere attends more to left hemispace than right hemispace, whereas the left hemisphere attends *only to right hemispace*.[14] A right-sided lesion would then deprive the brain of attention to left hemispace, whereas a left-sided lesion would still allow some attention to right hemispace.

Left   Right

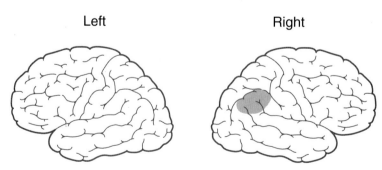

Figure 16–1. Hemispatial neglect. Schematic shows a right posterior parietal lesion, the most common site of damage in patients with hemispatial neglect.

Differential Diagnosis

Although hemispatial neglect is a spatially directed disorder of attention, its visual component looks clinically like a hemianopia. The distinction between these two disorders is important. Although hemispatial neglect tends to improve more than hemianopia, it is much more disabling. Hemianopic patients are, in some regions, permitted to drive a car, as they can usually "work around" their hemianopias. Even the mildest hemispatial neglect is dangerous because patients are unaware of what they are missing. Hemispatial neglect is differentiated from hemianopia by the following findings (Boxes 16-1, 16-2; Table 16-2).

EXTINCTION TO DOUBLE SIMULTANEOUS STIMULATION IN MORE THAN ONE SENSORY MODALITY

Extinction occurs if a stimulus goes unrecognized when an identical stimulus is presented concurrently in the opposite hemispace. Perhaps the rival stimulus draws on the marginal attentional reserve available to the affected hemispace.[8] *Visual extinction occurs in patients with either hemispatial neglect or subtotal hemianopias,* so one must demonstrate it in at least one other sensory modality (auditory, tactile) to make a diagnosis of neglect.

EXTINCTION IN HEMISPACES RATHER THAN HEMIFIELDS

Because visual fields and attentional hemispaces have different coordinates, they can be dissociated by shifting the eyes out of straight-ahead gaze. Double simultaneous static stimulation is serially performed in gaze forward, gaze right, and gaze left positions. If patients have left hemispatial neglect (from a right parietal lesion), they should be able to identify fingers displayed in the left hemifield much better when the eyes are in right gaze than when they are in left gaze.[15,16] This technique is not perfectly reliable.

Box 16–1

HEMIANOPIA OR HEMISPATIAL NEGLECT? DOUBLE SIMULTANEOUS STIMULATION TESTS

1. Perform standard confrontation field testing with single fingers (Chapter 7). If patients fail to identify fingers in one hemifield, go to Step 4 to test for tactile and auditory neglect. If all fingers are identified, go to Step 2.

2. Present single or double fingers simultaneously on either side of the vertical fixational meridian. If patients detect all fingers, hemianopia and neglect are very unlikely. If patients fail to detect the fingers in one hemifield, go to Step 3.

3. With the patient's eyes first in right gaze, then in left gaze, repeat double simultaneous testing as before. If extinction is consistently less with the eyes deviated toward the intact hemispace than with the eyes deviated toward the affected hemispace, the diagnosis of hemispatial neglect is likely.

4. Test for neglect in the tactile and auditory modalities. Position your hands in front of both ears and rub together the fingers of one hand or the other to create sound. Then rub fingers of both hands together simultaneously. With the patients' eyes closed or gaze averted, touch an extremity on one side or the other, then simultaneously. To enhance the sensitivity of this maneuver, touch the face (stronger stimulus) on the intact side and an extremity on the affected side simultaneously. Consistent lack of hearing or tactile awareness on one side suggests multimodal neglect.

Box 16–2

HEMIANOPIA OR HEMISPATIAL NEGLECT? CONSTRUCTION TESTS

1. *Line cancellation.* Draw 30 evenly spaced line segments 2 cm in length in various orientations on a blank page. Instruct patients to "cancel" each segment once by drawing a perpendicular line through it. A consistent failure to cross out lines in a hemifield suggests hemispatial inattention.

2. *Letter cancellation.* Scatter different alphabet letters across a blank page, interspersing a particular letter (A, for example) more frequently.[70] Instruct patients to cancel all the A's. This is a somewhat more demanding test of attention than line cancellation.

3. *Line bisection.* Draw a single 20 cm line segment horizontally across a blank page. Display it to patients by sequentially touching its extremes. Instruct them to draw a short perpendicular line through its midpoint to divide it in half. Repeat this sequence four times. Consistent unidirectional deviation of the mark away from the midpoint suggests hemispatial inattention.[71] Repeat the same sequence after having placed the patient's index finger on the two margins of the line. With this proprioceptive cueing, line bisection usually becomes more accurate in hemispatial inattention.

4. *Copying figures.* Instruct patients to copy a simple line drawing of a house, flower, or a box. Displacement of elements into a hemispace suggests hemispatial neglect.

5. *Picture interpretation.* Select a magazine or newspaper photograph that contains interacting elements. Ask patients first to identify the components. If they consistently miss components in left hemispace, they have either hemispatial neglect or a hemianopia. Point out the missed components and emphasize that they lie in left hemispace. Show them another image. Marked improvement suggests a hemianopia, because patients with neglect usually continue to ignore one hemispace, whereas patients with hemianopia, once cued, correct their error.

Table 16–2. **Hemispatial Neglect versus Hemianopia**

Test Result	Hemispatial Neglect	Hemianopia
Extinction to double simultaneous visual stimulation	++	+
Extinction to double simultaneous tactile stimulation	++	−
Extinction to double simultaneous auditory stimulation	++	−
Extinction altered by using hemispaces instead of hemifields	+	−
Extinction reduced by priming	++	+
Items in hemispace omitted in line/letter cancellation	++	−
Bisection of line segment biased toward intact hemispace	++	−
Eyes more often gaze toward intact hemispace	++	−
Misreaching toward intact hemispace	++	−
Component in affected hemispace left out of drawing/copying	++	−

EXTINCTION REDUCED BY PRIMING

Hemispatial neglect can be attenuated by previewing the task, drawing attention to the weak side by intermittently pointing out the stimulus, and motivating the patient to perform the task. If these maneuvers markedly reduce the hemifield loss, the deficit is more likely to be neglect.

SPATIAL BIAS IN LINE CANCELLATION, LINE BISECTION, AND OTHER DIRECTIONALLY BASED MOTOR ACTIVITY

Patients with hemispatial neglect generally bisect lines ipsilesional to the midpoint,[17] fail to cancel arrays of lines and letters in the neglected hemispace, and leave out components in drawing and copying that fall into neglected hemispace.[18,19] They have horizontal gaze and gestural preference, misreaching, and ambulation in the direction of the lesion. *Patients who have hemianopia without neglect never behave this way.*

BILATERAL SPATIAL NEGLECT: THE BALINT-HOLMES SYNDROME

A lesion that involves both posterior parietal lobes may give rise to a spectacular and mystifying constellation of neurologic signs and symptoms known as the Balint-Holmes syndrome. In its complete form, this syndrome has four components: (*1*) bilateral visual inattention; (*2*) ocular motor apraxia, an impairment of volitional eye movements; (*3*) optic ataxia, a disorder characterized by visually guided misreaching for objects, and (*4*) impaired spatial relations. Minor forms of this syndrome are recognized if one or more components are present (see below).

Our understanding of this syndrome is due to sequential contributions by a Hungarian, English, German, and Russian scientist. In 1909, the Hungarian neurologist Rezso Balint[20] described a patient who had suffered biparietal and left frontal strokes. The patient paid little attention to stimuli on the left side of visual fixation—an example of hemispatial neglect. But he also failed to move his eyes to eccentric visual stimuli displayed in either hemifield, misreaching for these stimuli.

Ten years later in England, Gordon Holmes[21,22] reported seven World War I veterans who had sustained biparietal gunshot wounds and displayed the findings of Balint's patient, together with a failure to identify the absolute and relative size and shape of objects. In applying the term "visual disorientation" to this complex, Holmes emphasized the patients' disordered perception of spatial relations.

Several years later in Germany, Isaac Wolpert[23] pointed out that patients with similarly placed lesions could identify the components of a scene but not integrate them into an understanding of what was going on. Wolpert called this deficit "simultanagnosia." Three decades later, the Russian neuropsychologist Alexander Luria[24,25] interpreted simultanagnosia as a basic inability to recognize more than one object at a time.

"Visual disorientation" prevailed as a collective term to describe this symptom complex until recently, when a greater focus on the object recognition aspects led to a reemphasis of "simultanagnosia." In this chapter, the term "bilateral visual inattention" is used instead of simultanagnosia or visual disorientation because it places the emphasis on the underlying deficit, *a failure to attend to more than one component of a visual array* ("searchlight vision").

Most acute cases of Balint-Holmes syndrome derive from lesions lying in the dorsal occipital (cuneus, Brodmann's areas 19, 39) and occipitoparietal regions (precuneus, Brodmann's area 7) (Fig. 3-2). They are principally the result of hypotension or hypoxia and, less often, bilateral posterior cerebral artery occlusions, sagittal sinus thrombosis, demyelination, tumor, or trauma (Fig. 16-2).[26] Evolving visuospatial manifestations are increasingly recognized in Alzheimer's disease (Fig. 16-2*d*).[27–29]

Small lesions can produce minor versions of the Balint-Holmes syndrome that display only one or two components.[30–34] We turn now to a discussion of each, starting with the most important, bilateral visual inattention.

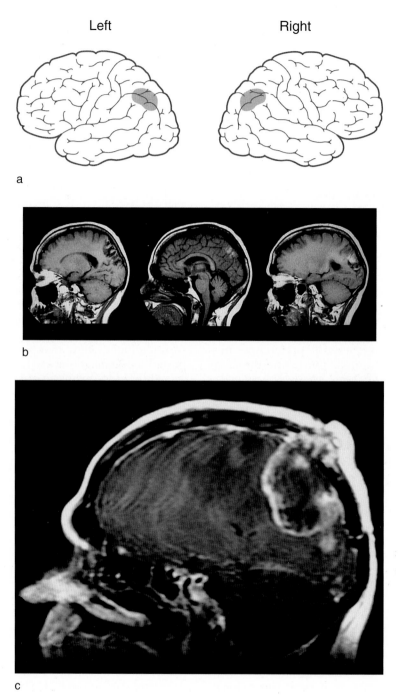

Left   Right

a

b

c

Figure 16–2. Balint-Holmes Syndrome. (*a*) Schematic shows bilateral posterior parietal lesions. (*b*) T1-weighted sagittal MRI sections show biparietal watershed hemorrhagic strokes in a 65-year-old woman who suffered a myocardial infarction. (*c*) T1-weighted sagittal MRI in a 50-year-old man with parafalcine meningioma.

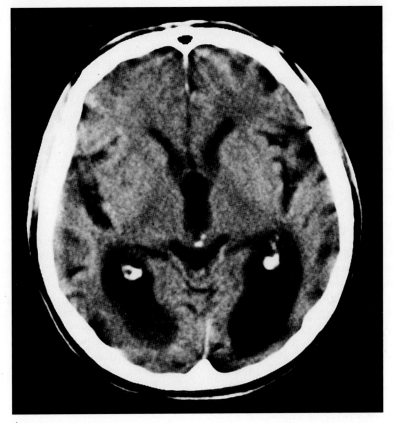

d

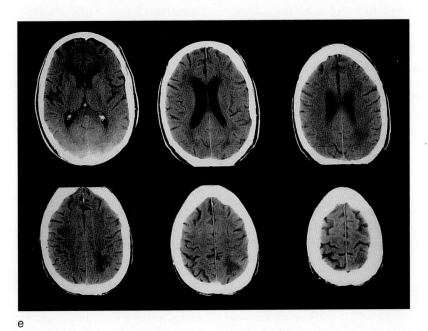

e

Figure 16–2. (*continued*) Balint-Holmes Syndrome. (*d*) CT shows marked parieto-occipital cerebral volume loss in a patient with Alzheimer's disease. (*e*) CT shows biparietal hypodensities in a 70-year-old man who had undergone a coronary artery bypass graft and developed hypotension. His principal difficulties were impaired puzzle construction, wayfinding, and optic ataxia (misreaching) of the right hand.

Bilateral Visual Inattention

Patients with bilateral visual inattention have a reduced response to stimuli presented on either side of visual fixation, reduced ability to detect more than one visual object at the same moment, and reduced ability to combine several viewed objects into a meaningful composite.

CHIEF COMPLAINTS

Patients complain of tunnel vision, objects fading in and out of sight, bumping into obstacles, and trouble reading and interpreting pictures. A minority report difficulty judging spatial relations (see "Impaired Spatial Relations," below), and loss of three-dimensional depth perception.

VISUAL FUNCTION TESTS

Visual acuity and color vision are intact. In severe cases, the visual field is dramatically constricted. One of Holmes's patients did not flinch as the examiner's hand was thrust at his face from either side, yet reacted briskly when the patient's own hand was waved at him.[21] In more moderate cases, a stimulus may be detected on one exposure and missed on the next, even when its position does not change. Visual stimuli may suddenly disappear from fixation even as the eyes continue to stare at them.[35]

In the mildest cases, the visual field is normal, but only if one eccentric stimulus is displayed at a time. When two eccentric stimuli are introduced into the visual field at the same time, patients are likely to see only one stimulus initially; the second may come into view moments later. But when the second stimulus is finally seen, the first has disappeared. Multiple stimuli are more likely to be seen simultaneously if stimulus presentation is preceded by a warning that they are about to be displayed (priming, cueing) (Box 16-3).

At all levels of severity, peripheral fields will be larger if the fixation target is removed and the patient asked to stare straight ahead into featureless space. Apparently, an interesting fixation target consumes enough central attention that peripheral attention cannot compete. Thus formal automated perimetry, which uses a central fixation target, invariably produces an inconsistent and severely constricted field. An important clue to diagnosis of this condition is the large discrepancy between relatively intact visual fields to cued, single-finger confrontation without an interesting fixation target and depressed visual fields to uncued, standard multiple-finger confrontation or automated field testing.

READING

Patients typically make no errors when asked to read letters. But as the letters are combined into words and the words into sentences, the errors grow. They are not phonemic errors, as patients with aphasia would make, but errors of leaving out and inserting parts or entire words and phrases. As they read, patients will report that words seem to jump around or disappear. The term "spatial alexia" has been applied to this deficit.[36]

INTERPRETING PICTURES

Even single objects are often misidentified because of a failure to "take in" all relevant features. Shown a picture of a baseball, a patient of mine was distracted by the seam and called it "railroad tracks" (Fig. 16-3). Handed a dollar bill, another patient's attention was drawn to the picture of George Washington in its center; he identified the man, not the money.[30] The more detailed the picture, the more likely the patient will be misled by an internal element and make an error in identification.

Challenged to interpret the action or meaning of a scene, patients ploddingly but correctly identify the components, but then cannot describe their interactions. Their searchlight vision haphazardly scans the scene and fails to incorporate material from each sighting. Although standard pictures are used in formal evaluations, magazine photographs will serve to bring out this deficit. Less severely affected patients may appear to interpret pictures correctly yet complain that they do not always understand what they are seeing. Their inattention deficit may appear as an abnormal delay in identifying multiple objects displayed simultaneously on a tachistoscope.

Box 16–3

BALINT-HOLMES SYNDROME: SCREENING FOR BILATERAL VISUAL INATTENTION

Whereas standard visual field testing (Chapter 7) is designed to detect form and luminance deficits of the retinocortical pathway, the following techniques aim to detect visual attentional deficits of the integrative visual pathway.

1. *Presenting multiple static stimuli within a field quadrant.* Perform standard confrontation field testing with single fingers first (Chapter 7). If patients identify all single fingers, present two fingers in a single quadrant. If patients consistently fail to notice the second finger, keep varying the relative positions of the fingers to eliminate position as a variable. Persistent failure to notice both fingers suggests inattention within the quadrant, a sign of Balint-Holmes syndrome.

2. *Eliminating the fixation target in confrontation field testing.* Instead of having patients fixate your eye or nose, have them peer straight ahead into as featureless a space as is possible (white wall). Repeat finger confrontation as in Step 1. If peripheral stimuli are more consistently detected when there is no competing fixation target, the diagnosis is likely to be bilateral visual inattention.

3. *Counting arrays of objects.* Display a single coin or pen and instruct patients to identify the object and how many are present. If they are successful, display five coins or pens and instruct the patients to count them by sight. If they consistently make errors, allow the patients to pick up each item as they are counting them. If tactile contact clearly improves the counting accuracy, visual inattention is likely.

4. *Reading.* Given a paragraph to read, patients with Balint-Holmes syndrome typically make no lexical errors, but they compress words, omit words or parts of words, and jumble word order. These errors reflect attentional and spatial relations disorders.

5. *Interpreting pictures.* Select a magazine or newspaper photograph that contains interacting elements. Ask patients first to identify the components. If they correctly identify the components of a scene, instruct them to describe the action. A failure to do so suggests bilateral visual inattention.

COUNTING ARRAYS

A second object may go unnoticed unless it is small enough to share the fixational space with the first object. A valuable diagnostic test that brings out this phenomenon is a display of a horizontal array of coins or pens. Instructed to tote them up, most patients will miscount unless they are allowed the proprioceptive input of running the items through their fingers.[21]

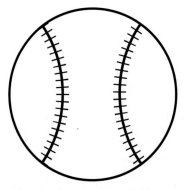

Figure 16–3. Searchlight vision in Balint-Holmes syndrome. The patient identified this picture as "railroad tracks."

AMBULATION

Patients with bilateral visual inattention often walk very cautiously and haltingly. Holmes and Horrax said of one patient that "he progressed with short, slow steps, his hands held out in front of him like a man groping his way in the dark. When asked to go across the ward, he invariably walked into any obstacle in his way, even though it was large and prominent and he had observed it before he started."[22(p 400)]

EYE MOVEMENTS

Patients cannot move their eyes to targets in extrapersonal visual space. Holmes and

Horrax wrote evocatively about an affected patient that

> he moved his eyes to order readily and accurately in every direction, but . . . if spoken to suddenly, he first stared in a wrong direction and then moved his eyes about until they fell, as if by chance, on the observer's face; he was extremely slow and inaccurate in his attempts to fix or bring into central vision any object when its image fell in the periphery of his retinae. . . . When, however, requested to look at his own finger or to any point of his body which was touched he did so promptly and accurately . . . he succeeded in keeping his eyes on the fixation point . . . but if they deviated from it for even a moment he was slow and awkward in finding it again. When an object at which he was staring was moved at a slow and uniform rate, he could keep his eyes on it, but if it was jerked or moved abruptly, it quickly disappeared from his central vision.[22]

PATHOPHYSIOLOGY

Single-cell recordings in monkeys affirm that the parietooccipital junction is activated during visual attentional tasks.[11,37] The behavior of patients with Balint-Holmes syndrome can be attributed to various disorders of attention. For example, difficulty seeing peripheral targets when there is an engrossing fixation target may represent delayed disengagement of attention.[8] An impaired ability to see more than one item at a time, together with the spontaneous disappearance of viewed objects, is best explained by an inability to sustain attention across a spatial array.[38] In a well-documented experiment, a biparietally lesioned patient disengaged attention normally but, in staring at a display of twinkling lights against a dark background ("starry night"), did not notice the appearance or disappearance of stationary lights, especially when the array was dense.[38] Dubbed the "cocktail party effect," this phenomenon is based on the fact that competing stimuli so overwhelm the attentional system that no sensory information is registered.

The lesions of bilateral visual inattention are in the same territory as those of hemispatial neglect.[39,40] Indeed, a patient who initially had right hemispatial neglect following a left parietal stroke later developed bilateral visual inattention when the nearly equivalent right parietal region was infarcted.[41] Objects were recognized only at fixation. The lesions were centered at the posterior intraparietal sulcus (Fig. 16-4). Interestingly, many patients with Balint-Holmes syndrome—including Balint's own patient—have had asymmetric deficits, and the greater the asymmetry, the more the patients look like they suffer from hemispatial neglect. Patients with hemispatial neglect resemble those with bilateral visual inattention in extinguishing one of two stimuli presented simultaneously *within* the affected hemispace.[42]

LESIONS

Bilateral visual inattention is encountered in two principal settings: (*1*) hypoxic-ischemic encephalopathy following systemic hypotension or respiratory compromise; or (*2*) Alzheimer's disease. In either setting, patients or their caregivers must be advised that crossing streets or driving a car could be dangerous because the patients' useful field of view (attentional field) is much narrower than standard testing indicates. There is firm evidence that the size of the attentional field is the best predictor of car crashes in the elderly.[43–45]

DIFFERENTIAL DIAGNOSIS

Bilateral visual attention is sometimes misdiagnosed as bilateral homonymous hemianopia with macular sparing. But within their narrow field, patients with bilateral hemianopia reach accurately, count arrays of objects correctly, and interpret pictures properly. In other words, their tiny visual field eventually gathers in all the findings. Their mobility may be impaired, but if given the time to look about, they can interpret visual scenes without difficulty.

Alternatively, patients with bilateral visual inattention may be called malingerers. After all, they have normal visual acuity, single-finger visual fields, and an otherwise intact neurologic examination. Yet they grope as they walk, miscount arrays of objects, misinterpret pictures, and make inaccurate eye movements. Such a combination of findings is bound to tax the physician's credulity.

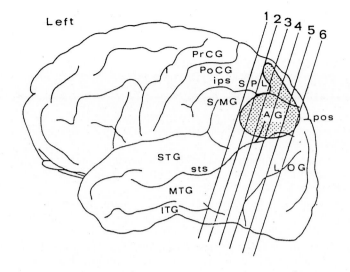

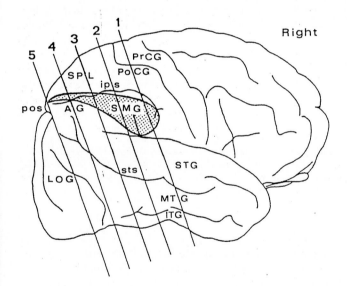

Figure 16–4. Balint-Holmes syndrome: the smallest lesions. This patient suffered consecutive infarctions, first in the angular gyrus (AG) of the right hemisphere causing hemispatial neglect, and then in the supramarginal gyrus (SMG) of the left hemisphere, causing the Balint-Holmes syndrome. (From Pierrot C, Gray F, Brunet P. Infarcts of both inferior parietal lobules with impairment of visually guided eye movements, peripheral visual inattention and optic ataxia. *Brain* 1986;109:81–97.)

Ocular Motor Apraxia

The second component of Balint-Holmes syndrome is a profound disorder of eye movements that cannot be explained by visual inattention. Called "ocular motor apraxia," it is a deficit of volitional saccades and pursuit eye movements, in the face of preserved spontaneous saccades, saccades to suddenly appearing eccentric visual targets (reflexive visually guided saccades), quick phases of nystagmus, and oculocephalic slow eye movements (Box 16-4, Table 16-3).[46]

All saccades except quick phases of nystagmus are triggered in the cerebrum, but reflexive and spontaneous saccades are of a lower order because they require no planning. These lower-order, but cerebrally mediated, saccades are preserved in patients with ocular motor apraxia, distinguishing it from "supranuclear gaze palsy," in which no cerebrally mediated eye movements can be generated.[47,48]

Ocular motor apraxia may be congenital or acquired. In congenital ocular motor apraxia, there is an absence of horizontal pursuit and saccades as long as the head is immobile. Horizontal saccades can be initiated with head thrusts; reflexive visually guided saccades are sometimes present. All

Box 16–4

BALINT-HOLMES SYNDROME:
SCREENING FOR OCULAR MOTOR APRAXIA

Balint-Holmes syndrome selectively impairs visually guided eye movements subserved by the posterior parietal cortex. This is a limited form of a supranuclear gaze palsy. Testing is designed to determine the nature of the eye movement disturbance.

1. *Fixation.* Instruct patients to fixate your nose directly ahead. Note whether they can bring their eyes to straight-ahead position accurately and maintain them there for 5 seconds. A lateral gaze deviation or gaze preference suggests the presence of hemispatial neglect.

2. *Pursuit.* Instruct patients to follow your penlight (or fingertip) as it is slowly moved (15 degrees/sec) to the extremes of horizontal and vertical gaze. Note whether the eyes keep up with the target with a smooth motion or with small catch-up movements (saccadic pursuit).

3. *Visually guided saccades.* With patients fixating a target straight-ahead, instruct them to gaze from straight-ahead to a visual target (penlight, fingertip) sequentially placed midway between fixation and the extremes of horizontal and vertical gaze in all directions. If they are unable, start them in straight-ahead gaze but without a fixation target. Removing the target may help to disengage the eyes from the "sticky" fixation that is a feature of bilateral visual inattention. Test patients in a featureless visual space. Visually guided saccades, like pursuit, are typically lost in patients with biparietal disease.

4. *Nonvisually guided saccades.* Repeat Step 3, instructing patients to look into the extremes of gaze or at body parts (shoulders, toes, top of head). Do not use a visible eccentric target. Nonvisually guided saccades are lost in patients with bifrontal or diencephalic disease.

5. *Oculocephalic maneuver.* If all saccades are absent, move the head in directions to test the integrity of the oculocephalic (doll's head or doll's eye maneuver) eye movements which should be opposite in direction from the head movement. Their preservation indicates that the brainstem eye movement centers and their outflow to extraocular muscles is intact. When all voluntary eye movements (saccades and pursuit) are absent and the oculocephalic eye movements are present, the patient has a full "supranuclear gaze palsy."

voluntary vertical eye movements are spared. The pathogenesis of this congenital form, which usually regresses by adolescence, is unknown. No consistent pathologic abnormalities have been found.

In acquired ocular motor apraxia, vertical as well as horizontal voluntary eye movements are impaired. Head thrusts are absent or less pronounced. The extent of gaze impairment is variable, depending on the size, nature, and location of the lesions, which lie in the frontal or parietal lobes, basal ganglia, and diencephalon, and are primarily caused by infarct or tumor.[46]

When lesions are restricted to the parietal lobes, pursuit and visually guided saccades are impaired, but saccades to command, to remembered targets, and to sounds are preserved.[21,33,41,49] Obliteration of all voluntary saccades requires that lesions damage not

only the posterior parietal lobes but the frontal eye fields and supplementary motor areas.[50] Sparing of the supplementary motor area allows preservation of spontaneous saccades.

In the form of acquired ocular motor apraxia associated with Balint-Holmes syndrome, saccades not dependent on vision are generally spared, in keeping with the fact that the lesions are usually confined to the parietal lobe.

PATHOPHYSIOLOGY

The selective impairment of visually guided eye movements in the ocular motor apraxia of patients with biparietal dysfunction fits with experimental evidence showing that the posterior parietal cortex generates both pursuit and visually guided saccades in mon-

Table 16–3. **Supranuclear Gaze Disorders**

Eye Movement	Congenital Ocular Motor Apraxia	Parietal Acquired Ocular Motor Apraxia[†]	Frontal Acquired Ocular Motor Apraxia	Frontoparietal Acquired Ocular Motor Apraxia[‡]	Supranuclear Gaze Palsy[§]
Voluntary saccades to visual targets	Absent*	Absent	Sometimes present	Absent	Absent
Voluntary saccades to nonvisual targets	Absent*	Present	Absent	Absent	Absent
Spontaneous saccades	Present	Present	Sometimes present	Sometimes present	Absent
Reflex saccades to visual targets	Usually present	Present	Present	Usually present	Absent
Quick phases of nystagmus	Present	Present	Present	Present	Present
Pursuit	Usually absent	Absent	Present	Absent	Absent
Oculocephalic	Present	Present	Present	Present	Present

*Horizontal voluntary saccades absent with head still; these saccades can sometimes be generated with a head movement.
[†]Commonly associated with Balint-Holmes syndrome.
[‡]Sometimes associated with Balint-Holmes syndrome.
[§]Most commonly associated with diencephalic lesion.

keys.[50,51] The frontal lobes preferentially trigger voluntary nonvisually guided saccades. In cases where hypoxic-ischemic lesions extend to the frontal lobes, nonvisually guided voluntary eye movements have been lost.[41,52]

An unsettled issue is whether a loss of voluntary eye movements could be based on inattention alone, as Balint believed in calling it "psychic paralysis of gaze."[20] Also, Holmes pointed out that patients with biparietal lesions execute volitional eye movements much more readily once a fixation target is removed and they are forced to peer at a featureless environment.[21] Could this phenomenon simply suggest an impaired disengagement of attention? Not likely, because bilateral visual inattention can exist without abnormal eye movements,[21,35] and abnormal eye movements can occur without inattention.[41] Therefore, both attentional and motor components probably contribute to acquired ocular motor apraxia.

Ocular motor apraxia is a parietal form of supranuclear gaze palsy in which low-level cerebrally triggered saccades are preserved. Alternative localizations for supranuclear gaze palsy are the diencephalon or bilateral frontal eye movement generating centers. Diencephalic lesions impair all voluntary eye movements equally; frontal lesions preferentially impair nonvisually guided eye movements.

Optic Ataxia

The third component of the Balint-Holmes syndrome is optic ataxia, or inaccurate reaching for a stationary target in extrapersonal space that is *more pronounced under visual than proprioceptive guidance* (Box 16-5).

Optic ataxia usually occurs in bilateral posterior parietal lesions[53,54] caused by infarcts. However, it may rarely occur in association with unilateral parietal lesions.[55–58] Bilateral optic ataxia is usually seen with other features of Balint-Holmes syndrome but may oc-

Box 16–5

BALINT-HOLMES SYNDROME: SCREENING FOR OPTIC ATAXIA

Testing is designed to differentiate between visually guided misreaching (posterior parietal lobe lesions), proprioceptively guided misreaching (anterior parietal lobe), and cerebellar system incoordination.

1. *Visually guided versus proprioceptively guided reaching.* Position your index finger or a vertically oriented pen or pencil at arm's length directly in front of the patient and instruct him to fixate it and touch its superior tip with the index finger of his right hand and then to touch the tip of his nose. Compare the patient's accuracy in touching the object in extrapersonal space (visually guided reaching) versus personal space (proprioceptively guided reaching). If visually guided reaching is consistently worse, consider the diagnosis of optic ataxia.[55]

Repeat these steps with the object positioned 30 degrees to the right and also to the left of straight-ahead. Note if there are any differences between the accuracy of reaching between hands and hemifields.

2. *Proprioceptively guided reaching into extrapersonal space.* Repeat the same sequence of reaching into extrapersonal space, but this time use the vertically extended index finger of the patient's other hand as the target, and instruct patients to close their eyes. If reaching is more accurate with eyes closed than with eyes open (Step 1), the patient may have optic ataxia. If reaching is less accurate with eyes closed, the patient has either a proprioceptive or cerebellar system incoordination, depending on other clinical features.

cur without them.[55] Unilateral optic ataxia often occurs as an isolated finding.

In bilateral lesions, both arms misreach for targets at fixation and in the peripheral fields. In unilateral cases, the manifestations depend on which hemisphere is lesioned. If it is the right hemisphere, both arms misreach into the contralesional hemifield; if it is the left hemisphere, only the right hand misreaches, but into both hemifields (Fig. 16-2e).[55]

The misreaching movement is made up of two components, a proximal part involving poor aiming of the arm and a distal part involving improper positioning of the fingers. The terminal movement is not necessarily an oscillation, as it is in patients with proprioceptive or cerebellar ataxia, but an inaccurate positioning which may improve with unidirectional or multidirectional corrective movements.

PATHOPHYSIOLOGY

Optic ataxia cannot be explained as a proprioceptive, perceptual, or attentional deficit because it occurs without any evidence of integrative somatosensory defects (aster-

eognosis, tactile extinction, graphesthesia, loss of two-point tactile discrimination), visuospatial misperception (see "Impaired Spatial Relations," below), or hemispatial neglect. It may be due to an inability to convert visual field coordinates into head-centered spatial coordinates, a transformation accomplished by the posterior inferior parietal cortex. Alternatively, information from the visual cortex may never reach the motor cortex via the superior longitudinal fasciculus, the major white matter tract connecting the occipital and frontal lobes. In monkeys, optic ataxia has been produced by cutting the superior longitudinal fasciculus at the parietooccipital junction[59] or by lesioning the posterior parietal cortex.[60]

DIFFERENTIAL DIAGNOSIS

Optic ataxia is often mistaken for lack of coordination due to cerebellar system or proprioceptive deficits. However, cerebellar and proprioceptive ataxia are unaffected or slightly improved under visual guidance; *optic ataxia is present only under visual guidance.* Therefore, the best way to differentiate optic ataxia from its mimickers is to observe that reaching is much less accurate when the patient directs a finger at a target in extrapersonal space than at the tip of his own nose (Box 16-5). Unlike patients with cerebellar and proprioceptive ataxia, those with optic ataxia do not manifest oscillations as the finger approaches the target. Rather, the hand reaches out smoothly, misses the target, and gropes about, sometimes landing on it, sometimes remaining suspended in space.

Impaired Spatial Relations

The fourth component of Balint-Holmes syndrome is impaired spatial relations, a disordered perception of space manifested either verbally by misestimates of the size, distance, shape, and orientation of objects in space, or motorically by impaired drawing, copying, block construction, dressing, and maze completion (Box 16-6).

Holmes first drew attention to this problem in six World War I soldiers who had sustained biparieto-occipital missile wounds.[21] They collided with furniture and misreached for objects. But they also complained of not being able to judge how far away or how large objects were, both in relation to themselves and other objects. When tested with two objects placed at different distances away from them, they incorrectly estimated their

separation even when it was as much as 15 centimeters. Yet the patients insisted that they perceived objects as having three-dimensional features. They often could not tell the difference in length of two line segments, even when one line was twice as long as the other. Sometimes they mistook the longer line for the shorter one. They had no trouble reading single words but stumbled through sentences, misplacing and leaving out syllables and words. One patient reported: "I start to read a column, but soon skip some lines; I get on to another column and I lose the place."[21(p 452)]

PATHOPHYSIOLOGY

Since Holmes's description, a vast number of patients with hemispheric damage have been tested for impaired spatial relations with a consensus that the posterior parietal lobe is the common site of the lesion. While bilateral lesions are typical, right parietal damage alone can account for it.[61]

Impaired spatial relations cannot be explained entirely by attentional or visuomotor abnormalities. For example, a patient with biparietooccipital injury following carbon monoxide poisoning misperceived the orientation of objects yet reached for them accurately.[62] How the parietal lobe integrates visuospatial information is still un-

---

Box 16–6

SCREENING FOR IMPAIRED SPATIAL RELATIONS

Assessing impaired spatial relations is complex. The following tests allow a crude impression.

1. *Clock numerals.* Draw a large circle and instruct patients to place the clock hour numerals in their proper places. Instruct them to draw the two hands to indicate 3:30.

2. *Copying.* Instruct patients to copy a simple line drawing of a house, flower, or a box.

3. *Maze completion.* Draw a simple maze on paper. Indicate the starting point and the destination and instruct the patient to mark a path toward the destination along the shortest possible route, keeping the pencil on the paper and staying within the corridors.

4. *Line orientation.* Draw a series of line segments radiating in a spokelike fashion at orientations differing by 15 degrees. Immediately below this sample, draw a single line at an orientation equivalent to that of one of the lines in the sample. Instruct the patient to match the single line to the line in the sample with the same orientation. In some cases, there will be two correct choices. In normal subjects, there should be no errors. A detailed, standardized version of this simple test[68] has been shown to be very sensitive in detecting right parietal lobe disease.

known, but the primacy of the right hemisphere in processing spatial information may be analogous to that of the left hemisphere in processing linguistic information.

DIFFERENTIAL DIAGNOSIS

The diagnosis of impaired spatial relations by motor-free perceptual tests may be confounded by inattention, poor comprehension, or psychiatric illness. For motoric tests, confounders are apraxia, visuomotor disconnection, and impaired planning.

AKINETOPSIA

Akinetopsia, an inability to detect motion, is not considered part of the Balint-Holmes syndrome. In fact, it is a surprisingly uncommon complaint, in view of the frequency with which lesions in parieto-occipital regions cause visual illusions of altered size, shape, and motion (Chapter 4) and deficits in pursuit and saccades to moving targets.

Clinical Features

In 1983, Zihl and colleagues[63] described a woman who, in recovering from bilateral convexity infarctions following superior sagittal sinus thrombosis, complained that when she poured water it looked frozen. People walking near her "were suddenly here or there but I have not seen them moving." She feared crossing streets because as she stepped off the curb, cars that initially seemed far away suddenly appeared to be next to her.[63]

Testing of this patient confirmed a failure to perceive objects as moving when their speed exceeded 10 degrees per second. She had impaired pursuit eye movements above those target velocities. The intriguing feature of this case was that there was no evidence of visual inattention or other cognitive deficits.

Pathophysiology

The lesions in akinetopsia have involved both parietooccipitotemporal junctions corresponding to V5 (MT), a region in macaque containing neurons sensitive to motion but not to orientation or wavelength (Fig. 16-5).[64–66] In view of the large size of the lesions, the absence of inattention or impaired spatial relations is surprising.

Whether akinetopsia is merely a manifestation of inattention or a separate disorder remains unresolved. Some patients with bilateral visual inattention report that they perceive moving objects only at successive points along a path,[31,32] a visual illusion called "polyopia for moving objects" (Chapter 4).[67]

SUMMARY

Lesions of the parietal vision-related cortex and its incoming pathways cause visual illusions and deficits related to the distribution of visual attention and the perception and manipulation of items in space. Patients fail to notice parts of objects. As a result, objects may not be recognized, even though their features may be correctly perceived. Unilat-

Left   Right

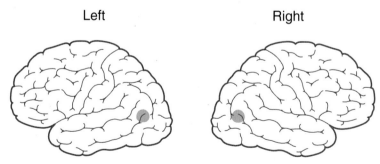

Figure 16–5. Akinetopsia. Schematic shows site of bilateral lesions at temporo-parieto-occipital junction reported to cause a lack of appreciation of motion.

eral posterior parietal lesions cause hemispatial neglect; bilateral posterior parietal lesions cause the Balint-Holmes syndrome.

Hemispatial neglect consists principally of reduced responsiveness to multimodal stimuli in the hemispace contralateral to the lesion. The damage affects attentional centers in posterior parietal cortex or its ipsilateral brainstem or subcortical inputs.

Patients with hemispatial visual neglect can be distinguished from those with hemianopia by their impaired performance on double simultaneous stimulation, line bisection, line and letter cancellation, drawing, and copying.

The Balint-Holmes syndrome has four components: bilateral visual inattention, ocular motor apraxia, optic ataxia, and impaired spatial relations. The full syndrome contains all four components; minor variants contain one or more component.

Bilateral visual inattention gives rise to narrowed attentional fields on both sides of ocular fixation, an inability to recognize more than one visual item at a time, an inability to integrate visual components into an understanding of a scene, and reduced eye movements to eccentric visual targets.

Ocular motor apraxia is a limited type of supranuclear gaze palsy. It consists of absent voluntary eye movements with preservation of spontaneous and reflex saccades. The acquired form is caused by diencephalic or bihemispheric frontal, parietal, or frontal and parietal lesions. Diencephalic lesions impair all voluntary saccades and pursuit. Frontal lesions impair nonvisually guided voluntary saccades, whereas parietal lesions, such as those most typical of the Balint-Holmes syndrome, impair visually guided saccades and pursuit.

Optic ataxia consists of inaccurate reaching that occurs under visual rather than proprioceptive guidance. It reflects either a loss of parietal transformation of retinotopic to craniotopic spatial coordinates or a disconnection between visual and motor cortex.

Impaired spatial relations represents a misperception of spatial items that results principally from right parietal lesions. It is manifested verbally by misestimates of the size, distance, shape, and orientation of objects in space, and motorically by errors in drawing, copying, block construction, dressing, and maze completion.

Akinetopsia is an inability to detect motion. An infrequently documented deficit not usually considered part of the Balint-Holmes syndrome, it is diagnosed by verbal report and by impaired pursuit eye movements. The lesion is located in V5 (MT), at the occipitoparietotemporal junction, an area identified in monkey as responsible for motion detection.

REFERENCES

1. Heilman KM, Valenstein EW, Watson RT. Neglect and related disorders. In: Heilman KM, Valenstein EW, eds. *Clinical Neuropsychology.* 3rd ed. New York: Oxford University Press; 1993:279–336.
2. Bisiach E, Luzzatti C, Perani D. Unilateral neglect, representational schema, and consciousness. *Brain.* 1979;102:609–618.
3. Baynes K, Holtzman JD, Volpe BT. Components of visual attention: alterations in response pattern to visual stimuli following parietal lobe infarction. *Brain.* 1986;109:99–114.
4. Andersen RA, Essick GK, Siegel RM. Encoding of spatial location by posterior parietal neurons. *Science.* 1985;230:456–458.
5. Butter CM, Kirsch N. The effect of lateralized kinetic visual cues on visual search in patients with unilateral spatial neglect. *J Clin Exper Neuropsychol.* 1995;17:856–867.
6. Riddoch MJ, Humphreys GW. The effect of cueing on unilateral neglect. *Neuropsychologia.* 1983;21:589–599.
7. Karnath H-O. Subjective body orientation in neglect and the interactive contribution of neck muscle proprioception and vestibular stimulation. *Brain.* 1994;117:1001–1012.
8. Posner MI, Walker JA, Friedrich FJ, Rafal RD. Effects of parietal lobe injury on covert orienting of visual attention. *J Neurosci.* 1984;4:1863–1874.
9. Levine DN, Warach JD, Benowitz L, Calvanio R. Left spatial neglect: effects of lesion size and premorbid brain atrophy on severity and recovery following right cerebral infarction. *Neurology.* 1986;36:362–366.
10. Mountcastle VB, Anderson RA, Motter BC. The influence of attentive fixation upon the excitability of the light sensitive neurons of the posterior parietal cortex. *J Neurosci.* 1981;1:1218–1245.
11. Wurtz RH, Goldberg ME, Robinson DL. Brain mechanisms of visual attention. *Sci Am.* 1982;246:124–135.
12. Mesulam M. Attention, confusional states, and neglect. In: Mesulam M, ed. *Principles of Behavioral Neurology.* Philadelphia: FA Davis; 1985:125–168.
13. Weintraub S, Mesulam M. Right cerebral dominance in spatial attention. *Arch Neurol.* 1987;44:621–625.
14. Weintraub S, Mesulam M. Neglect: hemispheric specialization, behavioral components and antomical correlates. In: Boller F, Grafman J, eds. *Handbook of Neuropsychology.* Vol 2. Amsterdam: Elsevier Science Publishers; 1989:357–374.

15. Kooistra CA, Heilman KM. Hemispatial visual inattention masquerading as hemianopia. *Neurology*. 1989;39:1125–1127.

16. Nadeau SE, Heilman KM. Gaze-dependent hemianopia without hemispatial neglect. *Neurology*. 1991; 41:1244–1250.

17. Ishiai S, Furukawa T, Tsukagoshi H. Visuospatial processes of line bisection and the mechanism underlying unilateral neglect. *Brain*. 1989;112:1485–1502.

18. Critchley M. *The Parietal Lobes*. New York: Hafner; 1953.

19. Weintraub S, Mesulam M. Visual hemispatial inattention: stimulus parameters and exploratory strategies. *J Neurol Neurosurg Psychiatry*. 1988;51: 1481–1488.

20. Balint R. Seelenlähmung des "Schauens," optische Ataxie, räumliche Störung der Aufmerksamkeit. *Monatschr Psychiatr Neurol*. 1909;25:51–81.

21. Holmes G. Disturbances of visual orientation. *Br J Ophthalmol*. 1918;2:449–468, 506–518.

22. Holmes G, Horrax G. Disturbances of spatial orientation and visual attention with loss of stereoscopic vision. *Arch Neurol Psychiatry*. 1919;1:385–407.

23. Wolpert I. Die Simultanagnosie: Störung der Gesamtauffassung. *Z Gesamte Neurol Psychiatrie*. 1924;93:397–415.

24. Luria AR. Disorders of "simultaneous perception" in a case of bilateral occipitoparietal brain injury. *Brain*. 1959;83:437–449.

25. Luria AR, Pravdina EN, Yarbuss AL. Disorders of ocular movement in a case of simultanagnosia. *Brain*. 1963;86:219–228.

26. Damasio AR, Geschwind N. Anatomic localization in clinical neuropsychology. In: Vinken PJ, Bruyn GW, Klawans HL, eds. *Handbook of Clinical Neurology*. Vol 45. Amsterdam: Elsevier Science Publishers; 1985:7–22.

27. Butter CM, Trobe JD, Foster NL, Berent S. Visual symptoms in Alzheimer's disease are related to visual spatial deficits. *Am J Ophthalmol*. 1996; 122:97–105.

28. Hof PR, Bouras C, Constantinidis J, Morrison JH. Balint's syndrome in Alzheimer's disease: specific disruption of the occipito-parietal visual pathway. *Brain Res*. 1989;493:368–375.

29. Graff-Radford NR, Bolling JP, Earnest F, Shuster EA, Caselli RJ, Brazis PW. Simultanagnosia as the initial sign of degenerative dementia. *Mayo Clin Proc*. 1993; 68:955–964.

30. Tyler HR. Abnormalities of perception with defective eye movements (Balint's syndrome). *Cortex*. 1968;3:154–171.

31. Girotti F, Milanese C, Casazza M, Allegranza A, Corridori F, Vanzaini G. Oculomotor disturbances in Balint's syndrome: anatomoclinical findings and electrooculographic analysis in a case. *Cortex*. 1982; 18:603–614.

32. Godwin-Austen RB. A case of visual disorientation. *J Neurol Neurosurg Psychiatry*. 1965;28:453–458.

33. Hecaen H, Ajuriaguerra JU. Balint syndrome (psychic paralysis of visual fixation) and its minor forms. *Brain*. 1954;77:373–400.

34. Pierrot C, Gautier JC, Loron P. Acquired ocular motor apraxia due to bilateral frontoparietal infarcts. *Ann Neurol*. 1988;23:199–202.

35. Rizzo M, Hurtig R. Looking but not seeing: attention, perception, and eye movements in simultanagnosia. *Neurology*. 1987;37:1642–1648.

36. Hecaen H, Albert ML. *Human Neuropsychology*. New York: John Wiley & Sons; 1978:215–227.

37. Lynch JC, Mountcastle VB, Talbot WH, Yin TCT. Parietal lobe mechanisms for directed visual attention. *J Neurophysiol*. 1977;40:241–251.

38. Rizzo M, Robin DA. Simultanagnosia: a defect of sustained attention yields insights on visual information processing. *Neurology*. 1990;40:447–455.

39. Vallar G, Perani D. The anatomy of unilateral neglect after right-hemisphere stroke lesions. *Neuropsychologia*. 1986;24:609–622.

40. Heilman KM, Valenstein E, Watson RT. Localization of neglect. In: Kertesz A, ed. *Localization in Neuropsychology*. New York: Academic Press; 1983:371–392.

41. Pierrot-Deseilligny C, Gray F, Brunet P. Infarcts of both inferior parietal lobules with impairment of visually guided eye movements, peripheral visual inattention and optic ataxia. *Brain*. 1986;109:81–97.

42. Rapcsak SZ, Watson RT, Heilman KM. Hemispace-visual field interactions in visual extinction. *J Neurol Neurosurg Psychiatry*. 1987;50:1117–1124.

43. Owsley C, Ball K, McGwin G, et al. Visual processing impairment and crash risk among older adults. *JAMA*. 1998;279:1083–1088.

44. Ball K, Owsley C, Sloane ME, Roenker DL, Bruni JR. Visual attention problems as a predictor of vehicle crashes in older drivers. *Invest Ophthalmol Vis Sci*. 1993;34:3110–3123.

45. Parasuraman R, Nestor PG. Attention and driving skills in aging and Alzheimer's disease. *Hum Factors*. 1991;33:539–557.

46. Leigh RJ, Zee DS. *The Neurology of Eye Movements*. 3rd ed. Philadelphia: FA Davis; 1999:542–547.

47. Sharpe JA, Johnston JL. Ocular motor paresis versus apraxia. *Ann Neurol*. 1989;25:209–210.

48. Devere TR, Lee AG, Hamill B, Bhasin D, Orengo-Nania S, Coselli JS. Acquired supranuclear ocular motor paresis following cardiovascular surgery. *J Neuro-ophthalmol*. 1997;17:189–193.

49. Tsutsui J, Takeda J, Ichihashi S, Kimura H, Shirabe T. Ocular motor apraxia and lesions of the visual association area. *Neuro-ophthalmology*. 1980;1:149–154.

50. Pierrot C. Cortical control of saccades. *Neuro-ophthalmology*. 1991;11:63–75.

51. Lynch JC, McLaren JW. The contribution of parieto-occipital association cortex to the control of slow eye movements. In: Lennerstrand G, Zee DS, Keller EL, eds. *Functional Basis of Ocular Motility Disorders*. Oxford: Pergamon Press; 1982:501–510.

52. Howard R, Trend P, Ross Russell MD. Clinical features of ischemia in cerebral arterial border zones after periods of reduced cerebral blood flow. *Arch Neurol*. 1987;44:934–940.

53. Damasio AR, Benton AL. Impairment of hand movements under visual guidance. *Neurology*. 1979; 29:170–178.

54. Denes G, Caviezel F, Semenza C. Difficulty in reaching objects and body parts: a sensory motor disconnexion syndrome. *Cortex*. 1982;18:165–173.

55. Perenin MT, Vighetto A. Optic ataxia: a specific disruption in visuomotor mechanisms: I. Different as-

pects of the deficit in reaching for objects. *Brain.* 1988;111:643–674.

56. Auerbach SH, Alexander MP. Pure agraphia and unilateral optic ataxia associated with a left superior parietal lobule lesion. *J Neurol Neurosurg Psychiatry.* 1981;44:430–432.

57. Rondot P, Recondo J, Ribadeau Dumas JL. Visuomotor ataxia. *Brain.* 1977;100:355–376.

58. Levine DN, Kaufman KJ, Mohr JP. Inaccurate reaching associated with a superior parietal lobe tumor. *Neurology.* 1978;28:556–561.

59. Haaxma R, Kuypers HGJM. Role of occipito-frontal cortico-cortical connections in visual guidance of relatively indepedent hand and finger movements in rhesus monkeys. *Brain Res.* 1974;71:361–366.

60. Lynch JC. The functional organization of posterior parietal association cortex. *Behav Brain Sci.* 1980;3:485–499.

61. DeRenzi E. Disorders of spatial orientation. In: Vinken PJ, Bruyn GW, Klawans HL, eds. *Handbook of Clinical Neurology.* Vol 45. Amsterdam: Elsevier Science; 1985:405–422.

62. Goodale MA, Milner AD, Jakobson LS, Carey DP. A neurological dissociation between perceiving objects and grasping them. *Nature.* 1991;349:154–155.

63. Zihl J, Von Cramon D, Mai N. Selective disturbance of movement vision after bilateral brain damage. *Brain.* 1983;106:313–340.

64. Zeki S. Cerebral akinetopsia (visual motion blindness). *Brain.* 1991;114:811–824.

65. Wurtz RH, Goldberg ME. The neurobiology of saccadic eye movements. In: Wurtz RH, Goldberg ME, eds. *Reviews of Oculomotor Research.* Vol 3. Amsterdam: Elsevier; 1989.

66. Marcar VL, Zihl J, Cowey A. Comparing the visual deficits of a motion blind patient with the visual deficits of monkeys with area MT removed. *Neuropsychologia.* 1997;35:1459–1465.

67. Bender MD. Polyopia and monocular diplopia of cerebral origin. *Arch Neurol Psychiatry.* 1945;54:323–338.

68. Benton AL, Varney NR, Hamsher K. Visuospatial judgment: a clinical test. *Arch Neurol.* 1978;35:364–367.

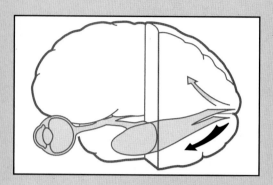

TEMPORAL VISION-RELATED CORTEX

Lesions of the temporal vision-related cortex and its incoming pathways (Fig. 1-30) cause complex hallucinations (Chapter 4), an inability to name and identify familiar objects, symbols, words, and colors, and difficulty recalling recently viewed items (Table 17-1)

The principal deficits are:
- **Visual object agnosia:** inability to demonstrate knowledge of a familiar object.
- **Visual anomia (optic aphasia):** inability to name a familiar object by sight despite being able to name it by touch or sound.

Table 17–1. **Temporo-Occipital Vision Disorders**

Condition	Impairment	Localization	Mechanism
Visual object agnosia*	Recognizing objects by sight	Bilateral (but left > right) occipitotemporal	Imperfect perception leads to loss of familiarity for items with verbalizable components
Prosopagnosia	Recognizing familiar faces	Right >> left occipitotemporal	Imperfect perception leads to loss of familiarity for items without verbalizable components
Pure alexia	Reading	Left occipito-temporal	Visual–verbal discon-nection
Cerebral achromatopsia	Identifying colors by hue	Occipitotemporal	Damage to cortical color processing center
Color anomia	Naming colors	Left occipito-temporal	Visual–verbal discon-nection
Visual amnesia	Learning new information by sight	Bilateral (but right >> left) occipitotemporal	Visual–limbic discon-nection

*Visual anomia, a closely related deficit, consists of an inability to name objects by sight but the capacity to name them by touch and describe their use.

- **Prosopagnosia (face agnosia):** inability to recognize familiar faces.
- **Pure alexia (alexia without agraphia):** acquired inability to read despite intact spelling and writing.
- **Cerebral achromatopsia:** inability to match or sort colors by hue as a result of a cortical lesion.
- **Color anomia:** inability to name colors despite being able to match or sort them by hue.
- **Visual amnesia:** inability to recall having seen a recently viewed object.

PITFALLS IN DIAGNOSIS

There are three important pitfalls in the diagnosis of these deficits.

Pitfall 1: Prerequisites are not met

An integrative vision disorder cannot be reliably diagnosed unless attention, global cognition, language, and elementary vision are reasonably intact. Thus the presence of toxic-metabolic delirium, low arousal state (including depression), aphasia, or advanced dementia precludes consideration of an agnosia. Yet only a profound deficit in visual acuity or visual field will stand in the way of such a diagnosis. For example, a visual acuity reduced to 20/100 and a visual field narrowed to 5 degrees do not impair recognition of familiar objects, provided the objects are large and unambiguous.[1]

Pitfall 2: Deficit involves more than one sensory modality

Agnosias are deficits limited to a single sensory modality. Visual object agnosia should be diagnosed only when an object not recognized by sight is recognized by touch or sound. Pure alexia ("word blindness"), which may be a visual agnosia for lexical symbols, should be diagnosed only when words cannot be read but can be spelled to dictation and understood by hearing. When a patient fails to recognize items in more than one sensory modality, global cognitive dysfunction is a more appropriate diagnosis.

Pitfall 3: Deficit involves naming rather than recognition

Patients who fail to name an object are more likely to have a naming disorder than a recognition disorder. Only those who cannot describe or mime the use of objects they cannot name qualify for a diagnosis of recognition disorder.

The distinction between naming and recognition disorders becomes complicated when patients are challenged with colors, which, unlike objects, have no inherent use. In analyzing a color disturbance, the physician must differentiate between an inability to sort or match colors (achromatopsia), an inability to name them (anomia), and a lack of understanding of their "meaning" (agnosia). Achromatopsia is diagnosed by a failure in color sorting and matching tasks. Color anomia is diagnosed when patients properly sort or match colors but cannot name them or, if given a color name, cannot point to the appropriate color. Color agnosia, an extraordinarily rare disorder, is diagnosed when patients can match, sort, and name colors, but cannot select the appropriate color to "color in" a line drawing of a familiar object (like a banana or tomato) or correctly answer questions such as "What color is a banana?" or "What are some things that are yellow?"

VISUAL OBJECT AGNOSIA

Clinical Features

Visual object agnosia is defined as impaired visual recognition of familiar objects that cannot be attributed to defective elementary vision, intellect, language, or attention.[2] Patients may misname objects, but they are visually agnosic only if they *cannot* describe or mime the use of an object presented visually, but they *can* name, describe, or mime the use of the object after touching it or hearing its sound. Inability to recognize objects is rarely the chief problem in this condition. Accompanying deficits—prosopagnosia, pure alexia, or loss of place familiarity—are typically more prominent.

In the most penetrating form of visual object agnosia, patients are unable, by sight alone, to recognize familiar three-dimensional objects such as a pen, ring, belt, tie, watch, or book, but they can identify them promptly if allowed to grasp them. These deficits often occur in the aftermath of a bilateral posterior cerebral artery infarction that initially caused cortical blindness. The most common form of visual object agnosia is less severe. Patients can visually recognize three-dimensional objects but cannot recognize photographs or line drawings, especially if they contain ambiguities—unclear borders, embedding, fragmenting, shading, a multiplicity of objects, or objects shown in nontraditional views. If patients fail to name two-dimensional (line drawing) objects but can describe their use, a diagnosis of visual object *anomia* is made. If they cannot describe the objects' use, a diagnosis of visual object *agnosia* is made.

Some patients who fail to recognize objects are also unable to copy line drawings or match drawings to samples.[3,4] Such patients are said to have a condition called "apperceptive visual agnosia."[5] Lesions are typically widespread across the occipital region, caused by carbon monoxide[3] or mercury[6] poisoning, Alzheimer's disease,[7,8] or bilateral posterior cerebral artery stroke.[9] The recognition defect is believed to rest on a failure to perform adequate feature analysis. However, visual acuity and visual fields are often so compromised that a diagnosis of agnosia is questionable (Pitfall 1).

On the other hand, there are many reports of patients who, despite intact elementary vision, copying, and matching, cannot visually recognize common objects.[10,11] They are said to have a condition called "associative visual agnosia."[5] More recent evaluations of such patients have shown that *they do not copy and match normally.* They compare individual features rather than making a "gestalt" impression.[12–14] For example, in copying a line drawing of a tea kettle, a patient of mine drew one short arc segment at a time, constantly referring back to the original drawing for accuracy. Even after he had produced a perfect replica, he had no idea what he had copied.[14]

The lesions causing the associative form of visual object agnosia appear to be similar in nature and extent to those causing the apperceptive form. Posterior cerebral artery occlusion is the most common mechanism, although one case was due to progressive multifocal leukoencephalopathy.[14] Lesions lie in the occipitotemporal regions, usually bilaterally, but sometimes unilaterally on either side.[2,12] A left hemisphere predominance is suggested by the majority of studies (Fig. 17-1).[15,16]

Most patients have prominent defects in visual recent memory (see "Visual Amnesia," below),[17] but there are notable exceptions.[13] Some combination of pure alexia, cerebral achromatopsia, and prosopagnosia is nearly always present.[2,11,12,18]

Patients recovering from visual object agnosia often display a deficit known as "visual anomia" or "optic aphasia,"[19] in which they cannot name objects by sight but can describe the use of the unnamed objects by sight and name them correctly if allowed to grasp

Left   Right

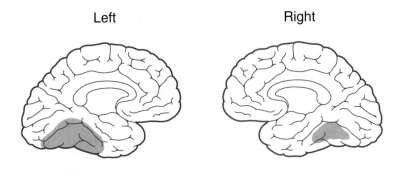

a

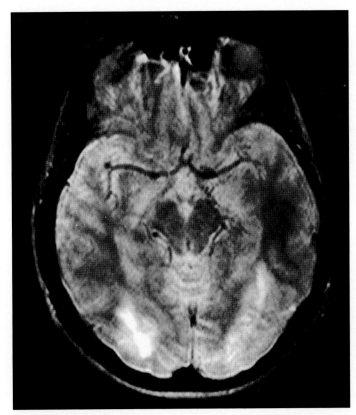

b

Figure 17–1. Visual object agnosia. (*a*) Schematic shows lesions in both occipitotemporal regions, involving the lingual, fusiform, inferior temporal, and parahippocampal gyri. There is a left hemisphere predominance. (*b*) MRI of a patient with proximal PCA occlusion causing visual object agnosia, pure alexia, and homonymous hemianopia. There is increased white matter signal in the inferior temporal and medial occipital regions.

them.[20,21] Some patients toggle between visual object agnosia and visual anomia.[12] As the deficit recedes, it can often be evoked by challenging the patient with pictures of objects that have ambiguous features.[22]

Pathophysiology

The process leading to disturbed object recognition is poorly understood. In visual object agnosia, perhaps a degraded perceptual stimulus fails to evoke widespread neural activation responsible for the sense of familiarity.[23] An amnestic component may also be involved, but it is unlike the standard amnestic syndrome, which impairs new learning rather than old memories.

Visual object agnosia and pure alexia commonly occur together, suggesting that objects and symbols are recognized when they have distinctive,[2] verbalizable[24] components, like the arm of a chair or the letter of a word.

In fact, lesions of the language-oriented left hemisphere predominate in patients with visual object agnosia or pure alexia. By contrast, faces are recognized without recourse to distinctive or verbalizable parts, and lesions of the space-oriented right hemisphere predominate in cases of face agnosia.

Differential Diagnosis

The examiner's challenge is to distinguish between naming and recognition disorders by presenting to the patient a simple sequence of tasks (Box 17-1; Fig. 17-2).

PROSOPAGNOSIA

Clinical Features

This condition is characterized by an inability to identify familiar faces (Greek *prosopon* =

Box 17–1

VISUAL OBJECT AGNOSIA, VISUAL ANOMIA, OR ANOMIC APHASIA?

Is an inability to name familiar objects by sight due to a recognition disorder (visual object agnosia), a visual naming disorder (visual anomia), or a language disorder that includes misnaming (anomic aphasia)? This is how to decide:

1. Instruct patients to name by sight some familiar three-dimensional objects such as a tie, glasses, watch, belt, or pen.

2. If they cannot identify the objects by name, ask them to describe or mime the objects' use. If they cannot do this, hand them the objects and ask them to name them by touch. If they are successful, the diagnosis is **visual object agnosia,** a recognition disorder limited to vision.

3. If they correctly describe or mime the objects' use, hand them the objects and ask them to name them by touch. If they are successful, the diagnosis is **visual anomia,** a naming disorder limited to vision. If they cannot name them after touching them, they have a naming disorder as part of an aphasia (**anomic aphasia**).

4. If they cannot name, describe, or mime the use of objects by sight or touch, they have a **global cognitive** or **sensorial disorder** that is not limited to vision.

5. To detect the more subtle—but more common—forms of visual object agnosia, display a series of magazine photographs of relatively isolated single objects with distinct borders. If these are correctly identified, select photographs containing multiple objects with indistinct borders. In seeking identification, ask for names first, and if the patients are unable to provide them, ask for use of the objects, in order to distinguish an anomia from an agnosia. The more ambiguous the forms, the more likely is elementary visual dysfunction to interfere with recognition. Therefore, always display large figures in good lighting with the patient's near correction in place. Many patients with subtle visual object agnosia will pass these tests. Their deficit can only be detected by testing them with standardized overlapping, embedded, or fragmented figures.

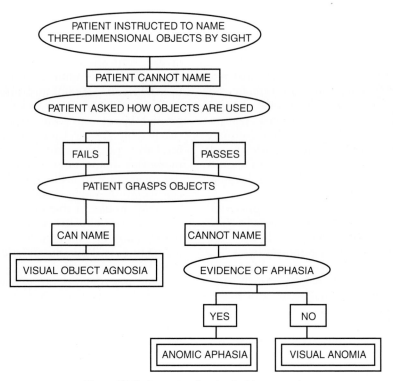

Figure 17–2. Screening for visual object agnosia.

face).[12,24–30] Patients cannot recognize a familiar face or learn to recognize a new acquaintance. They know that a face is a face, and whether it is a sad or happy face, but not whether they have seen it before.

Faces are not the only icons they fail to identify. They cannot make out the distinctive features that separate one representative of a class from another. Thus prosopagnosics can distinguish a knife from a fork, but not two knives that resemble one another. Face recognition becomes the most obvious deficit because faces are the most powerful images in daily life that lack *components that can themselves be easily distinguished.* Were other symbols to assume special importance in a person's daily living, they too would become a recognition issue. For example, an automobile aficionado lost the ability to differentiate among car models,[31] a birdwatcher the ability to recognize individual birds, and a farmer the ability to distinguish among his cows.[32]

As in visual object agnosia, patients are often affected after having suffered a posterior cerebral artery stroke that initially caused cortical blindness, visual hallucinations, and visual illusions. Within days to weeks of stroke onset, as positive visual phenomena recede and elementary sight and attention improve, patients develop a subdued awareness that they no longer recognize familiar faces. They may ludicrously introduce themselves as they look at their own reflection in a mirror!

Prosopagnosics fail to recognize photographs of celebrities and their own friends and relatives, provided they bear no distinctive (or verbalizable) facial characteristics such as an unusual hair style, beard, mustache, blemish, or clothing. Shown a series of pictures of five different unfamiliar faces, and rechallenged for recognition five minutes later with a new series containing one previously viewed face, they will be unable to pick out the previously viewed face unless it has distinctive features. The same fault pattern turns up when they are challenged to recognize members of any subclass. If they are briefly shown a key and minutes later shown an array of different types of keys containing the previously viewed key, prosopagnosics will be unable to identify the previously viewed key.

Prosopagnosics do not have normal perception.[12,24,29] They can discriminate between same and different unfamiliar faces, but only by pursuing a slow, slavish, feature-by-feature analysis, in which they compare mouths, ears, and hairstyles in order to tell the faces apart. Some patients fail to identify line drawings of objects whose outlines are ambiguous or fragmented.[24]

Most prosopagnosics also show profound impairments in visual memory tasks.[12,24,29,33] They can differentiate and match faces, but if those faces are briefly removed from view and then redisplayed, patients will fail to remember which ones they have already seen. The most debilitating daily aspect of this visual recent memory loss is impaired wayfinding. Stranded in an unfamiliar locale, patients will be unable to find their way home.[33,34] Verbal, auditory, and tactile memory are typically intact.

Other deficits accompany prosopagnosia, such as superior altitudinal visual field defects, pure alexia, and some degree of visual object agnosia. A blunted emotional response to visual stimuli is sometimes discovered. For example, sexually provocative pictures may fail to arouse libido yet galvanic skin responses indicate arousal on a subliminal level.[35,36] The galvanic skin response paradigm[37] and oculographic recordings[38] demonstrate that prosopagnosics are more aroused by famous than unfamiliar faces, indicating that they have greater familiarity than they acknowledge by verbal report.

The lesions causing prosopagnosia involve the lingual, fusiform, and parahippocampal gyri and subjacent bilateral white matter (Fig. 17-3). Right hemisphere lesions are consistently larger than left hemisphere lesions. In fact, right hemisphere lesions alone can produce prosopagnosia.[12,39–41] Stroke, tumor, demyelination, and degenerative atrophy are the principal causes of these lesions.

Pathophysiology

The mechanism of prosopagnosia is unclear. Poor perception alone cannot explain it because patients have a relatively intact ability to match identical yet unfamiliar faces. A reasonable hypothesis suggests that prosopagnosia results when a subtle visual perceptual disturbance is combined with a disconnection between occipital and inferior temporal cortex.[24,29] In other words, when a degraded image—an "underspecification of visual detail,"[30]—is transmitted over faulty lines to a putative center for stored visual memories in the inferior temporal cortex, the image fails to evoke familiarity.[42] A disconnection between visual and limbic motivational circuits in this or other nearby regions could explain why prosopagnosic patients are not consciously aroused by sexual pictures and not particularly troubled by their recognition deficit.

Some investigators are convinced that a specific brain region—perhaps in the right inferior temporal cortex—is allocated to face recognition. This hypothesis is based on functional MRI studies showing a discrete region of activity during face recognition tasks,[42a] cases in which faces are the only items that are not recognized,[43] and cases in which imaging shows a discrete right hemisphere lesion.[40] However, evidence from evoked potentials,[44] positron emission tomography,[45,46] and depth electrode[47] studies suggests that face recognition recruits wide areas of temporal cortex in both cerebral hemispheres.

Differential Diagnosis

Patients who claim not to recognize faces rarely have prosopagnosia. They usually have a psychiatric disturbance or an anterograde amnesia that prevents them from recognizing new faces but allows them to recognize celebrities or relatives. Another common error is to diagnose prosopagnosia when the deficit could be explained by a global sensorial or cognitive disorder (Pitfall 1).

Correct diagnosis of prosopagnosia depends on demonstrating a lack of recognition of familiar and famous faces (Box 17-2; Fig. 17-4). Those who believe that familiar persons have been replaced by imposters have Capgras syndrome, a psychiatric disturbance.[48]

Left   Right

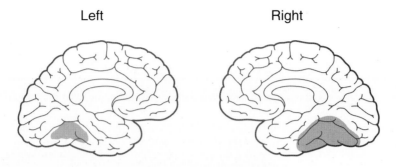

a

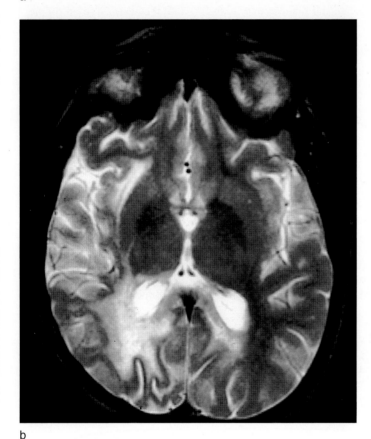

b

Figure 17–3. Prosopagnosia. (*a*) Schematic shows lesions are in the same location as those for visual object agnosia, but with right hemisphere predominance. A right-sided lesion alone can give rise to this manifestation. (*b*) MRI of a patient with progressive multifocal leukoencephalopathy showing increased signal in the inferior occipitotemporal regions, more on the right.

PURE ALEXIA

Clinical Features

Pure alexia (alexia without agraphia, pure word blindness) is an acquired reading disorder without other evidence of aphasia.[49–54] It must not be confused with dyslexia, a developmental reading disorder of childhood.

Patients with pure alexia complain of an abrupt loss of the ability to read, sometimes accompanied by loss of vision in the right hemifield. Testing typically shows normal visual acuity, a complete right homonymous hemianopia, and a variable deficit in reading words and letters. Some patients lose the ability to read numbers, musical notes, and other familiar symbols.[55] Apart from reading, all aspects of language are preserved, including spelling and writing spontaneously

Box 17–2

PROSOPAGNOSIA, AMNESIA, OR PSYCHIATRIC ILLNESS?

Is an inability to recognize faces due to prosopagnosia, an anterograde amnesia including faces, or a psychiatric illness? Here is how to decide:

1. Instruct patients to identify celebrities displayed from a magazine (politicians and actors are best). If they fail, ask them to tell you what the unnamed persons do or did. If they can do this, they have an **anomia** for faces. If they cannot do this, yet they have some general knowledge of celebrities, they may have **prosopagnosia**. Go to Step 2.

2. Instruct them to identify accompanying relatives or friends. Because they may do so on the basis of non–face attributes, arrange to have the companions leave the room and return in slight clothing disguise (for example, wearing a white physician's coat) without giving any verbal or behavioral cues as to their identity. Failure to recognize them under these circumstances suggests **prosopagnosia**.

3. An **amnestic disorder for new faces** is usually part of a more widespread anterograde amnesia. It does not extend to ancient celebrities or relatives. It can be demonstrated by displaying an array of objects, withdrawing them for an interval, then redisplaying another array containing one or more previously displayed objects and instructing the patient to identify which ones were previously viewed.

4. If prosopagnosia and amnesia are excluded, a **nonorganic** or **psychiatric disturbance** is likely.

and to dictation. After a distracting pause, patients will be unable to read what they have just finished writing. They may be able to read by tracing out the individual letters, thereby making use of intact proprioceptive input to the language cortex. Many patients can read individual letters but cannot combine them into words unless they read the letters out loud so as to recruit auditory language circuits. There is sometimes a deficit in color-naming (see "Color Anomia," below) and a visual object agnosia.

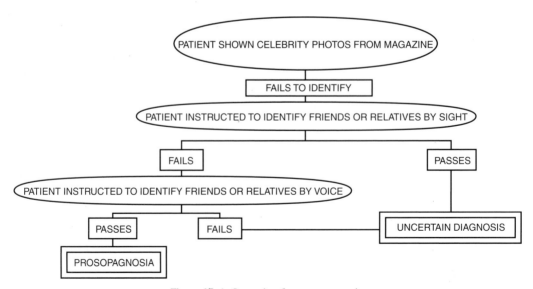

Figure 17–4. Screening for prosopagnosia.

Pure alexia usually improves spontaneously within months of onset; in some cases it disappears altogether. However, reading often remains labored, especially for long and complicated words. Patients learn to read aloud in a letter-by-letter fashion. The associated color anomia usually improves, but the hemianopia does not.

Pathophysiology

The offending lesion, nearly always caused by an occlusion of distal branches of the left posterior cerebral artery, lies beneath the occipital horn of the lateral ventricle, an important crossroad of visual–verbal traffic (Fig. 17-5). A lesion in this area interrupts the left optic radiations, causing right homonymous hemianopia, and the left forceps major carrying white matter connections from the contralateral primary visual cortex via the splenium (splenial alexia; Fig. 17-5a,b). In this way, the language cortex is cut off from visual input. A more laterally placed lesion in the white matter subjacent to the angular gyrus spares the optic radiations and the visual field but causes a pure alexia by disconnecting the angular gyrus from both visual cortices (subangular alexia; Fig. 17-5c).[54] Medial extension into the parahippocampal region brings about color anomia (see "Color Anomia," below).[51]

Pure alexia has been attributed to an interruption of neural information between the visual cortex and the language cortex—a visual–verbal disconnection.[56] But it may also be regarded as an agnosia for lexical symbols.[57] Nearly always present in the company of visual object agnosia and prosopagnosia,[2] it may also occur in isolation. Unlike other agnosias, pure alexia is caused by small, discrete, strictly left hemisphere lesions. Evidently the brain circuitry used for recognizing lexical material differs somewhat from that used for nonlexical material.

Differential Diagnosis

Pure alexia must be differentiated from two other important acquired reading disorders: aphasic alexia and spatial alexia (Box 17-3; Fig. 17-6). Aphasic alexia is diagnosed when other elements of aphasia are present, and the causative lesion localizes to the left angular gyrus region. Spatial alexia is diagnosed when the patient correctly reads letters and words but leaves out words in sentences or inserts words from other positions in the text. Evidence of spatial or attentional dysfunction should also be present (Chapter 16), localizing the lesion to occipitoparietal regions bilaterally.

CEREBRAL ACHROMATOPSIA

Clinical Features

This rare acquired inability to discriminate colors is usually caused by occlusion of the occipitotemporal branch of the posterior cerebral artery. As a result, the fusiform and lingual gyri become infarcted.[57a–h]

This condition is often misleadingly called "central achromatopsia," a term that would not exclude the far more common lesions of the retina and optic nerve, which are also parts of the central nervous system. There are two forms of cerebral achromatopsia: full-field and hemifield.

Full-field cerebral achromatopsia is caused by bihemispheric lesions. Loss of color vision can be debilitating. Patients suddenly announce that objects appear in shades of gray, as if the color knob on the television set had been turned off. They cannot select their clothing by color or tell green from red apples, ripe from unripe bananas.[58] One achromatopsic patient reported that she repeatedly washed her draperies because they looked dirty.[59] Lesions invariably extend into adjacent inferior primary visual cortex to cause bilateral superior quadrant achromatic visual field defects.

Hemifield cerebral achromatopsia, the more common form, is caused by a unihemispheric lesion. If the lesion lies in the left hemisphere, a right superior homonymous (achromatic) quadrantanopia will be present, as well as pure alexia. If the lesion lies in the right hemisphere, a left superior homonymous achromatic quadrantanopia will be present.

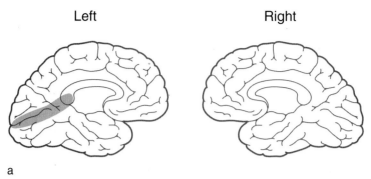

a

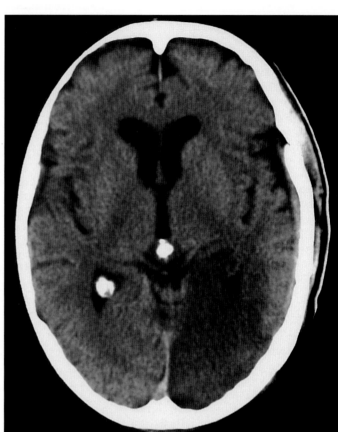

Figure 17–5. Pure alexia. (*a*) Splenial alexia. Schematic shows lesion involving left posterior optic radiations, splenium, and forceps major. (*b*) CT showing a posterior cerebral artery infarct affecting this territory (arrows). (*c*) Subangular alexia. Schematic shows a lesion in the region of the left angular gyrus which spares the optic radiations but disconnects visual input from the language center.

b

Left　　　　　　　　Right

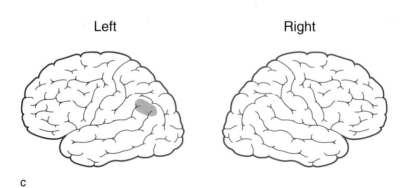

c

Box 17–3

DEVELOPMENTAL DYSLEXIA, APHASIC ALEXIA, PURE ALEXIA, OR SPATIAL ALEXIA?

There are three important lexical reading disorders—developmental dyslexia, pure alexia, and aphasic alexia. There is one spatial reading disorder—spatial alexia—that causes words and letters to be jumbled and omitted. Sort them out as follows.

1. Inquire if patients had unusual reading difficulty in childhood to rule out **developmental dyslexia**.

2. Instruct them to read paragraphs from a magazine or newspaper. If they make many errors or cannot read at all, present single words and, if performance is not normal, single letters. Test writing, spelling, spontaneous speech, comprehension, and repetition. If any of these elements is abnormal, the patients' reading difficulty is likely to be an **aphasic alexia**.

4. If there are no signs of aphasia, instruct patients to trace the letters and then try to identify them. If they can read by tracing, which draws on proprioceptive rather than visual input to language cortex, they probably have **pure alexia** (alexia without agraphia, pure word blindness). For further confirmation, instruct them to read what they wrote earlier. If they have pure alexia, they should fail this task.

5. If disordered reading consists of an omission of parts of words and a jumbling of word order, difficulty probably stems from visual spatial deficits—**spatial alexia**. It reflects a disordered perception of spatial elements, not a language disturbance.

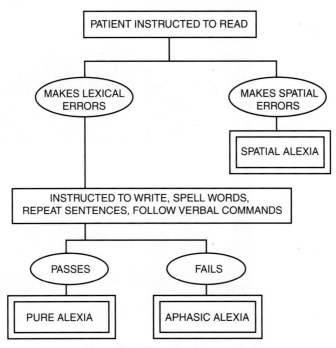

Figure 17–6. Screening for pure alexia.

Pathophysiology

During the performance of color tasks, functional MRI shows activation in the fusiform gyrus area bilaterally,[60] a region that corresponds anatomically to macaque V4 (Chapter 1). The lesion responsible for cerebral achromatopsia lies in this area (Fig. 17-7).[59,61] Unlike V1 and V2, which uncode achromatic stimuli for visual field quadrants, V4—with its small size and relatively large receptive fields—uncodes color for the entire hemi-

field.[61] As a result, when this area is lesioned, color vision is impaired across a hemifield. Because the lesion usually extends upward into a portion of V1, it also causes a superior quadrant achromatic visual field defect.

If a left hemispheric lesion extends far enough anteriorly to reach the underside of the occipital ventricular horn, it will interrupt the ipsilateral optic radiations and the connections between the splenium and the angular gyrus to cause a pure alexia (see "Pure Alexia," above). An equivalently

Left   Right

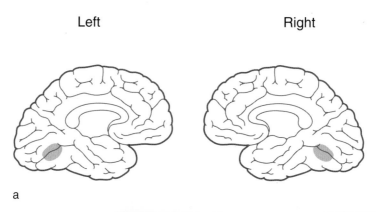

a

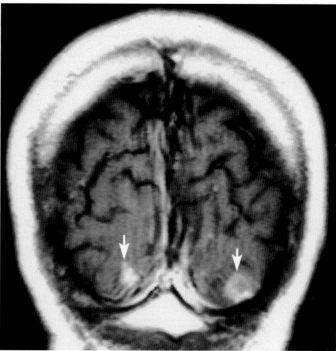

Figure 17–7. Cerebral achromatopsia. (*a*) Schematic shows lesions involving the fusiform-lingual gyri bilaterally, immediately inferior to the calcarine cortex. (*b*) Coronal T1-weighted MRI showing enhancement of these regions (arrows) in a patient with cerebral achromatopsia.

b

placed lesion in the right hemisphere may introduce deficits of face discrimination, figure-from-ground extraction, or line orientation judgment.[62,63] Bilaterally placed lesions in this area will produce prosopagnosia, visual object agnosia, and visual amnesia (see "Visual Amnesia," below) by interrupting both inferior longitudinal fasciculi carrying visual information to the inferior temporal cortex.

Differential Diagnosis

Cerebral achromatopsia is a very rare condition, and must be differentiated from the more common anterior visual pathway causes of color vision loss (Box 17-4). Unlike hereditary cone receptor dyschromatopsias, it arises suddenly. Unlike acquired retinopathies and optic neuropathies, it causes a symmetrical loss of color vision that may be restricted to a hemifield. Furthermore, it usually keeps company with other manifestations of occipital lobe lesions, such as achromatic hemianopias, hallucinations, and recognition disorders.

A firm diagnosis of *full-field* cerebral achromatopsia must fulfill four criteria:

1. Score on a color discrimination test is subnormal. The Ishihara isochromatic test will detect only the most severe cases;[58] Farnsworth tests are necessary to detect all cases (Chapter 6). Hereditary retinal dyschromatopsias may be separated by distinctive error patterns on the Farnsworth test.[64]

2. Bilateral superior quadrant achromatic visual field defects are present. Lesions that damage the small color-coding portion of cortex are likely to "spill over" into inferior primary visual cortex.

Box 17–4

IS THIS CEREBRAL ACHROMATOPSIA?

Cerebral achromatopsia, an acquired loss of color vision owing to damage in visual cortical area V4, occurs in two forms: hemifield and full-field. Screening is different for each type.

For **hemifield cerebral achromatopsia:**

1. Perform confrontation visual fields with fingers (Chapter 7) to determine if a homonymous superior quadrantanopia is present. If not, reject a diagnosis of hemifield achromatopsia, no matter what follows.

2. If homonymous superior quadrantanopia is present, test the inferior and superior quadrants ipsilateral to the defect with red test objects (red caps, match tips). Only if the patient fails to identify color in the entire hemifield can a presumptive diagnosis of hemifield cerebral achromatopsia be made.

3. With right hemifield cerebral achromatopsia, check for pure alexia, which should be present. With left hemifield cerebral achromatopsia, check for prosopagnosia or topographical agnosia, which are often present.

For **full-field cerebral achromatopsia:**

1. Perform confrontation visual fields with fingers to check for bilateral superior quadrantanopia, which should be present.

2. If so, check for achromatopsia in all field quadrants with red test objects. If present, confirm with Ishihara color tests. To detect subtle defects, perform Farnsworth hue test.

3. Confirm that visual acuity is normal; if not, bilateral retinal or optic nerve diseases could be causing achromatopsia.

4. Check for visual object agnosia, prosopagnosia, topographical agnosia, and pure alexia, which are often present.

3. Visual acuity is normal or near normal in both eyes. This excludes a bilateral retinal or optic nerve cause.
4. Visual object agnosia, prosopagnosia, or pure alexia is present.

A firm diagnosis of *hemifield* cerebral achromatopsia must meet two criteria:

1. Achromatic visual field loss is strictly limited to the superior quadrant in the involved hemifield. If the field loss also involves the inferior quadrants, the achromatopsia could simply be a reflection of primary visual cortex damage.
2. Color vision is totally absent in the superior and inferior quadrants of the involved hemifield. Partial loss could be attributable to damage to primary visual cortex (V1, V2) or its afferents.[65,66]

One should also hesitate to diagnose right homonymous hemiachromatopsia if pure alexia is not present.

Color anomia is a far more likely diagnosis than cerebral achromatopsia among patients who fail to name colors correctly on examination. A common accompaniment to pure alexia, color anomia is distinguished from cerebral achromatopsia by normal performance on color discrimination tests and a lack of complaints about color loss (Fig. 17-8).

COLOR ANOMIA

Clinical Features

This disorder is defined as an inability to name colors in the absence of achromatopsia or color agnosia (see below). In some cases, the deficit also involves an inability to point to examples of colors named by an examiner ("two-way defect"). Unlike patients

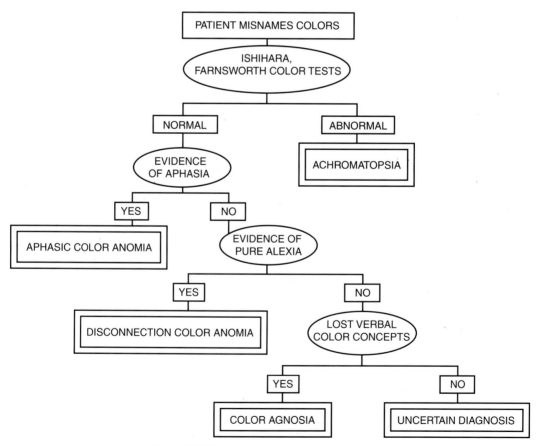

Figure 17–8. Screening for cerebral achromatopsia.

with cerebral achromatopsia, color anomics have no trouble identifying isochromatic plates or sorting Farnsworth color chips. They can discriminate between different hues but cannot name the colors that go with them. There are two forms:

- **Aphasic color anomia,** in which other signs of aphasia are present.[67,68] The causative lesion affects the left angular gyrus.
- **Disconnection color anomia,** in which anomia is limited to colors, and pure alexia is virtually always present. The causative lesion affects the left occipitotemporal white matter but also extends anteromedial to the region that is damaged in pure alexia.[51] There has been only one case report of color anomia without pure alexia;[69] it was caused by a lesion limited to the left parahippocampal white matter. Whereas nearly all color anomics have pure alexia, only 50% of pure alexics have color anomia.[70]

Pathophysiology

The pathways mediating disconnection color anomia and pure alexia are probably identical, as these deficits nearly always occur together.

Differential Diagnosis

Aphasic color anomia is diagnosed by discovering other evidence of aphasia. Disconnection color anomia must be distinguished from achromatopsia and color agnosia. Achromatopsia is ruled out by normal performance on color discrimination tests (Fig. 17-8). Color agnosia is ruled out by the patient's ability to demonstrate knowledge of verbal color concepts ("What color is blood?") and to select the correct color when instructed to "color in" line drawings of common objects.[12]

VISUAL AMNESIA

Clinical Features

This is an acquired loss of recent memory that differs from the more common amnestic syndromes in that only visual inputs are affected.[33] The causative lesion is usually a right medial posterior cerebral artery infarct.

Vision testing typically reveals normal acuity and often a left homonymous hemianopia. Verbal, tactile, and auditory recent memory are normal, but patients cannot learn new information presented in the visual domain. Although they can identify familiar objects, they fail to recall geometric figures shown briefly, withdrawn for three minutes, and then redisplayed. They also fail to recognize new faces and get lost in unfamiliar locales unless they cue themselves with written messages or maps. They may also discover that paths traveled during months that preceded the deficit are now unfamiliar (retrograde defect). Yet they display evidence of intact remote visual memory in being able to draw pictures of familiar icons such as the Eiffel Tower and the Statue of Liberty and floor plans of the home where they grew up.[33]

Cerebral achromatopsia, pure alexia, and visual object agnosia are variably present, but the strongest association is with prosopagnosia.[34] Some patients have bilateral occipitotemporal lesions, but right hemisphere lesions predominate (Fig. 17-9). Interestingly, some patients lose familiarity not merely for recently learned environments but also for topographical landmarks that have been a part of their lives for many years.[34,71]

Recovery is variable, depending on the cause. Patients must be equipped with maps and drilled in reciting directional phrases ("Turn left when I reach the intersection with the filling station . . .").

Pathophysiology

Are visual amnesia and prosopagnosia variants of the same dysfunctional process? The two conditions share lesions in the same area and some cases of visual amnesia involve loss of familiarity for remotely learned geographic landmarks. However, the two deficits also occur independently, and the gradient toward greater interruption of remote than recent memories in prosopagnosia is opposite to that found in visual amnesia.

Left   Right

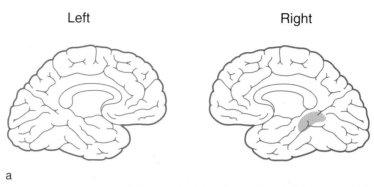

a

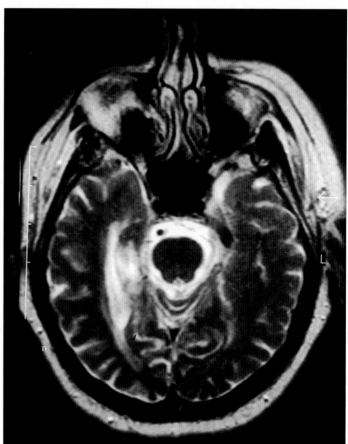

Figure 17–9. Visual amnesia. (*a*) Schematic shows the typical location of a lesion in the right parahippocampal gyrus. (*b*) MRI showing parahippocampal and optic radiation infarction (arrows) in a patient who had visual amnesia.

b

Differential Diagnosis

Visual amnesia often presents with topographical disorientation, but there are many other causes of this symptom (Table 17-2). The topographical deficit associated with visual amnesia is faulty recall of spatial landmarks. Individuals do not misreach or bump into furniture or doorways, problems typical of the visuospatial dysfunction of parietooccipital disorders (Chapter 16). They can find their way by using maps, indicating a

Table 17–2. **Manifestations and Causes of Topographical Disorientation**

Manifestation	Cause
Cannot learn routes in unfamiliar locales	Visual amnesia
Ignores one hemispace	Hemispatial neglect
Does not notice more than one object at a time	Bilateral visual inattention
Misreaches for objects	Optic ataxia
Misjudges distance and size of objects	Impaired spatial relations
Loss of directionality	Impaired spatial relations

preservation of topographical concepts. The loss of such concepts, assessed by indicating the position of cities on maps and running mazes, is associated with right parieto-occipital rather than temporo-occipital lesions.[16,72]

SUMMARY

Lesions of the temporal vision-related cortex and its incoming pathways cause complex visual hallucinations, an inability to name and identify familiar objects, symbols, words, and colors, and difficulty recalling recently viewed items. Posterior cerebral artery occlusions are the most common cause, although Alzheimer's disease, trauma, tumor, and demyelination play a role.

Recognition disorders, called "agnosias," are differentiated from naming disorders, called "anomias," by an inability to describe or mime the use of the item. Agnosias can be diagnosed only when elementary vision, global cognition, language, and attention are adequate to the task. They are confined to a single sensory modality (vision, hearing, or touch).

Visual object agnosia occurs rarely in its most severe form—a failure to recognize three-dimensional objects. More commonly, patients cannot recognize photographs or line drawings, especially if they contain ambiguous features. The responsible lesions are bilateral occipitotemporal; the left hemisphere lesion is predominant.

Visual anomia, or optic aphasia, consists of a failure to name objects by sight in the presence of intact naming by touch or sound. Visual anomia differs from visual object agnosia in that patients can describe or mime the use of visually misnamed objects. It is often found in the recovery stage of visual object agnosia.

Face agnosia (prosopagnosia) is more common than visual object agnosia; it results from bilateral lesions in the same region as those for visual object agnosia, except that right hemisphere lesions are predominant. Prosopagnosia shares with the standard amnestic syndrome a failure to learn to recognize newly presented faces. But it differs in that prosopagnosics do not recognize relatives and old friends. There is evidence that prosopagnosia is really a broad deficit in recognizing items that cannot be differentiated by distinctive, verbalizable components.

Visual object agnosia and face agnosia (prosopagnosia) are probably based on a combination of imperfect perception and visual–limbic disconnection that interferes with activation of neural circuits necessary to evoke familiarity. Whether faces are processed for recognition in a discrete brain region remains unsettled.

Pure alexia, also called alexia without agraphia or pure word blindness, is an acquired failure to read words in the absence of other signs of aphasia. Spelling and writing are intact. Right homonymous hemianopia is nearly always present; color anomia, hemiachromatopsia, and visual object agnosia are variably present. The lesion usually lies in the left occipitotemporal white matter below the occipital horn of the lateral ventricle. Pure alexia is considered a visual–verbal disconnection in which visual information never reaches the left angular gyrus language center. An alternative possibility is that it is an agnosia for lexical symbols. In many cases, the patient can read single letters and learn to read by spelling them out loud. Fortunately, the deficit often lessens over time.

Cerebral achromatopsia is an acquired loss of ability to discriminate colors owing to a lesion within the inferior occipitotemporal lobe. Most commonly of acute onset and caused by occlusion of the posterior cerebral artery, it usually consists of hemifield loss of color vision, and rarely full-field loss. This deficit is always accompanied by superior altitudinal achromatic visual field defects, and often by pure alexia or recognition disorders.

Color anomia is a failure to name colors or point to them, given their names. There are two forms: aphasic color anomia owing to lesions in the angular gyrus, and disconnection color anomia owing to left occipitotemporal lesions in the same location as for pure alexia but extending more anteromedially. Color anomia must be distinguished from achromatopsia by hue discrimination tests.

Visual amnesia consists of acute loss of ability to learn newly presented visual material, together with a short retrograde deficit. Topographical amnesia, an inability to learn new routes or remember recently learned routes, is a prominent feature. Bilateral occipitotemporal lesions are seen, but right hemisphere lesions predominate. In some cases, familiarity with remotely learned landmarks is lost as well. This condition is regarded as a visual–limbic disconnection.

REFERENCES

1. Trobe JD, Butter CM. A screening test for integrative visual dysfunction in Alzheimer's disease. *Arch Ophthalmol.* 1993;111:815–818.
2. Farah MJ. *Visual Agnosia: Disorders of Object Vision and What They Tell Us about Normal Vision.* Cambridge, Mass: MIT Press/Bradford; 1990.
3. Benson DF, Greenberg JP. Visual form agnosia: a special defect in visual discrimination. *Arch Neurol.* 1969;20:82–89.
4. Campion J, Latto R. Apperceptive agnosia due to carbon monoxide poisoning: an interpretation based on critical band masking from disseminated lesions. *Behav Brain Res.* 1985;15:227–240.
5. Lissauer H. Ein Fall von Seelenblindheit nebst einem Beitrage zur Theorie dersilben. *Arch Psychiatr Nervenkr.* 1890;21:222–270.
6. Landis T, Graves R, Benson DF, Hebben N. Visual recognition through kinaesthetic mediation. *Psychol Med.* 1982;12:515–531.
7. Mendez MF, Mendez MA, Martin R, Smyth KA, Whitehouse PJ. Complex visual disturbances in Alzheimer's disease. *Neurology.* 40:1990:439–443.
8. Benson DF, Davis RJ, Snyder BD. Posterior cortical atrophy. *Arch Neurol.* 1988;45:789–793.
9. Caplan LR. "Top of the basilar" syndrome. *Neurology.* 1980;30:72–79.
10. Rubens AB, Benson DF. Associative visual agnosia. *Arch Neurol.* 1971;24:304–316.
11. Albert M, Reches A, Silverberg R. Associative visual agnosia without alexia. *Neurology.* 1975;25:322–326.
12. Bauer RM. Agnosia. In: Heilman KM, Valenstein E, eds. *Clinical Neuropsychology.* 3rd ed. New York: Oxford University Press; 1993:215–278.
13. Riddoch MJ, Humphreys GW. A case of integrative visual agnosia. *Brain.* 1987;110:1431–1462.
14. Butter CM, Trobe JD. Integrative agnosia following progressive multifocal leukoencephalopathy. *Cortex.* 1994;30:145–158.
15. Warrington EK. Agnosia: the impairment of object recognition. In: Vinken PJ, Bruyn GW, Klawans HL, eds. *Handbook of Clinical Neurology.* Vol 39. Amsterdam: Elsevier Science; 1985:333–350.
16. Hecaen H, Albert ML. *Human Neuropsychology.* New York: John Wiley & Sons; 1978:215–227.
17. Newcombe F, Ratcliff G. Agnosia: a disorder of object recognition. In: Michel F, Schott B, eds. *Les Syndromes de Disconnexion Calleuse Chez l'Homme.* Lyon, France: Hôpital Neurologique; 1975:105–125.
18. Gomori AJ, Hawryluk GA. Visual agnosia without alexia. *Neurology.* 1984;34:947–950.
19. Freund DC. Ueber optische Aphasie und Seelenblindheit. *Arch Psychiatr Nervenkr.* 1889;20:276–297, 371–416.
20. Lhermitte F, Beauvois MF. A visual-speech disconnection syndrome: report of a case with optic aphasia, agnosic alexia and colour agnosia. *Brain.* 1973; 96:695–714.
21. Coslett HB, Saffran EM. Preserved object recognition and reading comprehension in optic aphasia. *Brain.* 1989;112:1091–1110.
22. Bisiach E. Perceptual factors in the pathogenesis of anomia. *Cortex.* 1966;2:90–95.
23. Damasio AR. Time-locked multiregional coactivation: a systems-level proposal for the neural substrates of recall and recognition. *Cognition.* 1989;33: 25–62.
24. Bauer RM, Trobe JD. Visual memory and perceptual impairments in prosopagnosia. *J Clin Neuro-ophthalmol.* 1984;4:39–46.
25. Meadows JC. The anatomical basis of prosopagnosia. *J Neurol Neurosurg Psychiatry.* 1974;37:489–501.
26. DeRenzi E, Scotti G, Spinnler H. Perceptual and associative disorders of visual recognition: relationship to the side of the cerebral lesion. *Neurology.* 1969;19:634–642.
27. Benton AL, Vanallen MW. Prosopagnosia and facial discrimination. *J Neurol Sci.* 1972;15:167–172.
28. Hecaen H, Angelergues R. Agnosia for faces (prosopagnosia). *Arch Neurol.* 1962;7:92–100.

29. Damasio AR, Damasio H, Van Hoesen GW, Cornell S. Prosopagnosia: anatomic basis and behavioral mechanisms. *Neurology.* 1982;32:331–341.

30. Levine DN. Prosopagnosia and visual object agnosia: a behavioral study. *Brain Lang.* 1978;5:341–365.

31. Lhermitte F, Chain F, Escourolle R, Ducarne B, Pillon B. Étude anatomo-clinique d'un cas de prosopagnosie. *Rev Neurol (Paris).* 1972;126:329–346.

32. Bornstein B, Sroka H, Munitz H. Prosopagnosia with animal face agnosia. *Cortex.* 1969;5:164–169.

33. Ross ED. Sensory-specific and fractional disorders of recent memory in man: I. Isolated loss of visual recent memory. *Arch Neurol.* 1980;37:193–200.

34. Landis T, Cummings JL, Benson DF, Palmer EP. Loss of topographic familiarity: an environmental agnosia. *Arch Neurol.* 1986;43:132–136.

35. Bauer RM. Visual hypoemotionality as a symptom of visual-limbic disconnection in man. *Arch Neurol.* 1982;39:702–708.

36. Habib M. Visual hypoemotionality and prosopagnosia associated with right temporal lobe isolation. *Neuropsychologia.* 1986;24:577–582.

37. Tranel D, Damasio AR. Knowledge without awareness: an autonomic index of facial recognition by prosopagnosics. *Science.* 1985;228:1453–1454.

38. Rizzo M, Hurtig R, Damasio AR. The role of scanpaths in facial recognition and learning. *Ann Neurol.* 1987;22:41–45.

39. Benton AL. Face recognition 1990. *Cortex.* 1990;26:491–499.

40. DeRenzi E. Prosopagnosia in two patients with CT scan evidence of damage confined to the right hemisphere. *Neuropsychologia.* 1986;24:385–389.

41. Sergent J, Villemure JG. Prosopagnosia in a right hemispherectomized patient. *Brain.* 1989;112:975–995.

42. Damasio AR, Tranel D. Disorders of higher brain function. In: Rosenberg RN, ed. *Comprehensive Neurology.* New York: Raven Press; 1991:639–657.

42a. Kanwisher N, McDermott J, Chun MM. The fusiform face area: a module in human extrastriate cortex specialized for face perception. *J Neurosci.* 1997;17:4303–4311.

43. McNeil JE, Warrington EK. Prosopagnosia: a face-specific disorder. *Q J Exp Psychol.* 1993;46:1–10.

44. Lu ST, Hamalainen MS, Hari R, et al. Seeing faces activates three separate areas outside the occipital visual cortex in man. *Neuroscience.* 1991;43:287–290.

45. Sergent J, Ohta S, MacDonald B. Functional neuroanatomy of face and object processing: a positron emission study. *Brain.* 1992;115:15–36.

46. Ishai A, Ungerleider LG, Martin A, Schouten JL, Haxby JV. Distributed representation of objects in the human ventral visual pathway. *Proc Nat Acad Sci.* 1999;96:9379–9384.

47. Seeck M, Mainwaring N, Ives J, et al. Differential neural activity in the human temporal lobe evoked by faces of family members and friends. *Ann Neurol.* 1993;34:369–372.

48. Alexander MP, Stuss DT, Benson DF. Capgras syndrome: a reduplicative phenomenon. *Neurology.* 1979;29:334–339.

49. Dejerine J. Contribution a l'étude anatomopathologique et clinique des différentes variétés de cécité verbaie. *Mem Soc Biol.* 1892;4:61–90.

50. Geschwind N, Fusillo M. Color-naming defects in association with alexia. *Arch Neurol.* 1966;15:137–146.

51. Damasio AR, Damasio H. The anatomic basis of pure alexia. *Neurology.* 1983;33:1573–1583.

52. Henderson VW. Anatomy of posterior pathways in reading: a reassessment. *Brain Lang.* 1986;29:119–133.

53. DeRenzi E, Zambolin A, Crisi G. The pattern of neuropsychological impairment associated with left posterior cerebral artery infarcts. *Brain.* 1987;110:1099–1116.

54. Greenblatt SH. Alexia without agraphia or hemianopia: anatomical analysis of an autopsied case. *Brain.* 1973;96:307–316.

55. Benson DF, Geschwind N. The alexias. In: Vinken PJ, Bruyn GW, eds. *Handbook of Clinical Neurology.* Vol 4. Amsterdam: North-Holland; 1969:112–140.

56. Mark VW. Could pure alexia be due to a disconnection syndrome? *Neurology.* 1998;50:835.

57. Benito-Leon J, Sanchez-Suarez C, Diaz-Guzman J, Martinex-Salio A. Pure alexia could not be a disconnection syndrome. *Neurology.* 1997;49:305–306.

57a. Verrey D. Hemiachromatopsie droite absolue. *Arch Ophthalmol Paris.* 1888;8:289–300.

57b. MacKay G, Dunlop JC. The cerebral lesions in a case of complete acquired colour-blindness. *Scottish Med Surgical J.* 1899;5:503–512.

57c. Meadows JC. Disturbed perception of colours associated with localized cerebral lesions. *Brain.* 1974;97:615–632.

57d. Albert M, Reches A, Silverberg R. Hemianopic colour blindness. *J Neurol Neurosurg Psychiatry.* 1975;38:546–549.

57e. Green GL, Lessell S. Acquired cerebral dyschromatopsia. *Arch Ophthalmol.* 1977;95:121–128.

57f. Pearlman AL, Birch J, Meadows JC. Cerebral color blindness: an acquired defect in hue discrimination. *Ann Neurol.* 1979;5:253–261.

57g. Damasio AR, Yamada T, Damasio H, Corbett J, McKee J. Central achromatopsia: behavioral, anatomic, and physiologic aspects. *Neurology.* 1980;30:1064–1071.

57h. Paulson HL, Galetta SL, Grossman M, Alavi A. Hemiachromatopsia of unilatreal occipitotemporal infarcts. *Am J Ophthalol.* 1994;118:518–523.

58. Meadows JC. Disturbed perception of colours associated with localized cerebral lesions. *Brain.* 1974;97:615–632.

59. Damasio AR, Yamada T, Damasio H, Corbett J, McKee J. Central achromatopsia: behavioral, anatomic, and physiologic aspects. *Neurology.* 1980;30:1064–1071.

60. McKeefry DJ, Zeki S. The position and topography of the human colour centre as revealed by functional magnetic resonance imaging. *Brain.* 1997;120:2229–2242.

61. Zeki S. A century of cerebral achromatopsia. *Brain.* 1990;113:1721–1777.

62. Benton A, Tranel D. Visuoperceptual, visuospatial, and visuoconstructive disorders. In: Heilman KM, Valenstein E, eds. *Clinical Neuropsychology.* 3rd ed. New York: Oxford University Press; 1993:165–213.

63. Mesulam M. Higher visual functions of the cerebral cortex and their disruption in clinical practice. In: Albert DM, Jakobiec FA, eds. *Principles and Practice*

of Ophthalmology. Vol 4. Philadelphia: Saunders; 1994:2640–2652.

64. Rizzo M, Smith V, Pokorny J, Damasio AR. Color perception profiles in central achromatopsia. *Neurology.* 1993;43:995–1001.

65. King-Smith PE. Cortical color defects. In: Drum B, Verriest G, eds. *Colour Vision Deficiencies.* Dordrecht, Netherlands: Kluwer Academic Publishers; 1989: 131–143.

66. Kolmel HW. Pure homonymous hemiachromatopsia: findings with neuro-ophthalmologic examination and imaging procedures. *Eur Arch Psychiatr Neurol Sci.* 1988;237:237–243.

67. Kinsbourne M, Warrington EK. Observations on color agnosia. *J Neurol Neurosurg Psychiatry.* 1964;27: 296–299.

68. Oxbury JM, Oxbury SM, Humphrey NK. Varieties of colour anomia. *Brain.* 1969;92:847–860.

69. Mohr JP, Leicester J, Stoddard LT, Sidman M. Right hemianopia with memory and color deficits in circumscribed left posterior cerebral artery territory infarction. *Neurology.* 1971;21:1104–1113.

70. Gloning I, Gloning K, Hoff H. *Neuropsychological Symptoms and Syndromes in Lesions of the Occipital Lobe and the Adjacent Areas.* Paris: Gauthier-Villars; 1968.

71. Aguirre GK, Zarahn E, D'Esposito M. Neural components of topographical representation. *Proc Natl Acad Sci USA.* 1998;95:839–846.

72. McFie J, Piercy M, Zangwill O. Visual-spatial agnosia associated with lesions of the right cerebral hemisphere. *Brain.* 1950;73:167–190.

Part V

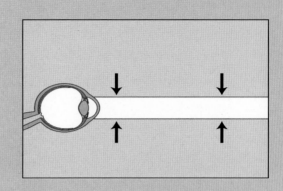

NONORGANIC VISUAL DISTURBANCES

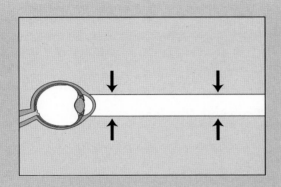

NONORGANIC VISUAL DISTURBANCES

Every symptom and nearly every sign described in this book has at one time been a manifestation of a nonorganic, or "psychogenic," condition. Nonorganic disturbances are indeed prevalent. In one study, they made up 10% of visits to general practitioners.[1] Among cases of fever of unexplained origin, 10% are artificial.[2] No prevalence data exist for nonorganic visual disturbances, but practitioners will affirm that they are not scarce.[3,4]

WHAT IS A NONORGANIC CONDITION?

A nonorganic condition is defined as one in which the clinical features are based on psychiatric or behavioral disorders rather than anatomic or biochemical abnormalities. This definition does not include psychosomatic illness, which is defined as organic illness triggered or exacerbated by psychologic factors (e.g., irritable bowel syndrome). The misleading term "functional" should be discarded as a synonym for "nonorganic" because it suggests that something is functioning.

To discover the nonorganic nature of a visual disturbance, one must develop finesse with a series of diagnostic maneuvers. To guide the patient properly once a nonorganic diagnosis is made, one needs a basic familiarity with the pertinent underlying behavioral and psychiatric conditions.

We turn first to the various manifestations of nonorganic visual disturbances and their diagnosis.

POSITIVE VISUAL MANIFESTATIONS

Hallucinations, illusions, and hypersensitive or aversive reactions to visual stimuli are important nonorganic visual symptoms. But nonorganic hallucinations and illusions so resemble those of organic illness that the diagnosis can be reached only by exclusion (Chapter 4).

Transient Hallucinations

Transient hallucinations, which may include flashes of light, geometric patterns, or formed images,[5] are relatively uncommon nonorganic visual manifestations (Chapter 4). Retinal and optic nerve disorders must be excluded as causes of monocular hallucinations. Substance abuse, toxic medication, metabolic or degenerative encephalopathies, migraine, transient ischemic attack, and seizure are the major causes of binocular hallucinations. The visual hallucinations of psychosis always consist of formed images, delusional, and often paranoid. Auditory hallucinations are usually integrated in these visual hallucinations.[6,7] One should not underestimate the power of childhood fantasy and trancelike states to induce vivid visual hallucinations.[8]

Persistent Hallucinations

Nonorganic persistent visual hallucinations usually take the form of twinkling lights around viewed objects. The organic causes are retinal photoreceptor dysfunction (digitalis, clomiphene toxicity, retinitis pigmentosa, choroidal inflammations), metabolic encephalopathy, encephalitis, Creutzfeldt-Jakob disease, and recent occipital stroke or excision of an occipital mass lesion (Chapters 4, 10, 15).

Transient Illusions

Transient visual illusions of distorted or discolored images are a rare manifestation of nonorganic illness, except in children. The same organic considerations apply as for episodic hallucinations (Chapter 4).

Persistent Illusions

Persistent illusions of altered shapes or sizes of images are also rarely nonorganic, except in psychosis. The common organic causes are (*1*) retinal disorders that distort the foveal photoreceptors and (*2*) refractive aberrations (Chapters 2, 4, 10). Monocular diplopia or polyopia due to an optical aberration disappears when the patient views visual targets through a pinhole occluder (Chapter 2). Metamorphopsia may be dismissed as a manifestation of foveal disease if there are no ophthalmoscopic abnormalities. Persistent illusions of cerebral origin occur chiefly in the setting of recent occipital stroke or excision of an occipital mass lesion, in which case a homonymous hemianopia will often be present (Chapter 4).

Sensitivity to Light

Excessive sensitivity to light, or photophobia—a painful, aversive reaction to a light that is not exceptionally bright (Chapter 2)—is often a manifestation of an anxiety disorder. Patients with this affliction avoid fluorescent lights, video display terminals, and car headlights. Their exaggerated photosensitivity may lead them to withdraw from all outdoor activities, dim the lights in the house, wear several layers of tinted eye shields, and shun all social activity. Extreme cases may proceed to involuntary eyelid closure (blepharospasm).

Photophobia may also be of organic origin, as when albinism or a dilated pupil allow too much light to reach the retina, when keratitis or uveitis cause light to trigger ciliary spasm, or when degenerating cone photoreceptors are unable to cope with ordinary amounts of light. Intracranial causes include migraine and inflammation of the meninges or basal cranial blood vessels.

Sensitivity to Patterns, Colors, or Moving Objects

Anxious, phobic, or obsessive patients may report that they feel unsettled, dizzy, anxious, or fearful when they gaze upon complicated, multicolored, or bright visual patterns or rapidly moving objects.

NEGATIVE VISUAL MANIFESTATIONS

Visual acuity and visual field loss are the most common nonorganic visual manifestations encountered in clinical practice.

Transient Visual Acuity Loss

Transient blackouts of vision are often manifestations of nonorganic disease, but it is impossible to prove this without excluding organic causes (Chapter 3). There is, however, one variant of transient visual acuity loss that is nearly always nonorganic: vision that fades with prolonged viewing. There is no organic mechanism for this "visual exhaustion," "visual fatigue," "asthenopia," or "visual burnout." *The closest organic simulation is presbyopia,* wherein patients strain to focus near objects with insufficient accommodation and eventually develop periocular pain and blurred vision from accommodative spasm (Chapter 2).

Persistent Visual Acuity Loss

Patients present with one of three patterns: (*1*) monocular acuity loss; (*2*) mild binocular acuity loss; and (*3*) severe binocular acuity loss merging into total blindness. To establish that these are nonorganic manifestations, the examiner must select from a series of maneuvers based on three strategies (Table 18-1).[9-16]

Table 18–1. **Techniques Used to Expose Nonorganic Visual Acuity Loss**

Strategy	Monocular Acuity Loss	Mild-moderate Binocular Acuity Loss	Marked Binocular Acuity Loss
Inducing the patient to "see normally" without realizing it (Gotcha!)	Fogging Polaroid test Duochrome test Pupil-splitting prism test	Snellen chart manipulation Optical aids	None
Demonstrating inconsistency	Pupillary reactions Ophthalmoscopy Stereopsis tests Base-out prism test	Optical aids Near–far discrepancies Potential acuity tests Stereopsis tests	Threat Mirror movement Optokinetic stimulus Ambulation Proprioceptively mediated tasks Inappropriate affect
Using objective measures	Swinging-light test VEP ERG	VEP ERG	VEP

1. **Inducing the patient to "see normally" without realizing it ("Gotcha!" maneuvers).** In this strategy, the objective is to have the patient exhibit normal acuity without being aware of it. In cases of monocular visual loss, the patient must believe that the acuity in the "good eye" is being tested. In cases of binocular visual loss, the examiner's demeanor must suggest that identifying ever smaller letters is not an admission of patient deception ("I know these are small letters and hard for you to see, but try and identify one of them; take a guess!"). This strategy is most successful if the patient is suggestible or unsophisticated.

2. **Demonstrating inconsistency.** In this strategy, the examiner attempts to elicit performance on corroborative vision tests that is incompatible with a depressed visual acuity. Unlike the "Gotcha!" maneuver, this strategy provides only indirect evidence that a complaint is nonorganic. Its advantage is that the patient is unaware of the relationship between test results and the veracity of the complaint. A major drawback is that even patients with organic visual loss may be inconsistent in their responses.

3. **Invalidating subjective responses with objective measures.** In this strategy, the examiner uses objective tests such as the swinging-light test, the ERG, and visual evoked potentials (VEPs) to contradict evidence from subjective tests. Each test has limitations. The swinging-light test is useful only when monocular or asymmetric visual loss is in question (Chapter 8). The standard ERG is insensitive to disease confined to the fovea (Chapter 9). The VEP can be deformed by deliberate defocusing (Chapter 9).

These three strategies should be deployed according to the pattern of the visual loss.

SUBNORMAL ACUITY IN ONE EYE

First try the following Gotcha! maneuvers, designed to induce the patient into believing that the "good eye" is reading the letters.

Fogging

Covertly place before the "normal" eye a high convex or astigmatic lens, which creates a blurred image for that eye.

Polaroid Filtered Spectacles

Place Polaroid spectacles over the eyes and instruct the patient to view a special (Project-O-Chart) slide, which will make some letters invisible to the right eye, others to the left eye.

Duochrome Test

Place a red spectacle over one eye, a green spectacle over the other and instruct the patient to view a special screen designed to make some letters invisible to the right eye, others to the left eye.

Pupil-Splitting Prism Test

Use a finger to block the vision in the eye with the alleged poor vision (Fig. 18-1). Place a 5 diopter prism base down so that it splits the pupil of the normal eye. Inquire if the patient sees two Snellen charts with the "good eye" (the pupil-splitting prism should create monocular diplopia). Tell the patient to begin reading the letters from the *bottom* chart. Once the patient has begun doing so, simultaneously slide the prism down so that its midportion is centered on the pupil and remove your finger from in front of the "bad" eye. The patient should be concentrating on reading the letters and will not notice that the bottom chart is now being viewed only by the "bad" eye!

If the Gotcha! maneuvers do not work, move on to maneuvers that bring out a pattern of inconsistent responses.

Pupillary Reactions

One can readily exclude an asymmetric optic neuropathy by finding normal pupillary reactions in the swinging-light test (Chapter 8). Cautions: subtle afferent pupil defects can be easily overlooked if technique is suboptimal. Also, recall that bilateral optic neuropathy, foveal disorders, and amblyopia will not display an afferent pupil defect.

Ophthalmoscopy

Examine the foveal region and optic disk for structural abnormalities to exclude many causes of subnormal acuity, bearing in mind that there are some rare conditions that pro-

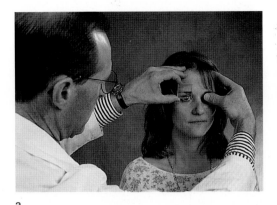

a

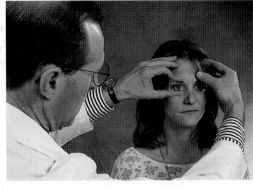

b

Figure 18–1. Pupil-splitting prism test. This test is used to unmask nonorganic monocular visual acuity loss. (*a*) Tell the patient to look at a distant Snellen chart. Place a 5-diopter prism base down over the "good eye" such that its lower border splits the pupil. Cover the "bad eye" with your thumb. The patient should see two sets of letters with the "good eye" as a result of the prism effect (monocular diplopia). (If the patient does not appreciate monocular diplopia, reposition the prism. If repositioning does not elicit diplopia, abort the test—it will not work!) Tell the patient to begin reading from the lower set of letters. (*b*) Move the prism down so that it no longer splits the pupil as you simultaneously uncover the "bad eye." The patient should not be aware that the visual scenery has changed, although the diplopia is now binocular. Tell the patient to continue reading letters from the bottom set. If all letters are correctly identified, the patient has done so with the "bad eye."

duce little or no structural alteration (see Table 10-2). Fluorescein angiography and electroretinography may be useful in the diagnosis of these cases, but they should be reserved for instances where skilled, high-magnification ophthalmoscopy has failed to disclose a diagnostic structural abnormality.

Stereopsis Tests

The ability to appreciate stereopsis on the Titmus Stereoacuity test (Fig. 18-2) is dependent on visual acuity in both eyes.[17,18] A nomogram has been developed that relates various degrees of subnormal monocular[17] and binocular[18] visual acuity to the ability to detect which of four circles stands up from the page. Achieving the maximum score—equivalent to a stereoacuity of 40 seconds of arc—requires a visual acuity of 20/20 or better in the poorer eye.

Base-Out Prism Test

After instructing the patient to fixate the 20/20 distant Snellen letter, introduce a 5 diopter base-out prism over the "bad" eye and observe for an inward deviation of that eye (Fig. 18-3). Then remove the prism and observe for an outward refixational movement of that eye. These refixational movements suggest there cannot be a substantial

central scotoma in the "bad" eye, and that visual acuity is therefore at least 20/50.

MILDLY-TO-MODERATELY SUBNORMAL ACUITY IN BOTH EYES

The maneuvers so useful for unmasking nonorganic monocular visual loss do not work in patients with symmetrical visual loss

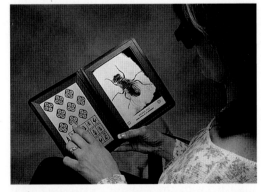

Figure 18–2. Titmus stereopsis test. This test is used to discover nonorganic monocular (or binocular) visual acuity loss. Wearing Polaroid glasses, the patient is instructed to look at each group of four circles and indicate which one of the circles appears to "stand up from the page." A patient who correctly identifies the "elevated circle" in the bottom right grouping has a stereoacuity of 40 seconds of arc, which demands an acuity of 20/20 in the poorer eye.[14]

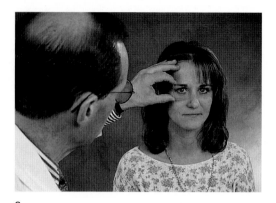
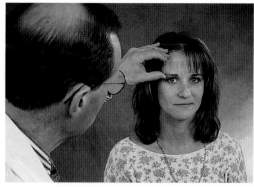

a   b

Figure 18–3. Five-diopter prism test for central scotoma. This test is used to cast doubt on the organic nature of monocular or binocular visual acuity loss. (*a*) Introduce a base-out 5-diopter prism over the eye with alleged poor vision, and observe if the eye makes an inward movement. (*b*) Remove the prism and observe for an outward movement. If these two movements occur consistently, the central 3 degrees of the visual field are functioning and the patient must have at least 20/50 acuity in that eye.

in both eyes. The best approach is to cajole and offer face-saving gestures. If that approach does not work, employ the following tests to develop a pattern of inconsistent responses.

Snellen Chart Manipulation

Display the smallest letters first (the 20/10 line) and offer the patient the chance to name only those letters that appear reasonably clear, even for a mere instant. Then work up to the larger letters, noting if the patient identifies the less recognizable letters rather than the more difficult ones. For those patients who may be practiced at reading the Snellen chart, display letters in columns rather than rows in order to disrupt their orientation.

Optical Aids

Place a 0.12 diopter lens before an eye being tested as a means of giving the patient a face-saving way to achieve a better acuity score. Offer the eyes a rest between attempts at identifying letters. Sometimes vision will improve with the pinhole. In testing near acuity, apply plus lenses that allow the patient to bring the reading material closer to the eyes. In organic visual loss, visual acuity improves as the reading material is brought closer because it plants a larger image on the fovea.

Near–Far Discrepancies

Test visual acuity at distance and at near and compare the scores. In nonorganic visual loss, these measurements often do not match. If patients cannot read distant Snellen letters perfectly, allow them to approach the chart, and note whether the improvement is appropriate for the shorter distance.

Potential Acuity Tests

Many patients are steadfast in claiming that they cannot see normally under ordinary viewing circumstances. But if tested under conditions that they consider inapplicable to ordinary life, they will see normally. For example, the pinhole occluder often dramatically restores vision. If it does not, try the Potential Acuity Meter, an optical device that allows patients to view Snellen letters in a "black box" (Fig. 18-4).[19] This device appears so artificial and complex to patients that they will often display normal visual acuity.[20]

MARKEDLY SUBNORMAL VISUAL ACUITY IN BOTH EYES

Among patients who claim severe vision loss, none of the maneuvers described thus far will work. However, the following tests are often successful.

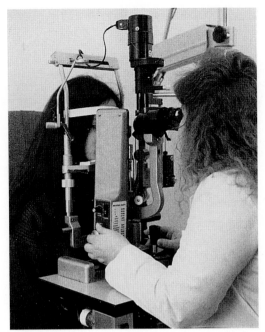

Figure 18–4. The potential acuity meter. This device may be used to detect nonorganic visual acuity loss. The rectangular box (arrow) attached to the slit-lamp biomicroscope, called a Potential Acuity Meter, allows patients to view Snellen letters through a "black box." Viewing through this instrument appears so artificial to patients that they will often allow themselves normal visual acuity even if they claim subnormal acuity on testing with the standard Snellen chart. (Reprinted with permission from Burde RM, Savino PJ, Trobe JD. Clinical Decisions in Neuro-ophthalmology, 2nd Ed. Mosby-Yearbook, St. Louis, 1992.)

Threat

Briskly wave your hand toward the patients' eyes, as if to strike them, being sure to avoid creating an air current on the cornea. An appropriately timed blink suggests at least some vision, but it may be rudimentary (Chapter 6).

Mirror Movement

Hold a mirror large enough to fill the patient's central field at a distant of about 6 inches from the eyes and rotate it from side to side. A patient who has vision will be unable to resist the temptation to move his eyes in pursuit of his reflected image.

Opticokinetic Stimulus

Rotate an opticokinetic drum or tape at a distance of 6 inches from the patient's eyes

and observe for nystagmus. Visual acuity of finger counting or better is necessary to mount this reflex response.

Unfortunately, the preceding measures require only rudimentary vision. More conclusive is a history from companions that the patient is performing activities incompatible with blindness, coupled with an examination of the following tasks.

Ambulation

Patients with severe organic visual acuity loss and preserved peripheral vision do not bump into door frames, furniture, or other obstacles. Even if they have lost both acuity and field, they will have learned to lead with their hands, take short steps, and walk cautiously. Those with nonorganic visual acuity loss often go out of their way to collide with obstacles, miraculously avoiding serious harm to themselves.

Proprioceptively Mediated Tasks

If proprioception is intact, organically blind patients should be able to bring their outstretched fingers toward one another and have them touch. They should also be able to sign their names legibly.

When the foregoing clinical maneuvers provide insubstantial evidence, one may resort to visual evoked potentials, with the acknowledgment that this test is subject to false-positive and false-negative results (Chapter 9). Despite attempts at monitoring fixation, fakers manage to defocus or look away from the target enough to degrade the signal.[21–23] Often VEPs have been perfectly intact in blind patients despite anatomic evidence of destruction of extrastriate visual cortex.[24–28] These tests evidently sample only a part of the pathway needed for seeing.[29] The ERG is valuable as a tool in detecting widespread retinopathies without ophthalmoscopic abnormalities, such as paraneoplastic retinopathy (Chapter 11). Recall, however, that the standard (full-field) ERG is not sensitive to focal retinal disorders; the newer multifocal ERG, not yet in wide clinical use, may fill this gap.

Persistent Visual Field Loss

Any visual field defect can be faked in any testing circumstance.[30] Central scotomas are hard to fake, but hemianopias, quadrantanopias (see Fig. 18-8), and altitudinal defects are relatively easy, particularly on the most commonly used automated instrument, the Humphrey Field Analyzer.[30,31] The reason for this is that the Field Analyzer's testing strategy is based on the patient's threshold visual sensitivity to targets displayed at the outset in each field quadrant. If the initial bright stimulus is not detected in a given quadrant, all subsequent stimuli displayed in that quadrant will be bright, allowing the patient to differentiate them from stimuli displayed in other quadrants, where initial sensitivity may have been higher.[31] The instrument's "reliability indices" will look perfectly acceptable in these contrived defects. Determined fakers can execute these deceptions without making errors in their responses related to "normal" parts of the visual field.[32]

A common misconception is that kinetic perimetry performed by an experienced perimetrist can uncover deceptions produced on the automated perimeters. When six subjects were instructed to fake defects on Humphrey and Goldmann perimetric testing, even the most practiced kinetic perimetrists mapped counterfeit defects.[30] In fact, the more experienced perimetrists unwittingly gave the subjects cues that aided in the deception.

The techniques used to diagnose nonorganic visual field loss are deployed in accordance with the type of visual field loss (Table 18-2).

CONSTRICTION

The visual field in patients with nonorganic disorders is usually shrunken to a central peephole (Fig. 18-5).[32] Two common organic causes of this pattern—retinitis pigmentosa and optic neuropathies—can usually be excluded because they typically produce obvious ophthalmoscopic abnormalities. However, beware of two conditions that display no such changes: bilateral visual cortex dysfunction with macular sparing (Chapters 7, 15) and toxic or paraneoplastic photoreceptor dysfunction (Chapter 11).

The nonorganic nature of constricted fields will emerge through one or more of the following techniques.

Testing at Two Distances

By finger confrontation, establish the limits of the visual field at 1/3 meter and at 1or 2 meters' distance from the patient (Fig. 18-6). If the constricted field is organic, the borders will markedly expand ("funnel field"). If the defect is nonorganic, the field borders will not expand ("tunnel field"). A related maneuver is to suggest to the patient that a finger displayed closer to the eyes will be easier to spot than one farther away, which is a physiologic untruth. That is, a finger displayed close to the lateral orbital rim is much

Table 18–2. **Techniques Used to Expose Nonorganic Visual Field Loss**

Constricted	Monocular Temporal Hemianopia	Bitemporal Hemianopia	Binasal Hemianopia	Homonymous Hemianopia
Test at two distances	Compare monocular and binocular fields; the defect should disappear with binocular field testing	Compare monocular and binocular fields; the defect should disappear with binocular field testing	Compare monocular and binocular fields; the defect should disappear with binocular field testing	No good methods
Convince patient that this is not a visual field test				
Demonstrate that field perimeter is not stable		Test for postfixational blindness	Test for prefixational blindness	
Use distracting verbal cues				

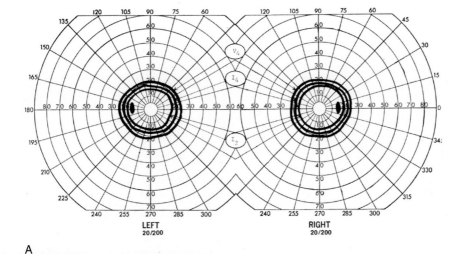

A

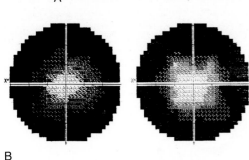

B

Figure 18–5. The constricted field. (*a*) Kinetic perimetry. All isopters are collapsed upon one another at 15 degrees eccentricity. (*b*) Static perimetry. Thresholds are marked elevated for stimuli displayed beyond 10 degrees. There are organic and nonorganic causes of this pattern.

harder to spot than one displayed a foot farther away at the same eccentricity.

Convincing the Patient That This Is Not a Visual Field Test

Tell the patient that the finger confrontation test is a test of "fast reflexes" or response latency. Then instruct him to reach for your stationary finger with his hand. Begin by displaying fingers well within the central peephole. Once the patient is lulled into responding, begin displaying fingers farther and farther from center. Distracted into believing this is a "reaching" test, the patient will forget the limits of his visual field.

Demonstrating That the Field Perimeter Is Not Stable

Display two vertically oriented fingers, one within the border previously acknowledged by the patient, the other finger outside that border. If the patient identifies only one finger, redisplay the two fingers in the horizontal plane with fingertips inside the acknowledged border. The patient with nonorganic field loss will usually report seeing only one finger.

Using Distracting Verbal Cues

Tell the patient that you will cue each presentation by announcing "Do you see it now?" and that she is to respond by saying "Yes" or "No." Present fingers well within the central peephole. The patient will be cautious about responding at first but will soon be drawn into a routine of answering "Yes" to centrally displayed fingers, as they lie well within acknowledged borders. Once the routine is established, introduce a finger outside the acknowledged border without cueing the patient. The unwary patient will quickly and sheepishly say "No!" You have demonstrated that the peripheral target was seen.

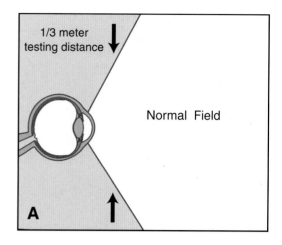

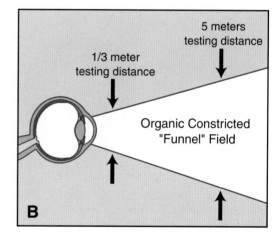

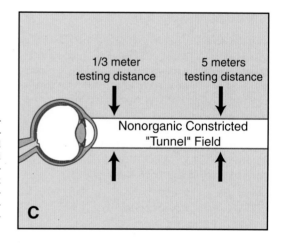

Figure 18–6. Funnel versus tunnel field. (*a*) The normal visual field. Its borders expand with increasing distance from the eye. (*b*) The organically constricted ("funnel") field. Arrows indicate points at which stimuli introduced from without are first detected at two different test distances. Although narrower at every point than the normal field, its borders expand with increasing testing distance from the eye. (*c*) The nonorganically constricted ("tunnel") field. Its borders do not expand with increasing testing distance from the eye.

Using Magical Remedies

Play on the patient's suggestibility by explaining that the constricted field comes from having pupils that are too small to admit all the light. Instill a "special dilating eyedrop" (in reality a standard mydriatic), inviting the patient to experience an expansion of the visual field. If it works, prescribe the topical nostrum for temporary instillation at home.

Many of the narrow fields produced on formal kinetic or static automated perimetry are due to testing artifact. For example, patients may be poorly positioned or incorrectly refracted. Others are tired, inattentive, confused, or under the false impression that they should withhold a response until they see the target clearly. When tested with kinetic perimetry, they must be told to signal upon first awareness of a moving stimulus. When tested with static perimetry, they must be reminded to pay attention and press the buzzer even if they are not certain they have seen a white dot.

MONOCULAR TEMPORAL HEMIANOPIA

A complete temporal hemianopia is a common accompaniment of nonorganic visual acuity loss in the ipsilateral eye.[33] Use the following two-step process to disclose a counterfeit defect: (1) test confrontation fields monocularly to establish that the hemianopia is limited to one eye; (2) test confrontation fields binocularly. The intact nasal field in the contralateral "good" eye should reduce an organic monocular temporal hemianopia to a tiny peripheral crescent. The faking patient will retain a complete temporal hemianopia.

Even if this maneuver yields equivocal results, be aware that an *organic* monocular temporal hemianopia has never been described without an afferent pupil defect.[34] A pseudo-hemianopic defect could, of course, arise from retinal disease (detachment, dysplasia, retinoschisis, inflammation, trauma) (Chapter 10).

BITEMPORAL HEMIANOPIA

This is a rare nonorganic manifestation. One way to unmask a nonorganic dense bitemporal hemianopia is to search for "postfixational blindness" (Fig. 18-7a). Instruct the patient to fixate on a small target at 1/3 meter from the eyes. A finger displayed 1/3 meter behind it will be invisible if the defects

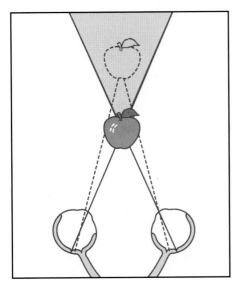
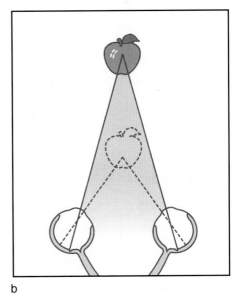

a   b

Figure 18–7. Postfixation and prefixation blindness. These tests are used to unmask nonorganic bitemporal or binasal hemianopias. (*a*) Postfixational blindness. When the patient with organic bitemporal hemianopia fixates on the closer apple, the more distant one becomes invisible because it falls within a triangular "postfixational" scotoma. (*b*) Prefixational blindness. When the patient with organic binasal hemianopia fixates on the more distant apple, the closer one disappears because it falls within a triangular "prefixational" scotoma.

are organic because it will be hidden within the absent temporal fields. An alternative way to expose these defects is to perform binocular perimetry. The intact nasal fields should overlap most of the defective temporal defects and erase them.

BINASAL HEMIANOPIA

Binasal hemianopia. Dense defects can be uncovered by looking for "prefixational blindness" (Fig. 18-7b). Instruct the patient to fixate on a target. A small target displayed between the patient and the more distant target will be invisible if the defects are organic because it will be hidden within the absent nasal fields.[35] Binocular perimetry can also be used to expose these defects, as with bitemporal hemianopia.

Binasal hemianopia with visual field defects that are aligned to the vertical meridian *is never caused by organic disease.* One might imagine that bilateral compression of the optic chiasm would selectively damage the noncrossing axons emanating from temporal retina, but this does not happen. Binasal nerve fiber bundle defects are, however, very common (ischemic, compressive, inflammatory, postpapilledema optic neuropathy). Whereas their borders may appear to "respect the vertical meridian," closer inspection reveals that there is "spillover" into temporal fields (Chapter 7).

HOMONYMOUS HEMIANOPIA

Counterfeit homonymous hemianopia or quadrantanopia (Fig. 18-8) is very difficult to expose. Fortunately, it is a rare nonorganic manifestation.

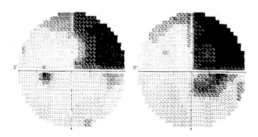

Figure 18–8. Nonorganic homonymous quadrantanopia. This field defect was a fake, an easy caper considering the test strategy of the instrument (see text). Counterfeit homonymous defects are very difficult to expose!

MANAGEMENT ERRORS

The management of patients suspected of having nonorganic visual disturbances is often marred by the following missteps:
1. Ordering expensive, misleading, or low-yield tests. Retinal fluorescein angiography, visual evoked potentials, electroretinography, and brain imaging are often ordered "defensively," even when the examiner has ample evidence that the manifestations are nonorganic. Not only do these tests create unnecessary expenses, they often turn up noncontributory abnormalities that compel further inappropriate tests and fortify the patient's sense that there must be a somatic disorder.
2. Failure to state unequivocally that the cause is nonorganic. Evasive and noncommital documentation propagate the misimpression of organic illness, invite therapies of dubious value, and establish a paper trail to support wasteful litigation.
3. Failure to differentiate between underlying psychiatric and behavioral disturbances. Most physicians are so angry at being manipulated by patients trying to "beat the system" or "get something for nothing" that they are reluctant to make distinctions between conscious and unconscious fakery. There is a tendency to consider everyone a malingerer. But some are not, and guiding them into the hands of the appropriate therapists leads to a more effective resolution of the underlying problem.

UNDERLYING BEHAVIORAL AND PSYCHIATRIC CONDITIONS

Nonorganic disturbances germinate within a spectrum of psychogenic conditions defined according to the patient's motivation and insight (Table 18-3).[36] At one end of the spectrum is malingering, which is based on conscious motivation and clear insight. At the other end is somatoform disorder, which is based on unconscious motivation and unclear or absent insight.

Malingering

Malingering is the feigning of illness in order to obtain monetary gain, narcotics, or

Table 18–3. **Behavioral and Psychiatric Disorders Underlying Nonorganic Visual Disturbances**

Condition	Risk Group	Pathogenesis	Disposition
Malingering	Mostly adult males	Conscious feigning of illness to secure material gains	In a nonconfrontative, affectively neutral manner say that exam fails to explain disturbance Medical treatment not indicated
Factitious disorder	Adults	Conscious feigning of illness to assume sick role	In a nonconfrontative, affectively neutral manner, say that exam fails to explain disturbance Psychologic care indicated
Somatization disorder	Children and young women	Unconscious feigning of illness for many reasons	*Adults:* reassurance and ritualistic aids *Children:* reassure parents; if problem is disruptive, recommend psychologic care; if child abuse is suspected, discuss with pediatrician
Conversion disorder	Young women	Unconscious feigning of illness to resolve conflicts	Discuss non-organic nature of disturbance with family or surrogate and arrange psychiatric care
Hypochondriasis	Adults	Exaggerated reaction to body signals and inappropriate fear of incapacity or death	Reassure that disturbance is not vision- or life-threatening but do not deny its existence; arrange periodic revisits to boost reasurrance

relief from unpleasant circumstances. Fully conscious of their goals, malingerers are engaging is antisocial behavior, not suffering from a psychiatric illness. Their interactions belong more with the law than with medicine.

Malingerers confront their examiners in an adversarial role, sometimes dangerously. The physician's most appropriate response ought to be emotionally neutral. One should explain calmly that the examination has not disclosed a clear explanation for the complaint, holding to that position despite entreaties from the patient for a more detailed explanation. The record should document unequivocally that the visual disturbance "has no organic basis." Psychotherapy has no role.

Factitious Disorder

Like malingerers, patients with factitious disorder are aware that they are creating a fake illness, but they have a poor understanding of why. In actuality, they are aiming for a sick role, but because they lack insight into this goal, they are considered to have a psychiatric illness.[36] Among the many underlying motivations proposed for assuming this role, however, most would be difficult to separate from malingering:[2]

- Control. Feeling downtrodden in other aspects of their lives, patients use illness to control the flow of events, even if only within a narrow sphere.
- Masochism. A heavy residue of guilt from childhood spurs the need for self-punishment.
- Reenactment of childhood parental abuse. Patients act out old scenarios, with caregivers playing the role of parents.
- Distraction. Attention is directed away from other emotionally traumatic situations.
- Regression. Primitive needs are met.
- Avoidance. The illness relieves the responsibility to fulfill difficult commitments.

The diagnosis of factitious disorder is particularly urgent when the examiner suspects Munchausen syndrome, an extreme variant wherein patients travel from caregiver to caregiver, fabricating illness and inducing potentially life-threatening interventions.[2] In managing factitious visual disturbances, the examiner should disclose the results in a nonconfrontative manner and direct the patient toward psychotherapy.[37]

Somatoform Disorders

Somatoform disorders differ from malingering and factitious disorders in that the patient believes that the physical symptoms and signs are organic. In other words, illness is not being deliberately faked. The three somatoform disorders with prominent visual manifestations are somatization, conversion, and hypochondriasis.

SOMATIZATION

Individuals typically complain of a multitude of symptoms, related mostly to pain and bodily malfunctions. Women outnumber men by 5- to 20-fold. Somatizers frustrate caregivers by reporting their symptoms vaguely and unconvincingly, histrionically and exhibitionistically. Antisocial behavior streaks through their history: crime, running away from home, truancy, substance abuse, poor employment record, marital difficulty, spousal abuse, and sexual promiscuity.[38] Given this profile, wouldn't caregivers assume that somatizers are deliberately faking illness?

According to most formulations, they are not. Their behavior is a form of depression or an expression of anger at a significant other. If the deficit is relatively mild and the patient appears suggestible, one can try reassurance and hope that the disturbance will eventually disappear. Alternatively, one can recommend health-promoting rituals (artificial tears, avoiding precipitating circumstances). In the long run, patients with visual impairment owing to somatization disorder have a high rate of spontaneous improvement.[39–41] The few who have persistent deficits are surprisingly unfettered in activities of daily living.[40] Counseling and psy-

chotropic medications are used to treat coexisting depression or anxiety. Socioeconomic woes must also be addressed.

Most nonorganic visual disturbances in children, especially in preadolescents and adolescents, are manifestations of a form of somatization disorder.[4,40,42,43] Conflicts or setbacks within the family or at school are often contributory.[42] Some children are high achievers who are having trouble meeting parental expectations; others are jealous of attention or favors bestowed on siblings. More troubling is evidence of current child abuse.[42] Visual disturbances may be chosen by children as a mode of expression because a parent or acquaintance has had visual difficulties.[42]

The examiner should review the nonorganic problem with the parents, but *without the child present*. In fact, the child should not be aware that this discussion is occurring. In this regard, a useful ploy is to take the child off to another room for a brief mock slit-lamp or visual field examination. In presenting the problem to the child's parents, the examiner may expect to encounter one of three reactions: (*1*) relief that the problem is nonorganic; (*2*) lack of acceptance of this explanation; (*3*) anger at the inference that there are "family problems" or at having been duped by the child. If the reaction is one of relief, the examiner should inquire whether the parents believe the visual problem is disruptive. If so, psychologic counseling is advocated; if not, the problem should be allowed to dissipate without undue attention. If the parents' reactions are a lack of acceptance or anger, the examiner must firmly recommend that no retribution be taken against the child. If an abusive situation is suspected, the examiner should discuss the matter with the child's pediatrician.

CONVERSION

In this disorder, patients have dramatic and immobilizing manifestations such as blindness, paralysis, involuntary movements, pseudoseizures, anesthesia, and mutism. As with somatization disorder, conversion affects mostly young, depressed women. But unlike somatization disorder, manifestations are not vague, changing, or multiple. They are discrete, immutable, and attached to one bodily function.

The psychodynamic explanation of conversion disorder is that the pseudo-neurologic manifestations derive from a maladaptive attempt to banish the anxiety of socially unacceptable impulses (anger, sexual desire)—the "primary gain." The "secondary gain" comes from attracting sympathy, avoiding obligation, and controlling other people's behavior.

Insight-oriented psychotherapy, hypnosis, anxiolytics, and relaxation techniques are the most effective therapeutic approaches. Patients are encouraged to explore intrapsychic conflicts, sometimes with the aid of "truth sera" such as parenteral amobarbital or lorazepam. Success depends on the duration of the disorder and on co-morbid conditions.

HYPOCHONDRIASIS

Patients with this condition misinterpret their normal body signals as a sign of disease. Morbidly preoccupied by a fear of illness, they are deaf to vehement denials of serious illness by their caregivers. Even if they can be temporarily disabused of their fears, they soon relapse with the same complaint—or a different one.

Hypochondriasis affects both sexes equally, and at all ages, with an estimated prevalence of 4%–6%.[1] The term is derived from the Greek word for "hypochondrium," or below the ribs—referring to the abdomen, the source of most complaints. Visual complaints are also common. Patients usually report vaguely impaired vision ("I just cannot see clearly," "There is something the matter with my eyes") and pain or discomfort about the eyes. These symptoms are often precipitated by an adverse interpersonal or job-related event. Visual function measures are usually normal—but only according to the examiner.

Hypochondriasis is variously believed to originate in a low tolerance for discomfort, a hypersensitivity to all body sensations, an abnormal propensity to lapse into dependency, or a perversion of feelings of guilt and low self-esteem. Patients resist psychotherapy because they refuse to accept their condition as psychologically based. They benefit most from periodic visits to caregivers who must assure them that their symptoms are medically respectable but not disabling. Diagnostic procedures should be avoided as much as possible, but the caregiver should not try to dissuade the patient of the physical basis of the symptoms. Hypochondriasis tends to be a lifelong mode of expression. Antidepressants and group therapy may be successful in easing the chronic despair.

Hypochondriasis may be an expression of chronic low-grade anxiety. An important visual manifestation of anxiety is sensitivity to light (see above). Patients with nonorganic photosensitivity often respond dramatically to a combination of desensitization strategies and anxiolytic medication.

SUMMARY

Nonorganic visual disturbances are defined as lacking a recognized anatomical or biochemical basis and having psychiatric or behavioral underpinnings.

Nonorganic visual disturbances may be transient or persistent; they include positive phenomena, such as illusions, hallucinations, and extreme sensitivity to visual stimuli, as well as negative phenomena, such as poor visual acuity and field loss.

Recognizing transient visual phenomena as nonorganic is very difficult. The best approach is to exclude organic disease.

Three strategies are used to disclose the nonorganic nature of persistent visual acuity loss: (1) fooling the patient into reporting normal acuity ("Gotcha!"); (2) demonstrating inconsistency between the alleged deficit and results on other subjective visual function tests; and (3) using objective measures of visual function, especially the swinging-light test, electroretinography, and visual evoked potentials, to invalidate the subjective test responses.

Nearly any pattern of visual field loss can be faked. The most frequently faked defect is the constricted visual field. Counterfeit hemianopias (monocular temporal, bitemporal, binasal, and homonymous) are also often encountered. These visual field defects are particularly easy to fake on the dominant automated perimeter, the Humphrey Field Analyzer, because of its testing protocol. A variety of tricks may expose the ruse.

The psychiatric and behavior disorders

underlying nonorganic visual disturbances include malingering, factitious, and somatoform disorders. Malingering is conscious dissembling of illness with a conscious goal of gaining money, narcotics, or relief from unpleasant circumstances. Factitious disorder involves a conscious effort to dissemble illness, but with an unconscious goal of playing the part of a sick person. In somatoform disorders—somatization, conversion, and hypochondriasis—the patient is unconscious of feigning illness and has little insight into the reasons for this behavior.

The management of patients with nonorganic visual disturbances requires finesse in disclosing the fact that the manifestations are not organic, and in addressing the underlying behavioral or psychiatric condition. Disposition depends on the nature of the visual disturbance, how disruptive it is, whether the patient is a child or an adult, and on some recognition of whether the underlying problem is malingering, factitious, or somatoform.

REFERENCES

1. Kaplan HI, Sadock BJ. *Concise Textbook of Clinical Psychiatry*. Baltimore: Williams & Wilkins; 1996:219–229.
2. Eisendrath SJ. Current overview of factitious disorders. In: Feldman MD, Eisendrath SJ, eds. *The Spectrum of Factitious Disorders*. Washington, DC: American Psychiatric Press; 1996:37–49.
3. Perley MJ, Guze SB. Hysteria—the stability and usefulness of clinical criteria. *N Engl J Med*. 1962;266:421–426.
4. Kathol RG, Cox TA, Corbett JJ, Thompson HS, Clancy J. Functional visual loss: I. A true psychiatric disorder? *Psychol Med*. 1983;13:307–314.
5. Vaphiades MS, Celesia GG, Brigell MG. Positive spontaneous visual phenomena limited to the hemianopic field in lesions of central visual pathways. *Neurology*. 1996;47:408–417.
6. Asaad G, Shapiro B. Hallucinations: theoretical and clinical overview. *Am J Psychiatry*. 1986;43:1088–1097.
7. Goodwin DW, Alderson P, Rosenthal R. Clinical significance of hallucinations in psychiatric disorders: a study of 116 hallucinatory patients. *Arch Gen Psychiatry*. 1971;24:76–80.
8. Sarbin TR, Juhasz JB, The social context of hallucinations. In: Siegel RK, West LJ, eds. *Hallucinations: Behavior, Experience, and Theory*. New York: John Wiley & Sons; 1975.
9. Smith CH, Beck RW, Mills RP. Functional disease in neuro-ophthalmology. *Neurol Clin*. 1983;1(4):955–971.
10. Keane JR. Neuro-ophthalmic signs and symptoms of hysteria. *Neurology*. 1982;32:757–762.
11. Miller NR, Keane JR. Neuro-ophthalmologic manifestations of nonorganic disease. In: Miller NR, Newman NJ, eds. *Walsh & Hoyt's Clinical Neuro-ophthalmology*. 5th ed. Vol 1. Baltimore: Williams & Wilkins; 1998:1765–1786.
12. Thompson HS. Functional visual loss. *Am J Ophthalmol*. 1985;100:209–213.
13. Kramer KK, LaPiana FG, Appleton B. Ocular malingering and hysteria: diagnosis and management. *Surv Ophthalmol*. 1979;24:89–96.
14. Weller M, Wiedemann P. Hysterical symptoms in ophthalmology. *Doc Ophthalmol*. 1989;73:1–33.
15. Keltner JL, May WN, Johnson CA, Post RB. The California syndrome: functional visual complaints with potential economic impact. *Ophthalmology*. 1985;92:427–435.
16. Miller BW. A review of practical tests for ocular malingering and hysteria. *Surv Ophthalmol*. 1973;17:241–246.
17. Levy NS, Glick EB. Stereoscopic perception and Snellen visual acuity. *Am J Ophthalmol*. 1974;78:722–724.
18. Donzis PB, Rappazzo A, Burde RM, Gordon M. Effect of binocular variations of Snellen's visual acuity on Titmus stereoacuity. *Arch Ophthalmol*. 1983;101:930–932.
19. Minkowski JS, Palese M, Guyton DL. Potential Acuity Meter using a minute aerial pinhole aperture. *Ophthalmology*. 1983;90:1360–1368.
20. Levi L, Feldman RM. Use of the Potential Acuity Meter in suspected functional visual loss. *Am J Ophthalmol*. 1987;114:502–503.
21. Bumgartner J, Epstein CM. Voluntary alteration of visual evoked potentials. *Ann Neurol*. 1982;12:475–478.
22. Tan CT, Murray NMF, Sawyers D, Leonard TJK. Deliberate alteration of the visual evoked potential. *J Neurol Neurosurg Psychiatry*. 1984;47:518–523.
23. Morgan RK, Nugent B, Harrison JM, O'Connor PS. Voluntary alteration of pattern visual evoked responses. *Ophthalmology*. 1985;92:1356–1363.
24. Bodis I, Atkin A, Raab E, Wolkstein M. Visual association cortex and vision in man: pattern-evoked occipital potentials in a blind boy. *Science*. 1977;198:629–631.
25. Spehlmann R, Gross RA, Ho SU, Leetsma JF, Norcross KA. Visual evoked potentials and postmortem findings in a case of cortical blindness. *Ann Neurol*. 1977;2:531–534.
26. Celesia GG, Archer CR, Kurosiwa Y, Brigell MG. Visual function of the extrageniculo-calcarine system in man: relationship to cortical blindness. *Arch Neurol*. 1980;37:704–706.
27. Hess CW, Meienberg O, Ludin HP. Visual evoked potentials in acute occipital blindness: diagnostic and prognostic value. *J Neurol*. 1982;227:193–200.
28. Aldrich MS, Alessi AG, Beck RW, Gilman S. Cortical blindness: etiology, diagnosis and prognosis. *Ann Neurol*. 1987;21:149–158.
29. Celesia GG, Bushnell D, Cone-Toleikis S, et al. Cortical blindness and residual vision: is the second visual system in humans capable of more than rudimentary visual perception? *Neurology*. 1991;41:862–869.

30. Thompson JC, Kosmorsky GS, Ellis BD. Fields of dreamers and dreamed-up fields. *Ophthalmology.* 1996;103:117–125.

31. Glovinsky Y, Quigley HA, Bisset RA, Miller NR. Artificially produced quadrantanopsia in computed visual field testing. *Am J Ophthalmol.* 1990;110:90–91.

32. Smith TJ, Baker RS. Perimetric findings in functional disorders using automated techniques. *Ophthalmology.* 1987;94:1562–1566.

33. Keane JR. Hysterical hemianopia: the "missing half" field defect. *Arch Ophthalmol.* 1979;97:865–866.

34. Gittinger JW. Functional monocular temporal hemianopsia. *Am J Ophthalmol.* 1986;101:226–231.

35. Pilley SFJ, Thompson HS. Binasal field loss and prefixation blindness. In: Glaser JS, Smith JL, eds. *Neuro-Ophthalmology.* Vol 8. St Louis: Mosby; 1975: 277–284.

36. American Psychiatric Association. *Diagnostic and Statistical Manual of Mental Disorders.* 4th ed. Washington, DC: American Psychiatric Association; 1994.

37. Eisendrath SJ, Feder A. Management of factitious disorders. In: Feldman MD, Eisendrath SJ, eds. *The Spectrum of Factitious Disorders.* Washington, DC: American Psychiatric Press; 1996:195–214.

38. Goodwin DW, Guze SB. *Psychiatric Diagnosis.* 5th ed. New York: Oxford University Press; 1996:117.

39. Sletteberg O, Bertelsen T, Hovding G. The prognosis of patients with hysterical visual impairment. *Acta Ophthalmol.* 1989;67:159–163.

40. Kathol RG, Cox TA, Corbett JJ, Thompson HS, Clancy J. Functional visual loss; follow-up of 42 cases. *Arch Ophthalmol.* 1983;101:729–735.

41. Barris MC, Kaufman DI, Barberio D. Visual impairment in hysteria. *Doc Ophthalmol.* 1992;82:369–382.

42. Catalano RA, Simon JW, Krohel GB, Rosenberg PN. Functional visual loss in children. *Ophthalmology.* 1986;93:385–390.

43. Kathol RG, Cox TA, Corbett JJ, Thompson HS, Clancy J. Functional visual loss: II. Psychiatric aspects in 42 patients followed for 4 years. *Psychol Med.* 1983;13:315–324.

Part **VI**

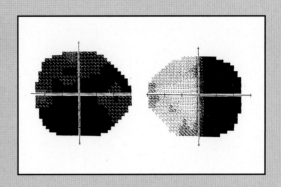

PROBLEM
CASES

Chapter 19

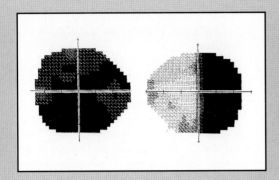

QUESTIONS

In each of the following cases, select the single best answer. The correct answers, and directions for where to get more information in the text, are found in Chapter 20.

1. A 70-year-old man is suddenly overcome by severe pain around his right eye, followed minutes later by foggy vision in that eye. An hour later, in the emergency room, his vision has returned to baseline and his eye pain has nearly resolved.

   The emergency room neurologist finds normal near acuity and visual fields in both eyes, normally reactive pupils, and a normal fundus examination.

   What might the diagnosis be?

   (*a*) Giant cell arteritis

   (*b*) Intermittent angle closure glaucoma

   (*c*) Internal carotid artery dissection

   (*d*) Ophthalmic artery aneurysm

2. A 50-year-old woman suddenly sees objects as distorted with both eyes, mainly in the right hemifield. Her only past medical history is a recent diagnosis of hypertension, treated with a beta blocker. She is going through a stressful divorce.

   She appears anxious and somewhat histrionic. Visual acuity and visual fields

are normal. Pupils are 5 mm in size and react normally without afferent defect. The fundi are unremarkable, as is the rest of the neurologic exam.

What is the diagnosis?

(*a*) Bilateral subtle retinopathy affecting foveal regions

(*b*) Posterior cerebral artery occlusion

(*c*) Nonorganic (psychogenic) visual disturbance

3. A 22-year-old woman awakens one morning to see a dark spot with her left eye just temporal to fixation. Over the next two days, the dark spot enlarges toward fixation and blurs her vision. The scotoma remains unchanged for several days. She denies any other symptoms except occasional tingling in her hands beginning upon awakening and clearing within minutes.

   Visual acuities are 20/15 in her right eye (OD), 20/40 in her left (OS). Objects appear slightly smaller and more distant when viewed with the left eye. Visual fields show no abnormality OD, and a suggestion of a central scotoma OS. The pupils are normal in size and reactivity, without afferent defect. Ophthalmoscopy shows no abnormalities of the optic disk or retinal vessels. The rest of the neuro-ophthalmologic examination is normal, including strength, gait, and deep tendon reflexes.

What does she have?

(*a*) Retrobulbar (optic) neuritis

(*b*) Retrobulbar tumor compressing optic nerve

(*c*) Central serous chorioretinopathy

(*d*) Nonorganic (psychogenic) visual loss

4. A 42-year-old woman notices poor vision in her right eye when she happens to cover her left eye. Two weeks later, she seeks your opinion, telling you that she's always had somewhat weaker vision in her right eye, but not this bad!

Visual acuities are best corrected to 20/50 OD, 20/20 OS. Her glasses are made up of a 2 diopter cylinder OD and a plano lens (window glass) OS. Pinhole does not improve her acuity OD. The visual field is normal OS; it shows a nerve fiber bundle defect OD. A large afferent pupil defect is present in the right eye. Ophthalmoscopy is normal in the left eye and shows mild optic disk edema in the right eye. A brain MRI shows no abnormalities.

What is causing her visual loss?

(*a*) Amblyopia

(*b*) Uncorrected refractive error

(*c*) Optic nerve sheath meningioma

(*d*) Optic nerve compression by internal carotid aneurysm

5. A 69-year-old man complains of headache, blurred vision, and metamorphopsia of one week's duration in both eyes.

Best corrected visual acuities are 20/25 in both eyes. Pupils, ocular ductions, and alignment are normal. Visual fields show markedly enlarged blind spots binocularly. Ophthalmoscopy shows moderate optic disk and macular edema bilaterally. Neurologic exam is otherwise normal.

A screening brain CT is normal and a lumbar puncture shows an opening pressure of 40 cm water with no cells and a protein of 105.

What is causing these findings?

(*a*) Idiopathic intracranial hypertension

(*b*) Meningitis with secondary optic neuritis

(*c*) Torcular obstruction by neoplasm

(*d*) Neuroretinitis in Guillain-Barré syndrome

6. A 20-year-girl develops fever, upper respiratory congestion, and mild headache. After a week, she notes persistent blurred vision in both eyes.

Visual acuities are 20/40 in each eye. Visual fields are shown in Fig. 19-1. Pupils, eye movements, and ocular alignment are normal. Ophthalmoscopy shows very subtle optic disk edema bilaterally.

What is her diagnosis?

(*a*) Bilateral retrobulbar neuritis

(*b*) Bilateral orbital inflammation

(*c*) Chiasmal lesion

(*d*) Bilateral visual cortex lesions

7. A 35-year-old woman has apoplectic onset of right hemiparesis, right hemisensory loss, complete right homonymous hemianopia, and aphasia. Visual acuity, pupillary reactions, and fundus examination are intact.

Where is the lesion?

(*a*) Left sylvian fissure

(*b*) Left splenio-occipital region

(*c*) Left posterior thalamus/internal capsule/root of optic radiations

(*d*) A single lesion cannot account for these findings

8. A 30-year-old surgical resident complains of the sudden onset of twinkling ameboid blotches in the field of vision of his left eye. The following day he develops mild left-hand weakness. Visual acuity is normal, but visual fields disclose small scotomas scattered throughout the

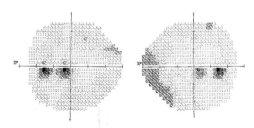

Figure 19–1

fields of both eyes. None of the scotomas has a border abutting the vertical meridian. Pupils react normally to light.

A brain CT is normal, and lumbar puncture shows a normal opening pressure with acellular fluid, normal glucose, and a protein of 69.

What is causing his visual symptoms?

(*a*) Optic neuritis

(*b*) Acute multifocal placoid pigment epitheliopathy

(*c*) Branch retinal artery occlusions

(*d*) Bilateral visual cortex infarctions

9. A 60-year-old man undergoes coronary bypass surgery but suffers an aortic dissection postoperatively. Following repair, he complains of difficulty judging distances and having objects disappear momentarily from view.

Visual acuity is normal. Pupils react normally to light. Ophthalmoscopy is normal. But when he is asked to pursue a visual target, his eyes wander. He can make saccades to parts of his body, but not to a stationary flashlight. When visual fields are tested to confrontation, they appear full. Finger–nose–finger testing is accurate to his nose but not to the examiner's finger.

Where does the damage lie?

(*a*) Bilateral parietal regions

(*b*) Bilateral occipital regions

(*c*) Bilateral frontal regions

(*d*) Bilateral temporal regions

10. A 37-year-old policeman has a 10 year history of episodic marching scintillations lasting 20 minutes and followed by headache. On the day before consulting you, he develops a scintillation in his left hemifield followed by persistent headache. He notices that since this episode, he is misreading license plates on moving vehicles; he consistently overlooks one or two numbers to the left of fixation.

An ophthalmologist finds 20/20 acuities and normally appearing globes. A standard 30 degree automated static perimetry test shows no abnormalities.

What's the problem?

(*a*) Status migrainosus

(*b*) Migraine followed by persistent anxiety

(*c*) A parietal lesion lying outside the retinocortical pathway

(*d*) Small visual field defects that have escaped detection with standard perimetric protocols

11. A 59-year-old retired music professor with new persistent low-grade headache has an episode in which objects in his left hemifield seem excessively bright for a period of ten minutes. Ten days later he experiences four episodes of left hemifield stationary pinwheel scintillations lasting about three minutes. He has a childhood history of ice cream headache and carsickness, but no severe headaches. Immediately before the onset of the visual hallucinations, he began using selegiline for early Parkinson's disease.

Visual acuity is normal, as are pupillary reactions. Eyes are perfectly aligned, and the fundus exam is normal.

What is his diagnosis?

(*a*) Migraine

(*b*) Selegiline-induced visual hallucinations

(*c*) Occipital lobe stroke

(*d*) Occipital lobe mass lesion

12. A 65-year-old man awakens with blurred vision in the nasal field of his left eye. He denies any constitutional or other systemic symptoms. Three years earlier he had suffered a similar episode involving his right eye that had been diagnosed as a "stroke of the eye." Visual loss in that eye has been stationary. A one-pack per day smoker, he has been told he has "white coat" hypertension that requires no medications.

Visual acuities are 20/20 in each eye. Pupillary reactions are normal. Fundus examination shows a pale disk in the right eye and a mildly swollen disk in the left eye. Visual fields are shown in Fig. 19-2.

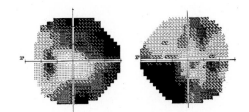

Figure 19–2

What is the diagnosis?

(*a*) Nonarteritic ischemic optic neuropathy

(*b*) Arteritic ischemic optic neuropathy

(*c*) Subfrontal mass compressing right optic nerve and causing increased intracranial pressure (Foster Kennedy syndrome)

(*d*) Optic neuritis

13. A 35-year-old welder crashes his motorcycle and spends a week in coma from a closed head injury. When examined three weeks later, he complains of persistent visual loss in the left hemifield since the accident. He denies earlier visual difficulties.

   Visual acuity is normal. A complete left homonymous hemianopia is present, as well as a subtle left afferent pupil defect. Fundus examination is normal. A review of his MRIs shows no abnormalities.

   What is the diagnosis?

   (*a*) Bilateral traumatic optic neuropathy

   (*b*) Right occipital lobe contusion injury together with a left traumatic optic neuropathy

   (*c*) Right optic tract injury

   (*d*) Right lateral geniculate body injury

14. A 25-year-old man has a generalized seizure. He has no neurologic complaints and has no history of visual difficulties.

   Neuro-ophthalmologic examination is entirely normal, except that formal visual fields disclose the defects shown in Fig. 19-3.

   Where does the lesion lie?

   (*a*) Lateral geniculate body

   (*b*) Optic tract

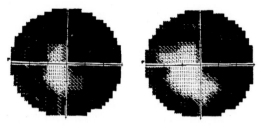

Figure 19–4

(*c*) Meyer's loop

(*d*) Occipital lobe

15. A 46-year-old man suddenly develops visual difficulty in both eyes. His past medical history is unrevealing. He has a conspicuous sick leave record from work on the assembly line at General Motors. He consults you eight months after onset, having been labeled a malingerer.

   He moves about the room tentatively, using his outstretched arms for guidance. Visual acuity is normal. Visual fields are severely constricted in both eyes to confrontation and on formal examination (Fig. 19-4). Pupillary reactions and fundus examination are normal.

   What is the problem?

   (*a*) Bilateral occipital infarction

   (*b*) Bilateral central retinal artery occlusions

   (*c*) Bilateral posterior ischemic optic neuropathy

   (*d*) Malingering

16. A 55-year-old woman complains of slowly progressive visual loss in both eyes of three months' duration. She has a long history of rheumatoid arthritis treated with prednisone and hydroxychloroquine. One year ago, she developed *Mycobacterium avium* intracellulare pneumonitis and has been treated with ethambutol 15 mg/kg/day for six months.

   Examination discloses 20/50 best corrected acuity in each eye. Pinhole fails to improve her acuity. Formal visual fields show cecocentral scotomas binocularly. Biomicroscopic examination shows moderate cataract in both eyes. Fundus examination, through slightly opaque media (because of cataract), is unremarkable.

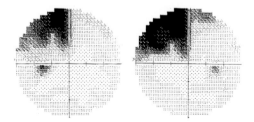

Figure 19–3

What is causing her subnormal acuity?

(*a*) Cataract

(*b*) Hydroxychloroquine maculopathy

(*c*) Ethambutol-induced optic neuropathy

(*d*) Pituitary tumor

17. A 60-year-old man consults you for visual blur that has been slowly progressing for several years with no explanation. His past medical history is utterly normal. High-resolution brain and orbit MRI have been negative, and multiple blood tests and lumbar punctures have given no helpful information.

His exam shows visual acuities are best corrected to 20/60 in each eye, having dropped about one Snellen line every year. Color vision is nearly absent when tested with the Ishihara plates. Pupils react normally. Visual fields show a suggestion of central scotomas. Fundus examination in both eyes discloses very mild temporal optic disk pallor, which could also be a variation of normal. The macular region shows subtle perifoveal depigmentation (Fig. 19-5*a*), more evident on fluorescein angiography as a white ring (Fig. 19-5*b*).

What's the problem?

(*a*) Cellophane maculopathy

(*b*) Cone dystrophy

(*c*) Stargardt's disease

(*d*) Malingering

18. A 68-year-old woman with progressive supranuclear palsy complains of blurred vision when she tries to read. Visual acuities are 20/20 at a distance target but only 20/200 at reading distance. Visual fields are full, and the fundus appears normal. She has nearly absent volitional vertical eye movements.

What is the cause of her symptom?

(*a*) Inability to use bifocals

(*b*) Uncorrected refractive error

(*c*) Pure alexia

(*d*) Accommodation weakness associated with PSP

19. A 70-year-old man develops sudden imbalance and blurred vision. At the bedside, visual acuity is 20/20 in both eyes and visual fields are full to confrontation. A jerk nystagmus is seen in extremes of horizontal gaze, but not in primary position (straight-ahead gaze). Ocular movements are of normal amplitude. He has bilateral appendicular and gait ataxia. MRI shows signal changes compatible with a small new stroke in the pons.

What is causing his blurred vision?

(*a*) Skew deviation

(*b*) Nystagmus

(*c*) Impaired vestibulo-ocular reflex

20. A 50-year-old truck driver complains of constricted vision that came on over a weekend three months ago and has not changed. It impairs his ability to drive, especially at night. There are no other symptoms.

Visual acuity is normal. Visual fields are shown in Fig. 19-6. Kinetic (finger-moving) confrontation visual fields show a diameter of 40 degrees in each eye when measured at a distance of 1 foot and 15 feet from the patient. Eye move-

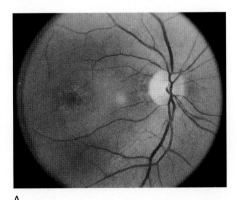

A

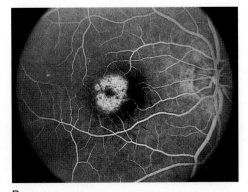

B

Figure 19–5

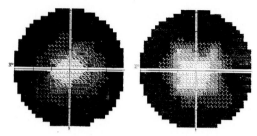

Figure 19–6

ments are full. Pupils react normally and the fundus exam is unremarkable.

What are his constricted visual fields caused by?

(*a*) Retinitis pigmentosa

(*b*) Bilateral occipital lobe infarctions

(*c*) Glaucoma

(*d*) Nonorganic visual field loss

21. A 45-year-old man notices a sudden cut in his field of vision. All aspects of his ophthalmic and neurologic examination are normal, except the visual fields shown in Fig. 19-7.

Where's the lesion?

(*a*) Optic nerves

(*b*) Optic tract/lateral geniculate body

(*c*) Meyer's loop of optic radiations

(*d*) Upper trigonal portion of optic radiations

(*e*) Primary visual cortex

22. A 50-year-old woman complains that for the past six months certain objects seem to shimmer. In particular, digital clocks and highly colored and patterned rugs arouse this sensation. Sometimes the shimmery objects are in peripheral vision and distract her from her main activity. Her past medical history is noncontributory; she is taking no medicines and denies use of hallucinogens.

Visual acuity is 20/20. Visual fields are full. The fundus examination is normal.

What's the problem?

(*a*) Occipital seizures

(*b*) Migraine

(*c*) Photoreceptor dysfunction

(*d*) Nonorganic visual disturbance

23. A 59-year-old man notes a curtain over the superior part of his vision in the left eye. He does not recall seeing it descend; one day it was just there. It stayed that way until six months later, when it seemed to descend farther to cover the entire top half of his sight in the left eye. Vision in that eye now appears distorted. Apart from moderately high myopia (5 diopters) in both eyes, he has had no previous visual problems. He denies any neurologic symptoms and has no arteriosclerotic risk factors.

Visual acuities are 20/20 OD, 20/50 OS. There is a trace afferent pupil defect in the left eye. The visual field of the right eye is normal; that of the left eye is shown in Fig. 19-8. Fundus examination through undilated pupils shows no abnormalities of the optic disks.

What is the cause of his vision loss?

(*a*) Posterior ischemic optic neuropathy

(*b*) Compressive optic neuropathy

(*c*) Retinal detachment

(*d*) Retinal arterial occlusion

24. A 10-year-old boy undergoes radical surgery and ventriculoperitoneal shunting for craniopharyngioma, leaving him with 20/25 best-corrected acuities with his −1.00 diopter myopia spectacle correction in each eye. Visual fields show partial bitemporal hemianopia. Fundus examination shows binocular optic disk pallor. A postoperative scan shows minimal residual tumor. Two years after the

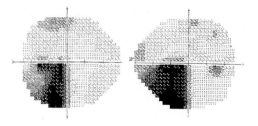

Figure 19–7

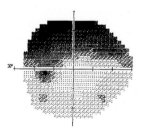

Figure 19–8

surgery, he complains of worsening vision in both eyes and headache.

Examination shows distance visual acuities of 20/40 in each eye with his current glasses. His near acuities are 20/25 in each eye with or without glasses. Visual fields show no change relative to the postoperative study. Pupils react normally to light. Fundus examination shows binocular optic disk pallor, as before.

What is the appropriate maneuver?

(*a*) Repeat MRI scan to look for tumor growth

(*b*) Assess shunt to rule out blockage

(*c*) Refract to rule out progressive myopia

25. A 70-year-old woman complains of the sudden onset of intermittent flashes of light in the extreme temporal field of her left eye. She can evoke the same sensation occasionally by moving her eyes rapidly from side to side.

Ophthalmic and neurologic examinations are normal.

Where are the scintillations coming from?

(*a*) Retina

(*b*) Optic nerve

(*c*) Optic chiasm

(*d*) Visual cortex

26. A 55-year-old hypertensive woman awakens to discover that she cannot read the newspaper.

Examination shows that the patient can read single letters and numbers, but not words. She can spell perfectly and write to dictation, but she is then unable to read what she has written. She has no other language disturbance. There is a right homonymous hemianopia, but otherwise the eye exam is normal. The rest of the neurologic exam is also normal.

Where does her lesion lie?

(*a*) Root of optic radiations

(*b*) Distal optic radiations

(*c*) Angular gyrus

(*d*) Supramarginal gyrus

27. A 25-year-old woman with relapsing-progressive quadriparesis from multiple sclerosis complains of blurred vision in both eyes for the past two months. She was recently started on an interferon drug in treatment of MS, amantadine for fatigue, oxybutynin for spastic bladder, and temazepam for sleeplessness. She has no previous history of visual difficulty and does not wear glasses.

An ophthalmologist has determined that visual acuities are 20/20 at distance, and that the structures of the eyes appear normal. Formal visual fields are normal.

What is causing her blurred vision?

(*a*) Depression

(*b*) Subtle bilateral symmetrical optic neuritis

(*c*) Subtle bilateral optic radiation lesions

(*d*) Cycloplegia

28. A 30-year-old woman slips on icy pavement at the entrance to her workplace, strikes her occiput, and is stunned for a few minutes. The next day she has headache and episodic blurred vision in both eyes. She has no prior ophthalmic history; an optometric exam one year earlier had shown 20/20 acuities without glasses.

Visual acuities are 20/50 in each eye at distance but 20/20 at near. Pupils measure 1.5 mm in dim illumination and react slightly to light. She has a comitant esotropia (convergent misalignment) and reduced abduction in both eyes. The rest of the ophthalmic and neurologic examination is normal.

What is the diagnosis?

(*a*) Accommodative spasm

(*b*) Traumatic increased intracranial pressure and occipital lobe contusion

(*c*) Traumatic bilateral optic neuropathy and sixth nerve palsy

29. A 25-year-old man develops painless loss of vision in his right eye over a five-day period. Ophthalmic examination shows 20/200 visual acuity in that eye and 20/20 in the asymptomatic left eye. An afferent pupil defect is present in the right eye. Fundus examination is normal, as is the rest of the ophthalmic and neurologic examination. He has no other complaints. His past medical history includes chronic renal failure on hemodialysis. Medications are limited to lisinopril 10 mg/day.

Vision does not improve in the right

eye, and six months later, the left eye develops the same problem. Visual acuities are now 20/400 in each eye. The visual fields consist of bilateral cecocentral scotomas. A pale disk is seen in the right eye, but there are no abnormalities in the left eye. The previously described afferent pupil defect is not found. Neurologic exam is otherwise normal, as before.

What is the diagnosis?

(*a*) Leber's hereditary optic neuropathy

(*b*) Optic neuritis

(*c*) Perichiasmal tumor

(*d*) Hypotensive ischemic optic neuropathy

30. A 40-year-old man complains of subnormal vision in his right eye of uncertain duration. He denies any prior ophthalmic problems. His past medical history is noncontributory.

Visual acuities are 20/40 OD, 20/20 OS. Pupils react normally without afferent defect. Visual fields are full to confrontation. Refraction with the retinoscope (which bounces light rays off the retina in order to calculate the optical power of the eyes) shows the following results: OD, +1.00 sphere with +3.00 cylinder; OS, +1.00 sphere with no cylinder. Fundus examination by a retinal expert is normal.

What is the appropriate intervention?

(*a*) MRI

(*b*) VEP

(*c*) ERG

(*d*) None of the above

31. A 45-year-old man undergoes partial surgical removal of a pituitary adenoma. After the surgery, he is treated with a standard course of 5000 cGy x-irradiation. At that point, his best corrected visual acuities are 20/20 in each eye, and visual fields disclose a residual bitemporal hemianopia. Three years later, he con-

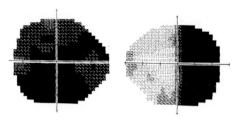

Figure 19–9

sults you for distorted vision in his left eye that has been slowly worsening for a year.

His best corrected acuities are 20/20 OD, 20/40 OS. Visual fields are unchanged. Pupillary reactions are normal. Pinhole examination does not improve visual acuity in the left eye. A new brain MRI scan shows a suprasellar mass abutting but not elevating the optic chiasm.

What is causing his recent vision loss?

(*a*) Optic nerve compression by recurrent pituitary tumor

(*b*) Optic nerve damage from radiation

(*c*) Cataract secondary to radiation

(*d*) Maculopathy

32. A 59-year-old man develops sudden painless visual loss in his right eye. He has no other complaints and has a noncontributory past medical history except heavy smoking.

Visual acuities are 20/400 OD, 20/20 OS. An afferent pupil defect is present in the right eye. Visual fields are shown in Fig. 19-9. The optic fundi are normal, as is the rest of the neurologic exam.

What is the diagnosis?

(*a*) Optic neuritis

(*b*) Posterior ischemic optic neuropathy

(*c*) Mass involving right optic tract

(*d*) Mass involving optic chiasm

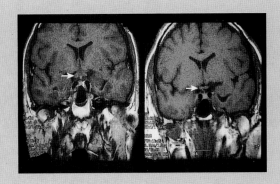

Chapter 20

ANSWERS

1. The correct answer is (b).

(a) Giant cell arteritis. No. Severe, remitting periocular pain is not typical, and the optic disk should be swollen, even if vision has apparently recovered. (p 219–222)

(b) Intermittent angle closure glaucoma. Yes. As the iris plugs the aqueous exit routes temporarily (Fig. 13-12d), the intraocular pressure goes sky high, causing severe periocular pain. The high pressure impairs ocular perfusion and produces foggy vision. If the pressure remains high long enough, the corneal endothelial metabolic pump will fail and the cornea will become edematous, producing persistent foggy vision. (p 59, 266)

(c) Internal carotid artery dissection. No. The pain usually persists and is more often localized to the neck and face. (p 58, 59)

(d) Ophthalmic artery aneurysm. No. Not an unreasonable guess, but foggy vision is not likely to clear so rapidly. An afferent defect is likely. (p 254–256)

2. The correct answer is (b).

(a) Bilateral subtle retinopathy affecting foveal regions. No. Admittedly, retinal causes of metamorphopsia may be hard to visualize with the ophthalmoscope. But here are two clues that the retina is unlikely to be the source: (1) retinal metamorphopsia is usually uniocular; (2) the patient reports that the distortion is perceived mostly in the right hemifield; this would be most unusual for retinal disease. (p 74)

(b) Posterior cerebral artery occlusion. Yes. MRI scan disclosed a occipitotemporal regions of gyral enhancement (Fig. 20-1). No visual field loss was found because the lesions lie just outside the retinocortical pathway. (p 77, 306–308)

(c) Nonorganic (psychogenic) visual disturbance. No. Although the patient's history of a stressful divorce, histrionic affect, and lack of findings on examination suggest a nonorganic cause, the persistent lateralization of the distortion to the right hemifield is a strong clue to an organic disturbance. (p 370)

3. The correct answer is (c).

(a) Retrobulbar (optic) neuritis. No. The lack of a relative afferent pupil defect excludes a uniocular optic neuritis. Uniocular micropsia suggests macular edema. (p 208)

(b) Retrobulbar tumor compressing optic nerve. No. For the same reason as answer (a). Moreover, compressive optic neuropathy rarely comes on acutely. (p 240–256)

(c) Central serous chorioretinopathy. Yes.

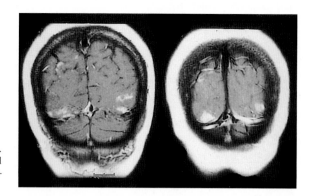

Figure 20–1. Posterior cerebral artery occlusion. Coronal T1-enhanced MRI shows gyral high signal in both inferior occipital regions, reflecting bilateral posterior cerebral artery occlusion.

Magnified ophthalmoscopy disclosed macular edema. Fluorescein angiography displayed a leak in the outer blood–retinal barrier (Fig. 20-2). The leak closed and vision resolved without treatment within two months. (p 162, 175, 181–185)

(*d*) Nonorganic (psychogenic) visual loss. No. Acute monocular visual loss with central scotoma and micropsia should demand exclusion of a maculopathy. (p 370)

4. The correct answer is (*c*).

(*a*) Amblyopia. No. Granted, she has a substantial difference in refractive errors in the two eyes (anisometropia) that could bring about amblyopia. But amblyopia will not explain her visual loss, for these reasons: (*1*) it

would not cause recent worsening; (*2*) it does not cause a large afferent pupil defect; and (*3*) it does not cause optic disk edema. (p 26, 291)

(*b*) Uncorrected refractive error. No. Her best corrected visual acuity, which indicated that all refractive errors have been accounted for, is subnormal. (p 6–8)

(*c*) Optic nerve sheath meningioma. Yes. The fact that a brain MRI is normal does not exclude an optic nerve sheath meningioma. To identify small orbital lesions, one must obtain a dedicated orbit study (high resolution, fat suppression). In this case, it showed typical imaging characteristics of a sheath meningioma (Fig. 20-3). (p 248, 249)

(*d*) Optic nerve compression by internal carotid aneurysm. No. The afferent pupil

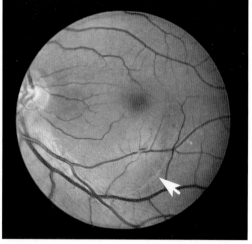

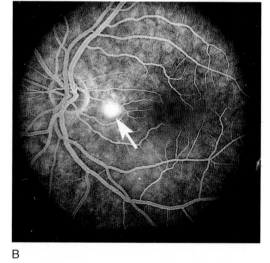

A   B

Figure 20–2. Central serous chorioretinopathy. (*a*) Fundus photograph shows large serous elevation of the sensory retina in the macular region (arrow points to the margin of the elevation) in the left eye. (*b*) Fluorescein angiography shows a small leak point (arrow) in the RPE between the optic disk and the fovea. Through this leak point, serum from the choroidal vessels, normally excluded from the retina by an intact outer blood–retinal barrier, has seeped into the retina and disturbed vision.

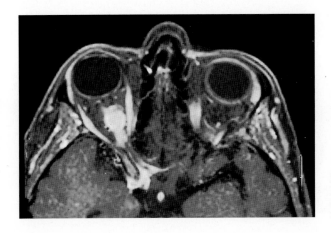

Figure 20–3. Optic nerve sheath meningioma. Fat-suppressed axial enhanced T1 MRI shows abnormal high signal and thickening of the right optic nerve.

defect suggests an optic neuropathy, but intracranial lesions do not usually cause optic disk edema. (p 253–256)

5. The correct answer is (*c*).

(*a*) Idiopathic intracranial hypertension. No. The elevated spinal fluid protein excludes that diagnosis. Besides, this diagnosis would be most unusual in a 69-year-old man! (p 229, 230)

(*b*) Meningitis with secondary optic neuritis. No. This is not an unreasonable choice, given that some meningitides can cause spinal fluid protein elevation without pleiocytosis. But such a high opening pressure would be unusual. (p 228, 229)

(*c*) Torcular obstruction by neoplasm. Yes. This patient has the ophthalmic features of papilledema: bilateral optic disk edema with minimal visual loss but metamorphopsia from macular edema. His age and male sex cast doubt on the diagnosis of idiopathic intracranial hypertension and suggest an underlying cause. Indeed, high-resolution MRI disclosed a torcular mass impairing venous outflow (Fig. 20-4). Biopsy showed carcinoma with prostatic specific antigen positivity. A primary prostatic cancer was found later. (p 226–228)

(*d*) Neuroretinitis in Guillain-Barré syndrome. No. The spinal fluid findings might be compatible, but intact deep tendon reflexes would not. (p 228)

6. The correct answer is (*a*).

(*a*) Bilateral retrobulbar neuritis. Yes. The visual field defects resemble bitemporal hemianopia, but are actually cecocentral scotomas. This distinction can be quite difficult. The binocular subnormal acuity helps

you realize that these are cecocentral rather than temporal hemianopic scotomas. The optic disk edema, which is not a feature of a chiasmal lesion, clinches the localization. (p 211–213)

(*b*) Bilateral orbital inflammation. No. Although orbital inflammatory disease can cause binocular optic neuropathy, it would be most unusual for this condition to cause acute, symmetrical field defects of this type. (p 211–215)

(*c*) Chiasmal lesion. No. This is a reasonable guess, given that the visual field defects look like bitemporal hemianopia. However, bilateral depression of visual acuity would be unusual in chiasmal disease causing such small field defects. Moreover, optic edema is not a feature of chiasmal disease. (p 203–208)

(*d*) Bilateral visual cortex lesions. No. The visual field defects are nerve bundle in shape, not hemianopic, and certainly not homonymous. (p 128)

7. The correct answer is (*c*).

(*a*) Left sylvian fissure. No—this would account only for the aphasia. (p 275–284)

(*b*) Left splenio-occipital region. No—this would account for hemianopia and pure alexia, but not the other findings. (p 308)

(*c*) Left posterior thalamus/internal capsule/root of optic radiations. Yes. A lesion here would explain all the findings. The visual field loss comes from damage to lateral geniculate or proximal optic radiations. CT showed a parenchymal hemorrhage, later traced to a ruptured MCA aneurysm (Fig. 20-5). (p 282–284)

(*d*) A single lesion cannot account for these findings. No. See answer (*c*). (p 282–284)

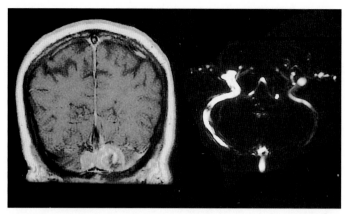

A

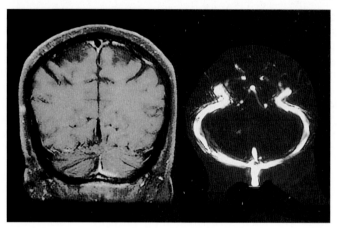

Figure 20–4. Torcular obstruction by neoplasm. (*a*) Coronal T1-enhanced MRI shows torcular mass (arrow) (*left*); MRA (*right*) shows that the mass obstructs flow in both transverse venous sinuses (arrows). (*b*) After radiation and hormone therapy, mass shrinks (*left*) and transverse venous sinus flow is reestablished (*right*, arrows).

B

8. The correct answer is (*b*).

(*a*) Optic neuritis. No. The scotomas of optic neuritis do not usually twinkle. (p 74, 75)

(*b*) Acute multifocal placoid pigment epitheliopathy. Yes. This inflammatory condition, which affects both the retinal pigment epithelium and photoreceptors, causes bloblike scotomas that scintillate because they irritate the photoreceptors. A similar process may rarely affect CNS vessels and cause meningitis, vasculitis, and stroke. Ophthalmoscopy disclosed scattered cream-colored opacities at the chorioretinal interface (Fig. 20-6*a*) and MRI disclosed a pontine stroke (Fig. 20-6*b*). (p 184)

(*c*) Branch retinal artery occlusions. No. Retinal arterial occlusions rarely cause persistent scintillations. (p 164–174)

(*d*) Bilateral visual cortex infarctions. No. Visual cortex lesions produce scotomas that have borders aligned to the vertical meridian. (p 134, 135)

9. The correct answer is (*a*).

(*a*) Bilateral parietal regions. Yes. He displays some of the elements of the Balint-Holmes syndrome, including optic ataxia, visual inattention, and impaired visually guided eye movements. He has suffered watershed infarcts in the inferior parietal lobules bilaterally (Fig. 20-7). (p 88, 89, 308, 331–342)

(*b*) Bilateral occipital regions. No—lesions confined to occipital regions generally cause more profound visual field defects than visual spatial problems and do not affect eye movements. (p 287–292)

(*c*) Bilateral frontal regions. No—frontal lobes receive visual integrative information, but lesions here do not cause visual spatial problems. (p 30–37)

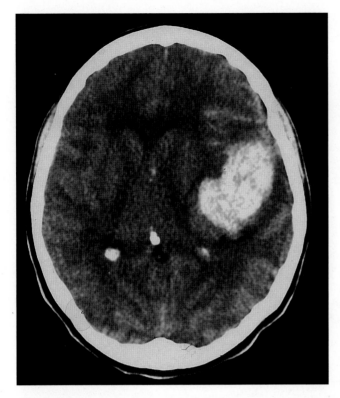

Figure 20–5. Intracerebral hemorrhage from ruptured aneurysm. CT shows left frontal hemorrhage damaging thalamus, internal capsule, and root of optic radiations. The lesion caused aphasia, right hemiparesis, hemisensory loss, and homonymous hemianopia.

(*d*) Bilateral temporal regions. No—temporal lobes deal more with recognition than spatial issues. (p 34–37)

10. The correct answer is (*d*).

(*a*) Status migrainosus. No. This could not explain his visual symptoms. (p 79–82)

(*b*) Migraine followed by persistent anxiety. No. See explanation in (*a*). (p 79–82)

(*c*) A parietal lesion lying outside the retinocortical pathway. No. See explanation in (*a*). (p 79–82)

(*d*) Small visual field defects that have escaped detection with standard perimetric protocols. Yes. The defect—homonymous paracentral scotomas—appears only with use of a special perimetric protocol that explores exclusively the central 10 degrees of

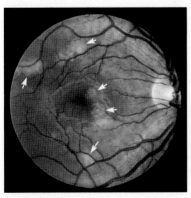

A

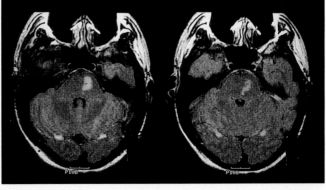

B

Figure 20–6. Acute multifocal placoid pigment epitheliopathy and pontine stroke. (*a*) Right optic fundus shows blotchy creamy spots (arrows) deep in the retina (under the blood vessels). This is inflamed retinal pigment epithelium. (*b*) FLAIR MRI shows left pontine infarct.

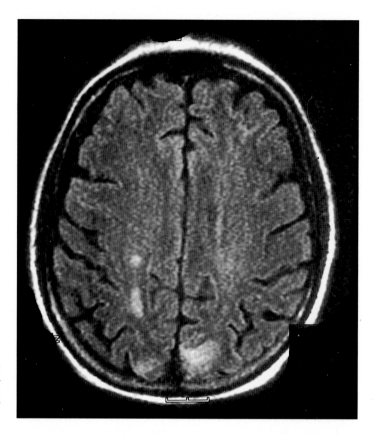

Figure 20–7. Balint's syndrome from parieto-occipital watershed infarcts. FLAIR MRI shows abnormal high signal foci over both posterior cerebral convexities.

the visual field (Fig. 20-8a). Even with this protocol, only one point in each hemifield is defective! But that is enough to cause symptoms because the defect is so close to fixation in both eyes. A high-resolution MRI (Fig. 20-8b) disclosed a small infarct in the right occipital pole. (p 28, 131, 132, 287, 288)

11. The correct answer is (d).

(a) Migraine. No. Although migraine is the most frequent cause of transient visual scintillations—even in older individuals—this patient's clinical features are so atypical that migraine would be a risky bet. The scintillations are stationary, last less than 20 minutes, their pattern changes, and the headache lingers between visual episodes. (p 79–82, 293–297)

(b) Selegiline-induced visual hallucinations. No. Visual hallucinations precipitated by medications or recreational drugs should not be lateralized to a hemifield. (p 71–74)

(c) Occipital lobe stroke. No. Not an unreasonable guess, but the visual hallucinations associated with acute stroke usually oc-

cur in a flurry immediately after the event. (p 80–83, 299–309)

(d) Occipital lobe mass lesion. Yes. These visual episodes represent partial seizures. MRI showed features of a right occipital glioblastoma (Fig. 20-9) confirmed on biopsy. Visual fields disclosed a congruous left homonymous hemianopia. (p 82, 83, 297, 298)

12. The correct answer is (a).

(a) Nonarteritic ischemic optic neuropathy. Yes. The event is new in the left eye, old in the right, as indicated by history and optic disk findings. The arcuate (nasal step) defects in both eyes are in keeping with an ischemic optic neuropathy, although not specific to it. The long interval (three years) between events, together with a lack of systemic symptoms, is strong evidence against arteritis. The combination of an old disk infarct in one eye and a new infarct in the other has been called the "pseudo Foster-Kennedy Syndrome." It is a hundredfold more common than the real Foster-Kennedy

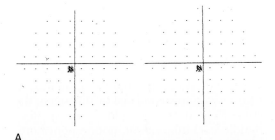

A

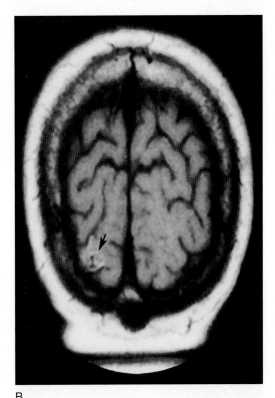

B

Figure 20–8. Small right posterior cerebral artery occlusion. (*a*) Static visual fields show left inferior homonymous paracentral scotomas. (*b*) Coronal T1-enhanced MRI shows a small posterior right occipital infarct (arrow).

syndrome caused by a mass lesion. See answer (*c*). (p 122–127, 215–223)

(*b*) Arteritic ischemic optic neuropathy. No. The long interval (three days) between events and the lack of systemic symptoms is strong evidence against arteritis. (p 215–223)

(*c*) Subfrontal mass compressing right optic nerve and causing increased intracranial pressure (Foster-Kennedy syndrome). No. The sudden but stationary vision loss the patient experienced in the right eye three years ago would be unlikely for compressive optic

neuropathy. Similarly, the sudden vision loss in the left eye would be unlikely in chronic papilledema. (p 202–204, 240–249)

(*d*) Optic neuritis. No. Although plausible, this is unlikely in a man of this age, who had painless loss of vision and did not recover any sight after the first attack. (p 203–211)

13. The correct answer is (*c*).

(*a*) Bilateral traumatic optic neuropathy. No. The field defects are retrochiasmal; the afferent defect must be explained in some other way. See answer (*c*). (p 264, 265)

(*b*) Right occipital lobe contusion injury together with a left traumatic optic neuropathy. No. A reasonable answer, but, you can explain all findings by postulating a single lesion. (p 264, 265)

(*c*) Right optic tract injury. Yes. This explains the combination of the homonymous hemianopia and afferent pupil defect. The characteristic bow-tie optic disk pallor in the eye ipsilateral to the field loss and temporal disk pallor in the eye contralateral to the field loss, reflecting dying back of injured right optic tract axons, would not appear until at least six weeks after the injury. A normal MRI is common in isolated optic tract injury. (p 278–280)

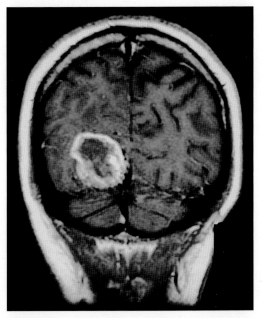

Figure 20–9. Posterior hemispheric glioblastoma multiforme. Enhanced coronal T1-weighted MRI shows ring-enhancing mass in right occipital lobe causing visual seizures.

(*d*) Right lateral geniculate body injury. No. A lesion here should not cause an afferent pupil defect. (p 280–282)

14. The correct answer is (*c*).

(*a*) Lateral geniculate body. No. Geniculate lesions produce complete hemianopias or sectoranopias. (p 280–282)

(*b*) Optic tract. No. Optic tract lesions produce either complete or incongruous homonymous hemianopias. (p 275–280)

(*c*) Meyer's loop. Yes. These are the typical pie-shaped wedges in the superior fields with one border aligned to the vertical meridian. MRI showed an anterior temporal lobe mass. (p 21–23, 129, 282–284)

(*d*) Occipital lobe. No—although occipital lobe lesions could cause these defects, their wedge shape is characteristic of Meyer's loop. Also, the combination of generalized seizure and these defects would make temporal lobe the first choice. (p 129–135)

15. The correct answer is (*a*).

(*a*) Bilateral occipital infarction. Yes. These are the keyhole defects of bilateral homonymous hemianopia with partial macular sparing. The infarct spares a portion of the caudalmost region of the primary visual cortex (Fig. 20-10). Normal visual acuity is based on this sparing. The patient had a presumed basilar apex "saddle" embolus that briefly occluded both posterior cerebral arteries. A source was found in the heart. (p 130, 134, 135)

(*b*) Bilateral central retinal artery occlusions. No. Although fundus examination could well appear normal at this stage, the visual field defects should be nerve fiber bundle in configuration, not homonymous, as here. (p 14–19)

(*c*) Bilateral posterior ischemic optic neuropathy. No. You would expect diminished pupillary reactions to light and visual field defects showing nerve fiber bundle defects. These defects are homonymous. (p 222)

(*d*) Malingering. No. Although constricted visual fields are a favorite way for malingerers to present, the formal visual fields are characteristic of another diagnosis. (p 376–379)

16. The correct answer is (*c*).

(*a*) Cataract. No. Certainly she has cataracts, and they might impair her vision if everything else were normal. But the fact that pinhole does not improve her acuity, and that she has cecocentral visual field defects, suggests a neural cause of visual loss. (p 6–10)

(*b*) Hydroxychloroquine maculopathy. No. This would cause central scotomas or pericentral scotomas (little rings around fixation), not cecocentral defects. (p 195, 196)

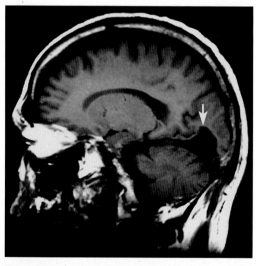 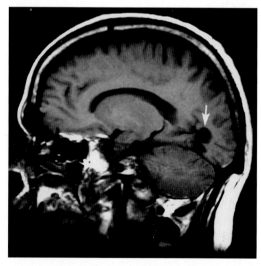

Figure 20–10. Bilateral posterior cerebral artery occlusions. Sagittal MRI shows encephalomalacia of both occipital lobes (arrows), nearly complete on the left (left), sparing the caudalmost area on the right (right). The caudal area decodes visual information from the central 10 degrees of the visual field, accounting for the spared center on field examination (macular sparing).

(*c*) Ethambutol-induced optic neuropathy. Yes. The cecocentral field defects are characteristic. Some individuals develop toxicity even at "safe" doses of ethambutol. (p 261, 262)

(*d*) Pituitary tumor. No. Cecocentral visual field defects often look bitemporal, but you can tell the difference by the fact that small bitemporal defects do not degrade visual acuity in both eyes. (p 240–252)

17. The correct answer is (*b*).

(*a*) Cellophane maculopathy. No. The fluorescein angiographic pattern is incompatible with that diagnosis. (p 191, 195)

(*b*) Cone dystrophy. Yes. This is one of the most frequent causes of progressive visual acuity loss without obvious structural abnormalities in the eyes. The devastated color vision is the clue. Although most cases are diagnosed earlier, the more indolent forms reach clinical threshold only in maturity. In this patient, an electroretinogram (ERG) showed defective responses of cones, with relatively intact rod function. (p 186, 187)

(*c*) Stargardt's disease. No. This degree of visual loss is usually reached much earlier in life. Color vision is not so badly damaged. Fundus abnormalities are usually evident by this time, and the fluorescein angiogram would fail to disclose normal choroidal vascular filling which is obscured by a pigment epithelium ballooned with opaque metabolites. (p 191)

(*d*) Malingering. No. Many patients with cone dystrophy are initially taken for malingerers. After all, their eyes appear normal. Their poor color vision is written off to a congenital condition. Without an ERG, they get no respect. (p 371)

18. The correct answer is (*a*).

(*a*) Inability to use bifocals. Yes. Her impaired downgaze means that she cannot move her eyes down into the range of her bifocals. She is reading through the distance portion of her glasses. Because of presbyopia, she cannot accommodate. A unifocal pair of spectacles empowered for near vision will solve the problem. (p 49)

(*b*) Uncorrected refractive error. No. Her normal distance acuity means she is properly refracted. (p 6–8)

(*c*) Pure alexia. No. She should have equal

difficulty with Snellen letters at distance and near. (p 353–355)

(*d*) Accommodation weakness associated with PSP. No. By the time patients develop PSP, they have lost all accommodation as part of the aging process (presbyopia). (p 8, 9)

19. The correct answer is (*a*).

(*a*) Skew deviation. Yes. A small vertical misalignment of the eyes caused by interruption of otolith–ocular motor connections is often misinterpreted by the patient as blurred vision. Because the misalignment is so small, the two images are too close together for them to be perceived as separate. Yet the patient cannot fuse them into one clear image. (p 50)

(*b*) Nystagmus. No. There is no nystagmus in straight-ahead gaze where the patient's eyes are most of the time. (p 50)

(*c*) Impaired vestibulo-ocular reflex. No. A unilateral impairment causes blurred vision only if there is nystagmus; a bilateral impairment causes blurred vision only if the head or body is moved. Small pontine strokes do not cause bilateral impairment of the VOR. (p 50, 66)

20. The correct answer is (*d*).

(*a*) Retinitis pigmentosa. No. He should have funnel rather than tunnel constriction. Funnel constriction means that the narrowed field expands as testing is carried out farther away from the patient. Tunnel constriction means that the diameter does not expand with more distant stimulus presentation. (p 135–137, 186–188, 376–378)

(*b*) Bilateral occipital lobe infarctions. No. Same argument as in (*a*). Also, formal perimeter should show central islands of different sizes in the two hemifields (see Question 15). (p 134, 135)

(*c*) Glaucoma. No. You should expect to see markedly excavated optic nerves. (p 265–269)

(*d*) Nonorganic visual field loss. Yes. The tunnel field is characteristic. The lack of findings to corroborate an organic diagnosis helps. But do not entirely exclude an organic diagnosis unless the patient's ambulation appears far better than it should be if visual fields were truly this narrowed! (p 376–378)

21. The correct answer is (*e*).

(*a*) Optic nerves. No. Whereas some optic nerve fiber bundle defects have borders aligned to the horizontal meridian, they should not have borders aligned to the vertical meridian. Homonymous defects with borders aligned to the vertical meridian must be caused by retrochiasmal lesions. (p 14–19, 123)

(*b*) Optic tract/lateral geniculate body. No. Quadrantic defects do not occur here because there is no anatomic split between axons conveying upper and lower visual field information. (p 20–23, 275–282)

(*c*) Meyer's loop of optic radiations. No. Lesions here cause pie-in-the-sky defects. (p 21–25, 282–284)

(*d*) Upper trigonal portion of optic radiations. No. Lesions here may be predominantly in the lower fields, but the field defect borders are not aligned to the horizontal meridian. (p 284)

(*e*) Primary visual cortex. Yes. The visual cortex is divided into upper and lower segments by the calcarine fissure. Each has a separate blood supply from posterior cerebral artery. In this case, the upper segment has been damaged on the left side. Strokes commonly cause such homonymous quadrantanopias. (p 25, 129–132, 289, 290)

22. The correct answer is (*d*).

(*a*) Occipital seizures. No. This is not the description of partial seizures, which should be intermittent with more discrete symptoms. (p 82)

(*b*) Migraine. No. Migraine auras can be like this, but they should not persist. (p 79–82)

(*c*) Photoreceptor dysfunction. No. Her symptoms would be unusual for this condition. Moreover, to present without field loss and fundus abnormalities would be strange. (p 74, 75)

(*d*) Nonorganic visual disturbance. Yes. This is a common visual complaint of patients with anxiety. (p 370, 371)

23. The correct answer is (*c*).

(*a*) Posterior ischemic optic neuropathy. No. The protracted, stuttering progression is not in keeping with ischemia. Other features against any optic neuropathy are (*1*) the visual field defect border has no real alignment to the horizontal meridian; (*2*)

the afferent pupil defect is too small for this degree of visual field loss; and (*3*) distorted vision is not part of an optic neuropathy. (p 203)

(*b*) Compressive optic neuropathy. No. Although the progression suggests it, other features militate against an optic neuropathy. See answer (*a*). (p 203, 240–252)

(*c*) Retinal detachment. Yes. Retinal detachments typically begin in the anterior retina (or peripheral visual field) and creep posteriorly (into the central field) as the two leaves of retina become unzipped. Metamorphopsia is typical once the detachment reaches the fovea. A subtle afferent pupil defect is a feature of large detachments. Even though the visual field looks like a nerve fiber bundle defect, it has no point of alignment to the horizontal meridian. In this patient, dilated ophthalmoscopy revealed a shallow detachment affecting the entire inferior retina. Watch out for this mimicker of optic nerve disease! (p 191–194)

(*d*) Retinal arterial occlusion. No. Although the configuration of the field defect might be compatible, the history is not. (p 164–169)

24. The correct answer is (*c*).

(*a*) Repeat MRI scan to look for tumor growth. No. The examination findings are compatible with progressive myopia. (p 6–8, 46)

(*b*) Assess shunt to rule out blockage. No. Same reason as given in answer (*a*). (p 6–8, 46)

(*c*) Refract to rule out progressive myopia. Yes. The discrepancy between poor distance and relatively preserved near acuities is characteristic of myopia. In this patient, a new refraction established that −1.75 diopters restored his acuity to 20/25 in each eye. (p 6–8, 46)

25. The correct answer is (*a*).

(*a*) Retina. Yes. Extreme temporal field flashes ("Moore's lightning streaks") are typical of vitreous detachment. As the vitreous fitfully tries to detach itself from the peripheral retina, it tugs on the photoreceptors and activates them. If the vitreous detachment does not go off perfectly, a piece of retina may be torn and the patient is then prone to a retinal detachment. (p 74, 75)

(*b*) Optic nerve. No. Lesions of the optic nerve rarely cause scintillations, and when

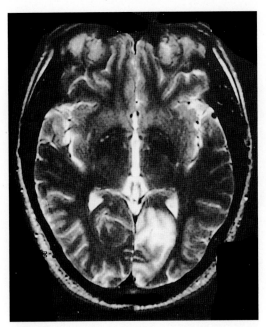

Figure 20–11. Posterior cerebral artery occlusion. T2 MRI shows left occipitosplenial lesion (arrow) in a patient with pure alexia and right homonymous hemianopia.

they do, it is usually in response to a noise (visual-auditory synesthesia). (p 75, 76)

(c) Optic chiasm. No. Lesions of the optic chiasm practically never scintillate. (p 72)

(d) Visual cortex. No. Episodic flashes can be a manifestation of occipital seizures, but such phenomena should not be evocable with rapid eye movement, which causes sloshing of the degenerating, semiliquid vitreous. (p 76–83)

26. The correct answer is (b).

(a) Root of optic radiations. No. This would account for the field loss but not the acquired (pure) alexia. (p 282–284)

(b) Distal optic radiations. Yes. This would explain both the hemianopia and disconnected input from the spared right cortex to the angular gyrus through the splenium (Fig. 20-11). (p 308, 353–355)

(c) Angular gyrus. No. This would create a more extensive language deficit. (p 353–355)

(d) Supramarginal gyrus. No. This would explain none of the deficits. (p 353–355)

27. The correct answer is (d).

(a) Depression. No. The explanation is elsewhere. (p 8, 9, 46–50)

(b) Subtle bilateral symmetrical optic neuritis. No. The explanation is elsewhere. (p 8, 9, 46–50)

(c) Subtle bilateral optic radiation lesions. No. The explanation is elsewhere. (p 8, 9, 46–50)

(d) Cycloplegia. Yes. She has lost some of her ability to accommodate because of the anticholinergic properties of oxybutynin. The ophthalmologist had failed to check her near vision, which was 20/100, and quickly restored to 20/20 with +2.00 diopter half-glasses. (p 8, 9, 46–50)

28. The correct answer is (a).

(a) Accommodative spasm. Yes. The clue is the discrepancy between normal acuity at near and subnormal acuity at distance. This suggests myopia. Given the normal optometric exam one year ago, and that fact that myopia does not normally progress at this age, the likelihood is that she has developed accommodative spasm. The presence of comitant esotropia and abduction deficit means that she has excessive convergence. Together with the small pupils (miosis), the excessive accommodative and convergence constitute spasm of the synkinetic near triad, or near response. The diagnosis is made by showing new myopia. This is nearly always a nonorganic disturbance. This patient was trying for a disability. (p 46–48)

(b) Traumatic increased intracranial pressure and occipital lobe contusion. No. See answer a. (p 46–48)

(c) Traumatic bilateral optic neuropathy and sixth nerve palsy. No. See answer (a). (p 46–48)

29. The correct answer is (a).

(a) Leber's hereditary optic neuropathy. Yes. The unremitting visual loss, the consecutive attacks in the two eyes within months, and the papillomacular nerve fiber bundle defects are characteristic. His blood disclosed one of the three mitochondrial DNA mutations. Eventually the left optic disk turned pale. (p 214, 256–259)

(b) Optic neuritis. No. The unremitting visual loss would be very unusual. (p 214)

(c) Perichiasmal tumor. No. The field defects are prechiasmal, not chiasmal. (p 240–256)

(d) Hypotensive ischemic optic neuropathy. No. Although patients on hemodialysis and ACE inhibitor antihypertensives are sub-

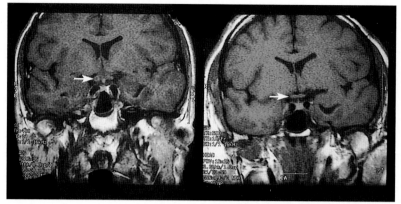

Figure 20–12. Chiasmal metastasis. MRI shows swollen chiasm (arrow) (*left*). Six weeks after radiation therapy, vision had returned to normal and the chiasm was of normal size (*right*).

ject to hypotensive ischemic optic neuropathy, this is not the likely explanation, for two reasons: (*1*) optic disk swelling is usually seen at the time of acute visual loss and (*2*) arcuate/altitudinal scotomas are more common than the centrocecal scotomas seen here. (p 215–222)

30. The correct answer is (*d*).

(*a*) MRI. No. The lack of an afferent pupil defect rules out a right optic neuropathy. Besides, there is a perfectly sound optical explanation for his subnormal vision—anisometropic amblyopia. (p 26, 291, 292)

(*b*) VEP. No. See answer (*a*). Besides, VEPs can give misleading information, especially in amblyopia. (p 153–155)

(*c*) ERG. No. There is no reason to believe he has a uniocular retinopathy that would be captured by a standard ERG. (p 149–153)

(*d*) None of the above. Yes. The refraction shows a large cylindrical correction in the right eye—enough to give him longstanding amblyopia. Why doesn't he own up to the fact that the vision in his right eye has been poor forever? Perhaps he is seeking a free ride. (p 26, 291, 292)

31. The correct answer is (*d*).

(*a*) Optic nerve compression by recurrent pituitary tumor. No. If so, you should expect a left afferent pupil defect. Besides, distorted vision (metamorphopsia) is not a symptom of optic neuropathy. Review of the postoperative MRI shows an identical amount of chiasmal compression. (p 203–207)

(*b*) Optic nerve damage from radiation. No—same reasoning as for (*a*). (p 203–207)

(*c*) Cataract secondary to radiation. No. Subnormal acuity due to cataract should improve with pinhole. Besides, distorted vision (metamorphopsia) is not a symptom of cataract. (p 9, 10)

(*d*) Maculopathy. Yes. Fundus examination shows cellophane maculopathy, a vitreoretinal interface disorder. It consists of crinkling of the inner retina as the result of a constricting surface membrane. The distorted vision should have been a tipoff. (p 191–195)

32. The correct answer is (*d*).

(*a*) Optic neuritis. No. The visual fields reflect a lesion at the junction of the optic nerve and chiasm. Mass lesions usually cause this, especially at his age. (p 19, 20, 123–128)

(*b*) Posterior ischemic optic neuropathy. No. Same reasoning as in answer (*a*). (p 19, 20, 123–128)

(*c*) Mass involving right optic tract. No. Nothing fits. (p 275–280)

(*d*) Mass involving optic chiasm. Yes. This is a junctional visual field loss pattern. The lesion must lie at the interface of the right optic nerve and chiasm. MRI showed a swollen chiasm (Fig. 20-12 left) and adenocarcinoma was eventually harvested from a lung lesion. Radiation to the chiasm completely reversed the vision loss within ten weeks and MRI showed a normal-sized chiasm (Fig. 20-12 right). The presumptive diagnosis is chiasmal metastasis. (p 19, 20, 123–128, 252, 253)

INDEX